Surgical Treatment of Primary Brainstem Hemorrhage

Gang Chen • Chao You
Editors

Surgical Treatment of Primary Brainstem Hemorrhage

Springer

PMPH
PEOPLE'S MEDICAL PUBLISHING HOUSE

Editors
Gang Chen
Department of Neurosurgery
Zhuhai People's Hospital (The Affiliated Hospital of Beijing Institute of Technology, Zhuhai Clinical Medical College of Jinan University)
Zhuhai, China

Chao You
Department of Neurosurgery
West China Hospital, Sichuan University
Chengdu, China

ISBN 978-981-95-8941-8 ISBN 978-981-95-8942-5 (eBook)
https://doi.org/10.1007/978-981-95-8942-5

Jointly published with People's Medical Publishing House, PR of China

This Springer imprint is published by the registered company Springer Nature Singapore Pte Ltd.
The registered company address is: 152 Beach Road, #21-01/04 Gateway East, Singapore 189721, Singapore

Foreword

Brainstem hemorrhage, a subtype of hemorrhagic stroke, is associated with the highest mortality and worst prognosis. It has long been regarded as a contraindication to surgical intervention, and conservative management has remained the mainstream strategy among clinicians worldwide. Unfortunately, this strategy is associated with an extremely high clinical mortality rate. In 1982, O'Laoire and colleagues reported that surgical intervention for brainstem hemorrhage could yield favorable clinical outcomes, sparking interest among a small number of neurosurgical specialists. Research on the surgical management of brainstem hemorrhage gradually began in the 1980s, with the main procedures including external ventricular drainage via burr hole and hematoma evacuation via posterior fossa craniotomy. However, the number of such operations and their therapeutic efficacy remained unsatisfactory. In recent years, minimally invasive neurosurgical approaches have advanced rapidly in China, prompting a growing number of specialists to adopt surgical interventions for brainstem hemorrhage, which has substantially increased the success rate in severe cases. Nevertheless, the number of hospitals and surgeons engaged in such research and practice remains limited, surgical procedures lack standardization, and no unified national or international guidelines have been established. Furthermore, no comprehensive monograph focusing on the surgical treatment of brainstem hemorrhage has been published to date. Therefore, this book is intended to fill the void in the literature concerning the surgical management of brainstem hematoma.

The editorial board of this monograph comprises leading domestic experts who were among the first to adopt and extensively perform a range of surgical interventions for brainstem hemorrhage, including craniotomy, microscope- and endoscope-assisted evacuation of brainstem hematomas, neuronavigation, and stereotactic puncture. These scholars have accumulated the largest clinical series of brainstem hematoma surgeries to date. Drawing on their substantial experience and insights gained from surgical management of brainstem hematomas, this volume serves as a comprehensive theoretical reference. Co-authored by distinguished experts and scholars from more than 20 major general hospitals across China dedicated to advancing the surgical treatment of brainstem hemorrhage, it stands as the first monograph worldwide entitled *Surgical Treatment of Hypertensive Brainstem Hemorrhage*. The content reflects the highest standards of clinical practice in brainstem hematoma surgery, represents an authoritative reference within China, and encapsulates the pinnacle of neurosurgical expertise in the country.

This monograph provides a comprehensive overview of surgical techniques for brainstem hematoma, addressing anatomical, pathophysiological, diagnostic, and differential diagnostic aspects, along with surgical approaches, indications, contraindications, operative methods, clinical experiences, and the management of postoperative complications. The content is thorough, technically advanced, and systematically organized. The breadth of surgical techniques described is unparalleled, and numerous novel concepts, insights, and technologies are presented in monograph form for the first time. It is anticipated that this work will serve as a valuable reference for clinicians worldwide involved in the surgical management of brainstem hemorrhage, contributing to enhanced clinical expertise and improved outcomes for patients with this severe condition.

Zhen Wu

Vice Chair of the Neuro-oncology Professional Committee
of the Neurosurgeon Branch of the Chinese Medical Doctor
Association; Department of Neurosurgery,
Beijing Tiantan Hospital, Capital Medical University
Beijing, China
October 2020

Preface 1

Severe hypertensive brainstem hemorrhage, characterized by an abrupt onset, critical clinical condition, and exceedingly high mortality and disability rates, has long been a major clinical challenge in neurosurgery. With the continuous development and widespread application of modern microsurgical techniques, minimally invasive neurosurgical concepts, and neuronavigation technology, a growing number of neurosurgeons have dedicated themselves to clinical research on the surgical treatment of this condition, yielding promising clinical outcomes. Compared with conventional conservative treatment alone, the mortality rate has seen a significant reduction. Nevertheless, a host of problems and deficiencies persist in the diagnostic and therapeutic process, including inadequate expertise in the diagnosis and differential diagnosis of hypertensive brainstem hemorrhage, inappropriate identification of surgical indications, suboptimal selection of surgical approaches, non-standardized surgical procedures, and improper management of postoperative complications. All these issues have severely impeded the treatment and rehabilitation of patients with hypertensive brainstem hemorrhage.

Although the neurosurgical management of hypertensive brainstem hemorrhage has advanced rapidly in China in recent years, no monograph dedicated to its surgical treatment has been published worldwide to date. It is therefore a great pleasure to see that, after more than three years of diligent work, a cohort of distinguished Chinese experts and professors—including Chen Gang and Yang Jinhua—who have long been committed to the clinical management and research of brainstem hemorrhage, have successfully completed this monograph entitled *Surgical Treatment of Hypertensive Brainstem Hemorrhage*. This book provides a detailed exposition of the anatomy and function of the skull base and brainstem. In particular, it offers a comprehensive and multi-perspective account of surgical indications and contraindications, preoperative preparation, surgical instruments, selection of surgical approaches, perioperative management, traditional Chinese medicine interventions, and rehabilitation therapy. It also presents and analyzes representative cases and key techniques, systematically summarizing the valuable experience and lessons accumulated by numerous experts in the treatment of brainstem hemorrhage. As an outstanding reference work for neurologists, neurosurgeons, emergency physicians, and other allied healthcare professionals, it boasts substantial academic merit and profound clinical significance. I am confident that the publication of this monograph will greatly support medical practitioners engaged in the treatment of brainstem hemorrhage, bring tangible benefits to society and patients afflicted with this devastating condition, and further elevate both basic and clinical research on severe hypertensive brainstem hemorrhage to an entirely new level.

Zhuhai, China
October 2020

Chao You

Preface 2

Hypertensive brainstem hemorrhage is characterized by sudden onset, rapid progression, critical condition, and high mortality. For patients with a hemorrhage volume exceeding 5 mL, the mortality rate of conservative treatment is nearly 100%. Surgery can directly and rapidly relieve the brainstem compression caused by hematoma, making it one of the first-choice treatments for massive hypertensive brainstem hemorrhage. Located in the posterior cranial fossa at the skull base, the brainstem is surrounded by a complex network of nerves and blood vessels with intricate anatomical relationships, which makes brainstem hemorrhage surgery extremely difficult and imposes stringent requirements on surgical methods and techniques.

Recent advances in neuroimaging, surgical instrumentation, and neural repair technologies have driven substantial progress worldwide in clarifying the pathophysiology and optimizing the clinical management of hypertensive brainstem hemorrhage. Innovations including simplified puncture and aspiration techniques, fiber tract-guided personalized surgical strategies, neuroendoscopic approaches, neural stem cell-based therapies, and research on post-hemorrhagic neural network remodeling have rendered brainstem hemorrhage a pivotal and intensively investigated topic in contemporary neuroscience.

Current therapeutic approaches for brainstem hemorrhage remain largely exploratory and experimental, with considerable divergence in treatment paradigms and marked interindividual variability in outcomes. At present, there is a scarcity of specialists worldwide devoted to the surgical management of brainstem hemorrhage. To better standardize clinical practice and foster engagement among researchers and clinicians committed to this field, we have convened leading Chinese experts—possessing robust theoretical knowledge and extensive clinical experience in brainstem hemorrhage—to compile this volume. The content is designed to closely align with clinical realities, with the aim of offering practical guidance and support to healthcare professionals involved in the diagnosis and treatment of brainstem hemorrhage. It is hoped that this work, particularly its discourse on surgical intervention and efficacy evaluation for hypertensive brainstem hemorrhage, will serve as a valuable reference and contribute to improved patient survival.

This book emphasizes the precise description, in-depth understanding, and proficient mastery of surgical techniques for brainstem hemorrhage, with a special focus on novel minimally invasive strategies that have emerged in recent years—including stereotactic puncture, keyhole craniotomy, and neuroendoscopic approaches for hematoma evacuation. We have endeavored to comprehensively gather and elucidate diverse and innovative surgical treatments for brainstem hemorrhage, integrating them into this volume. In addition, representative clinical cases are presented, together with practical insights and lessons learned from established surgical protocols for brainstem hematomas. Drawing on the authors' extensive expertise in skull base anatomy, this book also incorporates detailed anatomical fundamentals to enhance readers' comprehension and technical proficiency, thereby providing a reliable reference for optimizing surgical outcomes.

The compilation of this monograph has greatly benefited from the generous support and invaluable assistance of numerous distinguished experts and colleagues engaged in the field of brainstem hemorrhage management in China, to whom we extend our deepest and most sincere gratitude. It is our earnest aspiration that this volume will serve as a valuable educational resource and practical reference for professionals in neurology, neurosurgery, and critical care medicine who are involved in the diagnosis and treatment of brainstem hemorrhage. Owing to the constrained timeframe for its preparation and the limitations inherent in our own expertise and understanding, certain shortcomings may be present. We earnestly welcome constructive criticism and guidance from fellow experts, professors, and colleagues.

Zhuhai, China Gang Chen
October 2020

List of Editorial Board Members[1]

[1] Names are presented as Given name + Family name, arranged alphabetically by given name.

Contents

1 History of Surgical Treatment for Primary Brainstem Hemorrhage 1
Chuanyuan Tao and Chao You

2 History, Current Status, and Future Prospects of Surgical Treatment for Primary Brainstem Hemorrhage 7
Chuanyuan Tao and Chao You

3 Brainstem Anatomy and Function 11
Gang Chen, Xiaoan Wu, Yanming Chen, and Jiayan Li

4 Pathology and Pathophysiology of Primary Brainstem Hemorrhage 33
Chao Sun, Gangli Zhang, Qinxue Chen, and Dezhu An

5 Clinical Manifestations and Diagnosis of Primary Brainstem Hemorrhage 41
Zhouping Tang, Chaohui Li, Ping Zhang, and Haiquan Tao

6 Differential Diagnosis of Primary Brainstem Hemorrhage 47
Kai Shu, Ping Zhang, and Haiquan Tao

7 Surgical Treatment Principles for Primary Brainstem Hemorrhage 53
Gang Chen, Zhen Wu, and Chao Sun

8 Anesthesia Strategy for Brainstem Hemorrhage Surgery 71
Fan Zhang and Hong Chen

9 Surgical Evacuation of Brainstem Hematoma Via Subtemporal Approach 79
Hongtian Zhang and Haiquan Tao

10 Surgical Evacuation of Brainstem Hematoma Via Suboccipital Retrosigmoid Approach 89
Gang Chen, Yan Qu, Quan Zhou, Chao Sun, and Minfeng Sheng

11 Surgical Evacuation of Brainstem Hematoma Via the Posterior Median Approach 97
Gang Chen, Linsen Mu, Junfeng Huo, Xin Gao, and Zong Dai

12 Combined Microscopic and Endoscopic Surgical Treatment of Primary Brainstem Hemorrhage Via CPA Approach 111
Quan Zhou, Lihua Chen, and Zhiheng Jian

13 Surgical Treatment of Primary Brainstem Hemorrhage Via Keyhole Approach 119
Gang Chen, Chao Sun, and Junfeng Huo

14 Puncture Evacuation for Brainstem Hemorrhage Via Stereotactic Frame-Assisted Positioning 159
Fengqiang Liu and Chi Gu

15 Puncture and Aspiration Evacuation of Brainstem Hemorrhage Via Frameless Stereotactic Brainstem Hematoma . . . 173
Zefeng Wang and Fengqiang Liu

16 CT-Guided Bone Marker-Directed Puncture and Aspiration of Brainstem Hematoma . . . 179
Jinhua Yang, Yuxiong Wang, Shiji Wu, Shiquan Li, and Jieming Li

17 Cubical Stereotactic-Guided Puncture and Aspiration of Brainstem Hematoma . . . 197
Shujie Sun, Jinbiao Luo, Chao Liu, and Xuan Chen

18 Modified Directional Brainstem Hematoma Puncture and Aspiration . . . 209
Zhenchuan Liu

19 Puncture and Aspiration Evacuation of Brainstem Hematoma Via 3D Printing-Assisted Localization . . . 225
Zefu Li, Qingbo Wang, and Yu Li

20 Application of Lateral Ventricle Puncture with External Drainage in Brainstem Hemorrhage . . . 243
Yinqing Zhang, Jinhua Yang, Chao Sun, and Changhai Peng

21 Postoperative Intensive Care Treatment for Primary Brainstem Hemorrhage . . . 257
Yuhai Wang, Wenyan Zhuo, Huasong Wang, Xiaopeng Yang, and Jie Zhu

22 Surgical Complications and Countermeasures for Primary Brainstem Hemorrhage . . . 263
Hongtian Zhang, Jinhua Yang, Siying Ren, Guofeng Wu, and Junjun Liang

23 Postoperative Recovery and Traditional Chinese Medicine Treatment for Primary Brainstem Hemorrhage . . . 275
Zhiqiang Zhang, Yanling Gan, Jie Zhan, Yong Xu, Zhanneng Ren, Qibiao Weng, and Zeyu Li

24 Diagnosis and Treatment of Consciousness Impairment in Primary Brainstem Hemorrhage and Awakening Therapy . . . 297
Shizhong Zhang, Hongbo Zhang, Mengqi Gao, and Baoyan Wang

Postscript . . . 311

1 History of Surgical Treatment for Primary Brainstem Hemorrhage

Chuanyuan Tao and Chao You

The history of surgical treatment for primary brainstem hemorrhage (PBSH) is relatively short. Before the advent of computed tomography (CT), most research on brainstem hemorrhage (BSH) focused on clinical manifestations and pathological studies, with diagnosis often relying on autopsy to confirm the condition. As a result, the prognosis of BSH was considered extremely poor, with a mortality rate as high as 90% due to a lack of reliable imaging tools to accurately assess the extent and location of BSH. However, with the emergence of CT imaging in the 1970s, it became possible to visualize brainstem hemorrhages in vivo, revealing that the prognosis for some patients with BSH was not as bleak as previously thought. As research continued, the focus shifted to refining surgical techniques, understanding the indications for surgery, and improving postoperative care to further enhance outcomes for PBSH patients.

1.1 Discovery of Brainstem Hemorrhage

The discovery of BSH is traced back to 1812, when Cheyne first described stroke and somnolence in his research, later contributing to the identification of Cheyne-Stokes respiration [1]. In 1932, Dandy reported the first case of primary brainstem hematoma, marking an early step in understanding this condition [2]. Seven years later, in 1939, Környey provided a detailed description of a patient with pontine hemorrhage, from the onset of symptoms to death, followed by autopsy findings [3]. In 1973, Romanian neurosurgeon Arseni reported 2 cases of primary brainstem hematoma and reviewed 11 similar cases. He distinguished primary brainstem hematoma from brainstem hemorrhage, noting key differences: brainstem hematomas were localized, had a slow onset, and typically manifested as hemiplegia, facial paralysis, and mild consciousness impairment. In contrast, brainstem hemorrhage had a sudden onset, rapid progression, and presented with coma, high fever, respiratory disorders, and quadriplegia. Arseni emphasized that the treatment approaches for these two conditions were vastly different: While brainstem hematoma could be treated surgically, brainstem hemorrhage required conservative management [3]. This distinction laid the groundwork for the understanding of brainstem hemorrhage, although the term itself was not coined until 1988. In that year, Mangiardi clarified the concept of PBSH, differentiating it from other types of brainstem hemorrhagic diseases [4]. He described PBSH as a diffuse brainstem hemorrhagic condition that primarily affected elderly patients and was associated with severe and irreversible neurological dysfunction, leading to a very high mortality rate. Importantly, PBSH often coexists with systemic hypertension and needs to be distinguished from brainstem cavernous malformation, a key diagnostic consideration.

1.2 History of Surgical Treatment for PBSH

The development of surgical treatment for PBSH is deeply related to the clinical application of CT. CT, invented in 1972, began being used in clinical practice from 1974 to 1976, and by 1980, it became widely available. This technological advancement paved the way for more precise diagnosis and guided surgical interventions for brainstem hemorrhage, which gained surgical attention in the late 1980s, initially in Asian countries. The earliest form of surgical treatment for BSH involved stereotactic puncture and drainage. Stereotactic technology for treating brain hemorrhage was first reported by Backlund and other scholars in 1978 [5]. This technique utilizes CT guidance to accurately locate the hemorrhage within the brainstem. Once the hemorrhage is precisely identified, the next step involves remov-

C. Tao (✉) · C. You
Department of Neurosurgery, West China Hospital, Sichuan University, Chengdu, China

G. Chen, C. You (eds.), *Surgical Treatment of Primary Brainstem Hemorrhage*, https://doi.org/10.1007/978-981-95-8942-5_1

ing as much liquefied blood as possible, followed by the drainage of solid blood clots.

The advantage of this treatment method is that it does not require craniotomy, which reduces the damage to the important tissue structures within the brainstem. The operation steps of this method are relatively simple, the procedure duration is relatively short, and it allows precise localization of the hematoma. Therefore, it is particularly suitable for elderly, frail patients with brainstem hemorrhage who face high risks with craniotomy. In addition, the difficulty and technical requirements of stereotactic hematoma aspiration are relatively low, making it convenient for implementation and promotion in primary hospitals. However, there are notable disadvantages, such as slow clearance of the hematoma, the persistent toxic effect of the hematoma on brainstem tissue, and the incomplete dissolution and drainage of the hematoma. Stereotactic aspiration is typically performed after the hemorrhage has stabilized, as ultra-early hematoma puncture carries a high risk of rebleeding. Unlike craniotomy, stereotactic aspiration cannot address the responsible blood vessels, and the risk of postoperative rebleeding remains high. In 1989, Japanese scholar Takahama et al. first reported the effectiveness of stereotactic puncture and aspiration in treating PBSH. The study included nine patients with PBSH who underwent surgery, compared to a control group of 46 patients who received conservative treatment during the same period [6]. The surgery was performed 4 to 22 days after ictus, with an average of 7.7 days. The results showed that the prognosis of the surgical group was better than that of the conservative treatment group. Surgical treatment has also been shown to improve neurological function in patients with mild preoperative consciousness disturbance (Japanese Coma Scale, JCS score of 10–100) or those with unilateral basal-tegmentum-type and bilateral-tegmentum-type hematomas. In 1990, another Japanese scholar Shitamichi employed CT-guided stereotactic aspiration for treating pontine hematoma. He classified the prognosis into four levels: good, fair, poor, and death, and compared the prognosis of 20 surgical patients (average age 57.1 years, hematoma volume 6.5 mL) with 25 conservative treatment patients (average age 59.5 years, hematoma volume 10.5 mL). The results showed that nine surgical patients had a good recovery, four patients had a fair recovery, and seven patients had a poor prognosis [7]. Stratified analysis based on admission consciousness status showed that patients with semicoma (JCS score of 100) had a favorable prognosis regardless of the treatment approach. However, for patients in deep coma (JCS score of 200–300), the conservative group had a 90% mortality rate, whereas no deaths occurred in the surgical group. According to the stratified analysis of hematoma volume, the results indicated that patients with hematoma volume below 5 mL had a good prognosis in both groups. However, for patients with a hematoma volume of 5–10 mL, surgical treatment was more effective than conservative treatment. Surgical treatment showed poor efficacy for patients with a hematoma volume above 10 mL, though none survived under conservative treatment. This study demonstrated that surgical treatment could improve the prognosis of severe BSH. In 2001, Japanese scholar Hara et al. further validated the effectiveness of stereotactic aspiration for BSH. The study included 37 patients with BSH, with levels of consciousness ranging from somnolence to semicoma. Of these, 18 patients underwent CT-guided stereotactic aspiration between 1988 to 1990 and from 1995 to 1996, while 19 patients who received conservative treatment between 1991 and 1994 served as the control group. Three months post-treatment, 13 patients in the surgical group showed significant improvement in consciousness, while only 8 patients in the conservative group achieved good recovery [8].

In 1998, Korean scholar Hong JT explored the relationship between the timing of surgery and prognosis in patients with severe hypertensive pontine hemorrhage. The study included 13 patients with a preoperative Glasgow Coma Scale (GCS) score of 4–9 and a hematoma volume of 10 mL or more. The patients were divided into two groups: an early craniotomy group, which underwent surgery within 24 h of onset, and a late craniotomy group, which underwent surgery 6–20 days after the onset following a period of conservative treatment with worsening conditions [9]. The results showed early surgery provided no significant benefit. In contrast, in the late surgery group, three out of four patients experienced an increase in GCS score to 7–11 after surgery. Based on these findings, the authors suggested that surgery might be effective for some patients whose conditions deteriorate during conservative treatment. This conclusion contradicted the widely accepted belief that early surgical intervention for cerebral hemorrhage is necessary to relieve hematoma compression and reduce the toxic effects of the hematoma on brain tissues. Further research is required to clarify whether this discrepancy is due to the particularities of surgical treatment for pontine hemorrhage or the limitations such as the small sample size and potential sampling errors in the study.

In 2007, German scholar Rohde and colleagues reported their experience in treating 58 cases of spontaneous brainstem hematoma from a pathophysiological perspective [10]. They classified brainstem hematoma into two categories: arteriopathic and non-arteriopathic. The former is often associated with hypertension, while the latter is typically caused by cavernous malformations. For the arteriopathic type, they noted that the onset of severe unconsciousness, such as coma, immediately after the onset suggested direct damage to the reticular activating system. This primary damage was considered irreversible, and the recovery of consciousness was deemed unlikely, regardless of surgical intervention. Consequently, they recommended against surgical treatment for this type of patient. In the study, among the 15 patients with arteriopathic brainstem hematoma mentioned, 11 received conservative treatment, while 4 underwent external ventricular drainage for associated hydrocephalus; none of the patients survived. This viewpoint represents the mainstream opinion in Europe and the United States. Professor Lawton, chairman of the Barrow Neurological Institute in the United States and a prominent expert in cerebrovascular diseases, echoed this view in a commentary, stating that surgical treatment for PBSH is futile [10]. However, it is essential to recognize that this stance is influenced by Western cultural values, which often prioritize quality of life over life preservation. Therefore, treatment approaches should be tailored to local circumstances, considering cultural, social, and medical factors.

In 2011, Jang JH et al. reported the largest case-control study to date on surgical treatment of BSH [11]. The study included 86 patients who underwent one of three surgical interventions: stereotactic aspiration, craniotomy evacuation of hematoma, or external ventricular drainage alone. The results indicated that surgical treatment reduced the 30-day mortality rate but did not improve the 90-day neurological functional prognosis, regardless of the specific surgical modality employed, such as craniotomy, stereotactic aspiration, or external ventricular drainage. However, it is worth noting that the inclusion of patients who underwent external ventricular drainage alone may have biased the assessment of the effectiveness of hematoma evacuation.

The aforementioned studies primarily focused on patients with severe BSH, characterized by poor consciousness (GCS score < 12) and large hematoma volume (>5 mL). In contrast, mild cases of BSH often show good recovery with conservative treatment, and it remains uncertain whether surgery can further improve the prognosis for such cases. In 2018, Ichimura and colleagues reported the microsurgical treatment for five patients with mild PBSH, defined as hematoma volume < 5 mL and non-comatose state [12]. They observed significant improvement in neurological functional prognosis in all five patients, with three cases showing significant improvement in consciousness, four cases demonstrating improved motor function in hemiparetic patients, two of three cases with oculomotor nerve damage showing improvement, both cases with facial nerve dysfunction achieving complete recovery, and one case showing improvement in spontaneous breathing function. This study filled a gap regarding the surgical treatment of mild PBSH. However, it highlighted the technical demands of surgery for mild PBSH, which requires higher precision to avoid iatrogenic neurological impairments. Given the small sample size, further research with larger cohorts is needed to confirm the effectiveness of this treatment approach.

Surgical treatment for PBSH in China began in the late 1990s. In 1999, Zhuge Qichuan [13] reported on the use of CT-guided stereotactic aspiration via a supratentorial approach for treating PBSH. Among the 38 cases treated, 21 patients (55.3%) died. In 2003, Zhang Yuegao et al. [14] performed microsurgical treatment on four PBSH cases, with all patients achieving good postoperative outcomes. Notably, Prof. You Chao from West China Hospital of Sichuan University established the first sub-specialty group dedicated to the study of PBSH in China in 2005. Prof. You conducted systematic research [15–21] on surgical indications, strategies, and prognostic prediction for PBSH, making outstanding contributions to the advancing surgical treatment for this condition. The specific surgical indications proposed Prof. You's team [20] included: (1) hematoma volume > 5 mL, with a relatively concentrated hematoma; (2) GCS score < 8, accompanied by progressive deterioration of neurological function; (3) unstable vital signs, particularly in patients requiring mechanical ventilation; and (4) strong willingness for surgical treatment expressed by the patient's family. The key steps of the surgical procedure under microscopic visualization included "minimal traction on the brainstem, gentle suction of the hematoma, and delicate electrocoagulation of responsible vessels." The prognosis of patients undergoing surgery according to these indications revealed a 31.1% mortality rate within 1-month post-surgery, with 15.6% of patients showing good neurological recovery at 3 months. Multivariate analysis showed [19] that factors such as hematoma volume, GCS score at admission, and hemorrhage type were associated with mortality. Meanwhile, hematoma volume, GCS score at admission, and longitudinal extension of the hematoma were associated with neurological recovery. Subsequent comparative studies showed that surgical treatment (46 cases), compared to conservative treatment (240 cases), significantly reduced the 6-month mortality rate (30.4% vs. 70.4%), especially when performed within 6 h after onset, which demonstrated the most significant efficacy in the ultra-early stage. However, the results also indicated a higher rate of severe disability with surgery (32.6% vs. 8.8%) [21]. Thus, Prof. You Chao's team, for the first time in China, comprehensively elucidated the efficacy and outcomes of craniotomy evacuation of brainstem hemorrhage under the microscope from multiple perspectives.

In recent years, stereotactic aspiration has gained popularity in China as a treatment for brainstem hemorrhage. In 2005, Liu Fengqiang et al. [22] performed targeted puncture and catheter placement under stereotactic guidance, followed by aspiration and urokinase lavage drainage for pontine hemorrhage. The study included ten patients with an average hematoma volume of 9.5 mL and a mean time of 8 h from onset to surgery. The procedure was as follows: The center of the largest cross-section of the hematoma, determined by preoperative head CT, was selected as the target point. Entry points were chosen 2.5 cm below the superior nuchal line and 2.5 cm posterior to the mastoid process. A silicone tube with multiple side holes and an inner diameter of 2.0 mm was inserted into the guiding needle and was slowly inserted into the hematoma under stereotactic guidance. After removing the guiding needle, liquid blood was aspirated, and the hematoma cavity was slowly washed with saline solution and urokinase (5000–10,000 U). Postoperatively, urokinase was injected into the hematoma cavity every 6 h, and the drainage tube was opened 2 h after the procedure. The drainage tube remained open until most of the hematoma was cleared. Among the ten patients, seven survived, and five had good functional recovery. In 2009, Zhang Sai et al. from Tianjin Medical College of Armed Police used a similar method combined with lateral ventricle puncture, continuous intracranial pressure monitoring, and hypothermia treatment in 20 cases of severe PBSH. They reported that 18 patients survived, including 7 with good recovery. They concluded that the combination of postoperative hypothermia therapy and effective intracranial pressure monitoring could be beneficial for surgical treatment in severe PBSH. In 2015, researchers [24] compared the surgical outcomes of two different surgical approaches, the subtemporal approach and the suboccipital approach, for the treatment of BSH under stereotactic guidance. They found no statistically significant differences in the rates of favorable prognosis, severe disability, or mortality. The choice of surgical approach depended on the location of the hematoma. The subtemporal approach was suitable for hematomas located in the midbrain or upper pons, while the suboccipital approach was preferred for hematomas in the pons and the fourth ventricle. In 2019, Zhang Shaowei et al. [25] compared the clinical efficacy of stereotactic aspiration surgery with conventional conservative treatment for severe PBSH and concluded that stereotactic aspiration surgery had better efficacy for severe PBSH. In the same year, Liu Fengqiang et al. [26] from the Second Affiliated Hospital Zhejiang University School of Medicine used stereotactic aspiration to treat 47 cases of PBSH. They found that the average residual hematoma volume 1 day after surgery was 2.7 mL, with an average hematoma clearance rate of 75%. Urokinase was used for hemolysis in cases where the residual hematoma exceeded 3 mL. The results showed a 30-day mortality rate of 14.9%, and multivariate analysis indicated that hematoma extension was an independent risk factor for postoperative survival. The mortality rate significantly increased when the hematoma crossed the midline and exceeded three quarters of the brainstem. These findings have greatly promoted the application of stereotactic aspiration for PBSH, and currently, some primary hospitals in China have gradually started performing such surgeries.

The use of neuroendoscopy in neurosurgical procedures has become a research hotspot in recent years. Since 2016, some researchers have explored the application of neuroendoscopy for treating PBSH [27]. In their studies, neuroendoscopy was introduced via a midline suboccipital approach to treat patients with PBSH who had ruptured into the fourth ventricle. All patients presented with severe consciousness disturbance, ranging from semicoma to deep coma, and hematoma volumes ranging from 6 to 15 mL. During the operation, the hematoma within the fourth ventricle was initially aspirated through the fourth ventricle outlet using a microsuction device. Then, neuroendoscopy was introduced to identify the rupture site on the dorsal brainstem, followed by gently and slowly aspiration of the residual hematoma within the brainstem through the rupture site using the suction device. The adjunctive use of neuroendoscopy during microsurgery facilitates the identification of brainstem entry points and the bleeding sites, which allows for maximized hematoma evacuation while minimizing secondary damage and effectively achieving hemostasis. Postoperative cranial CT scans revealed a hematoma clearance rate of over 90%, and favorable recovery was observed during the follow-up period. The use of neuroendoscopy-assisted hematoma evacuation appears to be highly promising for the management of PBSH.

With advancements in intraoperative localization and monitoring techniques, the application of the ROSA robot has significantly enhanced the safety and precision of surgical treatment for PBSH. With its real-time navigation capabilities, the ROSA robot enables neurosurgeons to more accurately target hematomas, reducing the risk of injury to surrounding critical brain structures during surgery. Compared to conservative treatment, surgical intervention has been shown to significantly reduce mortality rates in PBSH patients. However, despite these improvements in survival rates, enhancing the quality of life for survivors after surgery remains a major challenge for neurosurgeons.

References

1. Cheyne J, Underwood T. Cases of apoplexy and lethargy. London: Thomas Underwood; 1821.
2. Arseni C, Staneiu M. Primary haematomas of the brain stem. Acta Neurochir. 1973;28(4):323–30.
3. KÖrnyey S, Hungary S. Rapidly fatal pontile hemorrhage clinical and anatomic report. Arch Neur Psych. 1939;41:793–9.
4. Mangiardi JR, Epstein FJ. Brainstem haematomas: a review of the literature and presentation of five new cases. J Neurol Neurosurg Psychiatry. 1988;51(7):966–76.
5. Backlund EO, von Holst H. Controlled subtotal evacuation of intracerebral haematomas by stereotactic technique. Surg Neurol. 1978;9(2):99–101.
6. Takahama H, Morii K, Sato M, et al. Stereotactic aspiration in hypertensive pontine hemorrhage: a comparative study with conservative therapy. No Shinkei Geka. 1989;17(8):733–9. Japanese.
7. Shitamichi M, Nakamura J, Sasaki T, et al. Computed tomography guided stereotactic aspiration of pontine hemorrhages. Stereotact Funct Neurosurg. 1990;54–55:453–6.

8. Hara T, Nagata K, Kawamoto S, et al. Functional outcome of primary pontine hemorrhage: conservative treatment or stereotactic surgery. No Shinkei Geka. 2001;29:823–9.
9. Hong JT, Choi SJ, Kye DK, et al. Surgical outcome of hypertensive pontine hemorrhages: experience of 13 cases. J Korean Neurosurg Soc. 1998;27:59–65.
10. Rohde V, Berns E, Rohde I, et al. Experiences in the management of brainstem hematomas. Neurosurg Rev. 2007;30(3):219–23. discussion 223–224
11. Jang JH, Song YG, Kim YZ. Predictors of 30-day mortality and 90-day functional recovery after primary pontine hemorrhage. J Korean Med Sci. 2011;26(1):100–7.
12. Ichimura S, Bertalanffy H, Nakaya M, et al. Surgical treatment for primary brainstem hemorrhage to improve postoperative functional outcomes. World Neurosurg. 2018;120:e1289–94.
13. Zhuge QC. CT monitoring and stereotactic aspiration therapy for hypertensive brainstem hemorrhage. Modern Diagnosis Treat. 1999:13–5. Chinese
14. Zhang YG, Wang J, Wang BH, et al. Microsurgical treatment of hypertensive brainstem hemorrhage. Pract J Med. 2003;20:323–4. Chinese
15. Li GP, Li H, You C, et al. Microsurgical treatment of hypertensive brainstem hemorrhage. West China Med. 2010;25:107–9. Chinese
16. Li H, Li GP, You C, et al. Clinical analysis of microsurgical treatment for hypertensive brainstem hemorrhage in 21 cases. Chinese J Neurosurg. 2007;23:944–5. Chinese
17. Li H, Liu WK, Lin S, et al. Discussion on the treatment of hypertension-related brainstem hemorrhage. Chinese J Neurosurg. 2013;29:339–41. Chinese
18. Liu X, Li H, Hu X, et al. Treatment discussion on spontaneous brainstem hemorrhage. J Clin Neurosurg. 2013;10:287–8. Chinese.
19. Tao C, Li H, Wang J, et al. Predictors of surgical results in patients with primary pontine hemorrhage. Turk Neurosurg. 2016;26(1):77–83.
20. Shrestha BK, Lu M, Zhigang L, et al. Surgical management of spontaneous hypertensive brainstem hemorrhage. Interdiscip Neurosurg. 2019;2:145–8.
21. Zhigang L, Seidu AR, Li H, et al. Spontaneous hypertensive brainstem hemorrhage: does surgery benefit the severe cases? Interdiscip Neurosurg. 2019;15:66–70.
22. Li FQ, Zhang XC, Zhao YZ, et al. Stereotactic surgery for pontine hemorrhage: a report of 10 cases. Chinese J Minimal Invasive Surg. 2005:1046–7. Chinese
23. Li JG, Wang P, Chen BY, et al. Stereotactic surgery for hypertensive brainstem hemorrhage. Chinese J Neurosurg. 2009;25:919–21. Chinese
24. Gao HX, Zhang WM, Xue ZS. Efficacy observation of two surgical approaches, temporal and suboccipital, for brainstem hemorrhage under stereotactic navigation. Acad J Hebei Medical Univ. 2015;36:579–81. Chinese
25. Zhang SW, Niu GM, Yuan JH, et al. Efficacy of stereotactic surgery versus conventional conservative treatment for severe brainstem hemorrhage. Chinese Pract Neural Disease J. 2019;22:853–8. Chinese
26. Liu FQ, Wang ZF, Yu XB, et al. Analysis of the efficacy and influencing factors of stereotactic precise aspiration treatment for primary brainstem hemorrhage. Chinese J Neurosurg. 2019;35:1094–8. Chinese
27. Feng X, Yingqun T, Xiao S, et al. Rosa-assisted stereotactic surgery for hypertensive brainstem hemorrhage. Chinese J Minimal Invasive Neurosurg. 2017;22:54–6. Chinese

2 History, Current Status, and Future Prospects of Surgical Treatment for Primary Brainstem Hemorrhage

Chuanyuan Tao and Chao You

Surgical treatment for primary brainstem hemorrhage (PBSH) has gradually evolved alongside the continuous understanding of pathophysiology, advancements in imaging technologies, and improvements in surgical techniques and monitoring systems. The primary surgical approaches include stereotactic hematoma aspiration and microsurgical hematoma evacuation with craniotomy. The former requires precise localization rather than technical complexity. In contrast, the latter necessitates proficient skills in deep brain operations, requiring close cooperation among surgical assistants, anesthesiologists, and electrophysiological monitoring specialists, as well as advanced facilities in the operating room. This chapter provides a concise historical overview of surgical treatment for PBSH, summarizes the status of surgical interventions, and discusses future prospects for surgical treatments in this challenging neurosurgical domain.

2.1 Historical Overview

Before the advent of computed tomography (CT), the diagnosis of PBSH primarily relied on clinical manifestations, with ventriculography and cerebral angiography via the internal carotid serving as artery auxiliary tools. Generally, differentiating PBSH from secondary causes such as cavernous malformations and occult vascular malformations was challenging, rendering surgical reports on PBH extremely rare. The emergence of CT scans enabled precise location and size determination of PBH, establishing the basic conditions for surgical interventions. Simultaneously, the development of CT-guided stereotactic systems laid the material foundation for accurate surgical procedures. Given the high prevalence of intracerebral hemorrhages in Asia, particularly in East Asian countries such as Japan and South Korea, the surgical management of PBSH originated from these regions.

C. Tao (✉) · C. You
Department of Neurosurgery, West China Hospital, Sichuan University, Chengdu, China

As discussed in the previous chapter, Takahama et al. [1] from Japan in 1989 first reported the application of CT-guided stereotactic systems for aspiration of brainstem hematomas, pioneering the surgical treatment of PBSH. For many years thereafter, CT-guided stereotactic aspiration became the primary surgical approach. In 1998, Hong JT [2], a South Korean scholar, reported craniotomy on 13 patients with severe PBSH. He found that early surgical interventions yielded unfavorable outcomes, while delayed surgery may benefit patients whose conditions deteriorated during conservative treatment. Subsequently, microsurgical hematoma evacuation emerged as a viable alternative. Compared to stereotactic aspiration, microsurgical intervention through craniotomy offered more thorough hematoma removal and hemostasis, significantly reducing the risk of postoperative rebleeding. However, this approach demanded superior microsurgical skills, meticulous neuroprotective measures, and advanced intraoperative management techniques.

2.2 Current Status and Future Prospects

2.2.1 Target Population

PBSH can be classified into four types based on hematoma extension: small unilateral tegmental, basal-tegmental, bilateral tegmental, and massive [3]. The corresponding survival rates were 94.1%, 26.1%, 14.3%, and 7.1%, respectively. Chinese researchers [4] have developed a novel prognostic scoring system for PBSH, incorporating the hematoma volume and level of consciousness at onset. Hematoma is scored as follows: 0 point (<5 mL), 1 point (5–10 mL), and 2 points (>10 mL). The level of consciousness is assessed using Glasgow Coma Scale (GCS) score: 0 point (8–15), 1 point (5–7), and 2 points (3, 4). Based on the scoring system, the 30-day mortality rates for patients with scores of 0, 1, 2, 3, and 4 are 2.7%, 31.6%, 42.7%, 81.8%, and 100%, respectively. These classifications clearly indicate that patients with

G. Chen, C. You (eds.), *Surgical Treatment of Primary Brainstem Hemorrhage*, https://doi.org/10.1007/978-981-95-8942-5_2

massive hematoma or scores above 2 face an extremely high mortality rate with conservative treatment. Consequently, these patients constitute the primary target population for surgical intervention.

2.2.2 Cultural Difference Between the East and West

Distinct cultural perspectives on life in Eastern and Western countries significantly influence the approach to the surgical treatment of PBSH. In Western countries such as the United States and Europe, severe disability or vegetative states following surgery for PBSH is considered an unacceptable outcome due to the profound burden it places on both patients and their families. Consequently, surgical interventions are rarely performed. Reflecting this stance, the guidelines [5] for the management of intracerebral hemorrhage published in 2015 by the American Heart Association and American Stroke Association (AHA/ASA) explicitly discourage surgical treatment for PBSH. In contrast, researchers in China have progressively adopted surgical management for PBSH since the late 1990s. Initially performed at major tertiary medical centers, this treatment has gradually expanded to municipal-level hospitals. A literature review of Chinese articles, since 2000 reveals nearly a hundred studies focusing on the surgical treatment for PBSH [6–9]. These studies explored minimally invasive techniques, surgical approaches, efficacy analyses, and complications. They also address intraoperative neurophysiological monitoring [10], robot-assisted localization [11], endoscopic hematoma evacuation [12], perioperative monitoring, and team coordination during surgery [13]. Collectively, these studies demonstrate substantial progress and clear benefits in reducing mortality through surgical intervention.

2.2.3 Surgical Approaches

2.2.3.1 Microsurgical Evacuation Via Craniotomy

Microsurgical craniotomy of PBSH for direct hematoma evacuation offers several advantages. It allows for precise, the maximum removal of the hematoma under visualization, facilitates identification and control of active arterial bleeding, and permits simultaneous clearance of hematomas extending into the fourth ventricle, thus restoring cerebrospinal fluid (CSF) circulation and reducing the need for secondary surgery for hydrocephalus management. Surgical approaches for PBSH typically include the midline suboccipital approach, the retrosigmoid approach, and the subtemporal approach [9, 14]. The midline suboccipital approach is commonly used for pontine tegmentum hematomas, particularly those extending into the fourth ventricle. After performing suboccipital craniectomy and partial C1 laminectomy, the cerebellomedullary cistern is opened to release CSF and lower intracranial pressure. The inferior vermis of the cerebellum is partially resected to expose the fourth ventricle, allowing for hematoma evacuation. Upon reaching the hematoma cavity, gentle aspiration using a No. 2 suction device is performed until the hematoma border is reached. If the hematoma is tough in texture, microsurgical scissors may be used for piecemeal removal. Arterial oozing is often identified in the brainstem cavity using higher magnification. If large perforating vessels are involved, bipolar coagulation is applied with minimal current. Alternatively, small gelatin sponge pieces followed by Surgicel gauze and saline irrigation can achieve hemostasis. It should be noted that initial entry into the hematoma cavity may cause transient bradycardia due to vagal stimulation. In such cases, the procedure should be temporarily paused until the heart rate normalizes. If preoperative hydrocephalus or cephalad hematoma extension into the midbrain is anticipated, and there is a high possibility of postoperative midbrain edema compressing the aqueduct and preventing the hydrocephalus relief, preemptive external ventricular drainage via the lateral ventricle's trigone can alleviate brainstem swelling and CSF outflow postoperatively. These procedures can be helpful for hematoma evacuation.

Through less commonly applied, the retrosigmoid approach is suitable for hypertensive brainstem hemorrhages, especially when the hematoma extends bilaterally in a basal-tegmental pattern. The cerebellar peduncles are accessed through the lateral cerebellum, allowing hematoma evacuation along its long axis with minimal disruption of fourth ventricular nuclei. Compared to cerebellopontine angle tumor surgeries, full exposure of the transverse and sigmoid sinuses is unnecessary in the retrosigmoid approach, simplifying craniotomy. However, the craniectomy should extend to the foramen magnum to facilitate adequate CSF release and surgical exposure.

The subtemporal approach is indicated for hematoma primarily involving the midbrain and extending into the thalamus. Key technical points include achieving optimal exposure through patient position, CSF drainage, and tentorial incision to avoid temporal lobe retraction. Intraoperatively, special attention must be given to preserving Labbé vein and trochlear nerve to prevent postoperative complications.

Lan et al. [15] conducted a retrospective cohort analyzing treatment outcomes of 286 patients with severe PBSH treated at West China Hospital of Sichuan University between 2005 to 2015. Of these, 46 underwent craniotomy with microsurgical hematoma evacuation, while 240 received conservative treatment. The mean follow-up period was 4.5 years. The study found that the mortality rate, moderate disability, and good functional recovery for the surgical group was 30.4%, 19.6%, and 13.1%, compared to 70.4%, 7.9%, and 5.9% in the conservative treatment group, respectively. However, the surgical group had a higher persistent vegetative rate (4.3% vs. 2.5%) and severe disability rate (32.6% vs. 13.3%). Further subgroup analysis revealed that patients undergoing extra-early within 6 h of symptom onset had significantly better neurological prognoses than those treated later. This study suggests that craniotomy can significantly reduce the mortality rate and increase the likelihood of functional recovery compared to conservative treatment. However, this benefit comes at the cost of a higher disability rate, reflecting a trade-off between survival and quality of life. This outcome underscores a fundamental divergence in Eastern and Western perspectives on life and healthcare ethics. Western nations prioritize the quality of life and dignified living, often opting against high-risk surgeries with uncertain functional recovery. Conversely, the traditional Chinese philosophy of "better a flawed life than a perfect death": emphasizes survival at all costs, advocating for aggressive surgical intervention as a form of respect for life and a moral imperative for treatment.

Stereotactic aspiration is another pivotal surgical modality for treating PBSH, including both framed and frameless stereotactic puncture. Due to its relatively low procedural complexity, it was among the earliest surgical interventions applied in this field. With the continuous advancement of imaging technology, hematoma localization has become increasingly precise. The introduction of thrombolytic agents such as urokinase has further facilitated hematoma clearance rates. Combined with its short operative time and ease of implementation, stereotactic aspiration has emerged as a principal treatment for PBSH in China. Professor Zhang Jianmin [16], from the Department of Neurosurgery at the Second Affiliated Hospital of Zhejiang University School of Medicine, has pioneered an innovative approach using computer-based imaging software for 3D hematoma reconstruction. This technique leverages the natural channels formed by hematoma expansion while avoiding critical neural pathways and densely packed verve nuclei, enabling a personalized surgical trajectory design. By evaluating the maximum deflection angle during preoperative path planning, irregularly shaped hematomas can be precisely evacuated from multiple orientations. In a cohort of 47 patients, 23 patients had preoperative hematoma volumes between 5 and 10 ml, while 21 had volumes exceeding 10 ml. At the 1-month postoperative follow-up, seven patients had died, yielding a mortality rate of 14.9%. These findings underscore the life-saving potential of stereotactic aspiration in managing severe PBSH while minimizing procedural risks.

With the rapid development of minimally invasive techniques, various keyhole approaches for PBSH have been explored in clinical practice, including the subtemporal keyhole, the retrosigmoid keyhole, and the posterior midline keyhole. Innovative stereotactic aspiration methods continue to emerge, such as frame-assisted stereotactic guidance, frameless navigation-assisted puncture, CT-guided puncture using osseous landmarks, cuboid stereotactic hematoma aspiration, modified stereotactic methods, and 3D printing-assisted navigation. The ongoing of these minimally invasive techniques promises greater precision and enhanced safety in the surgical hematoma evacuation.

2.2.4 Problems and Prospects

PBSH is relatively uncommon, accounting for only 5–10% of all intracerebral hemorrhages, making large-scale surgical data difficult to gather in a short time. Moreover, patients with PBSH present with severe symptoms; some patients succumb to brainstem failure before reaching the hospital. Even among hospitalized patients, unstable vital signs frequently necessitate respiratory and circulatory support, posing significant surgical risks. Postoperative complications, prolonged hospital stays, and high treatment costs often prompt families to opt for conservative treatment. Consequently, the evaluation of surgical outcomes lacks high-level evidence from large-scale clinical studies. Existing studies on surgical management, both domestically and internationally, face notable limitations, including retrospective design, inherent selection bias, relatively small sample size with insufficient statistical power, and yield inclusive results. Moreover, significant variability in surgical techniques and postoperative intensive care practices across centers results in inconsistent outcomes. The transformation of surgical experiences into reliable data and the subsequent upgrade of these data into compelling evidence remain substantial challenges.

The efficacy of surgical treatment for PBSH depends on multiple factors, including the timing and approach. Conducting corresponding clinical comparative studies with enrolled patients is highly challenging. Advances in clinical management require foundational research using animal models of PBSH. Investigations into optimal surgical timing and approaches can be guided by evaluating postoperative imaging (such as ultrahigh-field MRI assessing white matter fiber recovery and brainstem volume changes), histology (such as neuronal loss in the brainstem), and behavioral performance (including motor-sensory, cognitive, and memory functions) [17]. These assessments would provide multidimensional insights into surgical efficacy and pave the way for future clinical trials.

PBSH typically affects relatively younger individuals compared to other types of intracerebral hemorrhage, with onset commonly occurring between the ages of 40 to 60 [18]. Given the current poor functional prognosis despite both conservative and surgical treatments, preventive measures become especially critical. Proactive screening, early diagnosis, and strict management of risk factors such as hypertension and diabetes mellitus are of paramount clinical significance in reducing the incidence of PBSH.

Several key areas warrant further research to advance the surgical treatment of PBSH in China. First, it is imperative to generate high-level evidence demonstrating that surgical management is both safe and effective. Adopting international models for rare diseases, China could establish a "National Collaborative Group for Surgical Treatment of Hypertensive Brainstem Hemorrhage" by integrating qualified medical centers. This collaboration could prospectively enroll patients and conduct large-scale comparative studies of surgical versus conservative treatment, focusing on safety and efficacy. Second, efforts should be directed toward defining surgical indications and optimal timing. Employing advanced intraoperative monitoring techniques, postoperative intensive care strategies, and early-stage rehabilitation protocols could reduce mortality and disability rates while improving postoperative quality of life.

References

1. Takahama H, MorII K, Sato M, et al. Stereotactic aspiration in hypertensive pontine hemorrhage: comparative study with conservative therapy. No Shinkei Geka. 1989;17:733–9.
2. Hong JT, Choi SJ, Kye DK, et al. Surgical outcome of hypertensive pontine hemorrhages: Experience of 13 cases. J Korean Neurosurg Soc. 1998;27:59–65.
3. Chung CS, Park CH. Primary pontine hemorrhage: a new CT classification. Neurology. 1992;42(4):830–4.
4. Huang K, Ji Z, Sun L, et al. Development and validation of a grading scale for primary pontine hemorrhage. Stroke. 2017;48(1):63–9.
5. Hemphill JC, Greenberg SM, Anderson CS, et al. Guidelines for the management of spontaneous intracerebral hemorrhage: a guideline for healthcare professionals from the American Heart Association/American Stroke Association. Stroke. 2015;46(7):2032–60.
6. Chen LH, Wei Q, Xu RX, et al. Minimally invasive surgical treatment of primary hypertensive brainstem hemorrhage. J Clin Neurosurg. 2015:349–53. Chinese
7. Shi H, Zhou H, Wang FY, et al. Surgical treatment of hypertensive pontine hemorrhage via the transcerebellar vermis approach. J Clin Neurosurg. 2017;14:49–51. Chinese
8. Xu ZJ, Xu H, Yu DF, et al. Surgical treatment of hypertensive brainstem hemorrhage via the subtemporal pre-pontine approach. J Clin Neurosurg. 2019;16:497–99, 506. Chinese
9. Li H, Liu W, Lin S, et al. Treatment discussion of hypertensive brainstem hemorrhage. Chinese J Neurosurg. 2013;29:339–41. Chinese
10. Liang YH, Zhou Y, Xu TW, et al. Application of neurophysiological monitoring in surgery for brainstem hemorrhage. Chinese J Clin Neurosurg. 2014;19:229–30. Chinese
11. Xu F, Tao YQ, Sun X, et al. Rosa-assisted stereotactic surgery for hypertensive brainstem hemorrhage. Chinese J Minimal Invasive Neurosurg. 2017;22:54–6. Chinese
12. Liang JG, Dong J, Qu MQ, et al. Neuroendoscopic-assisted surgery for fourth ventricle penetrating brainstem hemorrhage. Chinese J Neurolog Med. 2013;12:197–9. Chinese
13. Li LY. Perioperative nursing care for patients with severe brainstem hemorrhage undergoing microsurgical treatment. Chinese J Pract Neurolog Diseases. 2014;17:105–6. Chinese
14. Liu X, Li H, Hu X, et al. Treatment discussion of spontaneous brainstem hemorrhage. J Clin Neurosurg. 2013;10:287–8. Chinese
15. Zhigang L, Seidu AR, Li H, et al. Spontaneous hypertensive brainstem hemorrhage: Does surgery benefit the severe cases? Interdiscip Neurosurg. 2019;15:66–70.
16. Liu FQ, Wang ZF, Yu XB, et al. Efficacy and influential factors analysis of stereotactic precise aspiration in the treatment of primary brainstem hemorrhage. Chinese J Neurosurg. 2019;35:1094–8. Chinese
17. Tao C, Zhang R, Hu X, et al. A novel brainstem hemorrhage model by autologous blood infusion in rat: white matter injury, magnetic resonance imaging, and neurobehavioral features. J Stroke Cerebrovasc Dis. 2016;25(5):1102–9.
18. van Asch CJ, Luitse MJ, Rinkel GJ, et al. Incidence, case fatality, and functional outcome of intracerebral haemorrhage over time, according to age, sex, and ethnic origin: a systematic review and meta-analysis. Lancet Neurol. 2010;9(2):167–76.

Brainstem Anatomy and Function

3

Gang Chen, Xiaoan Wu, Yanming Chen, and Jiayan Li

3.1 Overview

The brainstem is located in the posterior cranial fossa, adjacent to ventrally against the clivus. It consists of three anatomical segments arranged from inferior to superior: the medulla oblongata, pons, and midbrain. Superiorly, it connects with the diencephalon, while inferiorly, it transitions into the spinal cord. Internally, the brainstem comprises three primary components: gray matter, white matter, and reticular formation. It functions as the vital passageway for ascending sensory and descending motor pathways while also housing essential centers responsible for regulating key reflexes, including respiration, swallowing, sensation, and balance.

3.2 Learning Approach

3.2.1 Understanding the Brainstem: A Practical Perspective

3.2.1.1 Surface Anatomy

1. The brainstem resides in the posterior cranial fossa; a thorough understanding of its anatomical boundaries with the diencephalon, cerebellum, and spinal cord is essential for precise localization.
2. Familiarity with the boundaries of the three constituent parts of the brainstem—the medulla oblongata, pons, and midbrain—and their respective external morphological features, is crucial for accurate anatomical orientation (Fig. 3.1).
3. Ten pairs of cranial nerves emerge from the brainstem. It is necessary to be acquainted with the locations where these cranial nerves exit the brainstem.

3.2.1.2 Internal Subdivisions

1. Understanding the meanings of terms such as tegmentum, tectum, and basis.
2. Use the subdivisions of tectum, tegmentum, and basis to systematically map the distribution of sensory and motor pathways, somatic and visceral components, as well as fiber tracts and cranial nerve nuclei. This framework aids in precise localization diagnosis.
3. Through cross-sectional anatomy of the brainstem to deepen the understanding of the spatial relationships between its internal structures.

3.2.2 Rational Understanding of the Brainstem

3.2.2.1 Role of Neuroembryology

1. Understanding neuroembryonic development aids in comprehending the diverse functions of the brainstem.
2. Understanding the distribution of functional structures within the brainstem.

3.2.2.2 Familiarity with Functional Concepts

1. The concepts of the nervous system's functions are diverse, and understanding these functional concepts is a prerequisite for clear thinking due to the complex structural connections.
2. Unique functions of the brainstem compared to the spinal cord (e.g., special visceral sensation, special somatic sensation, special visceral motor functions).
3. Familiarity with the principles of the nervous system and the role played by the brainstem within it.

G. Chen (✉)
Department of Neurosurgery, Zhuhai People's Hospital (The Affiliated Hospital of Beijing Institute of Technology, Zhuhai Clinical Medical College of Jinan University), Zhuhai, China

X. Wu · Y. Chen · J. Li
Department of Neurosurgery, The Huangshan Changren Hospital, Huangshan, China

G. Chen, C. You (eds.), *Surgical Treatment of Primary Brainstem Hemorrhage*, https://doi.org/10.1007/978-981-95-8942-5_3

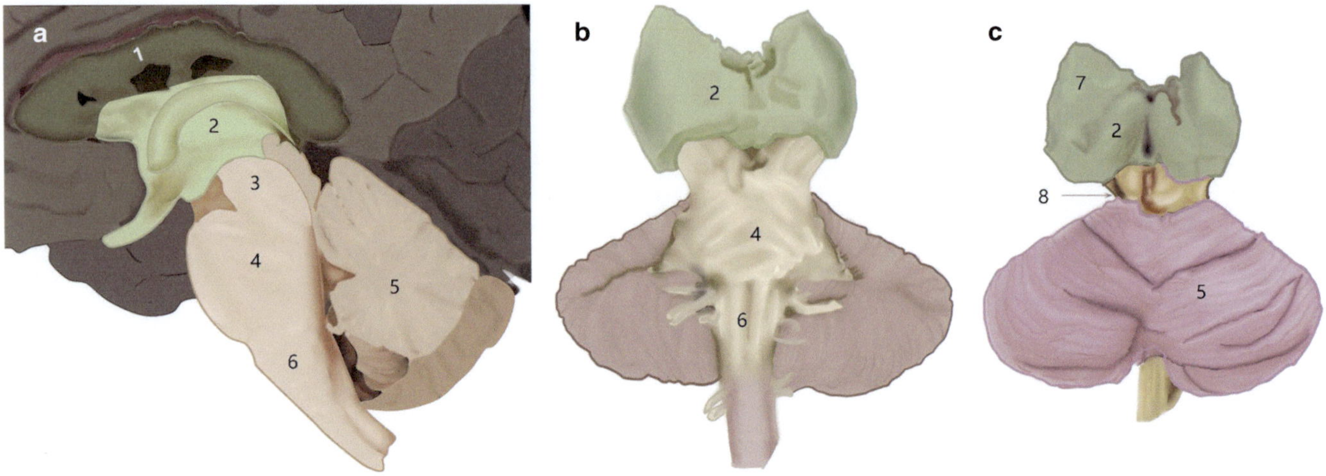

Fig. 3.1 Brainstem. Displayed in sagittal, ventral, and dorsal cross-sections, showing the three parts of the brainstem and their boundaries. (**a**) Sagittal view. (**b**) Ventral view. (**c**) Dorsal view. 1 corpus callosum. 2 diencephalon. 3 midbrain. 4 pons. 5 cerebellum. 6 medulla oblongata. 7 internal capsule. 8 tectum (corpora quadrigemina)

3.2.2.3 Conceptual "Stringing" Method

Once clear structural features and functional concepts are established in the mind, grouping and organizing the structures related to function facilitate anatomical memory and clinical localization and surgical positioning. This method is similar to stringing beads.

3.2.2.4 Blood Supply and Sectional Anatomy

The unique features of the brainstem's blood supply directly determine the manifestation of various syndromes in clinical settings. Combining the distribution characteristics of blood supply with sectional anatomy of the brainstem simplifies localization.

3.3 Neuroembryology

3.3.1 Tissue Origins of the Nervous System

The entire nervous system originates from the neural plate, which is ectoderm of the bottom of the amniotic sac. For clarity, the following sections describe the formation of the neural tube, spinal nerves, brain vesicles, ventricular system, and choroid plexus.

3.3.1.1 Neurulation

1. By the third week after fertilization, the neural plate forms paired neural folds that curve inward and fuse medially, creating the neural tube and neural canal (Fig. 3.2). The fusion process of the neural folds begins in the future cervical region of the embryo and extends bidirectionally the head and tail ends. The openings at the head and tail ends of the neural tube, called neuropores, close before the end of the fourth week. The formation of the neural tube from the ectoderm is called neurulation.
2. Cells at the edges of each neural folds migrate from the fusion line to form the neural crest along the neural tube. Neural crest-derived cells differentiate into various cell types, including spinal and autonomic ganglion cells, melanocytes, and Schwann cells of the peripheral nerves.
3. The two ends of the neural plate develop differently, with the rostral end of the neural tube developing into the brain, while the narrower caudal end grows rapidly, forming the spinal cord.

3.3.1.2 Spinal Nerves

1. The dorsal portion of the neural tube is referred to as the alar plate, while the ventral part is known as the basal plate (Fig. 3.3).
2. Neurons derived from the alar plate primarily serve sensory functions and grow into the dorsal nerve roots located in the spinal ganglia. Neurons originating from the basal plate primarily serve motor functions and form the ventral nerve roots. At the appropriate levels of the spinal cord, the ventral roots also contain autonomic nerve fibers. The combination of the dorsal and ventral roots forms the spinal nerves, which exit the vertebral canal through the gaps between the neural arches formed by mesenchymal vertebrae.
3. The neurons of the spinal (dorsal root) ganglia initially have a bipolar morphology. They transform into unipolar cells by the fusion of the two processes on one side of the parent cells.

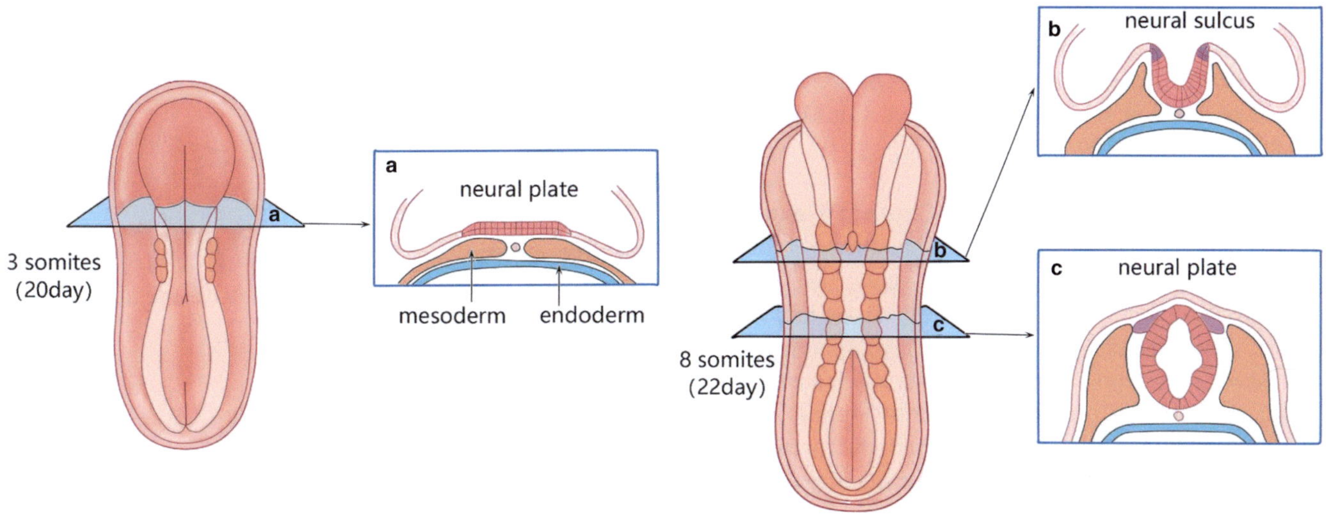

Fig. 3.2 Formation of the neural tube from the neural plate. (**a**) At 20 days of embryonic development, three somites are present. (**b**) At 22 days of embryonic development, 22 somites are present.(**c**) The neural plate, which is part of the ectoderm, folds inward to form the neural sulcus, which further folds in to form the neural tube. 1 neural plate. 2 mesoderm. 3 endoderm. 4 3 somites (20 days). 5 8 Somites (22 Days). 6 Neural Sulcus. 7 Neural Plate

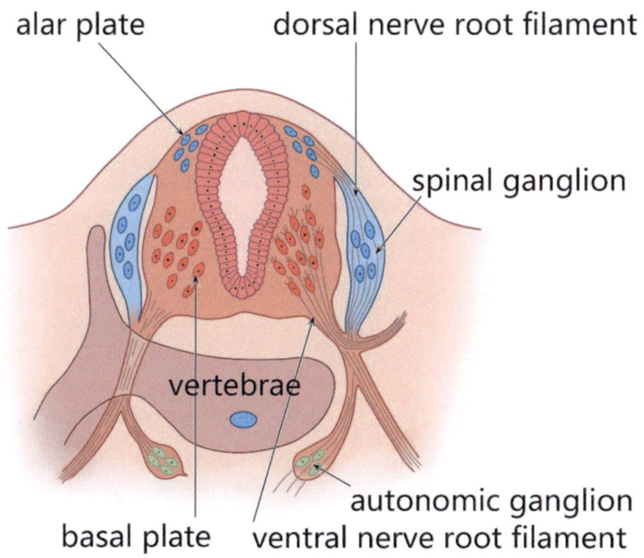

Fig. 3.3 Schematic representation of the neural tube and spinal nerves at 6 weeks of embryonic development. The basal plate on the ventral side of the neural tube develops into the ventral nerve roots responsible for motor functions, while the alar plate on the dorsal side develops into the dorsal nerve roots responsible for sensory functions. 1 alar plate. 2 dorsal nerve root filament. 3 spinal ganglion. 4 vertebrae. 5 basal plate. 6 autonomic ganglion. 7 ventral nerve root filament

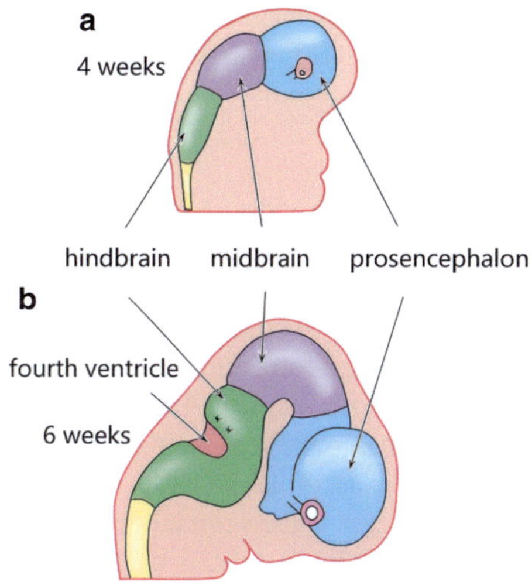

Fig. 3.4 Schematic representation of brain vesicle development. (**a** and **b**) show the development of brain vesicles at 4 and 6 weeks, respectively, with asterisks marking the initial sites of cerebellar development. 1. 4 weeks. 2. Hindbrain. 3. Midbrain. 4. Prosencephalon. 5. Fourth ventricle. 6. 6 weeks. 1 prosencephalon. 2 mesencephalon. 3 rhombencephalon. 4 telencephalon. 5 diencephalon. 6 diencephalon. 7 pons. 8 cerebellum. 9 medulla oblongata. 10 cerebral cortex. 11 corpus striatum. 12 thalamus. 13 hypothalamus

3.3.1.3 Development of Brain Vesicles into the Brain

By the end of the fourth week, the rostral part of the neural tube undergoes bending at the level of the future midbrain level (Fig. 3.4), forming the mesencephalon, with its slight constriction marking its connection with the prosencephalon and the rhombencephalon.

1. The alar plate of the prosencephalon expands laterally to form the telencephalon. The remaining basal plate gives rise to the diencephalon. The optic outgrowth of the diencephalon eventually forms the precursor of the retina and optic nerve.
2. The diencephalon, mesencephalon, and rhombencephalon together constitute the embryonic brainstem.
3. As the development progresses, the mesencephalon is brought to the rostral end of the brain. The rhombenceph-

alon undergoes folding, causing the alar plate to spread and form the diamond-shaped fourth ventricle. The rostral part of the rhombencephalon gives rise to the pons and cerebellum, while the caudal part forms the medulla oblongata (Fig. 3.5).

3.3.1.4 Ventricular System and Choroid Plexus

1. The neural canal, which develops into the cerebral hemispheres, expands to form the lateral ventricles. The lateral ventricles communicate with the third ventricle within the diencephalon. The two lateral ventricles are connected to the third ventricle through the interventricular foramen (Monro's foramina). The third ventricle and the fourth ventricle communicate through the cerebral aqueduct (aqueduct of Sylvius) within the midbrain (Fig. 3.6).
2. The thin roof of the forebrain and the hindbrain is penetrated by a cluster of capillaries, forming the choroid plexuses of the fourth ventricle. The choroid plexuses produce cerebrospinal fluid (CSF), which circulates within the ventricular system. The CSF exits the fourth ventricle through three openings in the roof of the fourth ventricle, facilitating its flow into the subarachnoid space (Fig. 3.7).

3.3.1.5 Summary

1. The nervous system initially develops from the neural tube, derived from the ectoderm, enclosing the neural canal. A cellular band migrates bilaterally from the neural tube, forming the neural crest on both sides. The caudal part of the neural tube forms the spinal cord. The neural crests form the spinal ganglia cells, which send sensory dorsal nerve roots into the sensory alar plate of the spinal cord. The basal plate of the spinal cord contains motor neurons that give rise to the ventral nerve roots, completing the spinal nerves by connecting the dorsal nerve roots.
2. The rostral end of the neural tube forms three brain vesicles. Among them, the prosencephalon forms the dorsal cerebral hemispheres (telencephalon) and the ventral diencephalon. The mesencephalon forms the midbrain, while the rhombencephalon becomes the hindbrain, including the pons, medulla oblongata, and cerebellum.
3. The rostral part of the neural tube expands to form the ventricular system. Cerebrospinal fluid is secreted by the choroid plexuses, which are invaginated capillary networks in the ventricular roof [1].

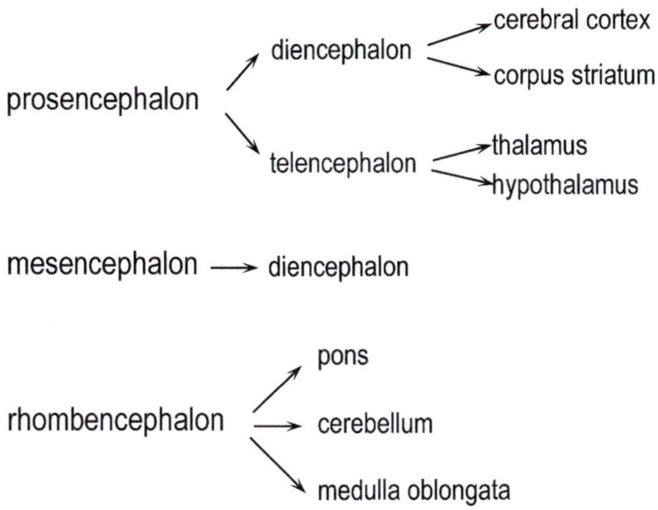

Fig. 3.5 Neural structures derived from brain vesicles. 1 Telencephalon. 2 Diencephalon. 3 Midbrain. 4 Rhombencephalon (hindbrain). 5 Spinal cord. 6 Lateral ventricle. 7 Choroid plexus. 8 Cerebral aqueduct. 9 Fourth ventricle. 10 Central canal

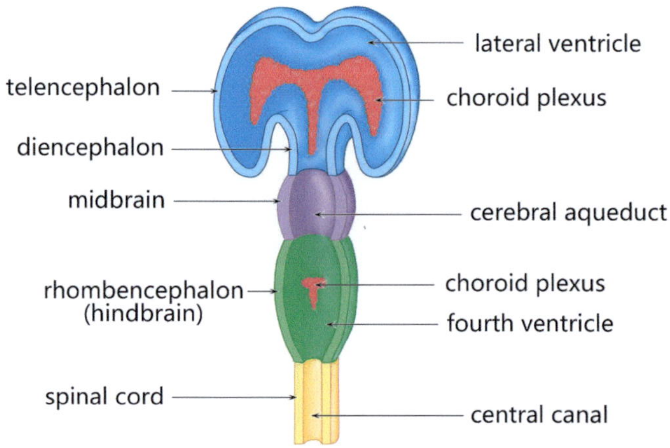

Fig. 3.6 Schematic representation of neural tube development into the nervous system. The entire nervous system develops from the neural plate, which folds to form the neural tube. The figure shows the development of the prosencephalon, diencephalon, mesencephalon, and rhombencephalon from the cranial part of the neural tube, as well as the development of the spinal cord from the caudal part. Simultaneously, the lumen of the neural tube develops into the ventricular system, cerebral aqueduct, central canal of the spinal cord, which are interconnected. 1 8 weeks. 2 Midbrain. 3 Roof(resected). 4 Cerebellum. 5 Rhombencephalon (hindbrain). 6 12 weeks. 7 Cerebellar hemisphere. 8 Foramen superior to the roof of the fourth ventricle. 9 Medulla oblongata. 10 Pons

3.3.2 Insights from Neural Embryonic Development

3.3.2.1 Sensory-Motor Distribution Patterns

1. During the development of the neural tube, there is a characteristic distribution of ventral motor and dorsal sensory functions, which is also observed in the adult spinal cord.
2. In the dorsal aspect of the brainstem, due to its openness (fourth ventricle), sensory nuclei are located bilaterally, while motor nuclei are positioned in the median sulcus. During development, the sulcus limitans demarcates sensory from motor nuclei.
3. In adults, the sulcus limitans can still be observed along the lateral wall of the fourth ventricle, separating the motor nuclei from the dorsal sensory nuclei on the ventral side.

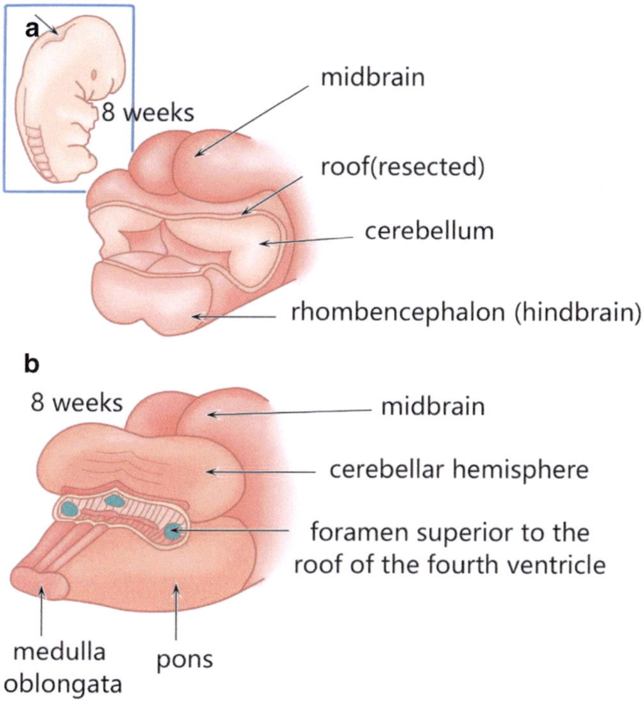

Fig. 3.7 Posterior view of developing hindbrain. (**a**) shows the development of the cerebellum from the dorsal aspect of the fourth ventricle at 8 weeks of gestation. (**b**) shows the ventral aspect of the cerebellum covering the fourth ventricle at 12 weeks of gestation, with three openings appearing in the roof of the fourth ventricle. 1 Primitive spinal cord. 2 Adult thoracic cord. 3 Dorsal sensory column. 4 Medium (lateral). 5 Visceral motor column. 6 ventral motor column. 7 Brainstem. 8 Special somatic sensory (vestibulocochlear nerve). 9 General somatic sensory. 10 Special somatic sensory (taste). 11 General visceral sensory. 12 General visceral motor. 13 Special visceral motor (innervate branchial arch-derived muscle). 14 General somatic motor. 15 Solitary nucleus

3.3.2.2 Understanding the Cellular Functional Columns of the Spinal Cord and Brainstem from a Developmental Perspective

1. Within the brainstem, neurons of the same functional category are clustered together to form cellular functional columns. In early embryonic development, these columns are arranged longitudinally as elongated gray columns. Later, the columns break apart, giving rise to various brainstem nuclei of different lengths (Fig. 3.8).
2. The seven types of cranial nerve fibers correspond to seven types of cranial nerve nuclei.
3. Due to the presence of special visceral sensory (taste) and general visceral sensory cells within the same cellular functional column (solitary tract nucleus), there are only six cellular functional columns in the brainstem.
4. The six cellular functional columns in the brainstem break apart to form 18 cranial nerve nuclei, but the arrangement of these nuclei still follows the distribution pattern of the functional columns (motor within the sulcus limitans and sensory outside the sulcus limitans) [2].

3.3.2.3 Characteristics of Brainstem Nuclei and Cranial Nerves

1. Brainstem nuclei are primarily associated with specific functions (one nucleus, one function).
2. Cranial nerves are primarily associated with the distribution or innervation of specific organs or regions (one nerve, one region).

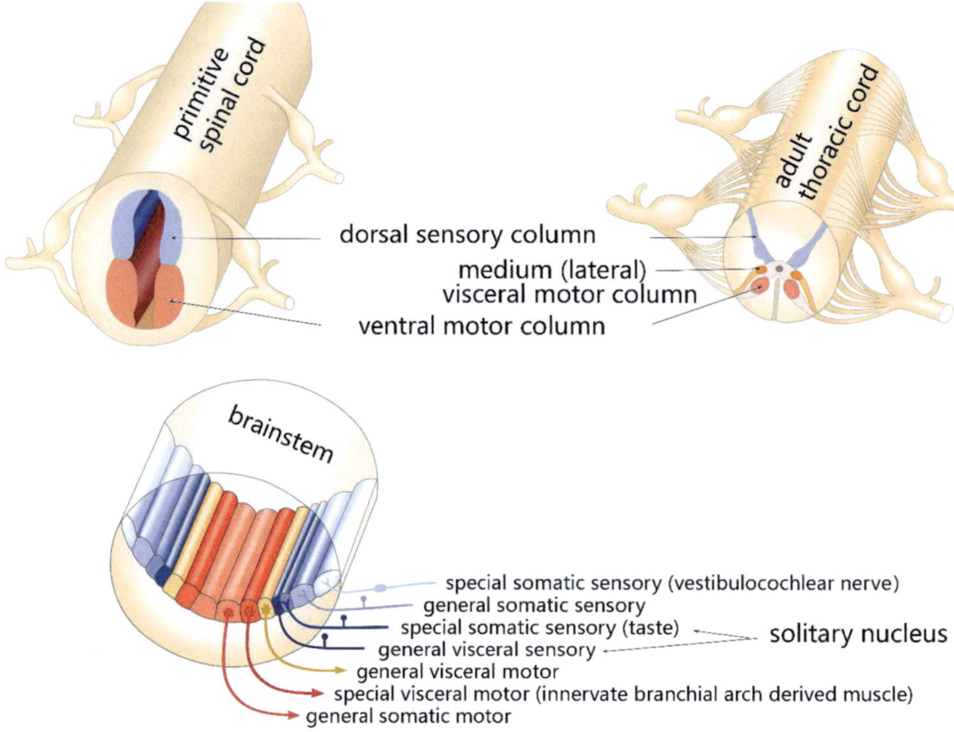

Fig. 3.8 Cellular functional columns in the embryonic and adult spinal cord and brainstem. Although the cellular functional columns in the embryonic and adult spinal cord and brainstem have their own characteristics, they share a common arrangement: ventral motor columns and dorsal sensory columns. Due to the dorsal splitting of the brainstem, the sensory columns are arranged on the outer side. 1 Oculomotor nerve. 2 Trochlear nerve. 3 Trigeminal nerve. 4 Facial nerve. 5 Intermediate nerve. 6 Vestibulocochlear nerve. 7 Olive. 8 Pons basis. 9 Pyramid of medulla oblongata. 10 Optic nerve. 11 Optic chiasma. 12 Optic tract. 13 Abducent nerve. 14 Glossopharyngeal nerve. 15 Hypoglossal nerve. 16 Vagus nerve. 17 Accessory nerve. 18 Pineal body. 19 Superior cerebellar peduncle. 20 Middle cerebellar peduncle. 21 Inferior cerebellar peduncle. 22 Striae medullares. 23 Hypoglossal nerve trigone. 24 Vagal nerve trigone. 25 Thalamus. 26 Corpora quadrigemina. 27 Median sulcus. 28 Nucleus ceruleus. 29 Sulcus limitans. 30 Facial colliculus

3.4 Surface of the Brainstem

3.4.1 Surface Anatomy of the Brainstem

From the ventral aspect, we can identify the boundaries between the brainstem and the diencephalon, cerebellum, and spinal cord, as well as the locations where cranial nerves III, V, VI, VII, VIII, IX, X, XI, and XII exit the brainstem. From the dorsal aspect, we can identify the trochlear nerve, tectum, and the fourth ventricle (Fig. 3.9).

3.4.1.1 Brainstem Overview: A Slingshot-Like Structure

1. At the top, there are two branches (cerebral peduncles of the midbrain).
2. In the middle, there is a thick handle (pons).
3. At the bottom, there is a slender tail (medulla).

3.4.1.2 Ventral Aspect of the Brainstem

3.4.1.2.1 Ventral Surface of the Brainstem (Midbrain, Pons, Medulla)

1. Boundary between midbrain and pons: On the ventral aspect, they are separated by the midbrain-pons sulcus, and on the dorsal aspect, they are separated by the upper limit of the rhomboid fossa.
2. Boundary between pons and medulla: On the ventral aspect, they are separated by the bulbopontine sulcus, and on the dorsal aspect, they are separated by the striae medullares within the rhomboid fossa.
3. Boundaries of the brainstem: It is bounded superiorly by the optic chiasm from the diencephalon and inferiorly by the decussation of pyramid from the cervical spinal cord.
4. There are nine pairs of cranial nerves that exit from the ventral aspect of the brainstem (except for the trochlear nerve, which emerges from the dorsal aspect).

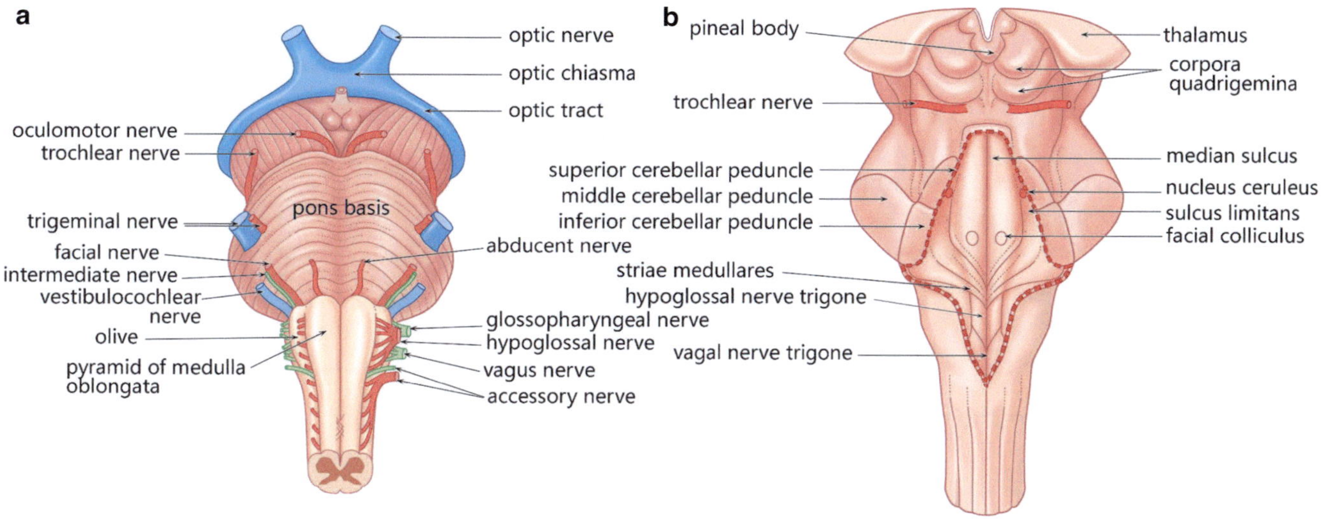

Fig. 3.9 Schematic diagram of key structures on the surface of the brainstem. (**a**) Ventral aspect of the brainstem, with the optic chiasm serving as the boundary with the diencephalon above and the pyramidal decussation serving as the boundary with the cervical spinal cord below. The diagram shows the nine pairs of cranial nerves entering or exiting the ventral aspect of the brainstem. (**b**) Dorsal aspect of the brainstem, showing the corpora quadrigemina, trochlear nerve, and the rhomboid fossa. 1 Median sulcus. 2 Sulcus limitans. 3 Striae medullares. 4 Medial eminence. 5 Facial colliculus. 6 Locus coeruleus. 7 Vestibular area. 8 Hypoglossal nerve trigone. 9 Vagal nerve trigone

3.4.1.3 Dorsal Aspect of the Brainstem

1. Tectum consists of the superior colliculus (center for visual reflexes) and the inferior colliculus (an important center in the auditory pathway). Together, they are referred to as the corpora quadrigemina.
2. Trochlear nerve emerges from the inferior border of the inferior colliculus.
3. Fourth ventricle is formed by the cerebellum, pons, and upper half of the medulla, surrounding it together.

3.4.1.4 Distinctive Structures of the Brainstem

3.4.1.4.1 Midbrain

1. Ventral Structures: The cerebral peduncles are two large columnar structures located on the ventral side of the midbrain. The space between the cerebral peduncles is known as the interpeduncular fossa, from which the oculomotor nerve emerges.
2. Lateral Surface: The lateral surface of the midbrain is adjacent to the uncus of the temporal lobe.
3. Dorsal Tectum: The dorsal surface of the midbrain consists of four colliculi. The superior colliculi, two upper colliculi, process visual information, while the inferior colliculi, two lower colliculi, process auditory information. The trochlear nerve emerges from the lower part of the dorsal surface of the midbrain, below the two inferior colliculi, then loops around the lateral side of the cerebral peduncles and travels forward between the peduncles and the uncus.

3.4.1.4.2 Pons

1. The majority of the pons is composed of transverse fibers known as the cerebellopontine tract. These fibers cause the surface of the pons to bulge, and in the midventral aspect of the pons, there is a shallow groove called the basilarsulcus, which accommodates the basilar artery. The pons gradually narrows on both sides and forms the middle cerebellar peduncles, which connect to the cerebellar hemispheres. At the junction between the middle cerebellar peduncles and the pons on each side, the trigeminal nerve enters the pons.
2. At the bulbopontine sulcus, the abduncent nerve, facial nerve, and vestibulocochlear nerve enter and exit the brainstem.
3. Cerebellopontine Peduncles: Located on the lateral side of the pontomedullary sulcus, it is the junction between the medulla/pons and the cerebellum. Clinically, it is referred to as the cerebellopontine angle, where the vestibulocochlear nerve is positioned.

3.4.1.4.3 Medulla Oblongata

1. Pyramids and olives: The pyramids are located on either side of the anterior median fissure. Just above the junction between the spinal cord and the medulla oblongata, the fibers from the decussation of pyramid fill the anterior median fissure. The olives are located on the lateral side of the pyramids, and behind the olives lies the inferior cerebellar peduncle.

2. Sulcus: The anterior median fissure is located between the pyramids. The groove between the pyramids and the olives is called the anterolateral sulcus, through which the hypoglossal nerve exits the brainstem. The groove between the olives and the inferior cerebellar peduncle is called the posterolateral sulcus, and within it, from top to bottom, the glossopharyngeal nerve, the vagus nerve, and the accessory nerve exit the brainstem. The spinal accessory nerve exits from the spinal cord and connects upward through the foramen magnum to join the cranial root of the accessory nerve.

3.4.1.4.4 Dorsal Surface of the Pons and Upper Medulla

The fourth ventricle is a cavity in the hindbrain, nestled within the rhombencephalon. It lies between the pons and medulla oblongata ventrally, and the cerebellum dorsally. The fourth ventricle is enclosed by a floor, a roof, and two lateral walls.

Roof: It has a tent-like shape, extending from the narrow head (near the cerebral aqueduct) to the wider apex (near the lateral recess). The roof is the widest and most expanded, where the tent-like shape is most pronounced. It descends, the roof narrows, and at the median aperture (foramen of Magendie), the space becomes very constricted, ending at the narrow tail of the ventricle. The apex of the roof divides it into an upper and lower part.

Floor: Due to its diamond shape, the floor of the fourth ventricle, named rhomboid fossa, is located on the dorsal aspect of the upper medulla and pons, beneath the cerebellum (Fig. 3.10).

1. Sulcus: A median sulcus divides the rhomboid fossa into left and right halves. Two sulcus limitans further divide each half of the rhomboid fossa into the inner medial eminence and the outer vestibular area.
2. Striae Medullares: They mark the boundary between the dorsal aspect of the pons and upper medulla. The anterior two-thirds of the rhomboid fossa corresponds to the dorsal aspect of the pons, while the posterior one-third corresponds to the dorsal aspect of the medulla.
3. Borders: The upper outer border is formed by the superior cerebellar peduncle. The lower outer border (from top to bottom) consists of the inferior cerebellar peduncle, the cuneate tubercle, and the gracile tubercle.
4. Important structures within the rhomboid fossa: The rhomboid fossa, or floor of the fourth ventricle, contains several important structures that are crucial for understanding brainstem function and for clinical neurology. These structures are related to sensory and motor nuclei, cranial nerve functions, and specialized centers. Medial eminence consists of facial colliculus (with the genu of the facial nerve and abducent nucleus deep within); hypoglossal triangle (with hypoglossal nucleus deep within); vagal triangle (with dorsal nucleus of vagus nerve deep within); separation stripe (a diagonal ridge at the lower outer border of the vagal trigone); last area (located between the funiculus separans and the gracile tubercle, considered part of the circumventricular organs); vestibular area (vestibular nucleus deep within); locus ceruleus (nucleus ceruleus deep within); and superior and inferior foveas (the sulcus limitans in the striae medullares form distinct concave regions known as the upper recess and lower recess)[3, 4, 5].

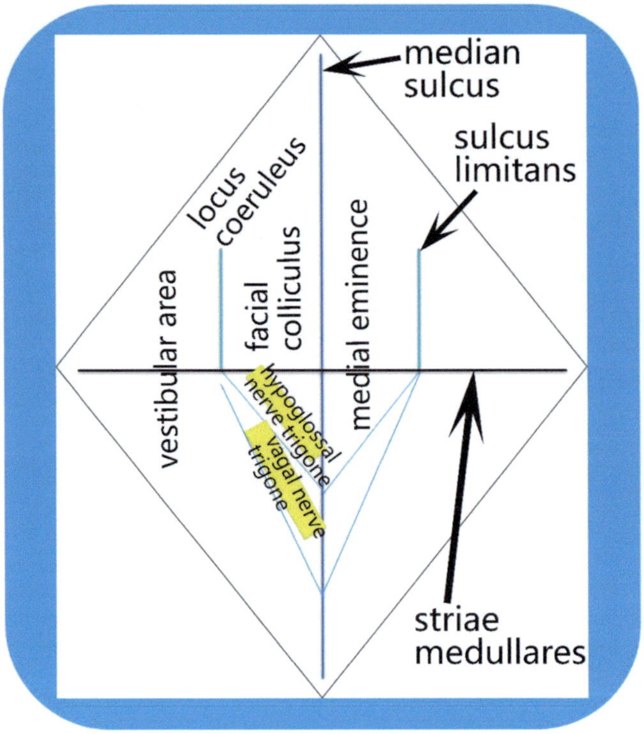

Fig. 3.10 Schematic diagram of important structures within the rhomboid fossa. 1 Olfactory tract (N I). 2 Optic nerve (N II). 3 Oculomotor nerve (N III). 4 Trochlear nerve (N IV). 5 Trigeminal nerve (N V). 6 Abducent nerve (N VI). 7 Facial nerve (N VII). 8 Vestibulocochlear nerve (N VIII). 9 Hypoglossal nerve (N XII). 10 Glossopharyngeal/vagus/accessory nerve (N IX/X/XI). 11 Observation of cranial nerve from ventral side of brainstem. 12 N I and ethmoidal foramen. 13 N II and optic canal. 14 NII, NIV, NVI, NV1, and superior orbital fissure. 15 NV2 and foramen ovale. 16 N V3 and foramen rotundum. 17 N VII and NVIII and porus acusticus internus. 18 N IX/X/XI and jugular foramen. 19 NXII and hypoglossal nerve canal. 20 Observation of the position of cranial nerves entering and exiting the skull base on the intracranial surface

3.4.2 Pairs of Cranial Nerves Emerging from the Brainstem and Their Exit Locations from the Cranial Cavity

Refer to (Fig. 3.11).

1. Interpeduncular fossa→oculomotor nerve→superior orbital fissure.
2. Lower of the inferior colliculus of the midbrain→trochlear nerve→superior orbital fissure.
3. Ventrolateral aspect of the middle cerebellar peduncle in the pons→trigeminal nerve→superior orbital fissure, foramen rotundum, foramen ovale.
4. Pontomedullary sulcus, from medial to lateral→abducens nerve→superior orbital fissure; facial nerve, intermediate nerve, vestibulocochlear nerve, cochlear nerve→internal acoustic meatus.
5. Posterolateral sulcus (between the olive and the inferior cerebellar peduncle), from top to bottom, glossopharyngeal nerve, vagus nerve, accessory nerve→jugular foramen.
6. Anterolateral sulcus (pyramidal olive sulcus) →hypoglossal nerve→hypoglossal neural tube.

3.4.3 General Layout of Internal Structures in the Brainstem

3.4.3.1 Cerebrospinal Fluid Pathways Within the Brainstem

Cerebrospinal fluid from the third ventricle flows through the cerebral aqueduct within the midbrain, enters the fourth ventricle in the dorsal aspect of the pons and upper medulla, communicates with the central canal of the spinal cord, and also flows into the subarachnoid space through the median aperture and lateral apertures of the fourth ventricle.

From an embryological perspective, the cerebral aqueduct, fourth ventricle, and central canal of the spinal cord are

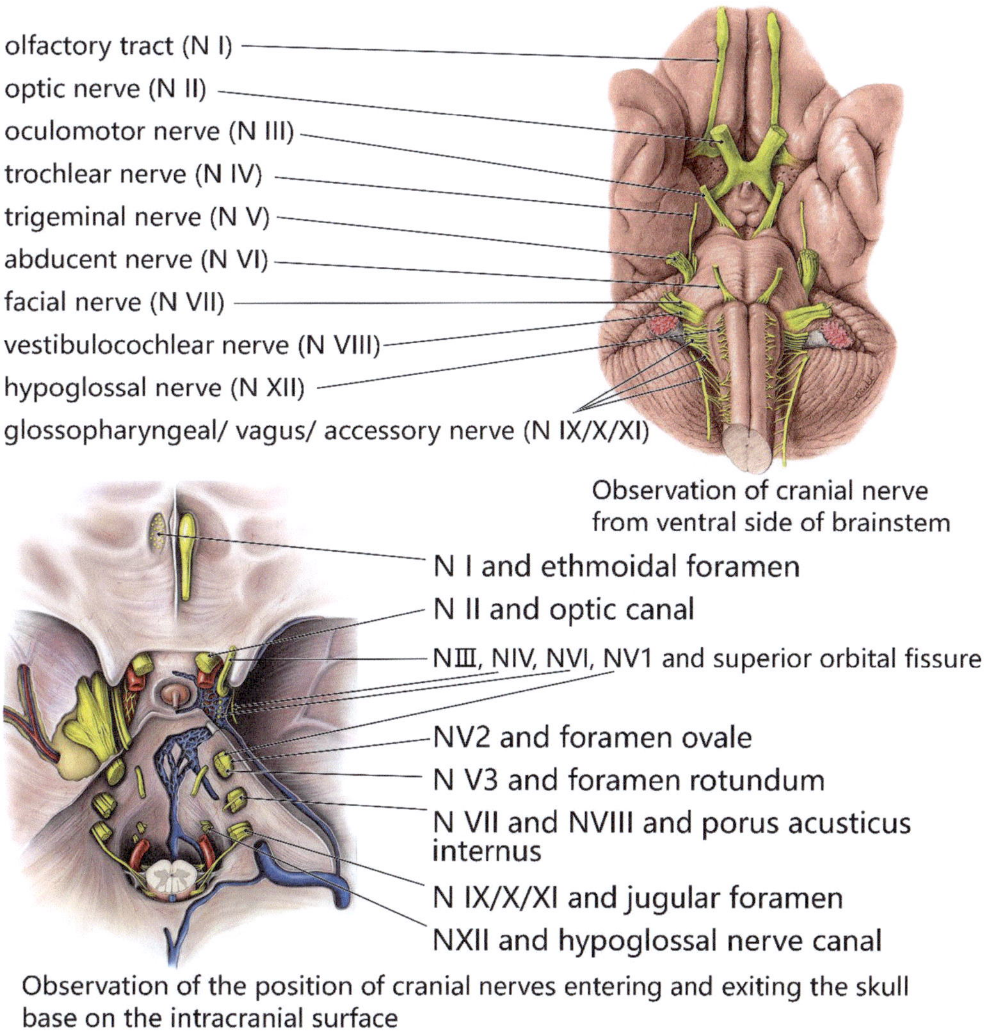

Fig. 3.11 Diagram illustrating the entry and exit points of cranial nerves in the brainstem and cranial cavity. 1 Tectum (corpora quadrigemina). 2 Tegmentum. 3 Basis

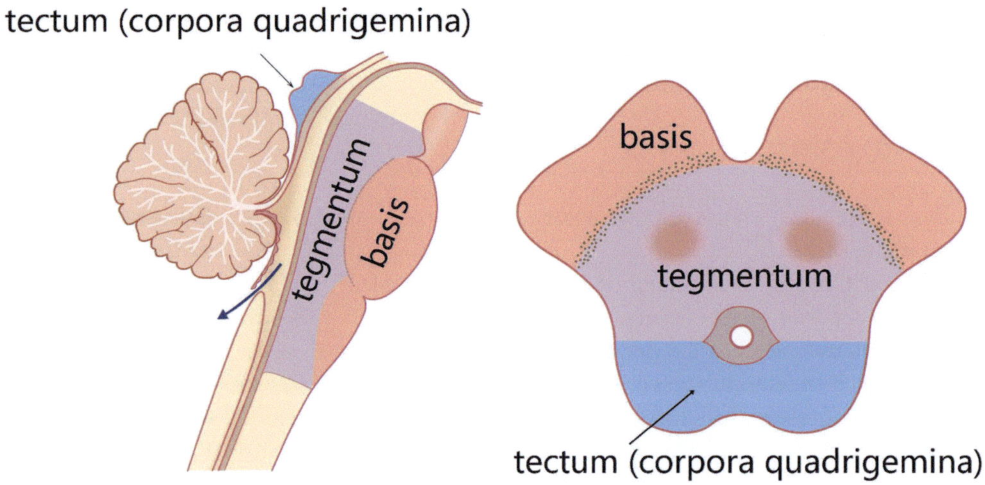

Fig. 3.12 Internal subdivisions of the brainstem. (**a**). Midsagittal view. (**b**) axial view. The brainstem is divided into tectum, tegmentum, and basis. 1 joint, skin, skeletal muscle. 2 somatic sensory nerve fiber. 3 afferent nerve. 4 visceral sensory nerve fiber. 5 viscus, blood vessel. 6 body. 7 central nervous system. 8 viscus. 9 skeletal muscle. 10 somatic motor nerve fiber 13 gland, smooth muscle, myocardium

all derived from the central canal of the embryonic neural tube, and they communicate with each other (see Fig. 3.4).

3.4.3.2 Naming of Brainstem Regions in the Anteroposterior Axis

When discussing the brainstem, three terms are commonly used: "tectum," "tegmentum," and "basis" (Fig. 3.12).

1. Tectum, meaning "roof" in Latin, is prominent in the midbrain and consists of the superior colliculi and inferior colliculi located on the dorsal aspect of the cerebral aqueduct.
2. Tegmentum, meaning "covering," is the middle region of the brainstem, located ventral to the cerebral aqueduct in the midbrain and ventral to the fourth ventricle in the pons and medulla. The tegmentum includes nuclei and the reticular formation.
3. Basis is the most ventral part, primarily composed of the corticospinal tracts and corticobulbar tracts. The anterior edge of the substantia nigra in the midbrain, the anterior edge of the medial lemniscus in the pons, and the posterior edge of the pyramid in the medulla mark the boundary between the basis and the tegmentum.

3.5 Key Functional Concepts of the Nervous System

3.5.1 Principles of Nervous System Operation

To fully understand the anatomy of the brainstem, it is best to comprehensively and systematically grasp the working principles of the nervous system, clearly delineating the specific roles played by the brainstem or the roles it assumes. The following simplified diagram (Fig. 3.13) will aid in understanding.

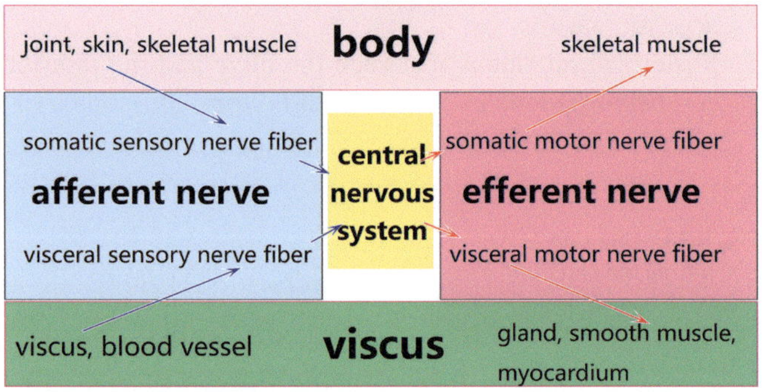

Fig. 3.13 Principles of the nervous system operation. 1 sensory cortex. 2 motor connectivity area of the prefrontal cortex. 3 motor cortex issuing instructions. 4 basal ganglia. 5 thalamus. 6 execution: influence of extrapyramidal system on posture, balance, and gait. 7 coordination and time selection: cerebellar input. 8 sensory afferent. 9 continuous feedback. 10 receptor. 11 play the role of uploading and issuing. 12 spinal cord. 13 execution: corticospinal tract to skeletal muscle. 14 muscle contraction and movement. 15 brainstem

3.5.2 Sensory and Motor Function Terms

3.5.2.1 Somatic and Visceral Functions

Somatic sensation refers to the response of receptors located in the body surface or deep tissues, including skeletal muscles, bones, and joints to external stimuli, enabling one to perceive their own position in relation to the surrounding environment.

Visceral sensation involves receptors located in the cardiovascular system, glands, and internal organs, which respond to changes in the internal environment, allowing for the perception of microenvironmental changes within the human body.

3.5.2.2 General and Special

1. Sensation and movement that occur in the head, face, trunk, and limbs are referred to as general (general) sensation and movement.

2. Sensation and movement that are exclusive to the head and face are termed special (special) sensation and movement [6].

3.5.2.3 Sensation

1. General somatic sensation includes two types: (1) surface sensation, which refers to the perception of external stimuli, and (2) deep sensation or proprioception, which pertains to the perception of one's own position and condition in the external environment.
2. General visceral sensation receives primary sensory fibers from the viscera and cardiovascular system, corresponding to the intermediomedial column of the spinal cord.
3. Special somatic sensation involves the eyes and ears, assisting in the perception of one's own position and condition, and is restricted to the head region.
4. Special visceral sensation includes taste and olfaction, which can influence the activities of certain visceral organs, glands, and blood vessels.

3.5.2.4 Movement

1. General somatic motor refers to the movement of most skeletal muscles throughout the body, including reflexive, voluntary, and rhythmic movements.
2. Visceral motor: (1) Special visceral motor controls the movements of the muscles of mastication, and (2) general visceral motor encompasses the sympathetic and parasympathetic nerve, regulating the activities of thoracic and abdominal viscera, blood vessels, glands, etc.

3.5.2.5 Upper Motor Neurons and Lower Motor Neurons

1. Upper motor neurons are the efferent neurons from the cerebral cortex to the nuclei involved in general somatic and special visceral motor functions of the cranial nerves, as well as the motor neurons in the anterior horn of the spinal cord.
2. Lower motor neurons are the motor neurons located in the nuclei responsible for general somatic and special visceral motor functions of the cranial nerves and the anterior horn of the spinal cord. Their cell bodies and axons constitute the final pathway for transmitting motor impulses, known as the "final common pathway."

3.5.2.6 Types of Motor Activity

1. Reflexive movement occurs at the spinal cord and brainstem levels but is modulated by higher central structures.
2. Rhythmic movement involves low central activity under higher-level control.
3. Voluntary movement originates from the cerebral cortex and requires conscious intent.

3.5.2.7 Role of the Brainstem in Voluntary Movement

The brainstem acts as a conduit for communication between the upper and lower structures, maintaining muscle tone and regulating posture (Fig. 3.14).

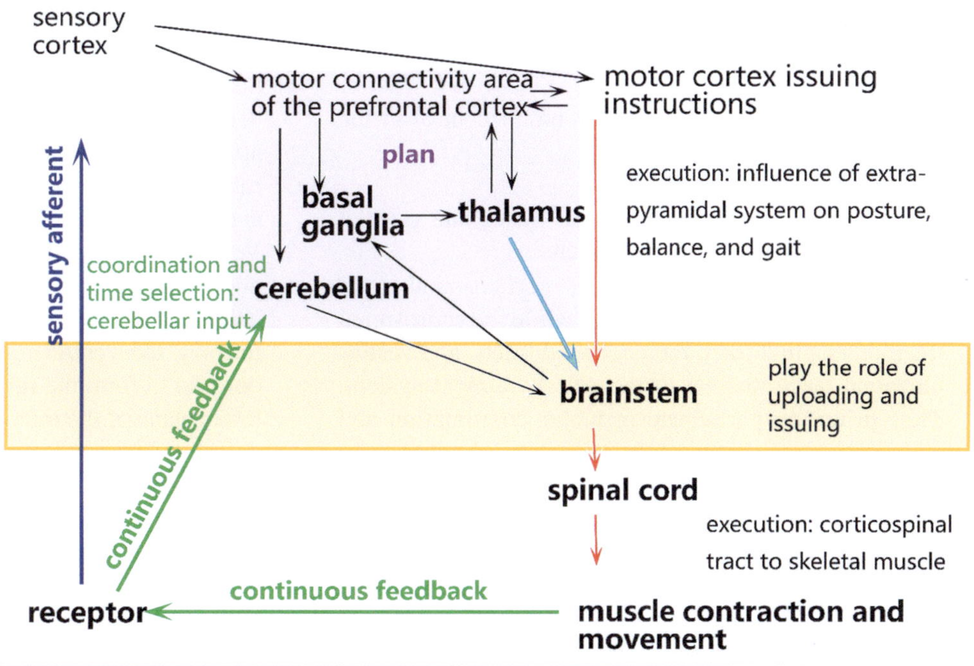

Fig. 3.14 Diagram illustrating the control of voluntary movement. 1 corticospinal tract. 2 corticonuclear tract. 3 dentate nucleus-thalamus tract. 4 pontocerebellar tract. 5 posterior spinocerebellar tract. 6 medial lemniscus. 7 spinal lemniscus

3.6 Functional Pathways and Related Nuclei Within the Brainstem

3.6.1 Overview of the Major Ascending and Descending Pathways

3.6.1.1 Major Ascending Pathways

1. From the spinal cord, there are two main pathways for superficial and deep sensations.
   (a) Dorsal column system (gracile fasciculus and cuneate fasciculus➔medial lemniscus) ➔deep sensation.
   (b) Anterolateral system (spinothalamic tract➔spinal lemniscus)➔superficial sensation.
2. Sensory pathways from cranial nerves (head and facial sensory receptors).
   (a) Trigeminal nerve➔trigeminal lemniscus➔head and facial somatic sensation.
   (b) Cochlear nerve➔lateral lemniscus➔audition.
   (c) Optic nerve➔visual pathway➔vision (does not pass through the brainstem, but visual fibers regulate eye movements via the superior colliculus).
   (d) Vestibular nerve➔vestibular pathway➔ equilibratory sensation.
   (e) Facial and glossopharyngeal nerves➔gustatory pathway➔taste.
   (f) Olfaction (does not pass through the brainstem).

3.6.1.2 Major Descending Pathways

1. Descending pathways for somatic motor control in the lateral system to the spinal cord.
   (a) Lateral corticospinal tract.
   (b) Rubrospinal tract
2. Descending pathways for somatic motor control in the medial system to the spinal cord.
   (a) Anterior corticospinal tract.
   (b) Tectospinal tract, reticulospinal tracts, and (medial and lateral) vestibulospinal tracts.

   Among these pathways, the corticospinal tract belongs to the pyramidal system, while the rubrospinal tract, tectospinal tract, reticulospinal tracts, and vestibulospinal tracts belong to the extrapyramidal system. They primarily participate in motor coordination and control, establishing close connections with the cerebellum.

3.6.1.3 Pathways for Cerebellar Input and Output Through the Brainstem

The cerebellum communicates with the brainstem, spinal cord, and cerebrum through its superior, middle, and inferior peduncles, enabling it to fulfill its unique functions.

3.6.1.4 Visceral Motor Functions of Cranial Nerves

The dorsal longitudinal fasciculus serves as a crucial pathway for the hypothalamus to regulate sympathetic and parasympathetic functions. The medial region of the anterior hypothalamic region promotes parasympathetic activity, while the lateral region of the posterior hypothalamic region stimulates sympathetic activity.

3.6.2 Major Crossings along the Axis of the Brainstem and Spinal Cord (Fig. 3.15)

1. Anterior white commissure of the spinal cord: Fibers carrying superficial sensory information cross and form the spinothalamic tract, ascending throughout the entire spinal cord.
2. Pyramidal decussation: The corticospinal tract crosses at the level of the medulla oblongata, specifically at the junction between the medulla and cervical spinal cord.
3. Medial lemniscus decussation: Fibers from the gracile and cuneate nuclei form an arch-shaped crossing, creating the medial lemniscus at the level of the medulla.
4. Trapezoid body: The majority of axons from the cochlear nucleus cross to the contralateral side, along with a small portion of fibers, forming the lateral lemniscus, which ascends to the inferior colliculus at the level of the pontomedullary junction.
5. Trigeminal lemniscus decussation: Axons from the trigeminal nucleus (spinal tract, principal, and mesencephalic) cross to the contralateral side, forming the trigeminal lemniscus at the level of the pons.
6. Superior cerebellar peduncle decussation: The track of dentate nucleus-red nucleus-thalamus cross each other after exiting the cerebellar superior peduncle➔ nucleus ruber pars parvocellularis ➔ventrolateral nucleus of the thalamus at the level of the midbrain.
7. Ventral tegmental decussation: Efferent fibers from the nucleus ruber pars magnocellularis cross to the contralateral side in the lower plane of the superior colliculus, forming the ventral tegmental decussation. They then descend to form the rubrospinal tract at the level of the lower plane of the inferior colliculus.
8. Dorsal tegmental decussation: Fibers from the superior colliculus cross the midline on the ventral side of the cerebral aqueduct in the midbrain and then descend to form the tectospinal tract at the level of the upper midbrain.
9. Crossing of two special corticonuclear tracts: The hypoglossal nucleus and the upper part of the facial nucleus are contralaterally innervated, while the rest are bilaterally innervated.

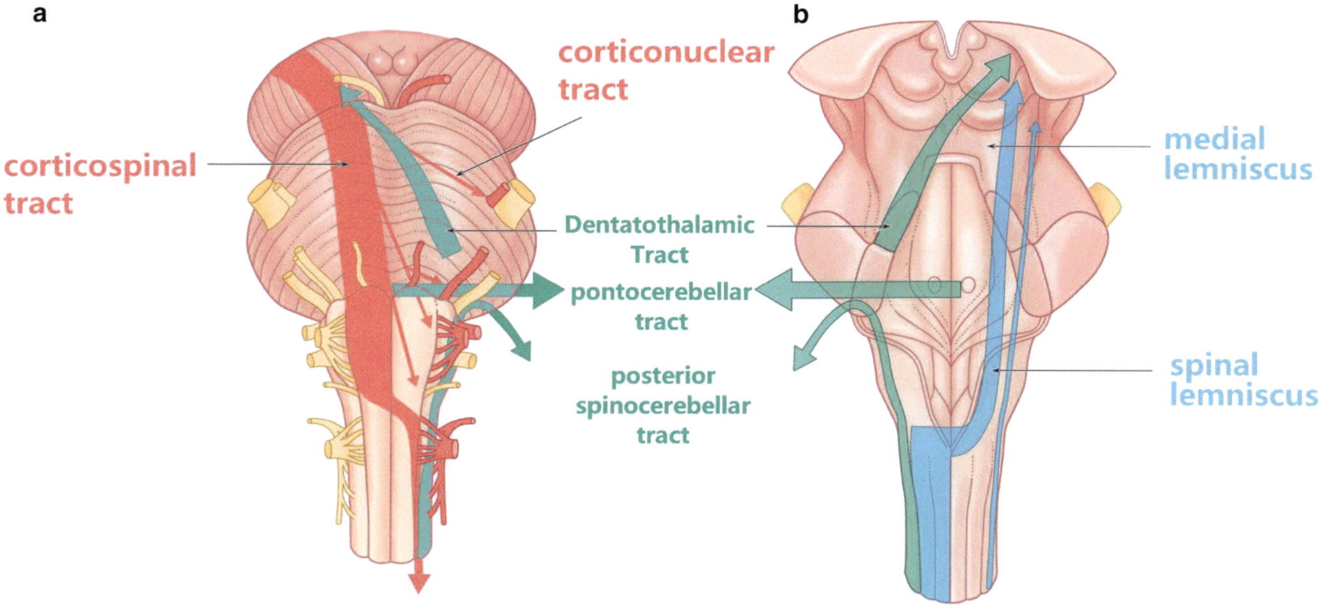

Fig. 3.15 Schematic diagram of the main conduction pathways and crossings in the brainstem. (**a**) The main conduction pathways on the ventral side of the brainstem are the pyramidal system for motor function (corticospinal and corticonuclear tracts). (**b**) The main conduction pathways on the dorsal side are the ascending sensory pathways (medial and lateral leminisci). The corticonuclear tract is mostly bilaterally innervated, while the corticospinal tract mostly crosses to the contralateral side. The gracile and cuneate nuclei cross in the medulla to form the medial lemniscus, which ascends. The cerebellum connects to the brainstem, vestibular nuclei, and spinal cord through fiber tracts, all of which cross within the brainstem. 1 Midbrain. 2 Superior pons. 3 Superior medulla oblongata. 4 Inferior medulla oblongata. 5 Cervical spinal cord. 6 Rostral reticular formation. 7 Caudal reticular formation

10. Decussation of the trochlear nerve: The only crossing of cranial nerves within the brainstem occurs in the midbrain.

3.6.2.1 Brainstem's 18 Cranial Nerve Nuclei

3.6.2.1.1 Pairs of Cranial Nerve Nuclei

1. Composition: Four pairs of general somatic motor nuclei (oculomotor, trochlear, abducens, and hypoglossal nuclei); four pairs of special visceral motor nuclei (trigeminal motor, facial, glossopharyngeal, and vagus nuclei); one pair of general visceral motor nuclei (E-W, superior and inferior salivatory nuclei, the dorsal nucleus of the vagus nerve); one pair of visceral sensory nuclei (solitary nucleus); three pairs of general somatic sensory nuclei (trigeminal midbrain, pons, and spinal nuclei); and two pairs of special somatic sensory nuclei (vestibular and cochlear nuclei).
2. Location: All 18 pairs of cranial nerve nuclei are located within the tegmentum of the brainstem, adjacent to the dorsal side of the cerebral aqueduct or the fourth ventricle.
3. Brainstem exits of cranial nerve fibers: The fibers connecting to the 18 pairs of cranial nerve nuclei remain within the brainstem, except for the trochlear nerve fibers, which cross and exit the brainstem on the dorsal side. The other fibers run to the ventral or lateral sides of the brainstem and do not cross within the brainstem.

3.6.2.2 Location of Cranial Nerve Nuclei and Cranial Nerves

1. Midbrain
   (a) Oculomotor nucleus and oculomotor accessory nucleus (➔oculomotor nerve).
   (b) Inferior colliculus level: trochlear nucleus (➔trochlear nerve).
2. Pons
   (a) Upper level of pons: Trigeminal motor nucleus (➔motor root of trigeminal nerve with mandibular branch exiting the brainstem). Trigeminal pontine nucleus (receives cutaneous touch-pressure sensation from the face).
   (b) Middle level of pons: Abducens nucleus (➔abducens nerve) located deep to the facial colliculus. Facial nucleus (➔facial nerve) is located vetrolateral to the abducens nucleus.
   (c) Lowest level of pons: Superior salivatory nucleus (➔facial nerve). Vestibular nucleus (receives vestibular nerve input) located deep to the vestibular area consisted of the superior, inferior, medial, and lateral vestibular nuclei. Dorsal cochlear nucleus and ventral cochlear nuclei (receives cochlear nerve input)

are located in the dorsolateral and ventrolateral side of the cerebellar peduncle, respectively.

3. Medulla Oblongata
   (a) Upper medulla: Nucleus ambiguus (sends fibers to join the glossopharyngeal nerve, vagus nerve, and accessory nerve) located within the reticular formation of the upper medulla. Inferior salivatory nucleus (sends fibers to join the glossopharyngeal nerve) is located in the upper olive of the medulla. Solitary nucleus is located in the upper medulla, the upper part of the solitary nucleus (receives taste input from the facial nerve, glossopharyngeal nerve, and vagus nerve), and the lower part of the solitary nucleus (receives general visceral sensory input from the glossopharyngeal nerve and vagus nerve). Hypoglossal nucleus (sends fibers to form the hypoglossal nerve) is located in the deep aspect of the hypoglossal nerve triangle in the upper medulla.
   (b) Solitary nucleus: Accessory nucleus (sends fibers to form the accessory nerve) located at the caudal end of the special visceral motor column, actually extending into the upper cervical spinal cord, specifically the dorsolateral aspect of the anterior horn of the upper five or six cervical segments.
   (c) Trigeminal sensory nuclei spanning the entire brainstem: Mesencephalic nucleus of trigeminal (receives proprioception input from the trigeminal nerve), pontine nucleus (receives touch-pressure sensation input from the trigeminal nerve), and spinal trigeminal nucleus (receives pain and temperature sensation input from the trigeminal nerve).

3.7 Reticular Formation of the Brainstem

3.7.1 Overview of the Reticular Formation

The reticular formation is a highly ancient neural network in terms of evolutionary development; it is a prominent feature of the brainstem in reptiles. It originates from a slow-conducting polysynaptic pathway and is closely linked to olfactory and limbic regions. In the human brain, the reticular formation remains significant in automatic and reflex activities and maintains connections with the limbic system.

The reticular formation is located within the tegmentum of the brainstem, and its definition has evolved over time. The term "reticular" was first applied to this area in the late nineteenth century, because conventional techniques could not distinctly differentiate its neural nuclei; furthermore, some neurons in the tegmentum of the brainstem have very widespread projections, giving the impression of a dispersed organization. However, with the application of more refined techniques, many specific nuclei and their neurotransmitters have been identified, revealing precise organizational projections. Additionally, some cranial nerve nuclei (such as the superior and inferior salivatory nuclei or the nucleus ambiguus) do not belong to reticular formation but are embedded within it, while areas such as the periaqueductal gray matter (associated with pain modulation) around the cerebral aqueduct and the chemotactic trigger zone (area postrema) within the medulla, which triggers nausea, are closely related to the reticular formation but are not part of it. Therefore, in the modern era, the term "reticular formation" is used for fewer structures, and instead, we generally refer to specific nuclei within the tegmentum of the brainstem. The term "reticular formation" is still used for the tegmental region of the brainstem because of the lower degree of cell nucleus identification.

3.7.2 Organization of the Reticular Formation of the Brainstem

1. Medial to the midline, the medial reticular formation consists of a series of raphe nuclei. These nuclei serve as the primary source of 5-serotonin projection throughout the entire neural axis.
2. The paramedian reticular formation constitutes a major efferent system. It plays a role in generating motor patterns of synapse within the nuclei of the cranial nerves.
3. The outermost layer is the lateral parvocellular (small-cell) reticular formation. The parvocellular cells exhibit long and regular dendritic branching, primarily in the horizontal plane, with long pathways traversing toward the thalamus. The lateral reticular formation is primarily involved in receiving inputs, receiving fibers from all sensory pathways.

3.7.3 Functional Anatomy of the Reticular Formation

3.7.3.1 Rostral Reticular Formation and Its Functions

The reticular formation spans the entire brainstem.

With its rostral end connecting to specific diencephalic nuclei and its caudal end merging into the intermediate zone of the spinal cord, this anatomical arrangement highlights two primary functional divisions: the rostral and caudal reticular formations. The rostral reticular formation, located in the midbrain and upper pons, works in concert with diencephalic nuclei to maintain the forebrain's state of arousal and consciousness. It plays a crucial role in regulating wakefulness, alertness, and attention, ensuring that the brain remains responsive to internal and external stimuli (Fig. 3.16).

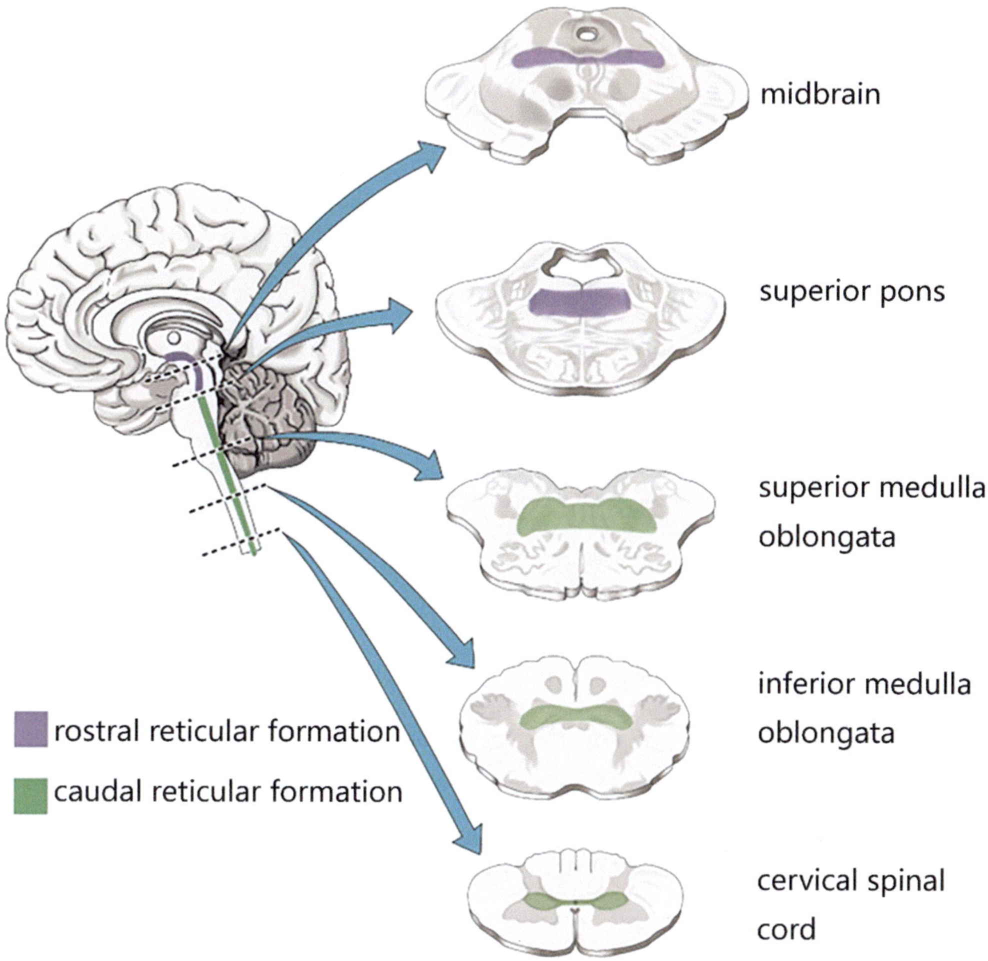

Fig. 3.16 Schematic diagram of the brainstem structures. The reticular formation spans the entire brainstem. The rostral portion of the reticular formation is connected to certain diencephalic nuclei, known as the rostral reticular formation (mainly responsible for maintaining wakefulness and consciousness of the forebrain). The caudal portion of the reticular formation merges into the intermediate zone of the spinal cord, known as the caudal reticular formation (involved in reflexes and motor functions) in collaboration with cranial nerve nuclei and the spinal cord, performing various important motor, reflex, and autonomic functions

3.7.3.2 Caudal Reticular Formation and Its Functions

The caudal reticular formation in the pons and medulla, in collaboration with cranial nerve nuclei and the spinal cord, is responsible for various essential motor, reflex, and autonomic functions. In summary, the rostral reticular formation is primarily associated with arousal functions, while the caudal reticular formation is primarily associated with reflexes and motor functions [7].

3.7.3.3 Summary of Functions of the Reticular Formation in the Brainstem

A summary of the specific functions and locations of the reticular formation in the brainstem can be found in Table 3.1.

Table 3.1 Functions of the brainstem

Generation of Motor Patterns	1. Vertical gaze center in the midbrain; horizontal gaze center in the pons
	2. Rhythmic chewing—motor trigeminal nucleus in the pons
	3. Swallowing, vomiting, coughing, yawning, and sneezing—medulla
	4. Pontine motor center initiates automatic walking
	5. Pontine center for micturition control
Respiratory Control	1. Dorsal (inspiration) and ventral (expiration) respiratory nuclei at the upper end of the medulla
	2. The parabrachial nucleus (surrounding gray matter surrounding brachium conjunctivum) is involved in the respiratory pattern during wakefulness
	3. Chemosensitive area around the lateral aperture of fourth ventricle in the dorsal part of the medulla is highly sensitive to the concentration of hydrogen ions in CSF
Cardiovascular Control	The solitary nucleus serves as the central processing site for baroreceptor inputs from the following:
	1. Carotid sinus-glossopharyngeal nerve
	2. Aortic arch-vagus nerve
Sleep and Wakefulness	The arousal-promoting systems in the posterior midbrain and rostral pons:
	1. Cholinergic pontine nuclei and the laterodorsal tegmental nucleus
	2. Sleep-inducing systems such as the raphe nuclei, the parafacial respiratory group, and the parabrachial nucleus, PAG in the midbrain and the GABAergic neurons in the caudal pons have a sleep-promoting effect
Sensory Gate Control	The nucleus raphe magnus serves as an important structure for supraspinal analgesia
	1 Tectum (corpora quadrigemina)
	2 Tegmentum (nucleus ruber)
	3 Basal cerebral peduncle (pyramidal tract)
	4 Basal ganglia of pons
	5 Olive nucleus of the superior medulla oblongata
	6 Gracile, cuneate body of inferior medulla oblongata
	7 Aqueduct
	8 Superior fourth ventricle
	9 Inferior fourth ventricle
	10 Fourth ventricle vanish

3.8 Transverse Anatomy of the Brainstem

3.8.1 Ten Key Transverse Sections of the Brainstem

1. Section of the First Cervical Segment of the Spinal Cord

   Apart from the accessory nucleus of the spinal cord, it is similar to other cervical segments. The spinal trigeminal nucleus is visible.
2. unction of the Medulla and Spinal Cord
   (a) The pyramidal decussation is the most prominent feature (located at the base of the medulla).
   (b) The reticular formation appears (located in the tegmentum of the medulla), and the posterior column is within the tegmentum of the medulla.
   (c) The anterior surface of the central canal of the spinal cord shows the medial and dorsal longitudinal fasciculi.
3. Middle Medulla
   (a) The gracile and cuneate nuclei appear within the tegmentum of the medulla, along with the medial lemniscus crossing, reticular formation, inferior olivary nucleus, nucleus ambiguous, and hypoglossal nucleus. The hypoglossal nerve emerges from between the pyramid and the olive.
   (b) The pyramid occupies the basis of the medulla.
4. Upper medulla
   (a) The uncrossed corticospinal tract occupies the base of the medulla.
   (b) Within the tegmentum, the olivary nucleus is a prominent structure at this level: the olivocerebellar tract crossing—the spinothalamic tract and medial lemniscus and reticular formation.
   (c) The hypoglossal nucleus, vestibular nucleus, solitary nucleus, and nucleus ambiguous are in the dorsal tegmentum.
5. Junction of the Pons and Medulla
   (a) The trapezoid body separates the basis from the tegmentum.
   (b) (Ambiguus/facial nucleus.
6. Mid-Pons
   (a) Four colliculi are visible (medial, lateral, spinal, and trigeminal colliculi).
   (b) Trapezoid body.
   (c) Facial genu and abducens nucleus.

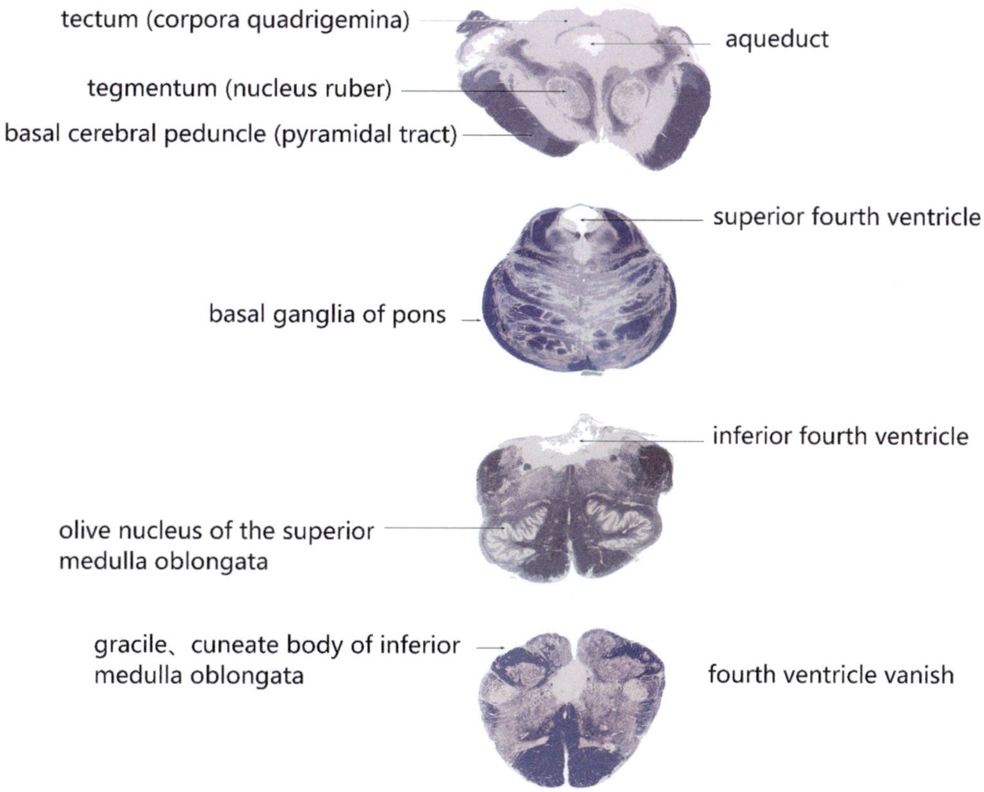

Fig. 3.17 Characteristic structures of the brainstem at key levels of section. 1 Decussation of the superior cerebellar peduncle. 2 Decussation of the medial lemniscus. 3 Decussation of the pyramid

7. Upper Pons
   (a) Pontine nuclei and transverse fibers (present throughout the entire pons).
   (b) The trigeminal nerve enters the ventrolateral aspect of the pons at the level of the middle cerebellar peduncle. Trigeminal colliculus crossing.
   (c) The cerebellopontine fibers of the corticospinal tract divide into many smaller bundles.
   (d) The superior cerebellar peduncles are visible on both sides of the roof of the fourth ventricle.
8. Lower Midbrain
   (a) Typical cerebral peduncle, substantia nigra, and decussation of the superior cerebellar peduncle. The only decussation of trochlear.
   (b) Ascending tracts are located in the tegmentum, and descending tracts are located in the basis. Inferior colliculus of tectum.
9. Upper Midbrain
   (a) The superior colliculus and substantia nigra appear simultaneously.
   (b) Dorsal and ventral crossings in the tegmentum.
10. Junction of the Midbrain and Thalamus
   (a) Thalamus, substantia nigra, nucleus ruber, and the internal and external geniculate body.
   (b) Habenular commissure.

3.8.2 Summary of Three Key Structures of the Brainstem

1. Key structures of the midbrain

   The midbrain is relatively short, and most axial sections pass through either the superior colliculus (closer to the head) or inferior colliculus (closer to the tail). These two levels of sections can be distinguished, because the axial section through the superior colliculus includes the oculomotor nucleus and the nucleus ruber, while the axial section through the inferior colliculus includes the trochlear nucleus and the brachium conjunctivum (superior cerebellar peduncle) crossing (Figs. 3.17 and 3.18).
2. Key Structures of the Pons

   The ventral pons consists of the basilar pons, which includes the corticospinal tracts and the corticobulbar tracts, as well as the pontine nuclei involved in cerebellar function. The pontine tegmentum contains many important nuclei and pathways. The fourth ventricle separates the pontine tegmentum from the cerebellum (see Fig. 3.17).
3. Key Structures of the Medulla Oblongata

   Like the midbrain, the medulla oblongata has rostral and caudal levels. In the rostral medullary section, the inferior olivary nucleus and the fourth ventricle are pres-

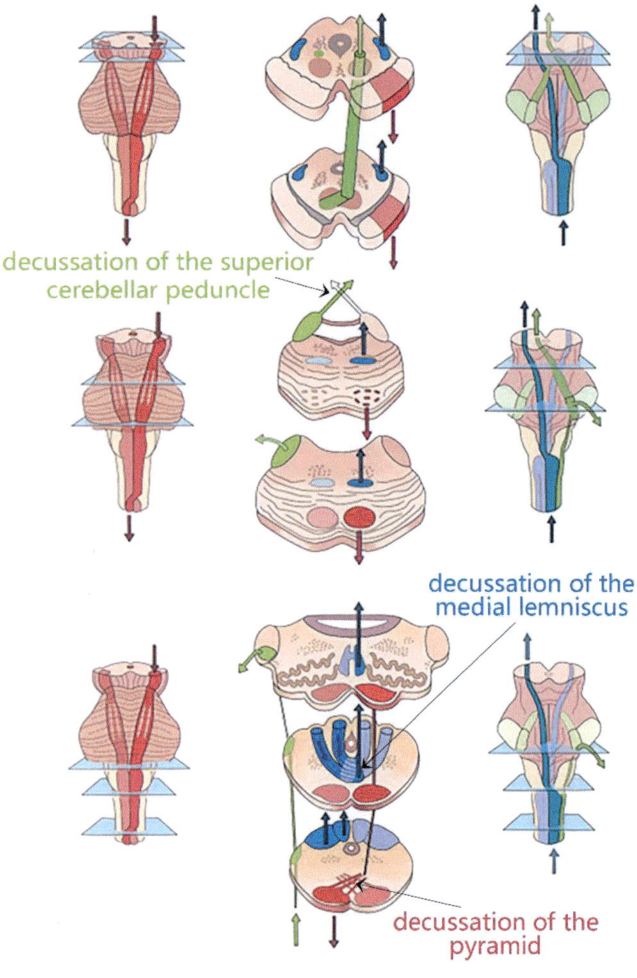

Fig. 3.18 Schematic representation of important crossings within the brainstem. 1 oculomotor nerve. 2 medulla oblongata. 3 trigeminal nerve. 4 abducent nerve. 5 vestibulocochlear nerve. 6 facial nerve. 7 glossopharyngeal nerve. 8 vagus nerve. 9 hypoglossal nerve. 10 left basilar artery. 11 midbrain. 12 pons

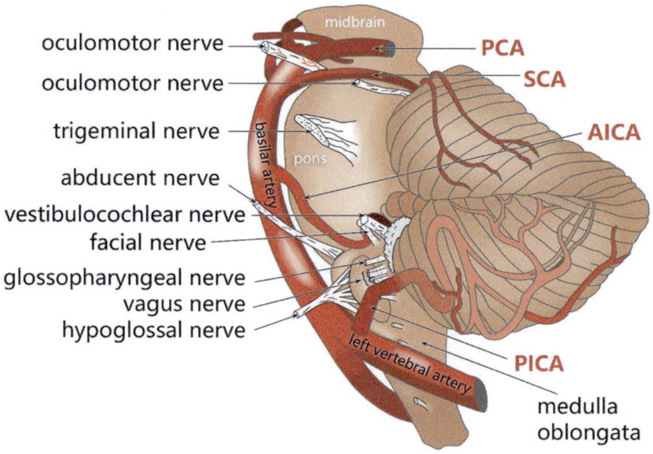

Fig. 3.19 Four major branches of the vertebral-basilar arterial system. The vertebral arteries on both sides converge to form the basilar artery. The posterior inferior cerebellar artery (PICA) arises from the vertebral artery and supplies the lateral medulla and the occipital surface of the cerebellar hemisphere. The anterior inferior cerebellar artery (AICA) arises from the basilar artery and supplies the pons and the petrosal surface of the cerebellar hemisphere. The superior cerebellar artery (SCA) arises from the basilar artery before it bifurcates and supplies the tentorial surface of the cerebellar hemisphere. The posterior cerebral artery (PCA) arises from the terminal bifurcation of the basilar artery and supplies the midbrain and the inferior surface of the cerebral hemisphere occipital lobe. Important cranial nerves entering and exiting the brainstem are labeled on the left side of the figure, and the four major branches of the vertebral-basilar arterial system are labeled on the right side of the figure: PCA, posterior cerebral artery; SCA, superior cerebellar artery; AICA, anterior inferior cerebellar artery; PICA, posterior inferior cerebellar artery. 1 short circumferential artery. 2 long circumferential artery. 3 paramedian perforating artery

ent. In the caudal medullary section, the inferior olivary nucleus and the fourth ventricle are absent, but the posterior column and posterior column nuclei are present. Other important landmarks include the inferior cerebellar peduncles, pyramidal tracts, anterolateral system, and medial lemniscus. The transition between the medulla oblongata and the spinal cord is marked by the pyramidal decussation. The upper cervical cord contains the spinal accessory nucleus (see Fig. 3.17).

3.9 Blood Supply of the Brainstem

Study Guide

Understand the arterial blood supply of the brainstem and the distribution of arterial branches: The blood supply of the brainstem comes from the vertebral-basilar arterial system. This arterial system gives rise to four major branches within the skull, which then give rise to the basal branch and dorsal lateral branches that supply the brainstem (Fig. 3.19).

Meanwhile, the basilar artery gives off small branches (paramedian, short circumferential, and long circumferential branches) to supply different regions of the brainstem.

3.9.1 Four Major Branches of the Vertebral-Basilar Arterial System

1. Posterior Inferior Cerebellar Artery (PICA)
   (a) Originating from the vertebral artery at the level of the medulla, the PICA wraps around the medulla to supply its lateral aspect and the inferior part of the cerebellum.
   (b) It forms a neurovascular complex with the posterior group of cranial nerves and enters the cerebellomedullary fissure.
2. Anterior Inferior Cerebellar Artery (AICA)
   (a) Arising from the proximal basilar artery at the level of the caudal pons, usually after the convergence of the vertebral arteries, the AICA supplies the caudal

aspect of the pons and a small portion of the cerebellar region.
   (b) It forms a neurovascular complex with the facial nucleus and vestibulocochlear nerve and enters the cerebellopontine fissure.
3. Superior Cerebellar Artery (SCA)
   (a) Originating from the top of the basilar artery at the level of the rostral pons, the SCA primarily supplies the upper small part of the cerebellum.
   (b) It forms a neurovascular complex with the trigeminal nerve and enters the cerebellomesencephalic fissure.
4. Posterior Cerebral Artery (PCA)
   (a) The posterior cerebral artery, also originating from the top of the basilar artery, immediately follows the superior cerebellar artery (SCA). The oculomotor nerve (CN III) usually courses between the SCA and PCA. The PCA wraps around the midbrain to supply it and provides blood supply to most of the thalamus, the medial aspect of the occipital lobe, and the inferomedial aspect of the temporal lobe.
   (b) PCA—to supratentorium region.

Additionally, the anterior spinal artery supplies the brainstem.

3.9.2 Branches of the Basilar Artery

The brainstem is primarily supplied by the main arteries branching into paramedian, short circumferential, and long circumferential arteries (Fig. 3.20).

1. Paramedian branches tend to run toward the midline, with individual branch providing blood supply to the right or left paramedian region.
2. There are also arteries extending different lengths from the ventral surface of the brainstem, with the longest branches reaching the ventricles. Short circumferential arteries and long circumferential arteries supply the lateral aspect of the brainstem.

3.9.3 Blood Supply Territories of the Brainstem

1. Medial medulla: Supplied by the paramedian branches of the anterior spinal artery on the ipsilateral side and the paramedian branches of the vertebral artery on the contralateral side.
2. Lateral medulla: Supplied by perforating branches from the vertebral artery and PICA.

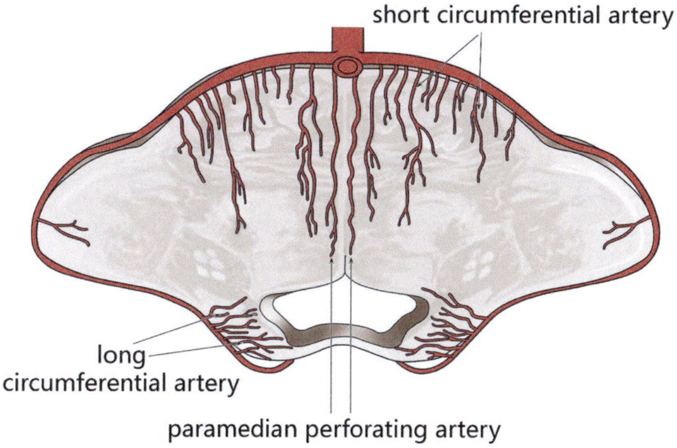

Fig. 3.20 Three types of perforating arteries in the brainstem. From ventral to dorsal, they are the paramedian perforating arteries (supplying the ventral paramedian region of the brainstem), the short circumferential arteries (supplying the lateral aspect of the brainstem), and the long circumferential arteries (supplying the dorsal aspect of the brainstem). 1 Midbrain. 2 Medial lemniscus. 3 Nucleus ruber. 4 Oculomotor nerve fiber. 5 Posterior cerebellar artery. 6 Peduncular syndrome (Weber's syndrome). 7 Pons. 8 Medial medullary syndrome (Dejerine syndrome). 9 Corticospinal tract. 10 Abducent nerve. 11 Anterior inferior cerebellar artery. 12 Medial pontine syndrome (Foville syndrome). 13 Basilar artery. 14 Medulla oblongata. 15 Posterior inferior cerebellar artery. 16 Hypoglossal nerve

3. Medial pons: Supplied by the paramedian branches of the basilar artery.
4. Lateral pons: Supplied by the circumferential branches of the basilar artery The lateral aspect of the pons, toward the caudal end, is supplied by the AICA. The internal auditory (labyrinthine) artery supplies the inner ear and usually arises as a branch of the AICA but sometimes directly from the basilar artery. The lateral aspect of the pons on the contralateral side is mainly supplied by the circumferential branches of the basilar artery known as the lateral pontine arteries. A small variable region in the upper dorsolateral pons receives some blood supply from the SCA. However, this artery primarily supplies the upper cerebellum rather than the brainstem.
5. Midbrain: Supplied by perforating branches from the top of the basilar artery and the proximal PCA. Arteries supplying the thalamus mainly arise from the top of the basilar artery and the proximal PCA. Paramedian branches from the top of the basilar artery enter the interpeduncular fossa, supplying the midbrain and thalamus. Sometimes, these arteries bifurcate after their origin, forming the so-called Percheron arteries, which supply both sides of the midbrain and thalamus. Occlusion before the bifurcation of the Percheron arteries can lead to bilateral medial midbrain or thalamic infarction [7].

3.10 Localization Diagnosis of Brainstem Dysfunction

3.10.1 Anatomical Basis

3.10.1.1 Pathways of Conduction

1. Four Major Lemniscus for Sensory Transmission
   (a) Medial lesmniscus—deep sensation.
   (b) Spinothalamic lesmniscus—superficial sensation.
   (c) Trigeminal lesmniscus—head and facialsomatic sensation.
   (d) Lateral lemniscus—auditory sensation.
2. Pyramidal Tracts in Descending Motor Pathways
   (a) Corticospinal tract—voluntary movement of the body.
   (b) Corticonuclear tract—eye movement, facial muscle movement, tongue activity, masseter swallowing, etc.
3. Four motor control pathways
   (a) Rubrospinal tract—function uncertain in humans.
   (b) Tectospinal tract—coordination of head and eye movements.
   (c) Reticulospinal tract—automatic postural and gait-related movements.
   (d) Vestibulospinal tract—head, neck position, and equilibrium.

3.10.1.2 Brainstem Nuclei

1. Nuclei associated with intraocular and extraocular muscle activity (oculomotor nucleus, E-W nucleus, trochlear nucleus, abducent nucleus).
2. Reticular structures involved in eye movement: vertical gaze center in the lower midbrain or upper pons; horizontal gaze center in the paramedian reticular formation in pons.
3. Trigeminal nerve for facial somatic sensation.
4. Facial nerve for facial expression muscles.
5. Vestibulocochlear nerve.
6. Nuclei of the lower cranial nerves involved in swallowing and chewing (solitary nucleus, salivatory nucleus—sensory; nucleus ambiguus, dorsal nucleus of the vagus nerve, hypoglossal nucleus—motor).

3.10.1.3 Relay Nuclei Within the Brainstem

1. Midbrain
   (a) Superior colliculus—center for visual reflexes, damage can lead to difficulty in upward gaze.
   (b) Inferior colliculus—center for auditory reflexes.
   (c) Nucleus ruber—regulates flexor muscle tone and coordinated movements; damage can cause contralateral limb dyskinesia.
   (d) Substantia nigra—synthesizes dopamine acting on the striatum, damage results in reduced movement.
2. Pons
   (a) Pontine nuclei—relay station connecting the cerebral cortex and cerebellar cortex.
   (b) Superior olivary nucleus—sends fibers to bilateral lateral lemniscus and is involved in sound localization.
   (c) Nucleus coeruleus is associated with sleep-wake cycles.
3. Medulla
   (a) Gracile and cuneate nuclei—deep sensation.
   (b) Inferior olivary nucleus—relay station from cerebral cortex to nucleus ruber and cerebellum, involved in cerebellar regulation of movement.
   (c) Respiratory nuclei in the medullary reticular formation—damage can lead to abnormal respiratory frequency or even respiratory arrest.

3.10.1.4 Overview of Brainstem Functions

The brainstem is involved in almost all critical functions of the central nervous system, including maintaining wakefulness and consciousness, regulating the sleep-wake cycle, controlling motor and sensory functions, and regulating visceral activities.

1. Functions of the midbrain: Receives visual input, governs eye movements, and participates in pupillary reflexes and control of extrapyramidal motor functions.
2. Functions of the pons: Receives input from head and facial sensations, auditory system, and vestibular system. Controls movements of the mouth, facial muscles, and extraocular muscles.
3. Functions of the medulla: Plays a vital role in maintaining basic life activities such as respiration and circulation. It is considered the vital center of life, involved in visceral movements and secretion of saliva and controls movements of the pharynx, larynx, and tongue [8].

3.10.2 Localization Diagnosis Approach

3.10.2.1 Brainstem Conductive Pathways as Diagnostic Clues

1. The ventral aspect of the brainstem contains the brainstem basis, mainly composed of the corticospinal tract. Therefore, syndromes affecting the ventral aspect of the brainstem will cause contralateral limb motor impairment.
2. The tegmentum contains the four thalamic systems for transmitting deep and superficial sensations, head and facial sensations, and auditory sensations. If the tegmentum is affected, the sensory pathways will be impaired.

3.10.2.2 Common Characteristics of Brainstem Lesions

Since the brainstem nuclei are primarily located in the dorsal tegmentum, but the associated cranial nerve fibers pass through the basis to enter and exit the brainstem (except for the trochlear nerve), lesions in either the basis or the tegmentum will result in cranial nerve paralysis symptoms and signs.

3.10.2.3 Differentiation Based on Nuclei Within the Midbrain, Pons, and Medulla

1. Midbrain: Oculomotor nucleus, E-W nucleus, and trochlear nucleus—cranial nerve palsy, pupillary changes, and trochlear nerve palsy.
2. Pons: Trigeminal, abducent, facial, and vestibulocochlear nuclei are present in the lower pons.
3. Medulla: Hypoglossal, vagal, and accessory nuclei; solitary nucleus, nucleus ambiguus, salivatory nuclei; involved in swallowing, chewing, tongue, and pharyngeal functions.

3.10.2.4 Clues from Reticular Formation

1. Midbrain: Vertical gaze center, ascending reticular activating system—dysfunction can cause vertical nystagmus and conscious impairments.
2. Pons: Horizontal gaze center, sleep-wake control, and sensory gating.
3. Medulla: Ventral and dorsal respiratory nuclei are crucial.

3.10.2.5 Clues from Medial and Dorsal Longitudinal Fasciculi

1. Medial longitudinal fasciculus: Head-eye reflex, conjugate eye movements, and ocularovestibular reflex.
2. Dorsal longitudinal fasciculus: It is the pathway connecting the hypothalamus with the brainstem and spinal cord, controlling visceral activities. Damage to this fasciculus can disrupt visceral functions.

3.10.2.6 Brief Summary of Localization Diagnosis in the Three Parts of the Brainstem

1. In the midbrain: Though the oculomotor and E-W nuclei are located in the midbrain tegmentum, theoretically not affected by basis lesions. The oculomotor nerve fibers travel forward, passing through the nucleus ruber and exiting the midbrain through the interpeduncular fossa. Therefore, lesions in the ventral aspect of the midbrain can also cause oculomotor nerve palsy (typically with dilated pupil, loss of direct and consensual light reflex on the same side, and impaired eye movements with ptosis). If the reticular formation in the tegmentum is also involved, it can lead to coma (see Fig. 3.21).
   (a) Contralateral hemiparesis + ipsilateral oculomotor nerve palsy = Weber's syndrome.
   (b) Contralateral hemiparesis + ipsilateral oculomotor nerve palsy + coma = uncal herniation (tentorial herniation).
2. In the pons: Similarly, although the trigeminal, facial, and abducent nuclei are located in the tegmentum of the pons, their fibers pass through the lateral aspect of the basis. If the lesions affect the slightly lateral aspect of the basis of the pons, these nerve fibers may be affected, resulting in trigeminal nerve palsy, facial nerve palsy, and abducens nerve palsy (see Fig. 3.21).
   (a) Contralateral hemiparesis + ipsilateral trigeminal nerve palsy = mid-pons lesion.
   (b) Contralateral hemiparesis + ipsilateral facial nerve palsy + abducent nerve palsy = lower pons lesion.
3. In the medulla, involvement of the respiratory nuclei in the reticular formation and the pressure-sensing central solitary nucleus can directly lead to respiratory and circulatory suppression, even respiratory and cardiac arrest. In patients with cranial brain diseases presenting with respiratory arrest and cardiac arrest, cerebellar tonsillar herniation should be considered first (see Fig. 3.21).

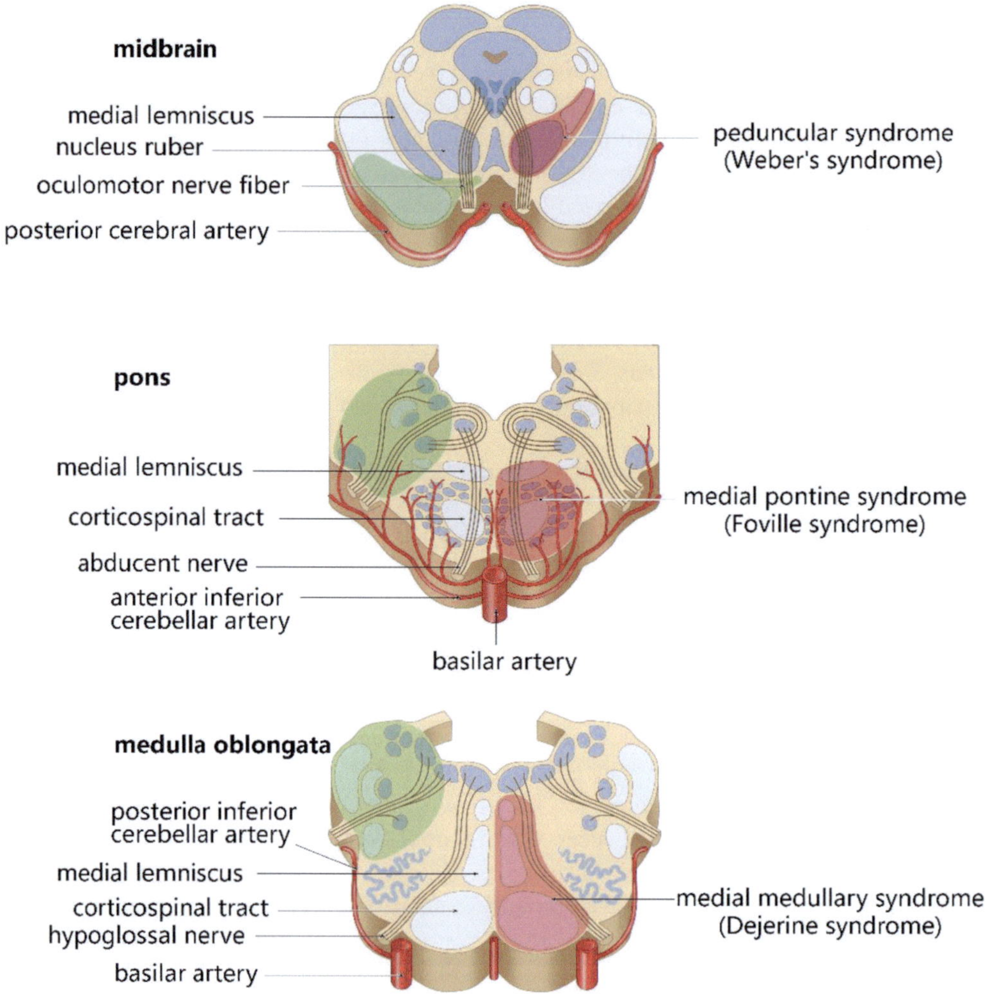

Fig. 3.21 Illustration of brainstem arterial syndromes. Weber's syndrome in the midbrain is caused by lesions involving the basis of the midbrain, primarily affecting the nucleus ruber and oculomotor nerve, sometimes involving the medial lemniscus. The medial pontine syndrome is caused by lesions involving the ventral aspect of the pons, primarily affecting the medial lemniscus, corticospinal tract, and abducens nerve. The medial medullary syndrome is caused by lesions involving the ventral aspect of the medulla, primarily affecting the medial lemniscus, corticospinal tract, and hypoglossal nerve

References

1. Mtui E, Gruener G, Dockery P. Clinical neuroanatomy and neuroscience. 7th ed. Philadelphia: Elsevier; 2015.
2. Standring S. Gray's anatomy. 41st ed. London: Elsevier; 2016.
3. Bai SL, Ying DJ. Systemic anatomy. 9th ed. Beijing: People's Medical Publishing House; 2018. Chinese
4. Zhu CG. Neuroanatomy. 2nd ed. Beijing: People's Medical Publishing House; 2009. Chinese
5. Zhang SX. Applied neuroanatomy. Beijing: People's Medical Publishing House; 2010. Chinese
6. Li ZP. Clinical central neuroanatomy. 2nd ed. Beijing: Science Press; 2017. Chinese
7. Blumenfeld H. Neuroanatomy through clinical cases. 2nd ed. Sunderland: Sinauer Associates; 2010.
8. Bai SL. Chinese medical encyclopedia: basic medicine: human anatomy. Beijing: China Union Medical University Press; 2015. Chinese

4 Pathology and Pathophysiology of Primary Brainstem Hemorrhage

Chao Sun, Gangli Zhang, Qinxue Chen, and Dezhu An

The exact mechanisms underlying the occurrence and development of PBSH have not been fully elucidated. While sharing common pathogenic mechanisms and pathophysiological foundations with other types of cerebral hemorrhage, PBSH presents unique challenges due to the complex morphology and concentrated functions of the brainstem. Following the onset of hemorrhage, the neurons in the brainstem suffer from the compressive and neurotoxic effects of the hematoma and its metabolic byproducts, leading to severe neurological deficits. Moreover, the subsequent pathophysiological changes after brainstem hemorrhage also exhibit certain differences.

4.1 Pathogenic Mechanisms

Sudden elevation of blood pressure serves as the basis for the development of hypertensive brain diseases. Clinical observations have shown that the arterial blood pressure in the majority of hypertensive brain disease patients is significantly elevated. However, there are currently two main theories regarding how elevated arterial blood pressure causes brain damage.

1. Cerebral Small Artery Spasm Theory

C. Sun (✉)
Department of Neurosurgery, The Second Affiliated Hospital of Soochow University, Suzhou, China

G. Zhang
Department of Neurosurgery, Shanxi Provincial People's Hospital, Taiyuan, China

Q. Chen
Department of Neurosurgery, Renmin Hospital of Wuhan University, Hubei General Hospital, Wuhan, China

D. An
Department of Neurosurgery, Zhuhai People's Hospital (The Affiliated Hospital of Beijing Institute of Technology, Zhuhai Clinical Medical College of Jinan University), Zhuhai, China

Early clinical observations have revealed that hypertensive encephalopathy often occurs when blood pressure is extremely and sharply elevated. At this time, due to the presence of cerebral blood flow autoregulation, the small arteries within the brain undergo intense contraction and spasm, resulting in ischemia of the capillaries and neuronal cells. This ischemia leads to increased capillary permeability, causing fluid to leak into the extracellular space and resulting in cerebral edema. Early animal experiments also support this theory. In renal vascular hypertensive rats, alternating contraction and dilation of small arteries on the dura mater were observed through a transparent cranial window when the blood pressure rapidly elevates, indicating that cerebral vascular spasm causes ischemia, leading to disruption of the blood-brain barrier and cerebral edema. Patients with hypertensive encephalopathy may also experience vascular spasms in organs other than the brain, such as retinal vascular spasm leading to transient blindness or peripheral vascular spasm causing ischemic necrosis. These findings support the theory of cerebral vascular spasm.

In the 1870s, Charcot and Bouchard first proposed the hypothesis of microaneurysmal-like dilatation, suggesting that hypertensive patients constantly exhibit microaneurysmal-like dilatations in the perforating artery supply area. Some of these dilatations can rupture under increased arterial pressure. For most patients, a sudden increase in blood pressure can cause rupture of small perforating arteries that were previously unaffected by vascular damage. The extravasated blood from these small vessels can exert sudden compressive effects on local capillaries or small arteries, leading to further rupture of more small vessels. As a result, the bleeding area gradually increases, resembling a snowball effect. Hypertension, along with this "snowball" effect, can expand the extent of bleeding. However, the local tissue pressure restricts the continuous expansion of the bleeding area. Primary

G. Chen, C. You (eds.), *Surgical Treatment of Primary Brainstem Hemorrhage*, https://doi.org/10.1007/978-981-95-8942-5_4

brainstem hemorrhage is predominantly located in the pons, accounting for more than 90% of cases, few in midbrain, and medullary hemorrhage is rare. Based on clinical case analyses, pontine hemorrhage is the most common, and the paramedian artery is generally considered the source arterial of pontine hemorrhage. The artery perpendicularly from the basilar artery has a blood flow direction opposite to that of the basilar artery, making it susceptible to rupture and bleed under the influence of blood pressure [1].

2. Breakthrough of Autoregulation Theory

   Under normal circumstances, human cerebral blood flow remains relatively stable; even when systemic blood pressure or cerebral effective perfusion pressure undergoes significant changes, cerebral blood flow remains relatively unchanged. This mechanism by which cerebral blood vessels maintain a relatively stable blood flow in the presence of variations in arterial perfusion pressure is known as cerebral autoregulation. When cerebral arterial perfusion pressure decreases, cerebral blood vessels dilate accordingly, and when perfusion pressure increases, cerebral blood vessels constrict, thus maintaining a stable cerebral blood flow. However, this regulatory mechanism has its limits. When mean arterial pressure fluctuates within the range of 8.0–21.3 kPa (60–160 mmHg), cerebral blood vessels can constrict or dilate to maintain a relatively stable cerebral blood flow. When mean arterial pressure falls below 6.7 kPa (50 mmHg), cerebral blood flow decreases by 40%, resulting in cerebral ischemia. If mean arterial pressure exceeds the upper limit of autoregulation at 21.3 kPa (160 mmHg), cerebral blood flow increases with the rise in systemic blood pressure. In hypertensive patients with extensive cerebral arteriosclerosis, both the upper and lower limits of autoregulation are shifted upward. This means that even if mean arterial pressure exceeds 21.3 kPa (160 mmHg) or even reaches 26.7 kPa (200 mmHg) during hypertension, it may not necessarily disrupt autoregulatory function. However, cerebral ischemia will occur when mean arterial pressure falls below 6.7 kPa (50 mmHg).

   Subsequent animal experiments have shown that during the early stages of rapid blood pressure elevation, the blood-brain barrier remains intact. Once the blood-brain barrier is disrupted, the cerebral blood flow in that area exceeds that of the region with an intact blood-brain barrier. The blood-brain barrier is more susceptible to damage in the vasodilated region than in the constricted region. This suggests that the main factor leading to blood-brain barrier disruption is vasodilation rather than spasm. Therefore, some researchers believe that the breakthrough of cerebral autoregulation or forced vasodilation is the true pathogenic mechanism of hypertensive brain diseases. The initial manifestation of cerebral autoregulation is the constriction of cerebral small arteries. When the rapidly elevated blood pressure exceeds the upper limit of cerebral autoregulation, the cerebral small arteries passively dilate instead of constricting, leading to the breakdown of autoregulatory function. This results in a passive increase in cerebral blood flow, cerebral tissue edema due to excessive perfusion, disruption of capillary walls, and subsequent development of secondary focal hemorrhage and infarction.

4.2 Pathophysiological Basis

1. Hyaline Arteriolosclerosis: Over time and with aging, arteriosclerotic changes in arterioles will cause degeneration and sclerosis of blood vessels. Sustained hypertension puts increased pressure on the walls of cerebral parenchymal arteries, perforating arteries, and capillaries, leading to structural changes such as hyalinization and other alterations in the vessel walls. These changes result in a loss of the original layered structure of the vessel walls, replaced by homogeneously stained collagen fiber changes.
2. Cerebral Atherosclerosis: In some patients with hypertensive cerebral hemorrhage, cerebrovascular atherosclerosis can be seen under the endothelium of the blood vessel wall in the surrounding tissue of hypertensive cerebral hemorrhage. Foam cells containing atherosclerosis and fibrous hyperplasia containing rhombic lacunae can be seen. Long-term hypertension leads to corresponding pathological changes in the blood vessel walls. It is generally believed that the endothelial cells of blood vessels are the first to be damaged during hypertension, leading to necrosis, detachment, and disintegration. The internal elastic lamina located in the intima undergoes degeneration, thinning, and bulging due to the lack of nutrition and protection from endothelial cells. The damage to endothelial cells allows monocytes and lipids to easily enter the subendothelial layer. Monocytes transform into foam cells and macrophages after phagocytosis of lipids. Both foam cells and macrophages, along with damaged endothelial cells, secrete growth factors that stimulate smooth muscle cell proliferation. Additionally, the decreased secretion of vasoconstrictors and vasodilators by damaged endothelial cells leads to the formation of atherosclerotic plaques in arterial walls, causing hypertension-related changes in the blood vessel walls. The main component of the external layer of cerebral small arteries is collagen, which undergoes degenerative thickening and decreased toughness due to prolonged hypertension. Under electron microscopy, the disorganized arrangement of smooth muscle myofilaments,

increased collagen content, and changes such as cellular hypertrophy, proliferation, and degeneration can be observed. Blood sinuses, typically seen in the external layer, can also appear in the middle layer, suggesting a result of vascular wall repair and reconstruction during the process of hypertension. All these changes increase the fragility of blood vessels and reduce their self-regulation and active contractile functions. Particularly, when the force-bearing layers of the vessel wall (internal elastic lamina and smooth muscle layer in the middle layer) undergo degeneration, local weakening or even rupture can occur. Due to the vessel's self-repair capability, proliferative tissue or surrounding structures (thrombi, atherosclerotic plaque tissue, etc.) replace and repair the force-bearing layers. However, the outcome of this repair process is the gradual loss of the vessel wall's normal self-regulatory physiological function and an increase in fragility [2].

3. Cerebral Amyloid Angiopathy: Cerebral amyloid angiopathy is also an important cause of cerebral hemorrhage. However, many patients with cerebral amyloid angiopathy also have a history of hypertension, and histopathological evidence confirms that more than 30% of cerebral amyloid angiopathy hemorrhages are mixed vascular lesions, with both hypertensive and cerebral amyloid angiopathy coexisting in many cases. Cerebral amyloid angiopathy is more common in the elderly, and under light microscopy, the walls of small arteries appear pale red under Congo red staining, with thickened walls and amyloid protein deposits in the middle and outer layers of the small arterial walls. In severe cases, the middle elastic layer can be completely replaced by amyloid substances. Since amyloidosis mainly affects brain lobe and meningeal blood vessels, its impact on perforating blood vessels is relatively small. Therefore, cerebral hemorrhage mainly manifests as lobar hemorrhage rather than deep brain tissue hemorrhage and often appears lobulated. Secondary intraventricular hemorrhage following lobar hemorrhage may be a characteristic of vascular amyloidosis, and bleeding tends to be multiple and recurrent.
4. Microaneurysms and Abnormal Vascular Clusters: The structure of cerebral blood vessel walls is relatively weak, with fewer medial muscle cells, a lack of external elastic lamina, and underdeveloped arterial adventitia. Particularly in cases of long-term chronic hypertension, localized dilation of small cerebral arteries can easily occur, forming granular microaneurysms. However, the reported incidence of microaneurysms in studies of cerebral hemorrhage varies among different scholars. Xie Fangmin and others in China found that among 38 stable cerebral hemorrhage cases, 5 cases (13.16%) had abnormal vascular clusters, while among 35 unstable cerebral hemorrhage cases, 26 cases (74.29%) had abnormal vascular clusters. The difference in the percentage of abnormal vascular clusters between the two groups was statistically significant.

4.3 Pathophysiological Changes in Brainstem Hemorrhage

1. Hematoma and early hematoma expansion refers to the continuous expansion of intracranial hematomas in patients with cerebral hemorrhage due to ongoing active bleeding. Hematoma enlargement generally occurs within 24 hours after the onset of the disease. The direct cause of hematoma enlargement is the presence of active bleeding in the affected blood vessels. Additionally, there is a certain correlation with the degree of elevated blood pressure, coagulation function, bleeding location, and even the morphology of the hematoma [3, 4, 5]. After the formation of the hematoma, there is often a surrounding zone of decreased density, previously referred to as the edema zone or the so-called semi-lucent zone. In recent years, based on pathological observations, it is believed that this circular low-density zone is not solely edema but rather represents typical necrotic changes. Therefore, some propose to rename the semi-lucent zone as the necrotic edema zone, which is more accurate. The necrotic edema zone in the surrounding tissue of the hematoma usually reaches its peak within 24–48 h [6]. Thus, from a clinical perspective, if the symptoms of a cerebral hemorrhage patient worsen progressively within 48 h, it often indicates the presence of active bleeding or hematoma enlargement [7].
2. Ischemic Changes in the Surrounding Brain Tissue of the Hematoma: After cerebral hemorrhage, the hematoma can directly compress the surrounding brain tissue, reducing the vascular bed and causing localized hypoperfusion. Furthermore, the release of vasoactive substances from the hematoma and surrounding tissues can induce vascular spasms and exacerbate cerebral ischemia [8].
3. Toxic Reactions of Hematoma Dissolution Products: After hematoma formation, its components dissolve quickly. The dissolved products can be classified into three major categories based on their physicochemical properties and effects: macromolecular substances, vascular substances, and cytotoxic substances. These dissolved products can cause cerebral vascular spasms, and cytotoxic substances can disrupt cellular metabolism, ultimately leading to cell death or cellular edema [9].
4. Edema in the Surrounding Tissue of the Hematoma: Animal experiments and dynamic CT observations have shown that perihematomal edema can appear as early as 1 h after intracerebral hemorrhage, and the severity of edema is proportional to the amount of hematoma.

Cerebral hemorrhagic edema is the combined result of interstitial edema, vascular-origin edema, and cytotoxic edema. In the ultra-early stage after cerebral hemorrhage, a large amount of protein from the hematoma cavity infiltrates into the interstitial space of the surrounding brain tissue, leading to increased osmotic pressure and the formation of interstitial edema. Therefore, the low-density area surrounding the lesion observed on early-stage MRI is mainly caused by clot retraction and plasma protein exudation. Coagulation thrombin is an important factor in causing early-stage (within 24 h) cerebral edema after cerebral hemorrhage. Clinical data indicate that thrombin released by the blood clot persists for about 2 weeks, which is equal to the duration of cerebral edema after cerebral hemorrhage. Early-stage thrombin may exert direct cytotoxic effects, while in the later stages, it disrupts the blood-brain barrier, leading to edema. Additionally, it has been found that intracerebral hemorrhage-induced inflammatory reactions, such as red blood cell lysis and activation of the complement system, significantly increase blood-brain barrier permeability, which is the primary cause of delayed cerebral edema. Although different types of cerebral edema have different evolving processes in theory, in reality, different forms of cerebral edema do not exist in isolation; they overlap in time and space and interact with other pathological processes. Restricted blood supply, ischemia, and hypoxia rapidly lead to mixed cerebral edema in normal brain tissue, further progressing to tissue necrosis and liquefaction. Therefore, although the perihematomal edema after cerebral hemorrhage is caused by different mechanisms, it has a common impact on secondary damage to the brain tissue and the ultimate outcome [9].

4.4 Molecular Factors in the Pathogenesis of the Brainstem Hemorrhage

1. Thrombin: Thrombin, a serine protease involved in coagulatin, plays a crucial role in activating coagulation factors and converting fibrinogen into fibrin. Thrombin is important in hemostasis after cerebral hemorrhage. However, thrombin can also contribute to brain damage induced by cerebral hemorrhage. After cerebral hemorrhage, blood clots and blood release a large amount of thrombin. Within 24 hours of cerebral hemorrhage, cytotoxic edema is caused by the release of thrombin. In the later stages, thrombin activates thrombin receptors, causing constriction of cerebral microvascular endothelial cells, increase of cell gap, and disruption of tight junctions, thereby disrupting the blood-brain barrier and resulting in vasogenic edema. High doses of thrombin injection result in infiltration of inflammatory cells, proliferation of interstitial cells, cerebral edema formation, and seizure activity. Thrombin can affect various cell types, including endothelial cells (blood-brain barrier disruption and edema formation), neurons, astrocytes, and microglia. Thrombin can also initiate potentially harmful pathways, such as programmed cell death and activation of SRE kinases, leading to increased vascular permeability, cytotoxicity, and inflammatory responses. Additionally, thrombin can damage the vascular basement membrane and disrupt the blood-brain barrier by inducing the expression of matrix metalloproteinases. Studies have shown that thrombin inhibitors can reduce the damage induced by cerebral hemorrhage. Further research has found that perihematomal edema is reduced when using the thrombin inhibitor argatroban. Although high concentrations of thrombin can mediate brain injury after cerebral hemorrhage, low concentrations of thrombin have neuroprotective effects. Therefore, the role of thrombin depends on the volume of the hematoma. There are also reports suggesting that thrombin plays a role in brain recovery and neurogenesis after cerebral hemorrhage.
2. Inflammatory Response: After cerebral hemorrhage, a significant inflammatory response occurs as a result of the activation of microglia, infiltration of leukocytes, and production of inflammatory mediators [10]. In animal models, microglial activation occurs early after cerebral hemorrhage, peaking at 3–7 days and lasting for 3–4 weeks. Experimental studies have used minocycline to inhibit microglial activation and suppress the inflammatory response. Neutrophils infiltrate the brain tissue early after cerebral hemorrhage and seem to contribute to tissue damage through the generation of reactive oxygen species. Monocytes also enter the brain tissue after cerebral hemorrhage, and Toll-like receptors on leukocytes appear to be important for the infiltration of neutrophils and monocytes. Two cell types that have received less attention in the past are mast cells and lymphocytes. Both cell types can contribute to brain damage following cerebral hemorrhage. In animal and human experiments, brain injury after cerebral hemorrhage has been associated with the upregulation of various inflammatory mediators, including cytokines such as tumor necrosis factor α and interleukin-1β, chemokines, adhesion molecules, and matrix metalloproteinases (MMP9, MMP3) [11]. There is evidence in animal experiments that these inflammatory mediators are involved in brain damage after cerebral hemorrhage and the disruption of the blood-brain barrier. This process may promote leukocyte infiltration but can also be a result of the inflammatory response. Leukocyte-derived reactive oxygen species, pro-inflammatory factors, chemokines, and matrix metalloproteinases all contribute to the destruction of the blood-brain barrier.

Animal studies have shown that inflammation not only damages brain tissue but also plays a role in brain tissue recovery. However, the role of inflammation in the repair of brain damage after cerebral hemorrhage is yet to be confirmed.

3. Complement After Cerebral Hemorrhage: The complement in the blood plasma enters the brain tissue. Complement activation occurs following cerebral hemorrhage, leading to the formation of membrane attack complexes. These complexes play a significant role in the lysis of red blood cells and are associated with the release of hemoglobin and iron, ultimately resulting in the destruction of neurons, glial cells, and blood vessels surrounding the hematoma. Complement cascade activation also generates C3a and C5a, which are potent leukocyte chemotactic factors, and activates microglia and mast cells, thereby enhancing the inflammatory response following cerebral hemorrhage. Inhibiting complement cascade reactions or gene knockout can reduce brain damage induced by cerebral hemorrhage. However, there is some controversy regarding the role of C5. While C5a inhibitors have a protective effect, rats with C5 knockout exhibit increased brain damage following cerebral hemorrhage. Complement activation in the early stages of cerebral hemorrhage can enhance brain tissue injury, but the complement cascade reaction also has beneficial aspects in long-term brain repair.
4. Hemoglobin and its degradation products; Numerous studies have indicated that hemoglobin (Hb) and its degradation products play a crucial role in cerebral edema following cerebral hemorrhage. Red blood cell lysis occurs 6–8 days after cerebral hemorrhage, releasing hemoglobin and globin. Hemoglobin eventually breaks down into iron ions, carbon monoxide (CO), and bilirubin, which are considered to have direct and indirect neurotoxicity. Xi et al. conducted experimental studies on cerebral edema after cerebral hemorrhage and found that concentrated red blood cells did not significantly induce cerebral edema. However, Bao et al. found that injecting Hb into the brains of rats caused noticeable cerebral edema within 24 h [12]. Hua et al. demonstrated that injecting iron ions into the rat brain significantly induced cerebral edema, while iron chelation with deferoxamine effectively reduced cerebral edema [13]. Hemeoxygenase inhibitor, an enzyme that releases iron from hemoglobin, or the absence of hemeoxygenase-1, also reduces brain damage following cerebral hemorrhage. The mechanism by which iron causes tissue damage is through the generation of free radicals. Free radical-mediated damage has been observed, and reducing free radicals can decrease brain damage caused by cerebral hemorrhage. Animal experiments have shown that the use of iron chelators can improve the prognosis of patients with cerebral hemorrhage. It has been demonstrated that the abundant production of bilirubin and CO after hemorrhage can cause severe brain tissue damage and lead to the occurrence of cerebral edema.
5. Matrix Metalloproteinases (MMPs): Matrix metalloproteinases, zinc-dependent proteases, are one of the most important extracellular matrix (ECM)-degrading enzymes. They increase vascular permeability, allowing large molecules such as fibrinogen to enter the brain tissue and trigger cerebral edema. Tejima et al. observed the role of MMPs in mice with cerebral hemorrhage and found that the brain tissue water content was significantly higher in wild-type mice compared to mice with MMP gene knockout [14, 15].
6. Glutamate: Glutamate-induced neurotoxicity plays a major role in cell death after cerebral ischemia, and some evidence suggests that glutamate is also involved in brain damage after cerebral hemorrhage.

4.5 Clinical Manifestations and Pathophysiological Basis

Primary brainstem hemorrhage is predominantly located in the pons, accounting for over 90% of cases, while midbrain hemorrhage is less common, and medullary hemorrhage is rare. Clinical analysis of medical records indicates that pontine hemorrhage is the most frequent. The paramedian arteries, which branch perpendicularly from the basilar artery, are considered the source of pontine hemorrhage. Due to the opposite blood flow direction to the basilar artery, these arteries are susceptible to rupture and bleeding under the influence of blood pressure. Based on the location of the hemorrhage, three types can be distinguished: (1) tegmento-basal type, (2) basal type, and (3) tegmental type. Depending on the specific pontine arteries involved, the resulting pontine hematoma can lead to different clinical syndromes. Primary pontine hemorrhage typically originates at the junction between the tegmentum and the base of the pons. These hematomas expand rapidly and often damage the central tegmental area and the basal portion of the pons. The hematoma frequently extends rostrally into the midbrain but rarely extends caudally into the medulla. Large hematomas often originate from larger penetrating vessels in the central pons and may rupture into the fourth ventricle.

1. Pontine Hemorrhage: The clinical manifestations of massive pontine hemorrhage include rapidly progressing coma, unstable vital signs, and severe bilateral neurological deficits (Table 4.1). In the early stages, patients may present with severe hypertension, arrhythmias, hyperthermia, respiratory failure, or cardiac arrest. Additionally, patients with massive pontine hemorrhage may exhibit

Table 4.1 Clinical manifestations of pontine hemorrhage

Massive pontine hemorrhage	Pinpoint pupils with extremely weak light reflex	Contralateral limb sensory loss
Coma	Inability for horizontal eye movements	Loss of sensation in the ipsilateral face
Quadriplegia, contralateral hemiplegia, or decerebrate rigidity	Ocular bobbing	Ipsilateral or bilateral limb ataxia
Dysarthria	Small amount of hemorrhage in the basal part of the brainstem	Ipsilateral facial nerve paralysis
Swallowing difficulties	Contralateral hemiplegia	Contralateral hemiplegia (rare)
Abnormal vital signs	Contralateral hemiplegia and ataxia	Neuro-ophthalmic symptoms
Slow and irregular breathing	Dysarthria	Gaze palsy on the same side
Irregular pulse	Ipsilateral facial paralysis	Internuclear ophthalmoplegia
		One and a half syndrome
		Ipsilateral miosis

Table 4.2 Clinical manifestations of midbrain or medullary hemorrhage

Small amount of hemorrhage in the midbrain	Contralateral hemisensory loss	Small amount of hemorrhage in the medulla
Cerebral peduncle	Contralateral hemibody tremor, ataxia, and bradykinesia	Ipsilateral soft palate paralysis
Contralateral hemiplegia	Tectum	Nystagmus
Ipsilateral oculomotor nerve paralysis	Unilateral or bilateral trochlear nerve paralysis	Ipsilateral limb ataxia (upper limb)
Tegmentum	Unilateral or bilateral hearing impairment	Ipsilateral half of the tongue muscle paralysis
Ipsilateral oculomotor nerve paralysis	Parinaud syndrome	Contralateral hemiplegia (upper and lower limbs)

quadriplegia and decerebrate posture. Neuro-ophthalmological abnormalities may include horizontal gaze palsy, pinpoint pupils with weak light reflex, and ocular bobbing. Although ocular bobbing can also be seen in extensive acute lesions of the cerebellum, it is relatively specific for acute pontine hemorrhage as a localizing sign. Small hemorrhages involving the basal portion of one side of the pons can present with unilateral signs (Table 4.1). Contralateral hemiparesis and dysarthria are the most common symptoms of pontine hemorrhage and resemble the presentation of pure motor lacunar infarction. If the hemorrhage involves the tegmentum of the pons, ipsilateral facial palsy and abducens nerve palsy may occur. Smaller hemorrhages can also be found in the dorsolateral aspect of the pons, causing clinical symptoms similar to infarctions in that region (Table 4.1). Although patients with hemorrhages in these locations may experience contralateral limb sensory and motor deficits or pain, they are usually conscious and complain of headache, dizziness, or visual symptoms. Physical examination reveals contralateral limb motor or sensory impairments, ipsilateral facial paralysis or sensory loss, and significant eye movement abnormalities. Ataxia or dysmetria may also be present with contralateral sensory deficits. Hemorrhage in the tectum region can cause eye movement abnormalities seen in Parinaud syndrome, hearing loss, or trochlear nerve palsy.

2. Midbrain Hemorrhage: Hemorrhage occurring in the cerebral peduncles, tegmentum, or tectum of the midbrain is less common than pontine hemorrhage. Bleeding in this region is often caused by ruptured vascular malformations or hypertension. The clinical manifestations of massive midbrain hemorrhage are similar to those of pontine hemorrhage, and when the aqueduct of midbrain becomes compressed, it can lead to acute hydrocephalus. Minor midbrain hemorrhage can result in localized neurological impairments, including ipsilateral oculomotor nerve palsy and contralateral limb paralysis (Weber syndrome), with the hemorrhage primarily located in the cerebral peduncles (Table 4.2). Hemorrhage in the tegmentum can cause oculomotor nerve dysfunction, ipsilateral or contralateral tremors, chorea, or ataxia, and contralateral sensory deficits. Hemorrhage in the tectum can lead to eye movement disorders seen in Parinaud syndrome, hearing loss, or trochlear nerve palsy.
3. Medullary Hemorrhage: Primary medullary hemorrhage is rare and presents with clinical symptoms such as headache, dizziness, swallowing difficulties, dysarthria, and balance disturbances. Posterior cranial nerve palsies may be accompanied by motor and sensory impairments (Table 4.2). Patients may exhibit symptoms of dorsal lateral medullary syndrome, also known as Wallenberg syndrome.

References

1. Anderson CS, Huang Y, Wang JG, et al. Intensive blood pressure reduction in acute cerebral haemorrhage trial (INTERACT): a randomised pilot trial. Lancet Neurol. 2008;7(5):391–9.
2. Wang DC, Li XL, Wang S, et al. Ultrastructural changes in cerebral small arteries of patients with primary intracerebral hemorrhage. Chinese J Neurol Psychiat. 2010;36(03):133–6.
3. Wang XW, Wang C, Wang YJ. Molecular biological markers of early hematoma expansion in intracerebral hemorrhage. Int J Cerebrovasc Diseases. 2008;16(1):31–4.
4. Lim JK, Hwang HS, Cho BM, et al. Multivariate analysis of risk factors of hematoma expansion in spontaneous intracerebral hemorrhage. Surg Neurol. 2008 Jan;69(1):40–5.
5. Naidech AM, Jovanovic B, Liebling S, et al. Reduced platelet activity is associated with early clot growth and worse 3-month outcome after intracerebral hemorrhage. Stroke.2009;0(7):2398–401.
6. Sun DY, Chen JF, Feng JC, et al. Morphological observations of perihematomal tissue in patients with primary intracerebral hemorrhage. J Stroke Neurolog Diseases. 2006;(05):555–7.
7. Dowlatshahi D, Demchuk AM, Flaherty ML, et al. Defining hematoma expansion in intracerebral hemorrhage: relationship with patient outcomes. Neurology. 2011;76(14):1238–44.
8. Ding HY, Dong Q, Shi LF, et al. SPECT study on Perihematomal hemodynamic changes in patients with basal ganglia intracerebral hemorrhage. Chinese J Neurol Psychiat. 2007;(05):285–8.
9. Pascual AM, López-Mut JV, Benlloch V, et al. Perfusion-weighted magnetic resonance imaging in acute intracerebral hemorrhage at baseline and during the 1st and 2nd week: a longitudinal study. Cerebrovasc Dis. 2007;23(1):6–13.
10. Dong Z, Shi Z, Wang L, et al. Characteristics of inflammatory reactions in the perihematomal tissue of patients with primary intracerebral hemorrhage during the acute phase. J Clin Neurol. 2007;(04):249–51.
11. Liang ZG, Liu ZK, Gao XL, et al. Expression of cell adhesion molecules in perihematomal brain tissue and its relationship with brain edema in a rat model of intracerebral hemorrhage. J Clin Neurol. 2006;(01):67–9.
12. Bao X, Wu G, Hu S, et al. Poly(ADP-ribose) polymerase activation and brain edema formation by hemoglobin after intracerebral hemorrhage in rats. Acta Neurochir Suppl. 2008;105:23–7.
13. Hua Y, Keep RF, Hoff JT, Xi G. Deferoxamine therapy for intracerebral hemorrhage. Acta Neurochir Suppl. 2008;105:3–6.
14. Tejima E, Zhao BQ, Tsuji K, Rosell A, van Leyen K, Gonzalez RG, Montaner J, Wang X, Lo EH. Astrocytic induction of matrix metalloproteinase-9 and edema in brain hemorrhage. J Cereb Blood Flow Metab. 2007;27(3):460–8.
15. Xie FM, Niu LJ, Zhang X, et al. Pathological observations of different hematoma morphologies in primary intracerebral hemorrhage. Chinese J Clin Neurosurg. 2010;15(01):29–31.

5 Clinical Manifestations and Diagnosis of Primary Brainstem Hemorrhage

Zhouping Tang, Chaohui Li, Ping Zhang, and Haiquan Tao

5.1 Overview

A brainstem hemorrhage is a neurological emergency with a sudden onset and serious consequences. Statistical data indicates that brainstem hemorrhage represents approximately 5.0–13.4% of clinical cases of cerebral hemorrhage, with an observed increase in incidence over recent years. The demographic most susceptible to brainstem hemorrhage is the middle-aged and elderly population, specifically those between the ages of 40 and 70. There is a notable trend toward younger individuals being affected, and the incidence is significantly higher in males than in females. The brainstem, situated within the brain in a relatively small volume, serves as the "life center," regulating vital signs such as body temperature, respiration, heart rate, and blood pressure. Consequently, brainstem hemorrhage frequently manifests with a sudden onset, a critical condition, a high risk of mortality, and a poor prognosis, with a mortality rate reaching as high as 70–80%. Prior to the advent of computed tomography (CT) and magnetic resonance imaging (MRI), this condition was challenging to diagnose and frequently identified only at the postmortem stage. With the advent of advanced imaging techniques, improvements in intensive care, and particularly in surgical techniques, brainstem hemorrhage is no longer a condition that is untreatable and instills fear. A considerable number of patients can survive, and many have a relatively good prognosis. Hypertension is an important cause of primary brainstem hemorrhage, and it is widely recognized that primary brainstem hemorrhage has a poor prognosis. Most studies indicate that a hemorrhage volume greater than 5 mL is an important factor contributing to increased mortality risk. This chapter provides an overview of the etiology, classification, clinical manifestations, imaging findings, and key points in the diagnosis of primary brainstem hemorrhage.

Z. Tang (✉) · P. Zhang
Department of Neurology, Tongji Hospital, Tongji Medical College, Huazhong University of Science and Technology, Wuhan, China

C. Li
Department of Neurology, Zhuhai People's Hospital (The Affiliated Hospital of Beijing Institute of Technology, Clinical Medical College of Jinan University), Zhuhai, China

H. Tao
Department of Cerebrovascular Diseases, Zhuhai People's Hospital (The Affiliated Hospital of Beijing Institute of Technology, Zhuhai Clinical Medical College of Jinan University), Zhuhai, China

5.2 Etiology and Pathogenesis

5.2.1 Etiology

Hypertension represents the primary etiological factor in cases of primary brainstem hemorrhage. Some patients may have a history of elevated blood lipids, coronary heart disease, diabetes, cerebral infarction, and other factors, all of which are related to cerebral arteriosclerosis [1]. In general, patients are older and have a history of hypertension. The hemorrhage is caused by the rupture of a long perforating artery that originates from the basal artery in the brainstem. Previous studies have identified multiple arterial aneurysmal changes in this region during autopsies, suggesting that they may be attributable to sudden elevations in blood pressure, hyaline degeneration of small arteries, or fibrinoid necrosis. It is possible that arterial sclerosis and occult vascular malformations may coexist as contributing factors.

5.2.2 Pathogenesis

The primary pathogenesis of primary brain hemorrhage is the rupture of small intracerebral arteries, which is caused by chronic changes resulting from long-term hypertension. Intracranial arteries are distinguished by a paucity of medial smooth muscle cells and external connective tissue, as well

G. Chen, C. You (eds.), *Surgical Treatment of Primary Brainstem Hemorrhage*, https://doi.org/10.1007/978-981-95-8942-5_5

as the absence of an external elastic lamina. Prolonged hypertension can precipitate hyaline degeneration and fibrinoid necrosis of small cerebral arteries and may even result in the formation of microaneurysms or dissecting aneurysms. Consequently, elevated blood pressure can readily give rise to vascular rupture and hemorrhage.

5.3 Classification of Primary Brainstem Hemorrhage

At present, there is no unified clinical classification for primary brainstem hemorrhage. However, the location of the hemorrhage, the volume of bleeding (excluding intraventricular hemorrhage), and the Glasgow Coma Scale (GCS) score at admission frequently serve as key determinants of prognosis in patients. Consequently, clinical scholars frequently utilize these factors as reference criteria for classification, as they possess considerable predictive value with regard to patient outcomes [2].

1. Classification based on the location of the hemorrhage, including midbrain hemorrhage, pontine hemorrhage, and medullary hemorrhage. Medullary hemorrhage is rare, midbrain hemorrhage is rare, and pontine hemorrhage is common.
   (a) Pontine hemorrhage: Accounts for 77.2–94.5% of brainstem hemorrhages. It is mostly caused by the rupture of pontine branches of the basilar artery, with the hemorrhagic focus often located between the basal and tegmental regions of the pons. A large hemorrhage (hematoma >5 mL) involving bilateral tegmental and basal regions commonly ruptures into the fourth ventricle, leading to rapid onset of coma, bilateral pinpoint pupils, coffee-ground emesis, central hyperthermia, central respiratory disturbances, ocular bobbing, quadriplegia, and decerebrate posturing. A small hemorrhage may not cause consciousness impairment but can manifest as crossed paralysis and ataxic hemiparesis, with bilateral gaze palsy toward the lesion on the ipsilateral or internuclear ophthalmoplegia.
   (b) Midbrain hemorrhage: Less common, often presenting with headache, vomiting, and consciousness disorders. Mild cases may exhibit unilateral or bilateral oculomotor paresis, disparate eye axes, and ipsilateral limb ataxia and can also manifest as Weber's syndrome or Benedikt's syndrome. Severe cases present with deep coma and flaccid quadriplegia, leading to rapid death.
   (c) (Medullary hemorrhage: Even rarer, clinically presenting as sudden consciousness impairment affecting vital signs such as respiration, heart rate, and blood pressure, ultimately resulting in death. Mild cases may exhibit atypical Wallenberg syndrome.
2. Classification based on hemorrhage volume (calculated using the Modified Tada Formula), Glasgow Coma Scale (GCS) score at admission, or level of consciousness:
   Type I: Hemorrhage volume < 2 mL, GCS score ≥ 13.
   Type II: Hemorrhage volume 2–5 mL, GCS score 9–12.
   Type III: Hemorrhage volume 5–10 mL, GCS score 6–8.
   Type IV: Hemorrhage volume ≥ 10 mL, GCS score 3–5.
3. Classification based on CT anatomical location tegmental type, central type, basal type, hemispheric type, and whole brainstem type, with better prognosis observed in the tegmental and hemispheric types. Some scholars also classify brainstem hemorrhage as central intraparenchymal hemorrhage or tegmental subependymal hemorrhage. The former is located deep within the brainstem, resembling a tumor, while the latter occurs in the subependymal space of the tegmentum, often rupturing into the fourth ventricle, presenting as subarachnoid hemorrhage and having a better prognosis than the former.
4. Classification of primary brainstem hemorrhage (based on the method proposed by Liu Fengqiang from the Second Affiliated Hospital of Zhejiang University School of Medicine) (Fig. 5.1).
   (a) Pontine hemorrhage accounts for 90% of primary brainstem hemorrhages. In the CT axial scan sequence, the largest section of the hematoma is selected, and the midline and the boundary between the brainstem/cerebellum on both sides are marked. Then, the midline is divided into left and right halves and named lines 1, 2, and 3, respectively.
      (i) If the hematoma is located in the fourth ventricle or around the pontine cistern, compressing the brainstem or blocking the cerebrospinal fluid circulation pathway, it is classified as type 0.
      (ii) If the hematoma involves line 1 or 3, without crossing line 2, it is classified as type 1.
      (iii) If the hematoma involves both lines 1,2 or 2,3, it is classified as type 2.
      (iv) If the hematoma involves all three lines, it is classified as type 3.

      For type 2 and type 3 hematomas, line 2 is evenly divided into three sections. Depending on the range of hematoma involvement in line 2, they are further classified into three subtypes: ventral (A), central (C), and dorsal (B).
   (b) Surgical Value
      (i) Type 0 hematoma: The brainstem is not directly damaged by the hematoma. Following the principles of brain hernia treatment, emergency treatment often leads to good outcomes.

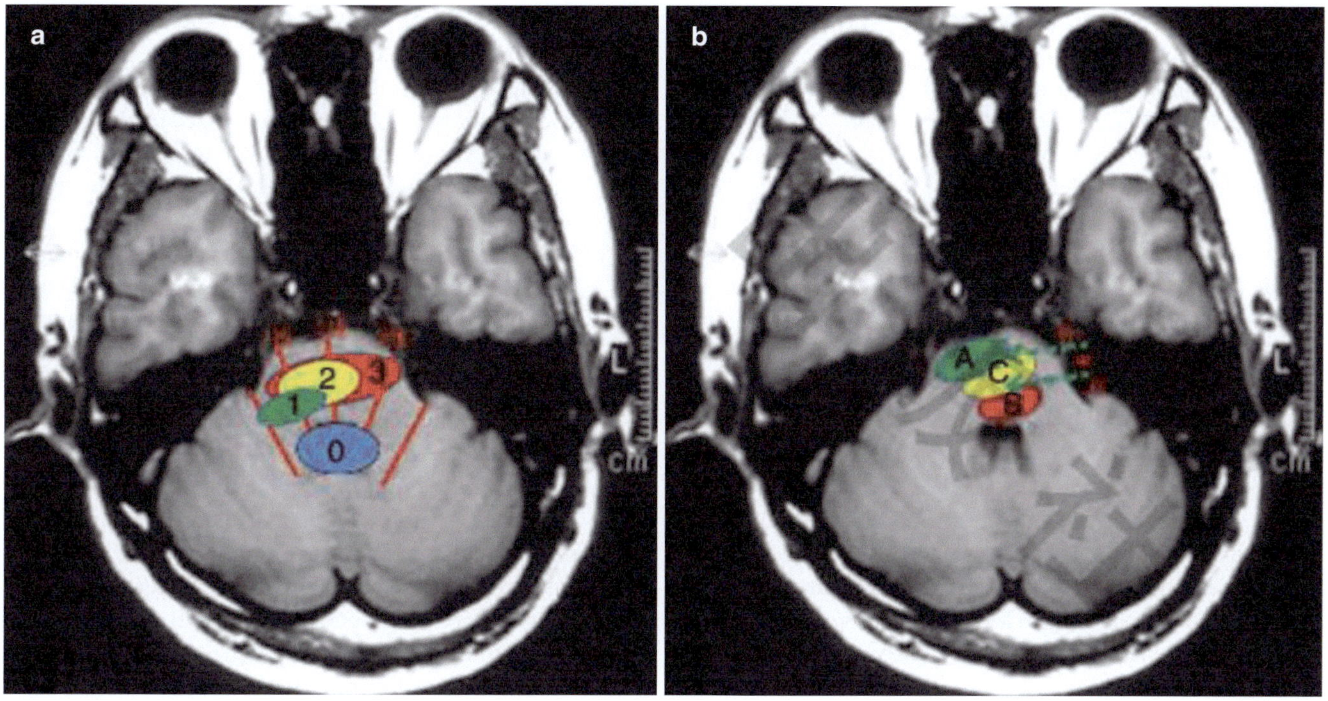

Fig. 5.1 Classification of brainstem hemorrhage

(ii) Type 1 hematoma: The primary damage to the brainstem is relatively small, and removing the hematoma can bring significant benefits.
(iii) Type 2 hematoma: The damage to one side of the brainstem is relatively mild, and removing the hematoma may be beneficial.
(iv) Type 3 hematoma: Bilateral brainstem is damaged, and removing the hematoma may benefit some patients.

Due to differences in the brainstem structures affected by the three subtypes, they often result in different consequences [3]:

A subtype: Relatively far from the brainstem reticular structure, with a high probability of postoperative recovery, but because it is easy to affect the cortical spinal tract, there is severe motor dysfunction. There are relatively more options for removing the hematoma.
B subtype: Adjacent to the brainstem reticular structure and dorsal nuclei, with more vegetative state and posterior cranial nerve impairments. Both craniotomy and puncture require special attention to the protection of residual functions.
C subtype: Involving the central area of the brainstem, when the hematoma volume is small (<5 mL), the damage to important functional areas is less severe than that of the B subtype, and removing the hematoma is more likely to be beneficial. However, when the hematoma volume is too large (>10 mL), it is difficult to benefit from any method.

5.4 Clinical Manifestation of Primary Brainstem Hemorrhage

5.4.1 General Manifestations

1. Often occurs during periods of activity.
2. Onset is sudden, progression is rapid, and clinical symptoms are severe, with most patients experiencing coma.
3. Irregular breathing, characterized by blowing-like, sighing-like, and Cheyne-Stokes respiration, indicating respiratory failure.
4. Pinpoint pupils.
5. Stress ulcers, mainly manifested as vomiting coffee-like material, with a higher incidence as the condition worsens.
6. Crossed paralysis, characterized by varying degrees of ipsilateral cranial nerve involvement and contralateral central hemiparesis.
7. Precise localization and qualitative diagnosis can be achieved through cranial CT scans or cranial MRI examinations.

5.4.2 Specific Manifestations

Depending on the location and extent of brainstem hemorrhage, various clinical syndromes may occur.

1. Primary Midbrain Hemorrhage

   Less common, characterized by sudden onset, coma or syncope, positive bilateral pyramidal tract signs, quadriplegia, unilateral or bilateral ophthalmoplegia, dilated pupils with weakened or absent light reflex, decerebrate rigidity, acute intracranial pressure elevation, respiratory disorders, and eventual death due to brainstem dysfunction.

   (a) Unilateral midbrain hemorrhage: Often manifests as ipsilateral oculomotor nerve paralysis and contralateral central hemiparesis.
   (b) Bilateral midbrain hemorrhage: Manifests as bilateral oculomotor nerve paralysis, bilateral central hemiparesis, elevated intracranial pressure, and coma. Consciousness loss and symptoms of increased intracranial pressure due to aquaeductus obstruction are common, indicating a critical condition.

2. Primary Pontine Hemorrhage

   The most prevalent form of brainstem hemorrhage is also the most complex in terms of clinical manifestations. It typically manifests abruptly, with a constellation of symptoms including severe headache, vomiting, dizziness, diplopia, dysarthria, ipsilateral facial numbness, and contralateral body numbness. Initially, the patient may remain conscious, but this is usually followed by a transition to a coma within a few minutes. In cases of minor hemorrhages, patients may not exhibit impaired consciousness but may present with signs of unilateral pontine damage, such as typical crossed paralysis, where the facial nerve on the hemorrhagic side is paralyzed along with contralateral limb paralysis and the head and both eyes turn toward the nonhemorrhagic side. In cases of substantial hemorrhages, the damage frequently propagates rapidly to the contralateral side, resulting in bilateral facial and limb paralysis. This may manifest as flaccid paralysis, though it can also present as spastic or decerebrate rigidity. Additionally, bilateral pathological reflexes may be observed.

   (a) Millard-Gubler Syndrome: A lesion on the ventral lateral side of the pons, resulting in impairment of the abducens nerve, facial nerve or its nucleus, and the pyramidal tract. It is characterized by an inability to abduct the ipsilateral eyeball, peripheral facial palsy, and contralateral central hemiparesis. If the medial lemniscus is affected, contralateral hemibody sensory impairment may occur.
   (b) Foville Syndrome: A lesion near the midline on one side of the pons, affecting the abducens nucleus and its interconnecting pathways, the facial nerve, and the pyramidal tract. It is characterized by the inability of both eyes to horizontally gaze toward the affected side, ipsilateral peripheral facial palsy, and contralateral central hemiparesis.
   (c) Locked-In Syndrome: A focal lesion in the bilateral basal pons, involving the bilateral corticospinal tracts and the corticonuclear tract below the trigeminal nerve. It is characterized by bilateral central hemiparesis. Apart from preserved eye movements controlled by the midbrain, the patient loses all motor and expressive abilities. Sensation and consciousness are generally intact, and communication can only be achieved through blinking or eye movements.

3. Primary Medullary Hemorrhage

   It is a rare occurrence that presents with sudden onset, coma, and death due to paralysis. In cases of small localized hemorrhages, when consciousness is clear, signs of medullary localization may manifest, including ipsilateral ninth, 10th, 11th, and 12th cranial nerve paralysis, contralateral hemiparesis, impaired pain and temperature sensation, hoarseness, choking during drinking, frequent hiccup, and dizziness. Extensive medullary hemorrhage is more likely to result in decerebrate rigidity, limb paralysis, true medullary paralysis, upper gastrointestinal bleeding, and loss of urinary and fecal control than medullary infarction. In some cases, minor hemorrhages in the medulla may not present any symptoms.

5.5 Radiological Imaging of Hypertensive Brainstem Hemorrhage

At present, the majority of scholars regard cranial CT scanning as the most appropriate method for diagnosing brainstem hemorrhage [4]. It can unambiguously determine the location and volume of the hemorrhage and provide a relatively accurate prognosis assessment. In certain cases, thin-slice CT scanning of the brainstem may be required.

5.5.1 Cranial CT Examination

Cranial CT scanning is the primary diagnostic method for cerebral hemorrhage. In the majority of cases of brainstem hemorrhage, CT scanning can ascertain the location, volume, and shape of the hematoma, whether it has invaded the ventricles and the presence of perihematoma hypodensity edema and mass effect. The lesion frequently manifests as a round or oval-shaped, uniformly high-density area with distinct boundaries. Due to the brainstem's location in the posterior fossa, there may be artifacts related to bone structure that can obscure small amounts of bleeding. In such cases, an ultrathin scan or cranial MRI may be employed. Furthermore, dynamic CT imaging following a brainstem hemorrhage can assess the progression of the bleeding and facilitate timely intervention, thereby reducing the impact of delayed treatment due to hematoma enlargement on the patient's outcome. Approximately 1 week following the hemorrhage, a ring enhancement may be observed around the hematoma. This subsequently becomes hypodense or cystic following absorption. The hemorrhage will gradually resolve within approximately 2 weeks and may completely disappear within 1–2 months [5, 6]. During the absorption process, the imaging of the hemorrhage may manifest as a ring-shaped, crescent-shaped, or irregular configuration.

5.5.2 Cranial MRI Examination

When CT diagnosis is challenging or when there are posterior fossa lesions, cranial MRI may be considered. Cranial MRI allows for multilayer cross-sectional scanning and provides clear visualization of posterior fossa lesions and lesions smaller than 1 cm. However, MRI scanning is time-consuming and relatively expensive, and some critically ill patients or those on mechanical ventilation may have difficulties completing the examination. MRI is superior to CT scanning in detecting brainstem hemorrhagic lesions and monitoring the evolution of the hemorrhage.

The pattern of MRI changes during cerebral hemorrhage is as follows:

1. Hyperacute phase (<24 h): Long T1 and long T2 signals, which are difficult to differentiate from cerebral infarction and edema.
2. Acute phase (2–7 days): Isointense on T1 and hypointense on T2 signals.
3. Subacute phase (8 days to 4 weeks): Hypointense on T1 and long T2 signals.
4. Chronic phase (>4 weeks): Long T1 and long T2 signals.

5.5.3 Cerebral Vascular Imaging

This includes CTA, MRA, and DSA, with DSA being the gold standard. Patients suitable for angiography should have relatively stable conditions, stable vital signs, and unclear clinical etiology.

5.6 Key Points in the Diagnosis of Hypertensive Brainstem Hemorrhage

In middle-aged and elderly patients, the abrupt onset of focal neurological deficits and symptoms of increased intracranial pressure, such as headache and vomiting, during activity or emotional excitement, should prompt consideration of the possibility of hemorrhage. In conjunction with a cranial CT examination, a prompt and definitive diagnosis can be reached [7].

The key points in the diagnosis are as follows:

1. Sudden onset with rapid progression, often presenting with severe symptoms and possible coma.
2. Irregular breathing patterns, such as blowing, sighing, or Cheyne-Stokes respiration, indicating respiratory failure.
3. Pinpoint pupils: Approximately 70% of cases exhibit pinpoint pupils that still react to light. This is due to sympathetic paralysis of the oculomotor nerve after damage to the pons and medulla, while the parasympathetic nerve remains intact or only mildly affected, resulting in pupil constriction with preserved light reflex. Damage to various oculomotor nerve nuclei, the medial longitudinal fasciculus, and the medial longitudinal bundle within the brainstem can lead to lateral gaze palsy, nystagmus, and abnormal eye movements.
4. Paralysis: After brainstem hemorrhage, disruption or damage to the ascending and descending conduction pathways and certain nuclei can result in varying degrees of impairment. This can manifest as ipsilateral peripheral cranial nerve palsy and contralateral central limb hemiparesis. Bilateral damage may cause quadriplegia or bilateral pathological signs.
5. Gastrointestinal bleeding: As the severity of the condition and level of consciousness impairment increase, the incidence of gastrointestinal bleeding also rises. This is associated with factors such as gastric and duodenal mucosal damage, decreased gastric mucosal barrier function, and increased intracranial pressure.
6. Elevated blood glucose and peripheral leukocytosis are not uncommon and are related to the severity of the patient's condition and the body's stress response. Higher blood glucose levels are associated with poorer prognosis.
7. Cranial CT scanning or cranial MRI examination provides accurate localization diagnosis and reliable basis for clinical diagnosis and prognosis assessment.

References

1. Jia JP, Chen SD. Neurology. 8th ed. Beijing: People's Medical Publishing House; 2018. Chinese
2. Wang ZC. Neurosurgery. Wuhan: Hubei Science and Technology Press; 2005. Chinese
3. Hemphill JC 3rd, Greenberg SM, Anderson CS, et al. Guidelines for the management of spontaneous intracerebral hemorrhage: a guideline for healthcare professionals from the American Heart Association/American Stroke Association. Stroke. 2015;46(7):2032–60.
4. Takeuchi S, Suzuki G, Takasato Y, et al. Prognostic factors in patients with primary brainstem hemorrhage. Clin Neurol Neurosurg. 2013;115(6):732–5.
5. Ding XQ, Li ZF. Current status and advances in surgical treatment of brainstem hemorrhage. Medical Rev. 2017;23(21):4252–5. Chinese
6. Huang YZ. Current diagnosis and treatment of brainstem hemorrhage. Pract Intern Med J. 2008;28(S2):146–9. Chinese
7. Zhang XJ, Li CY. Diagnosis and treatment of brainstem hemorrhage. Pract Heart Brain Lung J. 2006;14(4):266–9. Chinese

Differential Diagnosis of Primary Brainstem Hemorrhage

6

Kai Shu, Ping Zhang, and Haiquan Tao

6.1 Ruptured Intracranial Aneurysm Hemorrhage

Intracranial aneurysms are most frequently observed at the branching points of the basal arteries at the base of the skull. Posterior circulation aneurysms represent less than 20% of all cases [1]. Ruptured aneurysms frequently result in subarachnoid hemorrhage (SAH), intracerebral hematoma, or intraventricular hemorrhage. The clinical manifestations of this condition include severe headaches, nausea, and vomiting. In more severe cases, the patient may also experience impaired consciousness, coma, seizures, and focal neurological deficits.

Ruptured posterior fossa aneurysms present with subarachnoid hemorrhage (SAH), cerebellar hematoma, and, in some cases, brainstem hemorrhage. The clinical manifestations of ruptured aneurysms in the distal branches of the posterior cerebral arteries include thalamic infarction, contralateral limb weakness, and decreased sensation and may also involve ataxia or limb tremors. Rupture of aneurysms in the upper portion of the basilar artery results in damage to the midbrain and upper pons, manifesting as oculomotor nerve palsy, vertical gaze palsy, and nystagmus. Additionally, damage to the midbrain and cerebral peduncles leads to hemiparesis, quadriparesis, or bilateral paresis. Damage to the medial lemniscus and nucleus ruber may result in sensory deficits and impaired muscle tone. Impairment of the brainstem's ascending reticular activating system results in persistent coma, while damage to the midbrain can also cause decerebrate rigidity. Hemorrhage from aneurysms in the lower segment of the basilar artery affects the pontine level of the brainstem and extends upward to the medulla, resulting in the manifestation of corresponding symptoms. Rupture of aneurysms in the anterior inferior cerebellar artery results in a constellation of symptoms, including facial nerve palsy, hearing loss, tinnitus, and dizziness. Vertebral artery and its branches hemorrhage presents with symptoms of posterior group cranial nerve damage, including hoarseness and dysphagia, and may also involve hemiparesis, crossed paralysis, or quadriparesis. Additionally, symptoms of brainstem damage, such as a deep coma and dyspnea, may manifest. It is therefore essential to be able to distinguish between the clinical symptoms caused by ruptured posterior fossa aneurysms and those caused by brainstem hemorrhage. A head CT scan typically reveals either pure subarachnoid hemorrhage (SAH) or a combination of intracerebral hematomas in cases of ruptured intracranial aneurysm hemorrhage. Consequently, in cases of brainstem hemorrhage accompanied by SAH, the possibility of a ruptured posterior fossa aneurysm should be considered, and cerebral angiography should be performed to establish a definitive diagnosis of the underlying cause.

6.2 Ruptured Intracranial Arteriovenous Malformation Hemorrhage

Intracranial vascular malformations (ICVMs) are a group of cerebrovascular disorders that are characterized by an abnormal structure and function between the cerebral arteries and veins. This category encompasses a range of cerebrovascular disorders, including arteriovenous malformations (AVMs), venous malformations, capillary telangiectasias, cavernous angiomas, and vein of Galen aneurysmal malformations [2].

K. Shu (✉)
Department of Neurosugery, Tongji Hospital, Tongji Medical College, Huazhong University of Science and Technology, Wuhan, China
e-mail: kshu@tjh.tjmu.edu.cn

P. Zhang
Department of Neurology, Tongji Hospital,Tongji Medical College, Huazhong University of Science and Technology, Wuhan, China

H. Tao
Department of Cerebrovascular Diseases, Zhuhai People's Hospital (The Affiliated Hospital of Beijing Institute of Technology, Zhuhai Clinical Medical College of Jinan University), Zhuhai, China

G. Chen, C. You (eds.), *Surgical Treatment of Primary Brainstem Hemorrhage*, https://doi.org/10.1007/978-981-95-8942-5_6

As they age, AVMs tend to enlarge in a progressive manner, evolving from low-flow to high-flow lesions. In some cases, this enlargement may be accompanied by the formation of flow-related aneurysms. The overall incidence of AVMs is relatively low, with 60% of cases diagnosed before the age of 40 [3]. This makes AVMs the most common cause of spontaneous brain hemorrhage in young adults. The frontal and parietal lobes are the most common locations for AVMs, while those in the brainstem are less frequent. It has been demonstrated that infratentorial vascular malformations are more susceptible to bleeding, manifesting as subarachnoid hemorrhage (SAH) or deep posterior fossa hematomas [4]. The symptoms are similar to those of a brainstem injury. In cases of unruptured AVMs, occasional cluster-like or diffused curvilinear or punctate high-density shadows may be observed on head CT scans, or focal high-density, low-density, or mixed-density lesions may be seen. Contrast-enhanced CT imaging reveals irregular enhancement of the lesion, with tortuous and winding vascular shadows representing feeding arteries and draining veins. The presence of the malformation may be obscured by the ruptured AVM hematoma, rendering it difficult to discern on head CT scans. In some instances, however, tortuous vessels may be discernible on the surface, periphery, or deep regions of the hematoma, and magnetic resonance imaging (MRI) may reveal flow voids. In such cases, AVM hemorrhage should be considered as a potential diagnosis. In young patients presenting with a brainstem hemorrhage, the diagnosis of arteriovenous malformation (AVM) should be considered a highly probable possibility. The selection of the most appropriate imaging modality, including computed tomography angiography (CTA), magnetic resonance angiography (MRA), and digital subtraction angiography (DSA), should be based on the medical conditions of the patient [5]. Cerebral angiography is an effective method for establishing a definitive diagnosis of AVM. In patients with a high suspicion of cerebrovascular disease but a negative result from acute-phase angiography, a repeat angiography should be performed 3 months later to exclude false-negative results.

Cavernous angiomas are frequently observed in adolescents, and patients frequently lack a history of hypertension. The precise cause of the bleeding is unclear, but it may be attributed to the rupture and subsequent oozing of small or occult vascular malformations. Cavernous angiomas are most frequently observed in the cerebral lobes, brainstem, and cerebellum. Recurrent episodes of minimal bleeding are a common presenting feature of brainstem cavernous angiomas, which may ultimately result in progressive neurological deficits. Some patients may experience fluctuating neurological impairments, which may be associated with repeated small-volume bleeding from the cavernous angiomas. Brainstem cavernous angiomas are more frequently situated in the pons, and the resulting neurological irregularities have the capacity to serve as a means of diagnostic localization. In head CT scans, high-density or mixed-density lesions can be observed, and hemorrhages often appear as uniformly high-density shadows. Magnetic resonance imaging (MRI) demonstrates high specificity and sensitivity in the detection of cavernous angiomas, exhibiting a distinctive "popcorn" sign with a mesh-like mixed signal within the lesion, accompanied by a peripheral low signal on T2-weighted images. The absence of direct feeding arteries renders cerebral angiography an ineffective method for demonstrating cavernous angiomas. In cases of brainstem hemorrhage in young patients, a comprehensive investigation of the underlying cause is imperative. Typical imaging findings can assist in differentiating between hemorrhage from a brainstem cavernous angioma and primary brainstem hemorrhage.

6.3 Hemorrhage in Brainstem Tumors

The onset of symptoms in patients with brainstem tumors is often gradual, with symptoms developing over time and worsening in severity. The pathological diagnosis is typically glioma, although angioblastomas or metastatic tumors may also be observed. Brainstem gliomas are predominantly observed in pediatric and adolescent populations, with infrequent occurrences in middle-aged individuals. These tumors are predominantly low-grade astrocytomas, though they may also include glioblastomas or other highly malignant tumors. Tumors frequently demonstrate diffuse growth patterns, although some may exhibit relatively clear borders.

The classification of brainstem tumors is dependent on their location. There are three primary categories: midbrain, pons, and medulla oblongata tumors. The clinical manifestations of brainstem tumors are contingent upon their specific location. Tumors of the medulla oblongata typically manifest insidiously and exhibit a progressive deterioration. The clinical symptoms include dysfunction of the posterior group of cranial nerves, such as dysphagia, choking while drinking, hoarseness, and atrophy and fasciculation of the tongue muscles in some patients. In severe cases, alterations in respiratory rate, dyspnea, and cardiac arrhythmias may be observed. In many instances, the presence of increased intracranial pressure may not be readily apparent in these cases. However, some patients may present with symptoms such as neck pain, vomiting, and other manifestations. Patients with pontine tumors frequently present with diplopia and unsteady gait, which can result in a high incidence of falls. The majority of patients present with ipsilateral cranial nerve and facial nerve paralysis, accompanied by contralateral limb weakness and sensory impairments, impaired eye movements, strabismus, and episodes of excessive crying or laughing. Additionally, pontine tumors may present with symptoms consistent with Millard-Gubler syndrome and Foville syndrome. In patients with midbrain tumors, clinical symptoms typically indicate increased intracranial pressure, including headaches, vomiting, papilledema, and altered consciousness. Furthermore, psychiatric abnormalities and changes in intelligence may also be observed. Furthermore, there may be an oculomotor nerve palsy, pupillary dilation, anisocoria, and loss of the pupillary light reflex on the ipsilateral side, as well as contralateral limb hemiparesis and changes in hearing and vision. Midbrain tumors frequently manifest in conjunction with a constellation of visible syndromes, including Parinaud syndrome, Weber syndrome, and Benedikt syndrome.

In cases where a brainstem tumor is complicated by intratumoral hemorrhage, the patient's condition often deteriorates rapidly, necessitating a differential diagnosis between the two conditions. Primary brainstem hemorrhage is more frequently observed in the pons, while occurrences in the medulla oblongata and midbrain are less prevalent. A routine head CT scan may reveal a high-density hematoma, but an MRI examination is particularly valuable for distinguishing between hemorrhage in brainstem tumors and isolated brainstem hemorrhage.

6.4 Moyamoya Disease and Hemorrhage After Cerebral Infarction

The etiology of Moyamoya disease remains unknown. It is characterized by chronic progressive occlusion of the skull base vessels. The disease is characterized by a distinctive progression of occlusion of the intracranial arteries above the anterior perforated substance, including the anterior cerebral arteries and proximal middle cerebral arteries. This is followed by the gradual appearance of compensatory vessels, which are visible as smoky collateral vessels. In adolescents and children with Moyamoya disease, ischemic attacks and strokes are the predominant clinical manifestations, while hemorrhagic episodes are rare. The disease may manifest in a number of ways, including recurrent ischemic attacks, seizures, and, in severe cases, cerebral infarction. In adults with Moyamoya disease, the primary clinical manifestation is cerebral hemorrhage. The most prevalent clinical manifestation is intraventricular hemorrhage, followed by intracerebral hematoma and subarachnoid hemorrhage. Hemorrhage frequently manifests acutely, with patients presenting with symptoms such as headaches and vomiting. In severe cases, impaired consciousness may also occur. Hemorrhage typically occurs in the supratentorial region, with involvement of the posterior fossa being less prevalent. A head CT scan can differentiate this condition from brainstem hemorrhage; however, a definitive diagnosis requires cerebral angiography. Perfusion imaging can be employed to demonstrate the distribution of cerebral blood flow in patients with Moyamoya disease, thereby facilitating the guidance of treatment. It is not uncommon for patients to present with new neurological symptoms and signs during the treatment of cerebral infarction. In such cases, a head CT scan is performed to exclude hemorrhage after infarction. In instances where the quantity of bleeding is minimal, computed tomography scans may reveal scattered and uneven regions of high density within the low-density infarct lesion background, exhibiting a density that is lower than that of hematomas. In the event of a significant volume of bleeding, a high-density hematoma may be observed within the low-density area. Magnetic resonance imaging (MRI) reveals the presence of hemorrhagic signals within the infarcted region, manifesting as a low signal intensity on T1-weighted imaging (T1WI) and a high signal intensity on T2-weighted imaging (T2WI). The crucial aspect of distinguishing this phenomenon from primary brainstem hemorrhage is the presence of a documented history of brainstem infarction. The diagnosis can be established when the hemorrhage occurs in the infarcted region, based on this historical evidence.

Posterior circulation cerebral infarction primarily affects the brainstem, cerebellum, and thalamus, with a higher prevalence among middle-aged and elderly individuals. Cerebral infarction is characterized by a low signal intensity on T1-weighted imaging (T1WI) and a high signal intensity on T2-weighted imaging (T2WI). Diffusion-weighted magnetic resonance imaging (DWI-MRI) allows for the identification of alterations in lesion signals as early as 6 h following the onset of infarction. Diffusion-weighted magnetic resonance imaging (DWI-MRI) has the capacity to detect ischemic changes in the brain at an earlier stage than conventional T2-weighted imaging. In the case of fresh infarct lesions, both conventional T2-weighted imaging (T2WI) and diffusion-weighted MRI (DWI) demonstrate high signal intensity. Conversely, in chronic old infarct lesions, conventional T2-weighted imaging (T2WI) demonstrates a high signal intensity, whereas diffusion-weighted imaging (DWI) displays a low signal intensity. The term "hemorrhage after cerebral infarction" is used to describe secondary bleeding that occurs as a result of reperfusion in the infarcted area. The timing of this phenomenon is variable, and the morphology of the hematoma is frequently irregular.

6.5 Cerebral Amyloid Angiopathy Hemorrhage

Cerebral amyloid angiopathy (CAA), also referred to as Congo red angiopathy, is defined by the accumulation of amorphous Congo red-staining material within the walls of small- and medium-sized arteries. This disease frequently affects multiple cerebral blood vessels, with the most common involvement occurring in the occipital and parietal lobes, followed by the frontal lobe and cerebellum. The clinical course is typified by recurrent intracerebral hemorrhage, which most commonly occurs in the subcortical regions of the cerebral lobes. Magnetic resonance imaging (MRI) of affected patients frequently reveals multiple small, chronic hemorrhagic lesions, as well as small hemorrhagic foci distributed along the convex surface of the cerebral hemispheres. In cases of larger hemorrhages, supratentorial cerebral lobe hematomas may be observed, whereas hemorrhages in the posterior fossa are less common. Patients with concomitant cerebellar hemorrhage in the context of sporadic cerebral amyloid angiopathy often present with an acute onset, posterior occipital pain, and symptoms of brainstem involvement, such as pupillary changes, cranial nerve deficits, and pyramidal tract signs. A differential diagnosis of brainstem hemorrhage is essential, and head CT scans can accurately determine the location of the hemorrhage and assess the degree of brainstem compression, which is significant for diagnosis and treatment guidance.

6.6 Cerebellar and Thalamic Hemorrhage

Cerebellar hemorrhage represents 5–10% of all intracranial hemorrhages and is most commonly caused by hypertensive arteriosclerosis. In patients under the age of 40, cerebellar hemorrhage is primarily attributable to vascular malformations within the cerebellum. However, it can also occur in conjunction with the presence of aneurysms. Cerebellar hemorrhages are frequently situated in the cerebellar hemispheres and are predominantly caused by bleeding from the distal branches of the posterior inferior cerebellar artery and the superior cerebellar artery. Subsequent to this, bleeding occurs in the vermis, originating from the medial branches of the posterior inferior cerebellar artery or the superior cerebellar artery. All three blood vessels that supply the cerebellum have branches that also supply the brainstem. Additionally, approximately 25% of patients with cerebellar hemorrhage also have concomitant hemorrhages in the cerebral peduncles or pons. A cerebellar hemorrhage has the potential to result in secondary ischemic necrosis of the brainstem, which is associated with factors such as hematoma compression and elevated local pressure following the hemorrhage.

A cerebellar hemorrhage typically manifests acutely and is frequently accompanied by symptoms such as occipital pain, nausea, vomiting, dizziness, and unsteady gait. In cases of significant severity, there may be an impairment of consciousness or even a coma. In addition to the aforementioned symptoms, partial hemorrhages that involve or compress the brainstem may also present with changes in pupil size, conjugate eye deviation, facial paralysis, sensory disturbances, or pyramidal tract signs. In instances of extensive hemorrhage that ruptures into the fourth ventricle or compresses the fourth ventricle or cerebral aqueduct, acute obstructive hydrocephalus or even brain herniation may ensue. A differential diagnosis of brainstem hemorrhage is essential during the clinical assessment. Cranial CT scans are an effective method for determining the location and volume of the hemorrhage, identifying the source of bleeding, and assessing the involvement of the brainstem. This information is crucial for guiding treatment decisions and predicting prognosis.

Thalamic hemorrhage represents approximately 20% to 25% of all cases of cerebral hemorrhage, frequently resulting from hypertensive arteriosclerosis. Additional etiologies include arteriovenous malformations and aneurysms. The symptoms typically manifest as coma and hemiplegia, accompanied by impaired eye movement and constricted pupils. In instances where the bleeding is minimal, it tends to be localized, which results in a relatively stable condition and a favorable prognosis for recovery. In cases of extensive bleeding, the midbrain is often affected, resulting in a deep coma, decerebrate rigidity, high fever, accelerated pulse, elevated blood pressure, and other vital sign changes. Additionally, stress ulcers and pinpoint pupils may be observed. The clinical presentation of thalamic hemorrhage is not typical and can be similar to that of a brainstem hemorrhage, necessitating careful differentiation. In cases of significant thalamic hemorrhage, it is of particular importance to ascertain whether the bleeding has involved the brainstem, as this information is crucial for prognostication. A diagnosis can be confirmed through cranial CT scans. In cases suspected to be caused by intracranial aneurysms or arteriovenous malformations, cerebral angiography is also necessary.

6.7 Other Causes of Cerebral Hemorrhage

Hematological disorders frequently co-occur with coagulation dysfunction and a hypercoagulable state, rendering individuals more susceptible to both ischemic stroke and cerebral hemorrhage. In sickle-cell anemia, the presence of abnormal sickle-shaped cells can result in cerebral microcirculatory vessel blockage, which may lead to ischemic infarction and hemorrhagic changes. Conditions such as polycythemia vera, secondary erythrocytosis, and leukemia have been demonstrated to elevate blood viscosity, diminish cerebral blood flow, and facilitate the development of cerebral microthrombi, thereby contributing to both ischemic stroke and hemorrhage. Patients with leukemia may also present with decreased platelet counts and a tendency to bleed, rendering them susceptible to cerebral hemorrhage. Bleeding disorders resulting from platelet abnormalities are typified by an inability to halt the bleeding process once it has commenced, accompanied by a proclivity for recurrent bleeding. This can result in the occurrence of spontaneous hemorrhages within the central nervous system, including intracranial hemorrhage, brainstem hemorrhage, and spinal cord hemorrhage. Additionally, plasma cell dyscrasias, paroxysmal nocturnal hemoglobinuria, and hypercoagulable states are all considered high-risk factors for stroke. Moreover, specific genetic metabolic disorders, including familial hypercholesterolemia, multiple neurofibromatosis, homocystinuria, and MELAS syndrome, are associated with a considerable risk of ischemic and hemorrhagic strokes in young individuals. Patients with hematological diseases and genetic metabolic disorders frequently have pertinent medical histories and treatment records. Consequently, in the event of a stroke, it is imperative to consider the influence of the underlying disease. While the diagnosis may not be complex, a comprehensive and integrated treatment plan is essential to prevent systemic multi-organ complications. In instances where the medical history is ambiguous and the initial symptoms manifest as either ischemic or hemorrhagic stroke in young patients, it is crucial to distinguish them from cerebral complications resulting from systemic diseases. The performance of pertinent supplementary examinations can facilitate accurate diagnosis.

Additionally, intracranial infectious lesions have been linked to the development of cerebrovascular disorders and subsequent stroke. Spirochetal cerebral arteritis is an acute infectious disease caused by various spirochetes. From a pathological perspective, the disease presents extensive inflammatory changes in cerebral arteries, cerebral infarction, and lesions that primarily affect large-caliber intracranial arteries, including the internal carotid artery, middle cerebral artery, and vertebrobasilar artery. The severity of arterial stenosis caused by the lesions is most pronounced in the anterior and middle cerebral arteries, while the vertebrobasilar system is less affected. The clinical manifestations observed in patients include fever, chills, facial and conjunctival congestion, bleeding tendencies, and neurological signs such as limb weakness and aphasia. Hemorrhagic changes are less common. A differential diagnosis with brainstem lesions is necessary during the acute phase, and a head CT can distinguish between hemorrhagic and ischemic changes. Serological tests can be employed to diagnose spirochete infections, while cerebral angiography can be utilized to reveal intracranial vascular stenosis.

Neurosyphilis represents a central nervous system manifestation resulting from infection with the bacterium *Treponema pallidum*. Neurosyphilis primarily manifests as inflammatory changes in the meninges and blood vessels. These changes are characterized by tunica intima hyperplasia, which leads to luminal narrowing, and arachnoiditis, which obstructs cerebrospinal fluid circulation, resulting in hydrocephalus. During the acute phase, patients present with a range of symptoms, including severe headaches, vomiting, and signs of meningeal irritation. Additionally, they may exhibit manifestations of cranial nerve paralysis, such as impaired eye movement, facial paralysis, and hearing loss. The diagnosis of neurosyphilis is primarily based on a comprehensive history of high-risk sexual behaviors, cerebrospinal fluid examination, serological tests for syphilis, and thorough neurological examinations. In cases where neurological damage, such as cerebral infarction or hemorrhage, is present, the use of head CT and MRI scans can facilitate the diagnosis.

Patients who have been prescribed long-term oral antiplatelet and anticoagulant therapy for the purpose of disease or stroke prevention, such as those who have been taking aspirin, clopidogrel, or warfarin over an extended period of time, are at an increased risk of developing a cerebral hemorrhage [6]. These hemorrhages often occur in the supratentorial cerebral lobes and may present with multiple hemorrhagic foci. In some cases, patients may present with an isolated brainstem hemorrhage. The diagnosis of these patients is typically straightforward due to their long history of medication use. Treatment is primarily medical, with surgical intervention reserved for cases where it is necessary.

In cases of brainstem hemorrhage in young patients, it is crucial to inquire about the potential use of illicit substances, including cocaine, heroin, and amphetamines (methamphetamine). Cerebral infarction is more commonly observed in individuals with a history of heroin addiction, occurring either immediately after the administration of heroin or with a latency period of 6–24 h. Abuse of methamphetamine frequently results in necrotizing cerebral vasculitis and the occurrence of cerebral hemorrhage. Cocaine abuse has been linked to several adverse effects on the cardiovascular system, including vasoconstriction, a rapid increase in blood pressure, platelet aggregation, and cerebral arteritis. These effects contribute to a significantly higher incidence of brainstem infarction compared to other drug abusers. It is essential to exercise caution and differentiate between these conditions in clinical practice. Furthermore, in instances where drug abuse is concomitant with stroke, the response to vasoactive drugs may be suboptimal, and the effects of drug withdrawal can influence treatment outcomes.

References

1. Wang ZC. Neurosurgery. Wuhan: Hubei Science and Technology Press; 2005.
2. Lei T. Diagnosis and treatment guidelines for neurosurgical diseases. 3rd ed. Wuhan: Science Press; 2013.
3. Caplan LR. Caplan's stroke: a clinical approach. 5th ed. Cambridge, UK: Cambridge University Press; 2016.
4. Stahl SM, Johnson KP, Malamud N. The clinical and pathological spectrum of brain-stem vascular malformations Long-term course stimulates multiple sclerosis. Arch Neurol. 1980;37(1):25–9.
5. Kashiwagi S, van Loveren HR, Tew JM Jr, et al. Diagnosis and treatment of vascular brain-stem malformations. J Neurosurg. 1990;72(1):27–34.
6. Seiffge DJ, Curtze S, Dequatre-Ponchelle N, et al. Hematoma location and morphology of anticoagulation-associated intracere¬bralhemorrhage. Neurology. 2019;92(8):782–91.

7 Surgical Treatment Principles for Primary Brainstem Hemorrhage

Gang Chen, Zhen Wu, and Chao Sun

7.1 Overview

A brainstem hemorrhage represents 5% to 13.4% of clinical intracerebral hemorrhages, with a mortality rate of 70% to 80% [1]. The age group most susceptible to brainstem hemorrhage is between 40 and 70 years old, with a growing prevalence among younger patients [2]. The incidence rate is markedly higher in males than in females. The principal characteristics of a brainstem hemorrhage are its rapid onset, rapid progression, severe condition, and multiple complications. The intricate anatomy and vital functions of the brainstem render surgical intervention particularly challenging, with a high incidence of complications. Previously, the academic community viewed brainstem hemorrhage as a contraindication for surgical intervention, with the majority of scholars, both domestically and internationally, advocating for conservative treatment. In recent years, the advancement of microsurgical techniques and the application of intraoperative neuroelectrophysiology monitoring have led to improvements in the efficacy and prognosis of primary brainstem hemorrhage following surgical treatment [3]. This section provides an overview of the current status of surgical treatment and will discuss each aspect in detail.

G. Chen (✉)
Department of Neurosurgery, Zhuhai People's Hospital (The Affiliated Hospital of Beijing Institute of Technology, Zhuhai Clinical Medical College of Jinan University), Zhuhai, China

Z. Wu
Department of Neurosurgery, Beijing Tiantan Hospital, Capital Medical University, Beijing, China

C. Sun
Department of Neurosurgery, The Second Affiliated Hospital of Soochow University, Suzhou, China

7.1.1 Lateral Ventricular Puncture and External Drainage

In the event of a significant accumulation of brainstem hemorrhage, the majority of hematomas tend to rupture into the fourth ventricle. This results in the immediate disruption of cerebrospinal fluid circulation, which in turn precipitates a pronounced surge in intracranial pressure and a rapid expansion of the ventricles. The early puncture and drainage of the lateral ventricle can alleviate the rapid expansion of the ventricle, decrease intracranial pressure, and prevent the downward transmission of pressure from the brainstem hematomas in the posterior fossa, thus avoiding tonsillar herniation. The procedures of lateral ventricular puncture and external drainage are relatively straightforward yet yield substantial outcomes. These procedures have been demonstrated to reduce the mortality rate of patients with brainstem hemorrhage and are therefore suitable for implementation and promotion in primary hospitals.

7.1.2 Craniotomy with Microscopic Hematoma Evacuation

The majority of scholars concur that a craniotomy, which allows for direct visualization of the surgical site, represents the optimal surgical method for treating spontaneous massive brainstem hemorrhage. The advantages of craniotomy include direct visualization for hematoma evacuation and reliable hemostasis, with the possibility of simultaneous decompressive surgery. The disadvantages include the potential for significant surgical trauma, which could exacerbate the patient's condition if it affects the brainstem. At present, the advancement of microsurgical techniques has led to the development of sophisticated instruments and devices that facilitate enhanced visualization, thereby reducing the extent of surgical trauma. Enhanced comprehension of the safe zone within the brainstem and meticulous microsurgical

G. Chen, C. You (eds.), *Surgical Treatment of Primary Brainstem Hemorrhage*, https://doi.org/10.1007/978-981-95-8942-5_7

techniques ensure the removal of brainstem hematomas in the context of minimally invasive surgery [4, 5]. When surgical indications and timing are accurately identified, microsurgical techniques are skillfully employed, and surgical skills are exercised with elevated attention to detail; satisfactory results can be achieved with minimally invasive surgical treatment for brainstem hemorrhage.

7.1.3 Stereotactic Puncture and Aspiration

Since Backlund first successfully used stereotactic techniques to evacuate intracerebral hematomas in 1978, stereotactic evacuation for intracerebral hematomas has been widely used in neurosurgery. Subsequent improvements in surgical methods by Niizuma, Suzuki, Hondo, and others have achieved positive therapeutic effects [6]. Currently, the application of 64-slice CT imaging provides rapid scanning with minimal artifacts in the brainstem region, enabling three-dimensional reconstruction of brain tissue, which facilitates the identification of optimal puncture points and drainage paths [7]. The characteristics of stereotactic puncture and aspiration include no need for craniotomy, reducing the damage to vital structures in the brainstem and other areas caused by microsurgery with craniotomy. This method has relatively simple steps, shorter operation time, and precise localization of hematoma and is suitable for patients with brainstem hemorrhage who are unable to tolerate surgery with craniotomy or are elderly and frail. Stereotactic puncture and aspiration do not require high surgical skills or conditions, making it convenient for implementation and promotion in primary hospitals [8, 9]. With the widespread application of neuronavigation, the accuracy of stereotactic procedures has increased, significantly improving patient survival rates.

7.1.4 Endoscopic Brainstem Hematoma Evacuation

For brainstem hematomas, similar to surgical approaches for brainstem tumors, traditional surgical approaches include the retrosigmoid approach, subfrontal approach, Kawase approach, and others. These traditional approaches provide better exposure to lesions on the anterior-lateral aspect of the brainstem, but they pose challenges in exposing the midline and near-midline regions of the ventral surface of the brainstem. The combined use of neuroendoscopy allows for clear illumination of deep structures, eliminates surgical blind spots, enables close observation, improves hematoma evacuation rates, and reduces secondary damage to the brainstem [10]. The advancement of endoscopic techniques has led to a significant expansion in the applications of neuroendoscopy. It is no longer merely a supplementary observation tool for operations conducted under a microscope; rather, it has become a widely utilized technique in fully endoscopic surgeries. The endonasal endoscopic transsphenoidal-clivus approach, which utilizes the natural cavity, allows for the shortest distance to lesions on the ventral side of the brainstem. By capitalizing on the benefits of the diverse angles afforded by the nasal endoscope, the risk of brain tissue traction can be mitigated, and damage to cranial nerves can be prevented to the greatest extent possible. Sporadic literature reports from both domestic and international sources have described surgical experiences of resecting brainstem cavernous malformations and epidermoid tumors using the endonasal endoscopic clivus approach but with a relatively high incidence of cerebrospinal fluid leakage [11–13]. There are rare reports on hematoma evacuation via this approach. The endonasal space for surgical maneuvers is relatively limited, lacking three-dimensional visualization, and the light source may generate thermal damage. Therefore, the endonasal endoscopic transsphenoidal-clivus approach remains challenging and requires a thorough understanding of the anatomical region and proficiency in endoscopic techniques. Relying on comprehensive preoperative imaging evaluation, precise intraoperative localization, appropriate fenestration, and attention to the methods and details of skull base defect repair, satisfactory surgical outcomes can be achieved.

7.2 General Principles

7.2.1 Preoperative Preparation

Adequate preoperative preparation is often crucial for the success of the surgery, and the selection of the surgical approach is a major component of preoperative preparation.

7.2.2 Image Fusion and Navigation Techniques

Image fusion and navigation techniques serve as important references for selecting the surgical approach and determining the localization during brainstem lesion resection. When feasible in terms of the patient's condition and time, combining image-guided navigation with microscopic surgery can greatly enhance the efficiency and safety of the procedure.

7.2.3 Surgical Equipment and Instruments

Although the brainstem is small in size, its functionality is of utmost importance. The surgical corridor during the procedure is generally narrow and deep. To ensure safe manipulation, surgical microscopes, endoscopes, navigation systems, as well as specialized suction devices, bipolar coagulators, and microdissection instruments are required.

7.2.4 Intraoperative Brainstem Function Monitoring

Similar to patients undergoing resection of other brainstem lesions, intraoperative monitoring of somatosensory evoked potentials and motor evoked potentials is recommended for brainstem hemorrhage surgery. Depending on the location of the hemorrhage, selective monitoring of cranial nerves and neural nuclei function should be performed.

7.2.5 Technical Expertise of the Medical Team

The surgical treatment of brainstem hemorrhage is a complex undertaking that involves anesthesia, surgery, intraoperative electrophysiological monitoring, postoperative intensive care, and nursing. Each step is crucial, and just like the "weakest link" theory, any deficiency can impact the final outcome. Therefore, the establishment of a competent medical team and technical expertise are of paramount importance for the surgical treatment of brainstem hemorrhage. It is not recommended to perform brainstem hemorrhage surgery in hospitals without the necessary capabilities, especially at the primary hospitals.

7.2.6 "Two-Point Method" for Determining the Surgical Approach

This method is most commonly used to determine the surgical approach for brainstem lesion surgery. The surgical approach determined by the "two-point method" allows for convenient hematoma evacuation while minimizing damage to brain tissue [14].

7.2.7 Minimizing Coagulation and Traction

Appropriate positioning, precise selection of the craniotomy site, and judicious use of microsurgical instruments can help avoid unnecessary tissue traction during the procedure. The proper use of bipolar coagulation, suction devices, and microsurgical instruments allows gradual retraction of brain tissue, providing the surgeon with a clear surgical field and reducing brain tissue damage.

7.3 Indications and Contraindications

7.3.1 Surgical Indications

There is no unified standard for the surgical indications of brainstem hemorrhage both domestically and internationally. However, the following conditions are generally considered for surgical treatment:

1. Hematoma volume greater than 5 mL.
2. Hematoma is relatively concentrated, located near the surface of the brainstem or extending into the ventricles.
3. Patients with shallow to moderate coma, GCS < 8, with or without severe signs of life-threatening disturbances.
4. Strong surgical desire and risk awareness from the patient's family, with financial circumstances that can support long-term postoperative treatment.

7.3.2 Surgical Contraindications

1. Small brainstem hemorrhage (≤3 mL) without obvious obstruction of the ventricular system or consciousness impairment.
2. Large hemorrhage causing severe damage to the vital centers of the brainstem, with bilateral dilated pupils and extremely unstable vital signs.
3. Poor overall condition, unable to tolerate surgery.
4. Severe coagulation abnormalities.

7.4 Selection of Surgical Approach

7.4.1 General Principles for Selecting the Surgical Approach for Brainstem Hemorrhage

The selection of the surgical approach is of paramount importance for the success of the surgery. The selection of the surgical approach is dependent upon the location of the hematoma. The principles include the following:

1. The shortest surgical path.
2. Avoidance of important conducting tracts and nuclei of the brainstem, minimizing damage.
3. Alignment with the maximum diameter of the hematoma, facilitating complete evacuation of the intraparenchymal hematoma.
4. Simultaneous resolution of hydrocephalus and intracranial hypertension.

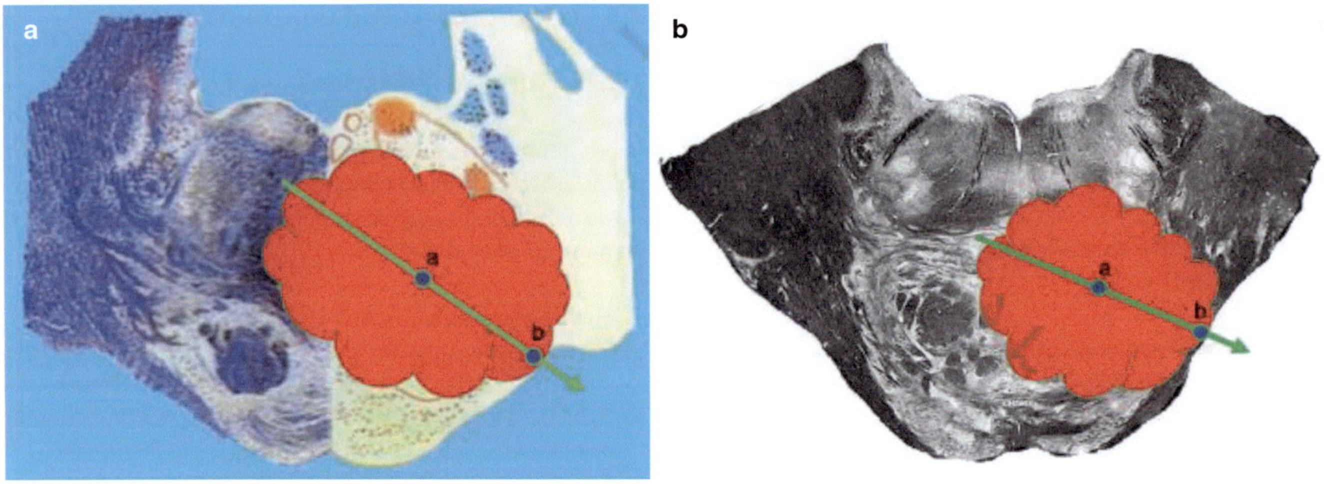

Fig. 7.1 Two-point method. The geometric center or midpoint of the long axis of the hematoma as point A and point B at the most superficial part of the hematoma or the safe operating area of the brainstem, the line connecting these two points can be extended to the skull, providing the required surgical path

Using Brown's two-point method to determine the surgical approach: The surgical approach determined by the "two-point method" allows for convenient hematoma evacuation while minimizing damage to brain tissue. This method is most commonly used to determine the surgical approach for brainstem lesion surgery. By reading CT or MRI scans, the geometric center or midpoint of the long axis of the hematoma is located as point A, while point B is positioned at the most superficial part of the hematoma or the safe operating area of the brainstem. The line connecting these two points is extended to the skull to obtain the desired surgical path (Fig. 7.1).

7.4.2 Safe Operating Areas of the Brainstem

Following the incision of several sites on the surface of the brainstem, no significant neurological deficits are to be expected. Such sites are designated as "safe operating areas" of the brainstem. In their study, Spetzler and colleagues identified a total of 13 safe areas, which are as follows:

1. Anterior mesencephalic zone (AMZ).
2. Lateral mesencephalic sulcus (LMS).
3. Intercollicular region (ICR).
4. Paratrigeminal zone.
5. Superior trigeminal nerve zone.
6. Lateral pons zone.
7. Superior collicular zone.
8. Inferior collicular zone.
9. Median sulcus of the fourth ventricle.
10. Anterolateral sulcus of the medulla.
11. Posterior median sulcus of the medulla.
12. Olivary zone.
13. Lateral medullary zone.

These 13 safe areas can be divided into 3 groups, corresponding to lesions in the midbrain, pons, and medulla. Here are the details:

7.4.2.1 Midbrain

1. Anterior Mesencephalic Zone (AMZ): Lesions in the anterior part of the midbrain can be accessed through this safe area. Its medial boundary is the oculomotor nerve bundle or nerve, the lateral boundary is the corticospinal tract (CST) (Fig. 7.2a, b), the superior boundary is the posterior cerebral artery (PCA), and the inferior boundary is the main branch of the superior cerebellar artery.
2. Lateral Mesencephalic Sulcus (LMS): Hidden in the deep surface of the lateral mesencephalic vein, it descends from the medial geniculate body to the pontomesencephalon sulcus (Fig. 7.2c). The anterior-lateral boundary of this safe area is the substantia nigra, the posterior boundary is the medial lemniscus, and the part where the oculomotor nerve fibers pass through the nucleus ruber toward the substantia nigra is the anterior-medial boundary. The average length of LMS is 9.6 mm (7.4–13.3 mm), and the average operable length is 8.0 mm (4.9–11.7 mm).
3. Intercollicular Region (ICR): Located between the superior and inferior colliculi on both sides, this area has few nerve fibers (Fig. 7.2d), making it a suitable entry point for surgery.

7.4.2.2 Pons

1. Paratrigeminal Zone (PTZ): This safe area is located in front of the region where the trigeminal nerve enters the brainstem, lateral to the corticospinal tract, and ventral to the motor and sensory nuclei of the trigeminal nerve. On

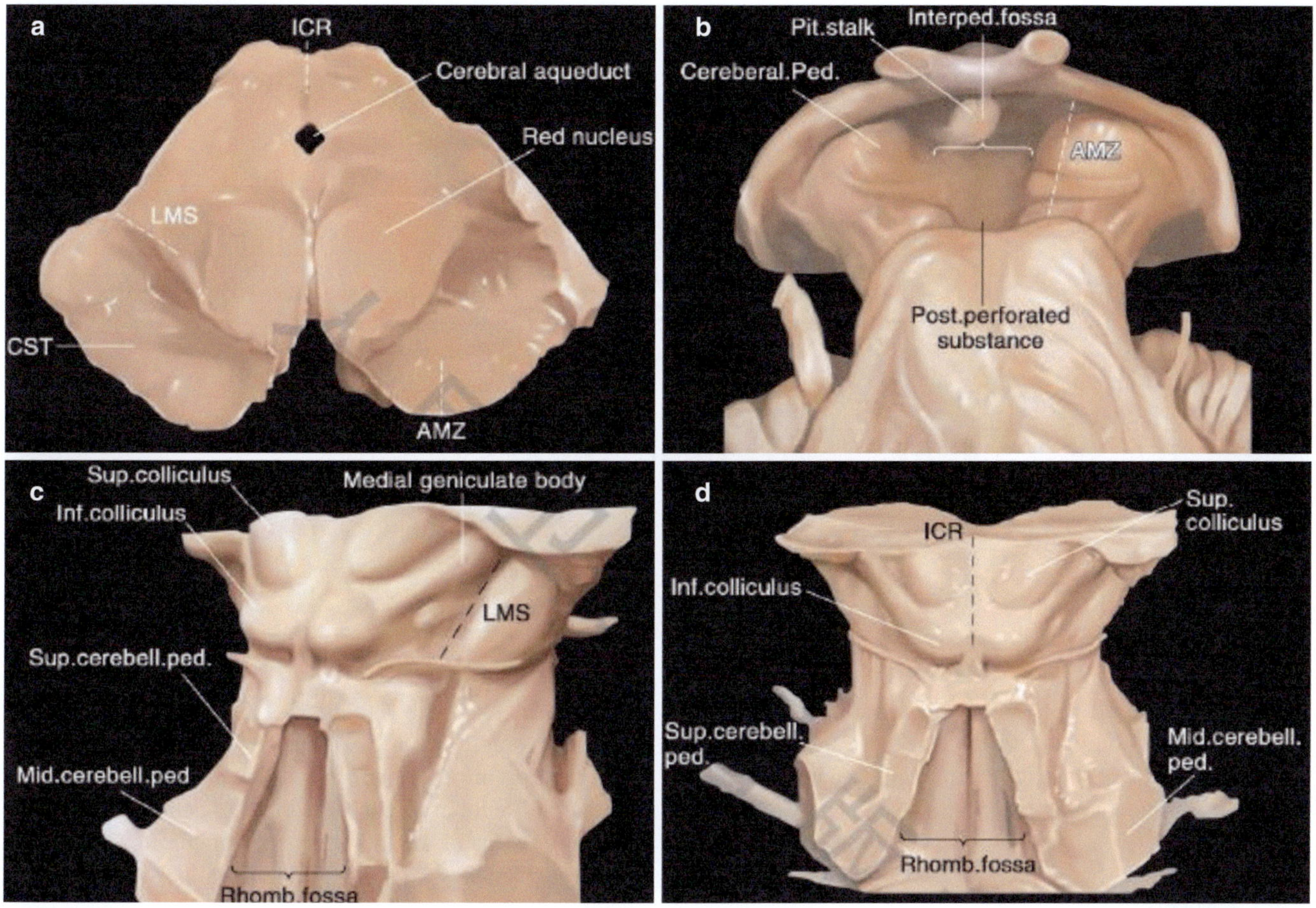

Fig. 7.2 Safe areas of the midbrain. (**a**) Transverse view of the cerebral peduncle. (**b**) Anterior view of the midbrain, illustrating the anterior mesencephalic zone (AMZ). (**c**) Right posterolateral view of the midbrain, illustrating the lateral mesencephalic sulcus (LMS). (**d**) Posterior view of the midbrain, illustrating the intercollicular region (ICR)

axial measurement, the average distance between the trigeminal nerve and the corticospinal tract is 4.64 mm (3.8–5.6 mm), and the average distance to reach the deep trigeminal nerve nucleus is 11.2 mm (9.5–13.1 mm). The descending fibers of cranial nerves VI, VII, and VIII all pass posterior to the trigeminal nerve nucleus, thus avoiding damage (Fig. 7.3a, b).

2. Superior Trigeminal Zone (STZ): This safe area is located above the region where the trigeminal nerve enters the brainstem, at the level of the middle cerebellar peduncle (Fig. 7.3c). Considering that the middle cerebellar peduncle is situated posterior-laterally to the pons, the pons arm fibers can be separated medially or anteromedially to enter behind the corticospinal tract.
3. Lateral Pons Zone (LPZ): This safe area is located between the middle cerebellar peduncle and the pons, extending superiorly to the region where the trigeminal nerve enters the brainstem and inferiorly to the region where the facial and auditory nerve enters the brainstem (Fig. 7.3c).
4. Superior and Inferior Collicular Zones (SCZ and ICZ): The rhomboid fossa contains many important structures, and damaging them can lead to severe consequences. Surface markers can help avoid injury to important structures deep within the fourth ventricle. The superior collicular zone is located between the facial colliculus and the trochlear nerve crossing, with a longitudinal length of 13.8 mm. Its medial boundary extends 0.6 mm from the midline, and its lateral boundary ends at the motor nucleus of the trigeminal nerve (adjacent to the midline) at 6.3 mm. The inferior collicular zone can be adjusted based on the projection of the facial nerve fibers onto the facial colliculus, with a 0.3 mm distance from the midline and the lower boundary being the hypoglossal nucleus and the dorsal nucleus of the vagus nerve. Its longitudinal extension can reach a length of 9.2 mm.
5. Median Sulcus of the Fourth Ventricle (MS): This area, located between the projection of the abducens nucleus and the projection of the trigeminal nerve in the pons through the posterior median approach (Fig. 7.3b), has

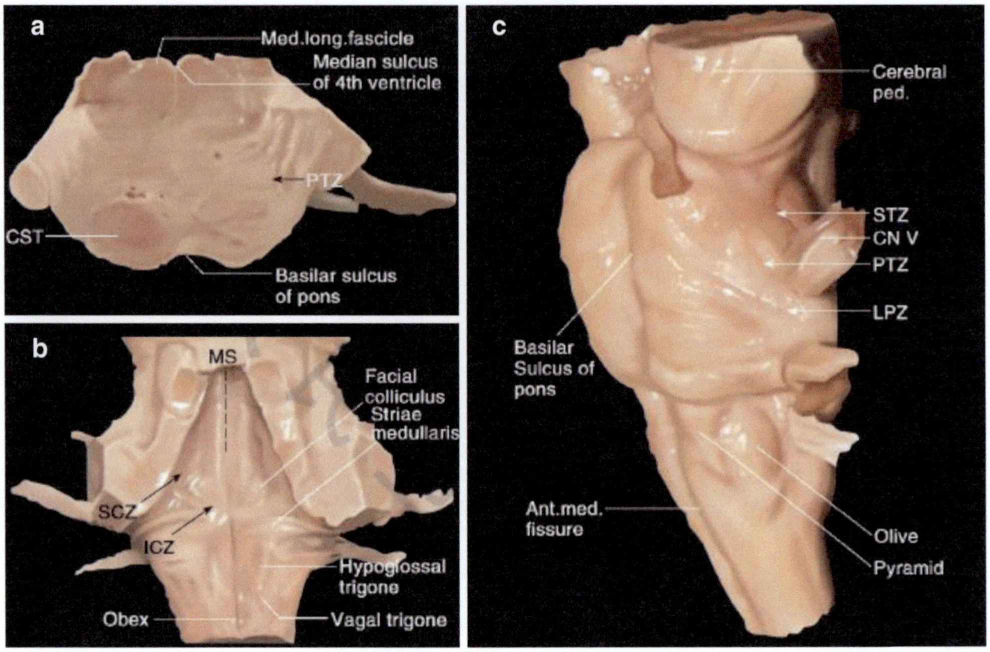

Fig. 7.3 Safe areas of the pons. (**a**) Transverse view of the pons showing paratrigeminal zone (PTZ). (**b**) Three surgical safe operating areas in the rhomboid fossa: superior collicular zone, inferior collicular zone, and median sulcus of the fourth ventricle. (**c**) Surgical safe operating areas on the lateral and anterolateral aspects of the pons: superior trigeminal nerve zone, paratrigeminal zone, and lateral pons zone

fewer distributed nerve fiber bundles. However, it is important to note that any traction outward may potentially cause damage to the medial longitudinal fasciculus and result in ocular motor disturbances.

7.4.2.3 Medulla Oblongata

1. Anterolateral Sulcus of the Medulla (ALS): Located lateral to the pyramidal decussation, the hypoglossal nerve emerges from the anterolateral sulcus of the brainstem. These nerve roots, along with the C1 nerve root, travel inward and converge at the pyramidal decussation. By performing oblique separation in this region, damage to the pyramidal tract can be avoided, allowing access to lesions located anterior to the lower medulla (Fig. 7.4a,b).
2. Posterior Median Sulcus of the Medulla (PMS): Separation through the posterior median sulcus of the medulla provides a pathway close to the middle portion of the medulla. Within the region shown in Fig. 7.4c, surgical procedures within the medulla can be performed similarly to the resection of intramedullary spinal cord tumors.
3. Olivary Zone (OZ): The olive nucleus is located on the anterolateral surface of the medulla, bordered medially by the anterolateral sulcus and the pyramids and inferiorly by the posterolateral sulcus. In the axial section of the lower olive nucleus, the hypoglossal nerve fibers separate the olive nucleus from the corticospinal tract within the pyramids. Its medial boundary is limited by the hypoglossal nerve fibers and the medial lemniscus, while its posterior boundary is defined by the roof and the spinothalamic tract. The safe zone of the olive nucleus has a vertical length of approximately 13.5 mm and a depth of separation inward ranging from 4.7 to 6.9 mm.
4. Lateral Medullary Zone (LMZ): For lesions in the dorsolateral region of the medulla, excision through the lateral medullary safe zone can yield favorable outcomes. By utilizing the retrosigmoid approach and opening the foramen of Luschka, the origin of the IX and X cranial nerves on the brainstem can be identified. A small vertical incision is made at the inferior cerebellar peduncle, inferior to the vestibulocochlear nerve nucleus, and posterior to the origin of the IX and X cranial nerves (Fig. 7.4a).

7.4.3 Surgical Approaches for Brainstem Hematomas

1. Subtemporal approach: In the subtemporal approach, the patient is positioned in lateral decubitus or supine position with the head tilted to the side to align the sagittal suture parallel to the ground. The surgical incision can be made as a preauricular question mark incision or a straight incision. The main steps are as follows: Dissect the temporal muscle and temporal muscle fascia, and expose a large portion of the temporal bone. Drill a hole at the root of the zygomatic arch, and grind the lower edge of the bone window as close to the skull base as possible. Incise the dura mater, and perform dissection at the base of the temporal lobe until the tentorial edge is reached. Confirm the mid-anterior incisure of the tentorial edge and open

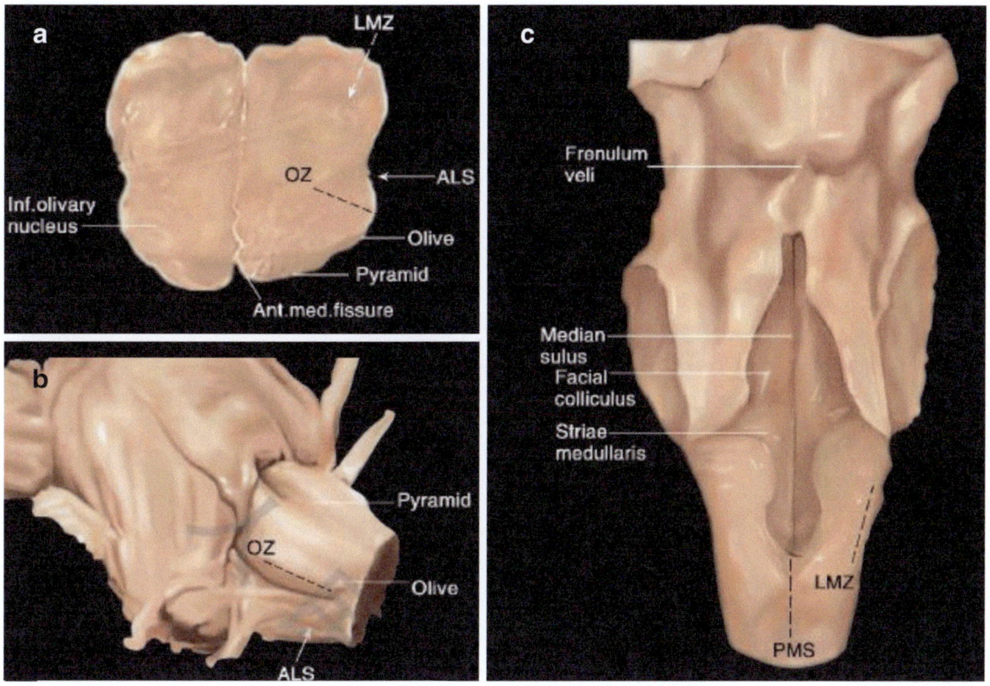

Fig. 7.4 Surgical safe zones in the medulla. (**a**) Transverse section of the medulla illustrating three surgical safe zones: anterolateral sulcus, olive zone, and posterolateral sulcus. (**b**) Anterolateral view of the medulla showing the region of entry into the olive zone and anterolateral sulcus, just below the hypoglossal nerve root. (**c**) Posterior view demonstrating the safe zones of the posterior median sulcus and posterolateral sulcus during surgery

the arachnoid membrane of the ambient cistern and the interpeduncular cistern. This exposes the lateral aspect of the midbrain and the pontomesencephalic junction, with a view of the posterior cerebral artery, posterior choroidal artery, and lateral mesencephalic vein. The drawback of this approach is that it provides suboptimal visualization of the upper part of the pons, requiring a 1 cm incision of the tentorial edge to expose the upper part of the pons (Fig. 7.5).

2. Subtemporal transtentorial approach: Building upon the subtemporal approach, the tentorial edge is incised approximately 1 cm anterior to the entry of the trochlear nerve into the tentorial edge, allowing for the tentorium to be pulled apart. This exposes the pontomesencephalic junction and the anterolateral region of the superior pons. By incising the tentorial edge in addition to the pure subtemporal approach, the surgical field of view can be expanded to expose the pontomesencephalic junction and the lateral part of the upper pons, as well as the superior cerebellar artery and the trochlear nerve. Further exposure can reveal the posterior cerebral artery, posterior communicating artery, oculomotor nerve, and trigeminal nerve. The disadvantage of this approach is that it provides suboptimal visualization of the midbrain, especially the lateral aspect of the midbrain peduncle. Excessive traction on the basal surface of the temporal lobe may cause contusion and hematoma of the temporal lobe (Fig. 7.6).
3. Temporooccipital approach: The intracranial exposure range of this approach is similar to the subtemporal approach. However, the surgical field of view in this approach is more posterior, and the Labbe's vein is located within the surgical area. Therefore, the range of traction on the base of temporal lobe is relatively limited, resulting in a smaller field of view and restricted operative space compared to the subtemporal approach. In the temporooccipital approach, the patient is placed in the lateral decubitus position, and the surgical incision is made as a horseshoe-shaped incision above the external auditory canal. The temporal muscle fascia is dissected, exposing a large portion of the temporal bone. Two holes are drilled, one 1 cm above the external auditory canal and the other 1.5–2 cm posterior to it. The bone flap is formed, and the lower edge of the bone window is ground as close to the skull base as possible. The dura mater is incised, and dissection is performed at the base of the temporal lobe until the tentorial edge is reached, taking care to protect the Labbe's vein. Confirming the mid-anterior incisure of the tentorial edge, the arachnoid membrane of the ambient cistern is opened, exposing the lateral aspect of the midbrain, the posterior cerebral artery, and the region below the tentorial edge where the trochlear nerve is located. By incising the tentorial edge, the surgical field of view is increased, revealing the lateral aspect of the pontomesencephalic junction and the upper pons, the trochlear nerve, and the superior cerebellar artery. Further dissection allows for the downward exposure of the trigeminal nerve and the petrosal vein, as well as the anterosuperior exposure of the posterior cerebral artery, oculomotor nerve, and posterior communicating artery (Fig. 7.7).

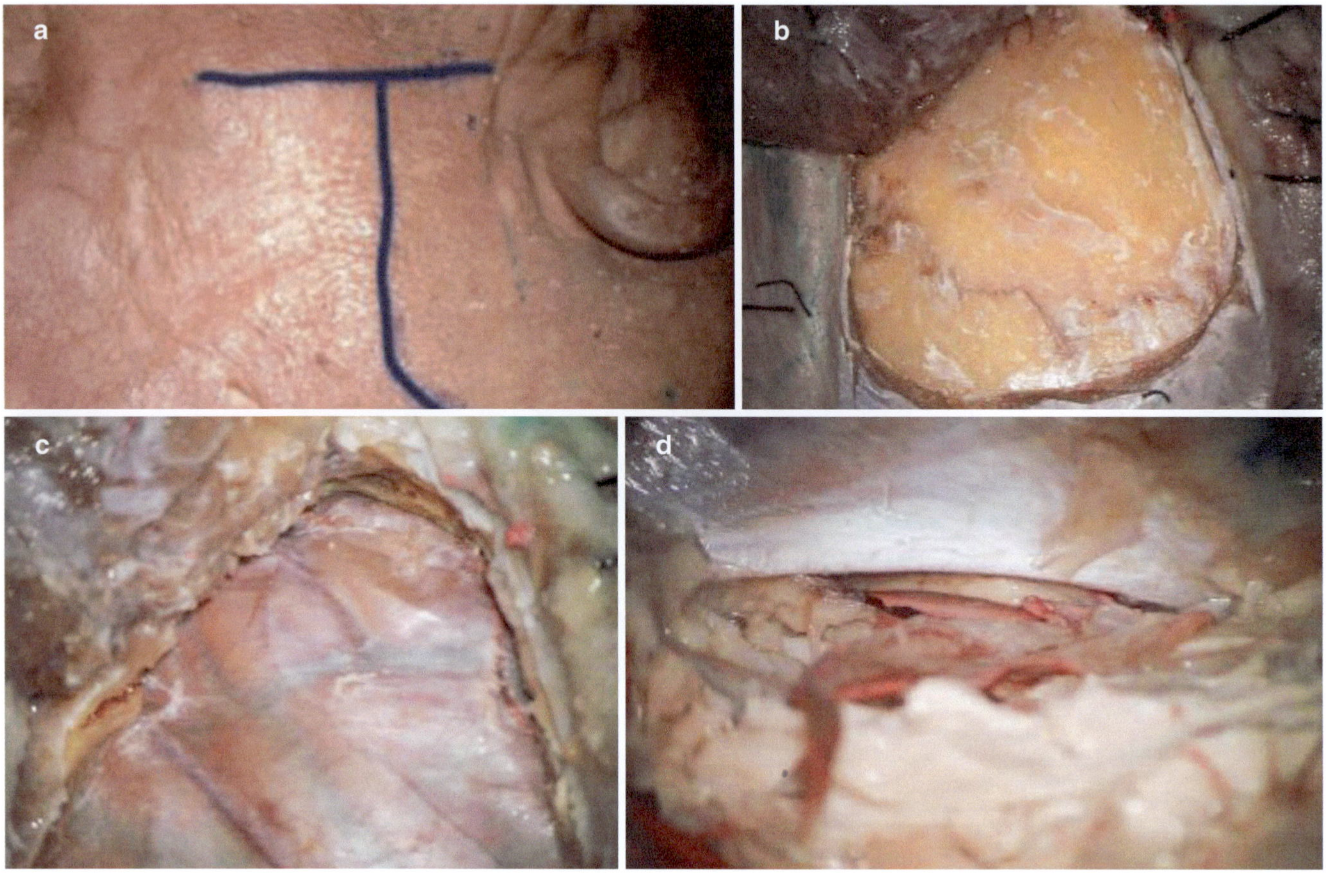

Fig. 7.5 Subtemporal approach. (**a**) Surgical incision for the subtemporal approach. (**b**) Formation of the bone flap, grinding the lower edge of the bone window to the middle cranial fossa floor. (**c**) Carefully separate the basal part of the temporal lobe and the tentorial edge, and open the arachnoid membrane of the ambient cistern. (**d**) This surgical approach exposes the anterior and lateral parts of the tentorial edge, as well as the lateral part of the midbrain

4. Transinferior temporal sulcus and transtemporal horn choroidal fissure approach: This approach is suitable for the lateral exposure of the midbrain cerebral peduncle, avoiding excessive traction on the base of temporal lobe, which can cause temporal lobe contusion and hematoma formation. The craniotomy technique is similar to the subtemporal approach. After the dura mater is incised, a cortical fistula is created in the temporal lobe through the inferior temporal fissure, entering the temporal horn of the lateral ventricle. Using the temporal angle choroid and its vessels as landmarks, the choroidal fissure below the choroid is dissected, entering the arachnoid membrane of the ambient cistern. This exposes the lateral aspect of the midbrain cerebral peduncle, and the field of view also includes the P2 segment of the posterior cerebral artery and the lateroposterior choroidal artery (Fig. 7.8).
5. Subtemporal prepetrosal approach: If it is necessary to expose the anterolateral aspect of the pons inferior to the exit of the trigeminal nerve from the brainstem, the prepetrosal approach or Kawase approach can be used. Based on the subtemporal approach, the bone in front of the petrous bone and the superoinner side of the internal auditory canal is further ground away, allowing for additional exposure of the anterolateral aspect of the pons (anterolateral pons below the brainstem end of the trigeminal nerve), as well as the anteroinferior cerebellar artery, abducent nerve, and basilar artery. The range of prepetrosal bone removal includes the V3 branch of the trigeminal nerve on the inner side, the anterior aspect is the greater superficial petrosal nerve, the outer side is the arcuate eminence, and the posterior aspect is the superior petrosal sinus. When grinding away the bone in front of the petrous bone, care should be taken to avoid injury to the aforementioned four anatomical structures, as well as the facial and auditory nerve, cochlea, and internal carotid artery within the internal auditory canal (Fig. 7.9).
6. Suboccipital retrosigmoid approach: This approach is suitable for the exposure of the lateral aspect of the pons and the middle cerebellar peduncle. The specific method involves placing the patient in a lateral decubitus position, making a straight incision behind the mastoid pro-

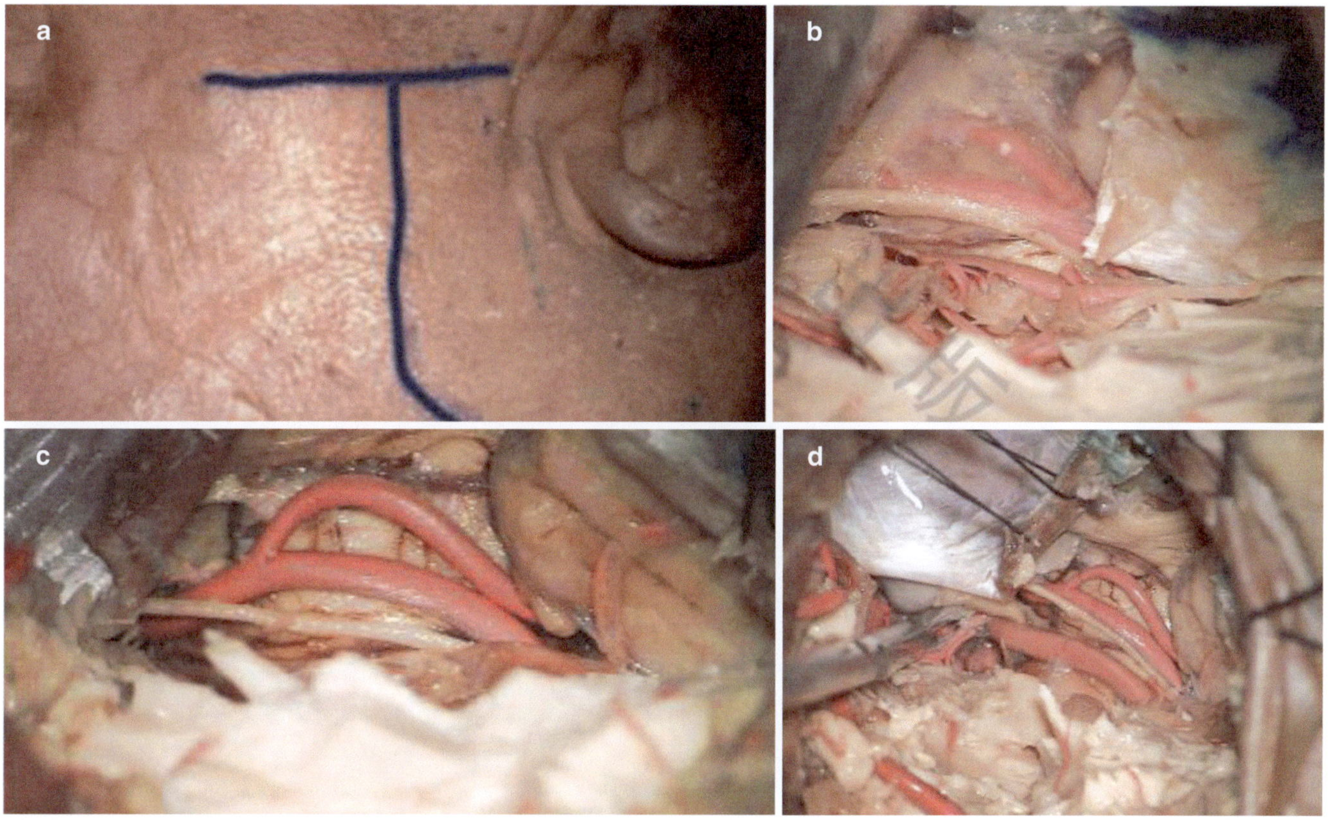

Fig. 7.6 Subtemporal transtentorial approach. (**a**) By incising the tentorial edge in addition to the pure subtemporal approach, the surgical field of view can be expanded. (**b**) Expose the pontomesencephalic junction and the lateral part of the upper pons, as well as the superior cerebellar artery and the trochlear nerve. (**c**). Further exposure can reveal the posterior cerebral artery, posterior communicating artery, oculomotor nerve, and trigeminal nerve

cess, approximately 6–8 mm in length. The scalp and muscles are incised, exposing the apex of the digastric groove. A keyhole is formed by drilling, and a bone flap with a diameter of approximately 3 cm is created using a milling cutter. The dura mater is arched incised, and the arachnoid membrane is gradually separated upward in the cerebellomedullary cistern. This allows for the visualization of the posterior group of cranial nerves and the facial and vestibulocochlear nerves above them. By gently retracting the petrous surface of cerebellar hemisphere to the cerebellopontine peduncle, the trigeminal nerve and the lateral aspect of the pons in the cerebellopontine peduncle can be exposed. By separating the arachnoid membrane downward in the cerebellomedullary cistern, the posterior group of cranial nerves, vertebral artery, posteroinferior cerebellar artery, and the lateral aspect of the medulla can be visualized. The retrosigmoid approach is more commonly used than other surgical approaches, and postoperative motor impairments are rare (Fig. 7.10).

7. Suboccipital transtelovelar approach: The patient is positioned in lateral decubitus or prone position. After selecting the appropriate site, a midline vertical incision is made, exposing the suboccipital region down to the posterior arch of C1. The bone flap is shaped, and a Y-shaped incision is made in the dura mater, revealing the bilateral cerebellar tonsils. The cerebellar tonsils and the posteroinferior cerebellar arteries are gently retracted on both sides, dissecting the choroidal frenulum and inferior medullary velum. This exposes the cisterna magna and the lateral recess, providing a safe surgical field near the facial colliculus (Fig. 7.11).
8. Far lateral approach.

The patient is placed in the lateral decubitus position. A reverse U-shaped incision is made, and the suboccipital muscles are dissected sequentially, exposing the suboccipital triangle. The superior oblique, inferior oblique, and rectus capitis posterior major muscles form the suboccipital triangle, which contains the V3 segment of the vertebral artery. If it is necessary to displace the vertebral artery, the C1 posterior arch may be removed. The extent of removal of the occipital condyle is determined by actual need. After cutting the dura mater, the arachnoid is dissected lateral to the cisterna magna and cerebellomedullary cistern to confirm the V4 segment of the vertebral

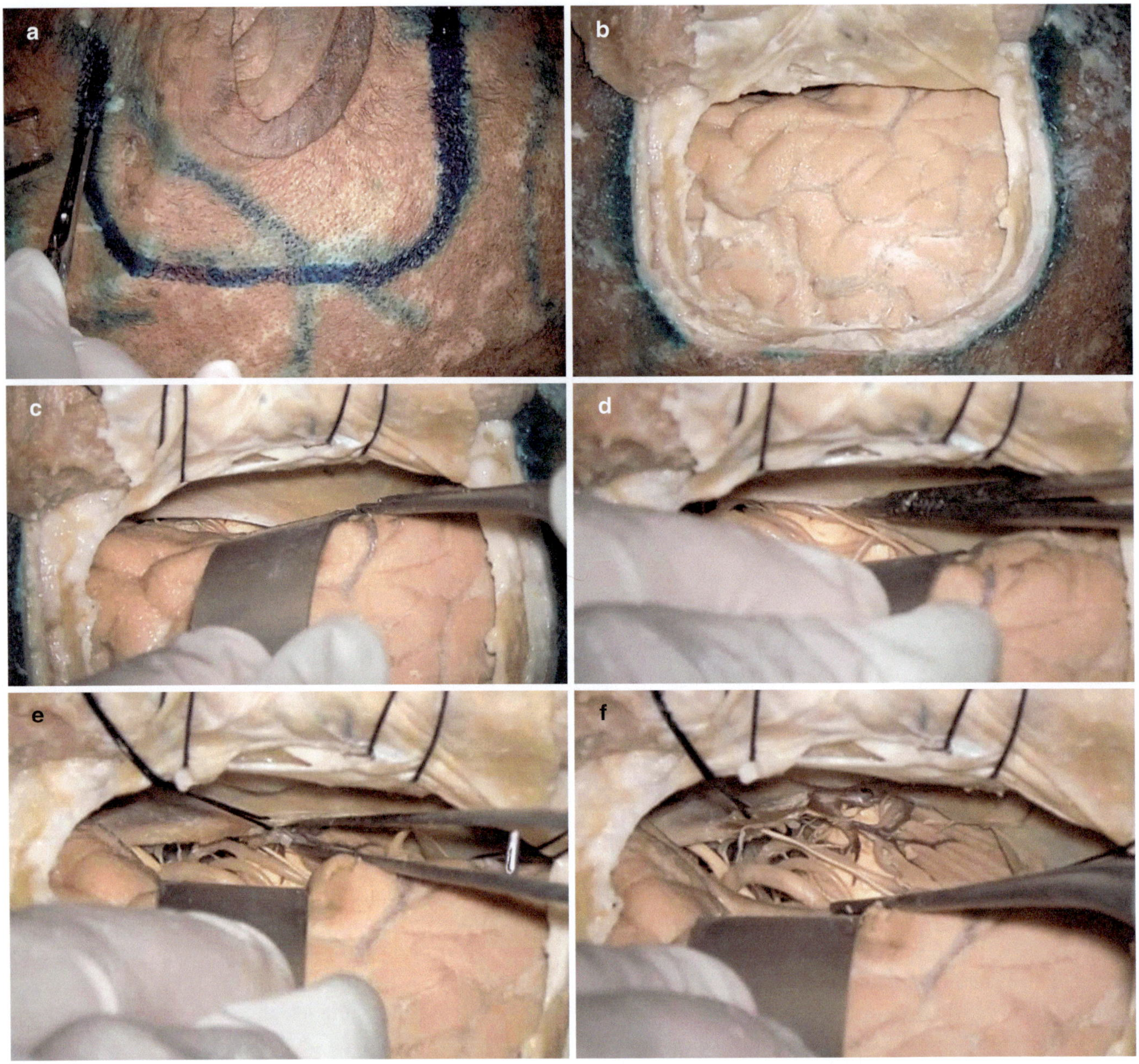

Fig. 7.7 Temporooccipital approach. (**a** and **b**) Incision and formation of the bone flap, grinding the lower edge of the bone window to the skull base. (**c** and **d**) Careful dissection of the basal part of the temporal lobe and the tentorial edge, opening the arachnoid membrane of the ambient cistern, exposing the tentorial edge, superior cerebellar artery, trochlear nerve, and the lateral aspect of the lower midbrain. (**e** and **f**) Incision of the tentorial edge, exposing the pontomesencephalic junction and the lateral aspect of the upper pons, as well as the trigeminal nerve. Further anterosuperior dissection allows for the exposure of the posterior cerebral artery, posterior communicating artery, and oculomotor nerve

artery, which lies lateral to the accessory nerve and anterior to the hypoglossal nerve root. This exposes the inferolateral side of the spinal cord and the junction between the spinal cord and the cervical spinal cord. In addition, dissection of the arachnoid of the cerebellopontine peduncle may expose the pons. By dissecting the anterior side of the medullary cistern toward the ventral side, the anterolateral fissure of the medulla oblongata and the olive can be reached (Fig. 7.12).

9. Endonasal Endoscopic Approach (for Ventral Brainstem Hematoma).

According to the two-point principle, the endonasal clivus approach is best suited for lesions at or near the midline of the ventral pons. Compared to other surgical

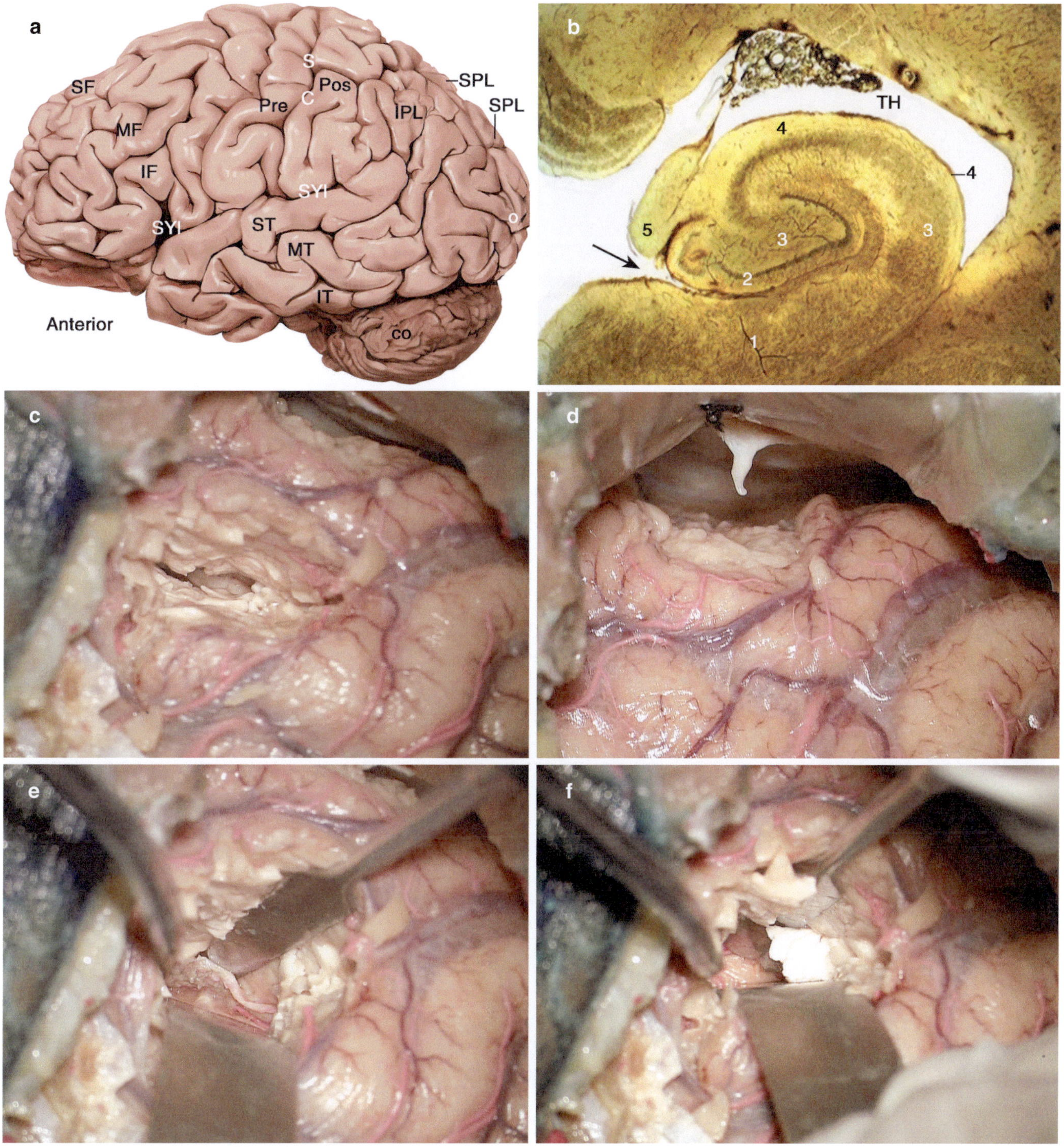

Fig. 7.8 Transinferior temporal sulcus and transtemporal horn choroidal fissure approach. The temporal lobe cortex is fistulated, entering the temporal horn of the lateral ventricle through the choroid. Using the temporal angle choroid and its vessels as landmarks, the choroidal fissure below the choroid is dissected, entering the arachnoid membrane of the ambient cistern. This exposure facilitates visualization of the lateral aspect of the cerebral peduncle

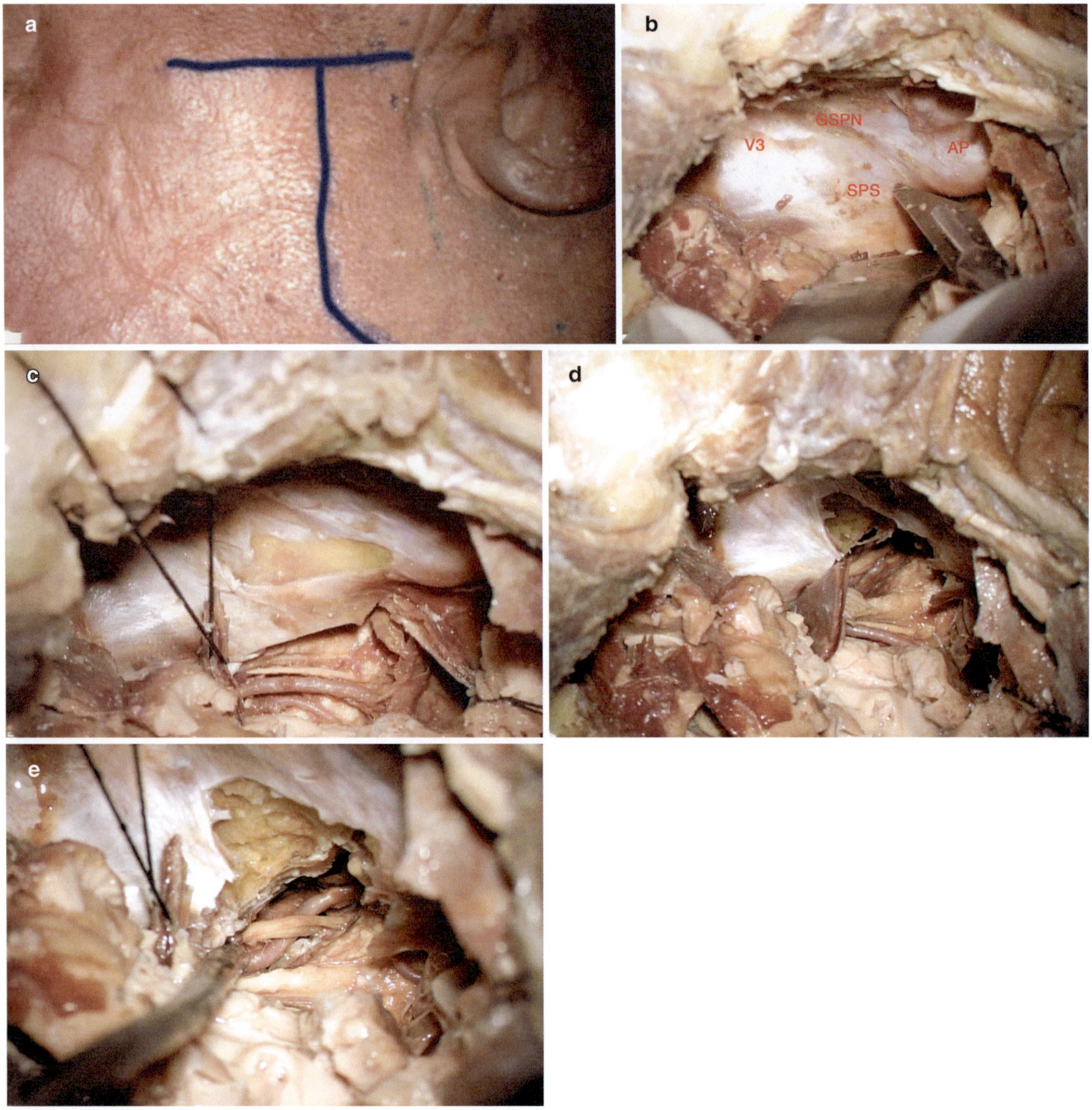

Fig. 7.9 Subtemporal prepetrosal approach. (**a**) Surgical incision for the right subtemporal prepetrosal approach. (**b**) revealing the four borders of Kawase's triangle in subdural space. (**c**) in addition to the simple subtemporal approach, opening the tentorial edge and craniotomy with prepetrous approach can increase the surgical field of view. (**d**) after drilling Kawase's triangle, the dura is incised 1 cm away from the superior petrosal sinus, exposing the pons. (**e**) the abducent nerve and the inferior petrosal sinus can be seen, with the abducent nerve originating from the inner side of the pons along the pontine sulcus. *AP* arcuate eminence; *GSPN* greater superficial petrosal nerve; *V3* V3 branch of the trigeminal nerve; *SPS* superior petrosal sinus

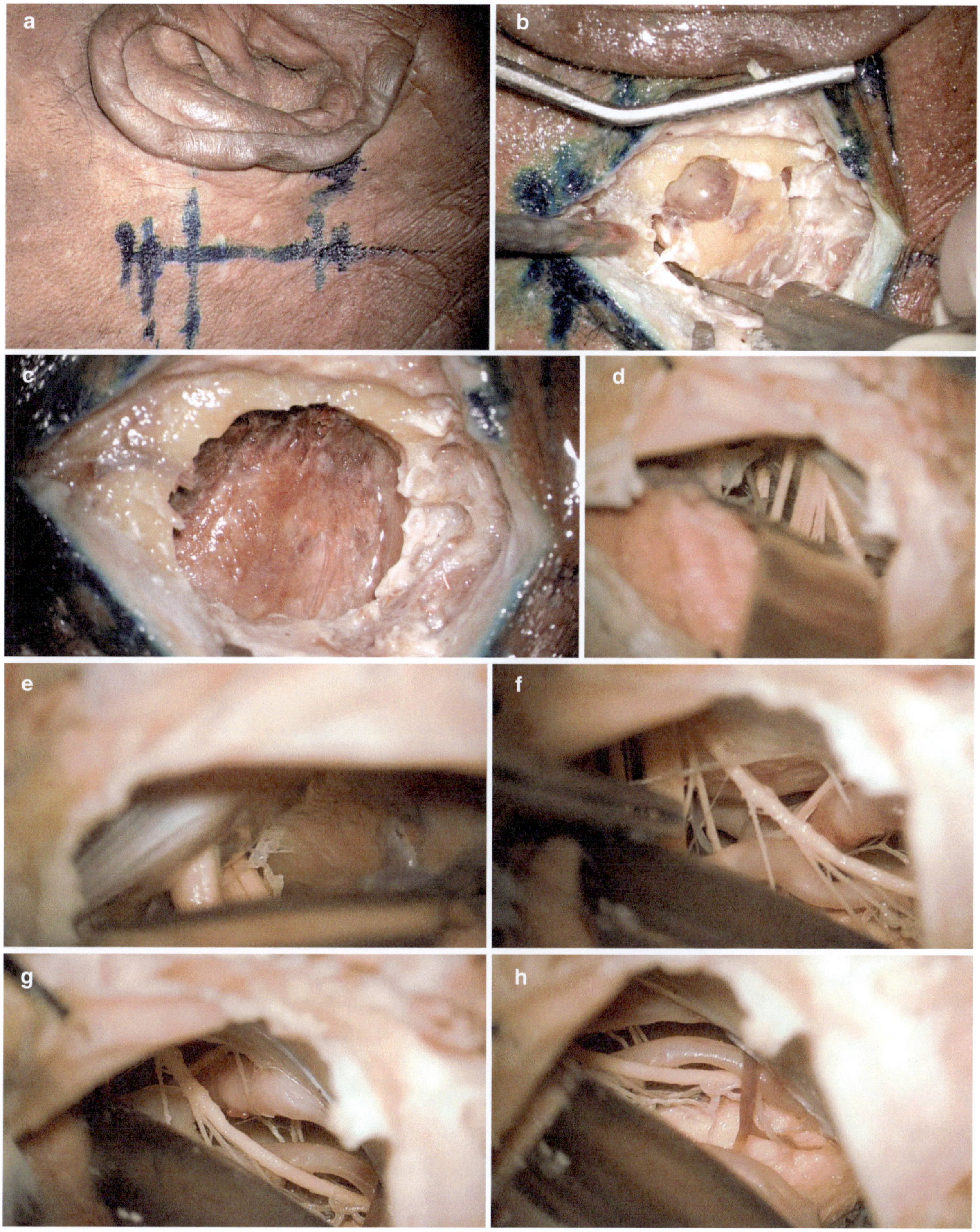

Fig. 7.10 Suboccipital retrosigmoid approach. (**a**) Position the patient in a lateral decubitus position, and mark the surgical incision site, approximately 6–8 cm in length, two fingerbreadths behind the earlobe. (**b**) Drill a hole at the key points, and create a 3 cm diameter bone flap. (**c**) Expose the posterior margin of the sigmoid sinus and the inferior margin of the transverse sinus. (**d**) Incise the dura mater, retract the petrous side of cerebellum, and expose the medullary cistern of the cerebellum. Separate the arachnoid membrane to reveal the posterior group of cranial nerves and the facial and vestibulocochlear nerves above them. (**e**) Dissect along the cerebellar petrous side upward to reach the trigeminal nerve in the cerebellopontine angle. (**f**) Continue dissecting along the cerebellar petrous side upward to expose the posterior group of cranial nerves and their adjacent vertebral arteries and posterior inferior cerebellar arteries. (**g**) Reveal the accessory nerve, hypoglossal nerve, and their adjacent vertebral arteries and posterior inferior cerebellar arteries. (**h**) Display the lateral aspect of the medulla, accessory nerve, hypoglossal nerve, and their adjacent posterior inferior cerebellar artery

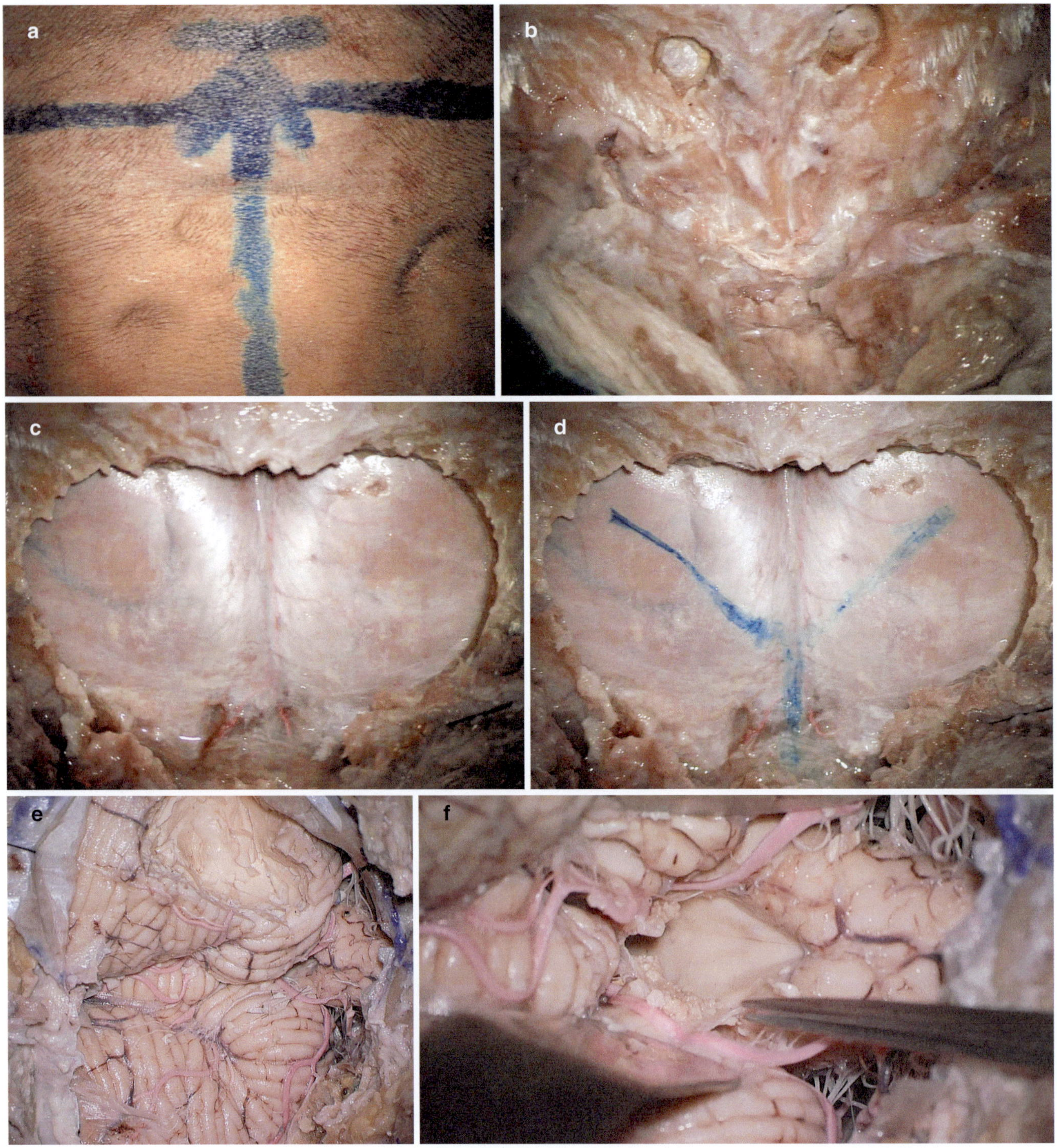

Fig. 7.11 Suboccipital transtelovelar approach. (**a**) Mark the surgical incision at the posterior midline. (**b**). Drill two holes on both sides of the external occipital protuberance, below the transverse sinus. (**c**) Open the C1 posterior arch, increasing the vertical view to the rhomboid fossa. (**d**) Y-shaped dural incision. (**e**) Open the midline foramen of the fourth ventricle, with the choroid plexus tissue on the outside, the tonsils of the cerebellum, and the posterior inferior cerebellar artery. (**f**) Separate the choroid plexus tissue and inferior medullary velum, exposing the rhomboid fossa. The gray area indicates the exposure of the brainstem dorsal region through the transtelovelar approach

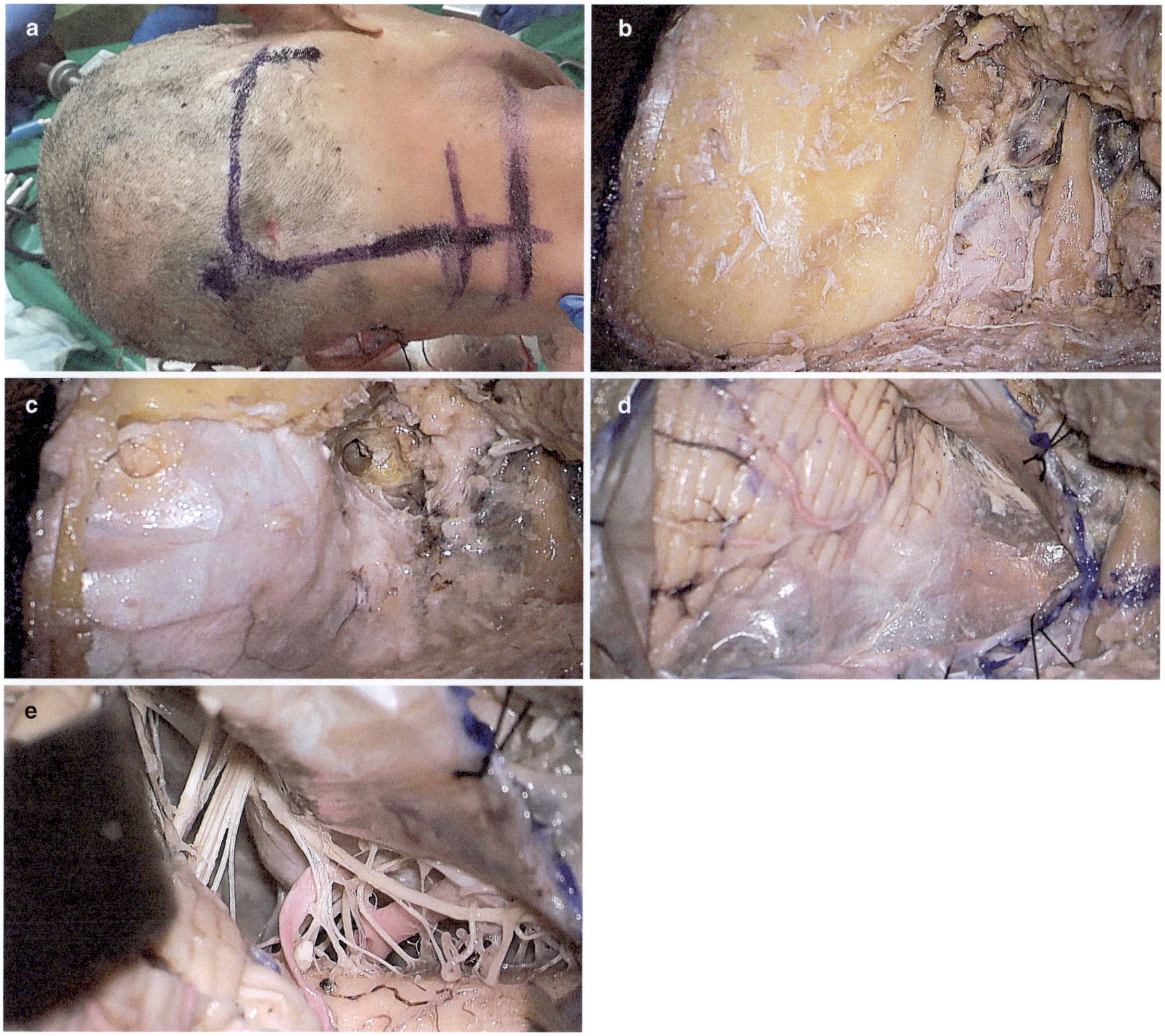

Fig. 7.12 Far lateral approach. (**a**) Position the patient in lateral prone position, and mark the surgical incision. (**b**) Sequentially dissect the posterior occipital muscle layer, exposing the lateral part of the occipital bone and the C1 vertebral lamina. (**c**) Form the bony flap of the lateral part of the occipital bone. Remove the C1 vertebral lamina as needed, and partially grind the occipital condyle. If necessary to manipulate the vertebral artery, the posterior arch of C1 can be ground. (**d**) Dura mater is flipped forward to expose the cerebellum and the cisterna magna. (**e**) Expose the posterolateral of the medulla oblongata, which can also expose the posterior group of cranial nerves to the jugular foramen, C1 spinal nerve root and CN XI spinal nerve root, vertebral artery, and posterior inferior cerebellar artery, upper cervical medulla, and cerebellar tonsil

approaches, the endonasal clivus approach provides the most direct route to address lesions in this area without the need to manipulate brain tissue, cranial nerves, or blood vessels. Surgical experience with resection of brainstem cavernous malformations and cholesteatoma using this approach has been reported in the literature, but the postoperative incidence of CSF leak is quite high. This may be due to the relatively thick bone and fascia in the clival region, the poorer blood supply compared to other areas of the skull base, and its close proximity to the prepontine cistern, which increases the likelihood of postoperative CSF leakage. During the surgical procedure, it is necessary to first create a mucosal flap on one side of the nasal septum and fully open the anterior wall of the sphenoid sinus. Using the bilateral internal carotid arteries as landmarks, the bone in the clival region is ground down according to the location of the hematoma, exposing the clival dura mater. The dura mater is incised

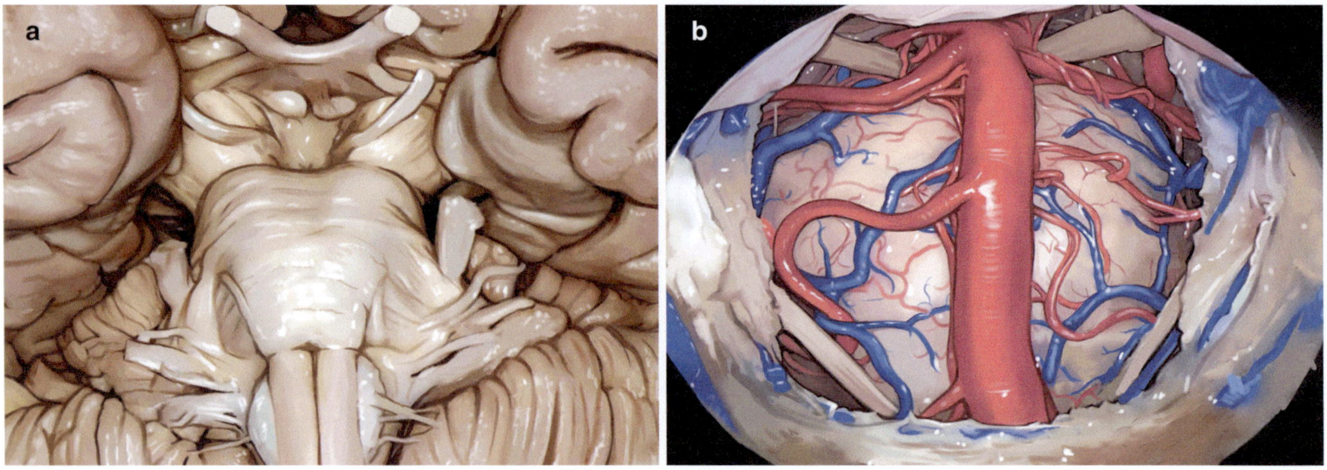

Fig. 7.13 Endonasal endoscopic approach. (**a**) Ventral brainstem. (**b**) Endoscopic view of the ventral brainstem

to expose the basilar artery and vertebral artery. Based on preoperative head CT or MRI localization, the site of local brainstem elevation or hematoma rupture is identified, and the hematoma is removed under intraoperative neuroelectrophysiological monitoring. The dural defect is filled with fat tissue, and the clival bone is reconstructed using nasal septal bone and finally covered with a mucosal flap. Depending on the postoperative situation, a lumber cistern drainage catheter may or may not be placed (Fig. 7.13).

7.5 Selection of Surgical Timing

PBSH causes primary damage to the brainstem, such as rupture of the brainstem parenchyma, acute expansion and enlargement of the hematoma, which compresses the brainstem, causing it to twist axially and shift longitudinally. These primary brainstem injuries, which are largely due to the hemorrhage itself, have a significant impact on the outcome of the disease. The hematoma compresses and obstructs the cerebrospinal fluid circulation, and the toxins from the hematoma's breakdown cause brainstem edema and ischemia, leading to increased intracranial pressure and even brain herniation. These secondary injuries can be minimized with modern neurosurgical techniques. After a brainstem hemorrhage, the hematoma or brainstem edema can directly compress the vital centers of the brainstem, leading to deterioration. The presence of the hematoma is the initiating factor in a series of subsequent pathological changes, and early evacuation of the hematoma is an important step in interrupting these secondary pathological damages. Surgical management should follow the principles of minimally invasive surgery to achieve the best surgical results with minimal trauma. Correct surgical indications and timing are critical to the success of surgery.

As brainstem hemorrhage often has an acute onset, early surgical evacuation of the hematoma to relieve the mass effect and prevent further damage to neurological function is highly beneficial to the patient's prognosis. From a pathophysiological perspective, brain tissue edema and necrosis of neurons and nerve fibres begin to appear around the hematoma approximately 6 hours after the brain hemorrhage and worsen with time. Theoretically, ultra-early surgery, i.e., within 6 hours of hemorrhage, is thought to result in better surgical outcomes and recovery of neurological function compared to mid- to late-stage surgery. Early reduction of the pressure of the hematoma on the brain tissue and interruption of the vicious circle caused by a series of secondary changes after hemorrhage may improve survival and prognosis.

References

1. Ding XQ, Li ZF. Current status and progress in the surgical treatment of brainstem hemorrhage. Medical Review. 2017;23(21):4252–5.
2. Liu X, Li H, Hu X, et al. Discussion on the treatment of spontaneous brainstem hemorrhage. J Clin Neurosurg. 2013;10(5):287–8.
3. Chen LH, Wei Q, Xu RX, et al. Minimally invasive surgical treatment of primary brainstem hemorrhage. J Clin Neurosurg. 2015;12(5):349–53.
4. Cavalcanti DD, Preul MC, Kalani MYS, et al. Microsurgical anatomy of safe entry zones to the brainstem. J Neurosurg. 2016;124(5):1359–76.
5. Yagmurlu K, Rhoton ALJR, Tanriover N, et al. Three-dimensional microsurgical anatomy and the safe entry zones of the brainstem. Neurosurgery. 2014;10(Suppl 4):602–19.
6. Li JG, Wang P, Chen BY, et al. Stereotactic surgical treatment for primary brainstem hemorrhage. Chinese J Neurosurg. 2009;10(25):919–21.
7. Gao JB, Li WD, Yu B, et al. Observation of the effects of two surgical methods for brainstem hemorrhage under stereotactic naviga-

tion through the temporal and occipital approach. China Medical Herald. 2018;15(18):175–7.

8. Zhang SW, Niu GM, Yuan JH, et al. Comparison of the efficacy of stereotactic surgery and conventional conservative treatment for severe brainstem hemorrhage. Chinese J Pract Neurolog Diseases. 2019;22(8):853–8.
9. Li X, Chen J, Zhong L, et al. Stereotactic surgery for severe primary brainstem hemorrhage. Chinese J Modern Neurolog Diseases. 2011;11(3):360–1.
10. Liang JG, Dong J, Qu MQ, et al. Neuroendoscopic-assisted surgical treatment of brainstem hemorrhage penetrating the fourth ventricle. Chinese J Neurolog. 2013;12(2):197–9.
11. Linsler S, Oertel J. Endoscopic endonasal transclival resection of a brainstem cavernoma: a detailed account of our technique and comparison with the literature. World Neurosurg. 2015;84(6):2064–71.
12. Zeng J, Qiu QH. A case of brainstem ventral lipoma surgery via the endoscopic transsphenoidal approach. Chinese J Otorhinolaryngol Head Neck Surgery. 2019;54(9):689–91.
13. Gao DK, Li SZ, Qi S, et al. Endoscopic removal of brainstem cavernous hemangioma. Chinese J Res Neurosurg Diseases. 2016;15(1):84–6.
14. Brown AP, Thompson BG, Spetzler RF. The two-point method: evaluating brain stem lesions. BNI Quart. 1996;12(1):20–4.

8 Anesthesia Strategy for Brainstem Hemorrhage Surgery

Fan Zhang and Hong Chen

8.1 Anatomical and Physiological Basis

8.1.1 Structure and Function of Brain Stem

The posterior cranial fossa is a critical region in the human body, housing essential nerve structures such as the brain stem, cerebellum, and fourth ventricle. The brain stem, a crucial pathway connecting the brain, cerebellum, and spinal cord, plays a vital role in transmitting nerve signals and maintaining basic life-sustaining functions. It contains both white and gray matter. The white matter in the brainstem is composed of ascending and descending conduction bundles, as well as nerve fibers originating from various parts of the brainstem. The gray matter houses various nerve nuclei, which are responsible for processing incoming sensory signals and facilitating the motor functions of the body. These nerve nuclei are integral to the regulation of vital physiological processes, including cardiovascular control, respiration, swallowing, vomiting, coughing, burping, chewing, and salivary secretion. They form reflex centers in the medulla oblongata and pons, which coordinate the body's automatic responses. Any damage to these centers can disrupt the regulation of heart rate, blood pressure, and other autonomic functions, often leading to severe, life-threatening conditions.

The medulla oblongata is located at the base of the brain, directly connecting with the spinal cord. Its primary function is to regulate essential involuntary processes, including breathing, heartbeat, swallowing, digestion, excretion, gastrointestinal, and other activities.

The pons is situated between the midbrain and medulla and contains white matter nerve fibers that transmit signals between the two cerebellar hemispheres. This allows for the coordination of muscle activities on both sides of the body. The pons is also involved in regulating sleep and plays a role in breathing control through its influence on the respiratory rhythm.

The midbrain is located above the pons, just the midpoint of the whole brain. It serves as the reflex center of vision and hearing and is responsible for controlling and dilation of pupils, and the coordination of eye muscles for visual tracking.

The reticular system, which runs through the core of the brainstem, is a network of neurons that extends throughout the brainstem. It is an unspecific, polysynaptic path involved in regulating the sleep-wake cycle, muscle tone, and various autonomic functions of human body.

8.1.2 Anesthesia Risk of Brain Stem Hemorrhage Surgery

In neurosurgical anesthesia, cerebellar hemorrhage surgery presents significant technical challenges due to the complex anatomy and physiology of the brainstem and surrounding structures.

The medulla oblongata and pons contain reflex centers that control vital functions, including cardiovascular regulation, respiration, swallowing, and other important physiological activities. Any hematoma or surgical injury in these areas can lead to severe disruptions in these functions, endangering the patient's life.

Surgical procedures near the brainstem nuclei are particularly risky, as they can cause imbalances in autonomic nervous system regulation, resulting in extremely unstable hemodynamics. These include hypotension, hypertension, bradycardia, tachycardia, and arrhythmia. Additionally, a severe vagal reflex can lead to cardiac arrest, while a subsequent sympathetic reflex may induce a hypertensive crisis and fatal tachycardia. These life-threatening conditions create extraordinary challenges for anesthesiologists, requiring precise and vigilant monitoring.

F. Zhang (✉)
Department of Anesthesiology, The First Affiliated Hospital of Harbin Medical University, Harbin, China

H. Chen
Department of Anesthesiology, Harbin Medical University Cancer Hospital, Harbin, China

G. Chen, C. You (eds.), *Surgical Treatment of Primary Brainstem Hemorrhage*, https://doi.org/10.1007/978-981-95-8942-5_8

The posterior cranial fossa, being a confined space with poor compliance, is directly connected to important tissues like the brain stem. Postoperative hypertension can exacerbate intracranial pressure by promoting intracranial edema or rebleeding, potentially damaging surrounding tissue structure. Patients may present with symptoms such as altered consciousness, hypertension, bradycardia, and irregular breathing or respiratory arrest. Anesthesiologists must anticipate the risk of worsening brain edema or rebleeding following tracheal extubation and, if necessary, reserve the endotracheal tube to ensure adequate airway protection and to manage hemodynamic stability.

8.1.3 Arterial Partial Pressure of Carbon Dioxide and Intracranial Pressure

Cerebellar hemorrhage induces significant changes in the central nervous system (CNS), affecting various physiological parameters, such as cerebral blood flow (CBF), cerebral oxygen metabolic rate ($CMRO_2$), cerebral perfusion pressure (CPP), and electrophysiological functions. A key factor in managing intracranial pressure (ICP) is arterial carbon dioxide partial pressure ($PaCO_2$). Each 1 mmHg change in $PaCO_2$ corresponds to a 4% change in CBF. Overventilation to $PaCO_2$ 25–30 mmHg is a well-established treatment method for acute or subacute intracranial hypertension. Reducing PaCO2 causes a rapid decrease in CBF and cerebral blood volume (CBV), which in turn lowers ICP and provides a better surgical field for the neurosurgeon.

Notes on anesthesia for $PaCO_2$ regulating the intracranial pressure are as follows:

(A) In cases of cerebral ischemia, trauma, tumors, and infections, the brain's response to CO_2 changes can be impaired due to vascular paralysis.
(B) Increasing $PaCO_2$ can lead to cerebral vasodilation, resulting in a temporary increase in CBF. However, this change usually normalizes within 6–8 h.
(C) Extended periods of hyperventilation can weaken or eliminate the brain's ability to regulate CBF. If hyperventilation is suddenly stopped (e.g., during transit), there is a risk of increased ICP and reduced CBF.
(D) When $PaCO_2$ falls below 25 mmHg, the oxygen dissociation curve shifts to the left, reducing the release of oxygen to tissues, which can lead to cerebral ischemia, metabolic acidosis, hemodynamic instability, or delayed anesthesia resuscitation.
(E) The difference between $PaCO_2$ and end-expiratory carbon dioxide partial pressure ($ETCO_2$) varies greatly during surgery, which could mislead clinical assessments. Therefore, blood gas analysis should be performed immediately after anesthesia induction to ensure accurate monitoring.

8.2 Influence of Surgical Position on Anesthesia Management

When performing surgery for brainstem hemorrhage, patient positioning is crucial for achieving optimal surgical exposure while minimizing complications. The most commonly used positions are prone or lateral prone. However, positioning must be managed carefully, especially under sedation, hypnosis, or general anesthesia, as the body loses muscle protection against bones, which can increase the risk of injury. Here are some key considerations when the patient's position changes:

(A) Fix the tracheal tube firmly to avoid falling off, folding or moving to bronchus.
(B) Avoid cervical joint or vocal cord injuries caused by excessive neck stretching, twisting or overpressure on the throat tissue.
(C) Prevent vision loss or skin damage caused by the eyes or ears compression.
(D) Pay attention to the position of head and limbs. The upper arm should bend less than 90°, and the knee is flexed to minimize stretching of the brachial plexus and sciatic nerves.
(E) Reduce the impact on intrathoracic and intra-abdominal pressure through the chest and hip supporting devices, achieving abdominal breathing and effective ventilation.
(F) Prevent accidental detachment of venous pathway, arterial access, urinary tube or gastric catheters, etc.

In particular, the obstruction of cervical venous reflux can increase intracranial pressure. Therefore, jugular vein compression should be avoided during the process of positioning.

8.3 Anesthesia Target and Preoperative Evaluation

8.3.1 Nesthesia Management Objectives

The anesthesia goals of craniotomy surgery, particularly in the context of brainstem hemorrhage, are critical in ensuring optimal outcomes and protecting brain function throughout the procedure. As a result, in addition to systemic hemodynamic stability, the following points are aiming to achieve:

(A) Intracranial pressure stability.
(B) Monitor systemic and cerebral hemodynamics, as well as manage CBF and CPP.
(C) Prevent cerebral ischemia injury and apply drugs with brain protective effects.

(D) Keep a relaxed state of brain tissue, improve surgical vision, and reduce traction.
(E) Maintain normal electrolyte, blood glucose, and plasma osmolarity within normal ranges.
(F) Minimize the interference of anesthetics on neural monitoring.
(G) Quick awakening for early postoperative neurological assessment.
(H) Stabilize the body temperature.

To achieve the best anesthetic effect, the above anesthesia maintenance goals must be comprehensively considered, and an appropriate amount of anesthetic drugs and agents should be selected and administered for combined application.

8.3.2 Preoperative Assessment

A thorough preoperative evaluation is crucial in ensuring a safe aesthesia process, especially for patients with brainstem hemorrhage, as they often present with underlying systemic diseases such as hypertension, diabetes, and coronary heart disease. Preoperative full understanding of the treatment above diseases is conducive to formulating a perfect intraoperative anesthesia scheme.

In addition to adequate preoperative evaluation, anesthesiologists should also thoroughly browse CT scans and other imaging data to determine any evidence of hydrocephalus and fourth ventricle compression or deformation before surgery.

For patients who are on diuretics, it is essential to assess electrolyte levels and blood volume to ensure hemodynamic stability during surgery.

Finally, a complete preoperative neurological examination should be performed and thoroughly documented as a baseline for postoperative comparison.

8.4 General Anesthesia Induction and Intraoperative Monitoring

8.4.1 Common Drugs for General Anesthesia Induction

The induction period of anesthesia is a critical phase. During this period, several factors can cause fluctuations in blood pressure, heart rate, and respiratory suppression, all of which can be further complicated in patients with brainstem compression due to cerebellar tonsil hernia.

Therefore, understanding the effects of various anesthetic drugs on both cerebral and systemic hemodynamics is essential for managing these patients safely. Except for ketamine, routine anesthesia-inducing agents, such as thiopental, midazolam, etomidate, and propofol, have neuroprotective effects by reducing ICP and oxygen consumption.

Usually, intravenous hypnotic drugs (propofol or etomidate) and opioids (fentanyl or sufentanil) are commonly used for induction to mitigate the cardiovascular response to laryngoscopy and intubation.

Before tracheal intubation, non-depolarizing muscle relaxants are recommended to ensure adequate muscle relaxation before tracheal intubation. This prevents acute coughing during intubation, which could lead to increased ICP. Preferred drugs include rocuronium and atracurium. Experienced anesthesiologists can achieve safe and effective anesthesia induction in brainstem hemorrhage patients, minimizing the risks of ICP increase, hemodynamic fluctuations, and respiratory complications by combining different doses of drugs.

8.4.2 Intraoperative Monitoring Items and Precautions

For patients undergoing complex neurosurgery, a comprehensive approach to monitoring is essential to ensure patient safety and optimize surgical outcomes.

Routine Monitoring Items
Electrocardiogram, blood pressure, pulse oxygen saturation, end-tidal carbon dioxide, urine volume, temperature, arterial blood gas analysis, etc.

Hemodynamic Monitoring Items
Invasive arterial blood pressure, central venous pressure, and precordial Doppler ultrasound (under risk of venous air embolism).

Brain Function Monitoring Items
Intraoperative neurophysiological monitoring indexes have become standard parameters for certain neurosurgical procedures (Table 8.1).

Taking SEP, BAEP, or EMG monitoring items as examples, the following points need to be achieved during anesthesia:

(A) Avoid using nitrous oxide (N_2O).
(B) Minimize the dosage of muscle relaxants.
(C) Keep volatile anesthetics below 0.5 MAC.
(D) Anesthesia maintenance mainly involves opioids combined with propofol infusion.

Therefore, complex neurosurgical operations such as brainstem hemorrhage greatly increase the difficulty of anesthesia management.

Table 8.1 Common neurological monitoring items and significance

Brain function monitoring project	Physiological significance
Electroencephalogram (EEG)	Monitor spontaneous brain activity to reflect cerebral ischemia status
Transcranial Doppler ultrasound (TCD)	Noninvasive monitoring of cerebral blood flow changes
Cerebral oxygen saturation (rSO_2)	Reflect brain oxygen balance
Electromyography (EMG)	Monitor the function of nerves and innervated muscles
Brainstem auditory evoked response (BAER)	Reflect the brainstem damage objectively and sensitively
Sensory evoked potential (SEP)	Monitor the integrity of ascending sensory motor pathway
Motor evoked potential (MEP)	Monitor the functional integrity of descending motor pathway

8.5 Anesthesia Mode Selection and Its Advantages or Disadvantages

Pain events in neurosurgery such as brainstem hemorrhage primarily occur at the beginning and end of the operation, such as laryngoscopy and tracheal intubation, headrest fixing, incision or suturing of skin, periosteum, and dura mater. However, pain stimulation is relatively mild during surgical manipulation of brain tissue. As a result, higher analgesics doses are required during dural incision and suturing, while hypnotics and muscle relaxants are more appropriate for intracranial operation.

8.5.1 Basic Anesthesia

Operation for brainstem hemorrhage with a short surgical duration and mild pain stimulation (e.g., drilling and drainage procedures) could be performed under local infiltration anesthesia. Commonly used anesthetic agents include lidocaine and ropivacaine. Sedative and analgesic medications (such as dexmedetomidine) can be administered as adjuncts in patients with stable vital signs [1].

8.5.2 Total Intravenous Anesthesia

At present, there is no consensus on the ideal method for the maintenance of anesthesia in neurosurgery. However, total intravenous anesthesia (TIVA) is gradually gaining popularity as an effective technique. Target-controlled infusion (TCI) technology enables precise administration of anesthetic drugs, thereby reducing overall drug dosages. Advances such as rapid-acting intravenous anesthetics (e.g., propofol), ultrashort-acting narcotic analgesics (e.g., remifentanil) and muscle relaxants (e.g., rocuronium), along with new pharmacokinetic and pharmacodynamic theories or models and computerized TCI systems, have revolutionized intravenous anesthesia and significantly advanced clinical anesthesia practices.

Meta-analysis indicates that TIVA offers certain advantages over inhalation anesthesia. Propofol has been found to be associated with a lower incidence of postoperative shivering and vomiting, as well as faster awakening, enabling early postoperative neurological assessment. Additionally, it has less interference with motor evoked potential, helps preserve the coupling of CBF metabolism, and maintains cerebrovascular response to changes in carbon dioxide levels.

Key points of intravenous anesthesia include the following:

(A) Administering a mixture of oxygen and air for inhalation.
(B) Adjusting the infusion rate of propofol based on EEG monitoring.
(C) Combining with opioids such as remifentanil for analgesia.
(D) Using nonpolarized muscle relaxants for neuromuscular blockade.

8.5.3 Inhalation Anesthesia

Inhalation anesthesia is one of the hallmarks of modern anesthesiology, and despite the growing popularity of TIVA, it continues to maintain a dominant position in general anesthesia.

At present, a common approach involves using inhaled anesthetics for anesthesia maintenance, with low-dose opioids and muscle relaxants administered intermittently based on intraoperative requirements. However, increasing the concentration of inhaled anesthetics might reduce cerebral metabolism and lead to cerebral vasodilation, which may make it challenging to maintain ideal CPP and pose a potential risk of increased ICP.

8.5.3.1 Advantages of Inhalation Anesthesia

(A) Comprehensive anesthetic effect

Inhaled anesthetics alone can achieve the ideal anesthesia states of sedation, analgesia, amnesia, and muscle relaxation.

(B) Convenience and waking up quickly
(C) Excellent anesthesia controllability

Inhaled anesthetics are excreted through respiration, bypassing liver or kidney metabolism. Increased mechanical ventilation can rapidly eliminate the anesthetic gases.

(D) Real-time monitoring and displaying the alveolar concentration of inhaled anesthetics in each breath

(E) Safer anesthesia induction

Inhalation induction maintains airway patency and allows patients to quickly enter an unconscious state.

8.5.3.2 Disadvantages of Inhalation Anesthesia and Countermeasures

(A) *Increased Intracranial Pressure*

Increase concentrations of inhaled anesthetic can reduce brain tissue metabolism and dilate cerebral vessels, leading to increased cerebral blood flow and volume, and ultimately raise ICP.

Solutions

1. Combination Medication

   The combined use of barbiturates, diazepam, or propofol during inhalation anesthesia can reduce brain metabolism, cerebral blood flow, and alleviate the impact on ICP.

2. Hyperventilation

   Maintaining $PetCO_2$ at about 30 mmHg can counteract ICP increases caused by inhaled anesthetics.

(B) *Postoperative Agitation*

Increasing minute ventilation can help expel residual anesthetic gases effectively. In addition, administering appropriate analgesics and sedatives allows for a gradual awakening, promoting the synchronous recovery of consciousness and cognitive function. This reduces adverse stimuli and psychological distress.

At present, no definitive evidence suggests that either propofol or inhaled anesthesia significantly improve the prognosis and survival rate [2]. Therefore, inhalation anesthesia remains a viable alternative for the maintenance of anesthesia during brainstem hemorrhage surgery.

8.6 Anesthesia Management of Perioperative High-Risk Events

8.6.1 Intraoperative Emergency Management

8.6.1.1 Acute Brain Swelling

The anesthesia coping strategies are as follows:

(A) Rapid Dehydration

Mannitol is the most commonly used diuretic in neurosurgery to alleviate intraoperative brain edema and achieve ideal ICP. Rapid infusion of mannitol within 20–30 minutes effectively reduces intraoperative brain swelling. However, it is worth noting that mannitol may increase CBF and ICP temporarily. The "rebound effect" should be considered when the dose reaches 0.5–1 g/kg. The combination of mannitol and loop diuretics enhances the dehydration effect, which requires close monitoring of urinary output and electrolyte imbalances.

(B) Controlled Hypotension

Maintaining systolic blood pressure at approximately 90 mmHg could effectively alleviate cerebral edema. However, the hypotensive time should be controlled strictly limited, and blood pressure must be gradually restored to baseline levels postoperatively to prevent cerebral ischemia.

(C) Hyperventilation

Reducing $PaCO_2$ to 25–30 mmHg causes cerebral vasoconstriction, which decreases CBF and rapidly reduces brain tissue volume.

(D) Postural Adjustment

The position of 30° head height is conducive to promoting venous reflux, reducing ICP, and minimizing brain edema.

(E) Restrict Liquid Infusion

Neurosurgical patients should avoid excessive infusion. The intraoperative fluids management should prioritize normal blood volume maintenance. The plasma osmotic pressure determines water movement across the blood-brain barrier. 0.9% saline solution is the preferred fluid to maintain blood volume. However, excessive use of hypertonic saline may cause hyperchloric metabolic acidosis. Hypotonic liquids such as a mixture of 5% glucose and 0.18% saline should be avoided, as they can increase ICP and worsen brain edema.

8.6.1.2 Cardiovascular Accident

Since the brainstem houses vital neural centers, surgical procedures like hematoma evacuation frequently lead to cardiovascular instability (Table 8.2). This is particularly critical in the case of intracranial hypertension, where the risk of cardiovascular events is significantly elevated.

Table 8.2 Common circulatory disturbance in brainstem surgery

Injury or operation	Cardiovascular manifestations
Early manifestations of brainstem injury	Sudden increase in blood pressure and alternating heart rate
Stimulate the bottom of fourth ventricle	Hypertension, bradycardia, tachycardia, arrhythmia
Separate or stimulate the cranial nerves and nuclei	Changes in blood pressure, heart rate, respiration, hiccups, or vomiting (irrelated to anesthesia depth)
Medulla oblongata and inferior pontine 1/3 reticular tissue	Excessive release of adrenaline leads to elevated blood pressure and heart rate
Direct or indirect stimulation of vagus nerve	Heart rate alternation
Direct stimulation of trigeminal nerve	Severe elevation of blood pressure
Separate the brain tissue around vagus nucleus	Acute sinus arrhythmia, bradycardia, or fatal ventricular arrhythmia

Abrupt hypertension and irregular heart rhythms are the early manifestations of brainstem injury caused by surgery. Surgical separation and stimulation of cranial nerves, nerve nuclei, or peripheral conduction pathways may lead to blood pressure changes, heart rate irregularities, respiratory disturbances, and reflexive hiccups or vomiting.

Acute sinus arrhythmia and sudden respiratory effort can occur when brain tissue near the vagus nucleus is manipulated. Severe bradycardia and ventricular arrhythmia can become life-threatening. The surgical stimulation must be interrupted immediately before any pharmacological intervention to control serious complications [3].

Although the specific mechanism is not yet clear, high-dose continuous intravenous infusion of short-acting opioids and propofol or benzodiazepines (midazolam) can suppress neuronal reactivity and reduce adrenergic activation during critical surgical periods like brainstem separation.

The application of high concentration inhaled anesthetics to control hypertension and tachycardia may pose hypotension and weaken cerebral autoregulation. In addition, high concentration of volatile anesthetics can also interfere with EEG monitoring, reducing its reliability.

Hypotension and bradycardia are easily induced by central anti-adrenergic drugs (clonidine). Specific central α_2-adrenergic antagonists are preferred, as they rarely cause hypotension and offer safer options for patients with brainstem hemorrhage [4].

8.6.1.2.1 Emergency Anesthetic Treatment

(A) Inform the neurosurgeon to immediately halt the surgical procedure to prevent further complications.
(B) Symptomatic pharmacological management.
   1. Administer atropine to counteract bradycardia, escape rhythm, and parasympathetic-induced low cardiac output.
   2. Use short-acting β-receptor blocker like esmolol to control severe tachycardia and hypertension.
   3. Employ specific agents like α_2-adrenoceptor antagonists to manage central nervous system-related autonomic dysregulation.

8.6.1.2.2 Anesthetic Precautions

(A) Administer high-dose opioids, short-acting intravenous anesthetics (e.g., propofol) or benzodiazepines (e.g., midazolam) to suppress neuronal response and adrenergic activation during surgery [5].
(B) Use opioid drugs such as fentanyl to enhance vagal efferent activity, thereby supporting baroreflex-mediated bradycardia and stabilizing heart rate [6].

8.6.1.3 Intracranial Pneumatosis

Intracranial air residue may occur in surgeries performed in a high head posture, making brainstem hemorrhage surgery particularly prone to intracranial pneumatosis. The use of N_2O is contraindicated during the dural suture process, as it can expand trapped gas within the intracranial space, leading to extensive damage to brain tissue.

Continuous intracranial pressure is recommended to detect real-time pressure changes and guide clinical interventions to optimize postoperative outcomes.

8.6.2 Anesthetic Management for Postoperative Complications

8.6.2.1 Cerebrovascular Accidents

Also known as strokes are classified into ischemic (such as cerebral infarction, cerebral thrombosis) and hemorrhagic types (such as cerebral hemorrhage, subarachnoid hemorrhage). These conditions significantly impact the quality of life and long-term survival rate of patients.

Ischemic stroke occurs when blood supply to the brain is disrupted, leading to cerebral ischemia and hypoxia. This results in brain tissue softening, necrosis, or cerebral infarction. In mild cases, recovery can occur gradually, while in severe cases, patients may experience long-term irreversible loss of consciousness and neurological dysfunction.

Due to the influence of anesthesia and analgesics, the early signs of intraoperative and postoperative cerebral ischemia are often covered up or ignored. Symptoms such as delayed awakening, disturbances in consciousness and speech, headache, frequent vomiting, or unilateral limb weakness following general anesthesia may indicate cerebrovascular accidents. These symptoms should raise concern for a potential ischemic event.

Preventing perioperative cerebrovascular accidents is complex due to the multifactorial nature of the disease. Anesthesiologists should remain vigilant in monitoring patients, particularly those with systemic underlying conditions, both during and after surgery. Early detection of complications can allow for timely intervention and treatment to improve patient outcomes.

(A) ***Preoperative Visit***
   1. Preoperative treatment of variable risk factors (such as hypertension and hyperglycemia) to improve patient's surgical tolerance and minimize perioperative complications.
   2. Monitor and evaluate the brain function of high-risk patients, including consciousness level and motor function, as comparison with postoperative status.

3. Create a comprehensive and stable perioperative anesthesia management plan tailored to the patient's needs.

(B) ***Anesthesia Induction and Maintenance***

During anesthesia induction, prudent medication and appropriate anesthesia depth could alleviate cardiovascular depression. Performing tracheal intubation and other anesthesia procedures gently to avoid causing arrhythmia and intracranial hypertension.

The key points of anesthesia maintenance are as follows:

1. Maintain appropriate blood pressure for patients and avoid significant fluctuations in blood pressure during operation.
2. Keep $PaCO_2$ between 25 and 30 mmHg to prevent CO_2 accumulation and ensure ICP stability.
3. Intraoperative liquid therapy.

Follow the principle of crystal to colloid ratio for infusion strictly, and control the total amount of fluid given. Avoid infusion of sugary crystalline fluid to prevent lactate accumulation from aggravating cerebrovascular damage.

(C) ***Anesthetic Treatments***

1. Specialist consultation and diagnosis according to clinical manifestations, cerebrospinal fluid, CT, or MRI.
2. Respiratory and circulatory support therapy.

   Oxygen inhalation, respiratory support, or assisted ventilation as needed.

   Prudent antihypertensive treatment to avoid worsening neurological deterioration. In cases of hypertensive crisis, opt for drugs with short-acting properties and minimal effect on cerebrovascular function.

   Blood volume supplement and arrhythmia correction.
3. Blood glucose control
4. Body temperature management

   In selective neurosurgery, mild hypothermia has not been shown to improve the prognosis of patients. Therefore, normal body temperature should be maintained during operation to avoid temperature extremes (hypothermia or hyperthermia).
5. Active brain protection therapy

   Use neuroprotective drugs such as calcium antagonists, excitatory amino acid antagonists, free radical scavengers, antioxidants, and anti-inflammatory agents to protect brain function during surgery [7].

8.6.2.2 Awakening Delay

Delayed anesthesia awakening is defined as a condition where the patient's consciousness has not yet recovered, and they are unable to follow commands more than 2 h after general anesthesia. This condition is common in patients with preexisting conditions such as stroke, hemiplegia, craniocerebral injury, and severe systemic [8].

For managing delayed recovery after general anesthesia, the following treatment measures should be considered:

(A) Ensure the patient is inhaling oxygen and maintain airway patency to provide adequate ventilation and oxygenation.

(B) Closely monitor the patient's vital signs, including blood pressure, heart rate, SpO_2, $PetCO_2$, and other indicators to assess the patient's respiratory and cardiovascular status.

(C) Review the patient's previous medical history, preoperative medication, and the type or dosage of narcotic drugs to identify potential causes of delayed recovery.

(D) Assess the status of muscle relaxation, and, if necessary, administer antagonists to reverse muscle paralysis (atropine 0.5 mg or neostigmine 1 mg) if necessary.

(E) Examine the retention effect of opioids or benzodiazepines.

Pupillary contraction and slow breathing are the main manifestations of opioids. Naloxone 200 μg can be administered intravenously in repeated doses if needed to reverse opioid effects. Flumazenil can be used to antagonize the effects of benzodiazepines such as diazepam or midazolam.

(F) Measure the patient's body temperature, and take appropriate measures to warm the patient and prevent complications from temperature extremes.

(G) Monitor blood glucose level. If blood glucose is found to be below 3 mmol/L, administer 50 ml of 50% glucose solution intravenously to correct hypoglycemia.

(H) Perform a blood gas analysis to check for potential electrolyte imbalances or acid-base disturbances.

8.6.2.3 Awakening Agitation

For patients exhibiting restlessness after general anesthesia, it is important to identify and address the underlying cause, remove any triggers, and prevent complications.

The following key points of anesthesia management are essential:

(A) Strengthen patient protection to prevent accidental injury, and reduce the risk of serious complications.

(B) Reduce adverse stimulation of endotracheal tube or catheter.

(C) The sedative and hypnotic drugs (such as diazepam or propofol) could be administered appropriately under the condition of stable respiration and circulation.

(D) Adequate postoperative analgesia. Intravenous analgesics are recommended to avoid central respiratory depression.

(E) Maintain respiratory circulation, electrolyte stability, and acid-base balance. Prevent agitation and delirium caused by hypoxemia, hypercapnia, and electrolyte disturbances [9].

8.6.2.4 Postoperative Nausea and Vomiting (PONV)

PONV are common complications, especially in patients with risk factors such as being female, nonsmokers, and a having history of opioid use. These issues can increase patient discomfort, lead to electrolyte imbalance, acid-base disturbances, and, in severe cases, aspiration pneumonia. In neurosurgical patients, frequent vomiting is particularly concerning, as it can raise ICP and cause adverse events [10].

Principles of PONV prevention and treatment:

(A) Implement fasting and drinking restriction before operation.
(B) Use physical methods (e.g., gastric tube) or medication (e.g., metoclopramide) to promote gastric emptying.
(C) Propofol used in total intravenous anesthesia has been shown to reduce the incidence of PONV by approximately 30%.
(D) Avoid postoperative factors that can trigger nausea, such as hypotension, hypoxia, and pain.
(E) Prophylactic use of antiemetic drugs. Intravenous dexamethasone administered after anesthesia induction or preoperative use of 5-HT3 receptor inhibitors can significantly reduce the risk of PONV.

References

1. Wu SX, Chen HQ. A prospective, randomised double-blind study on the anaesthetic effect of dexmedetomidine hydrochloride in brainstem tumour surgery. World J Surg Oncol. 2019;17(1):118.
2. Chui J, Mariappan R, Mehta J, et al. Comparison of propofol and volatile agents for maintenance of anesthesia during elective craniotomy procedures: systematic review and meta-analysis. Can J Anaesth. 2014;61(4):347–56.
3. Gruenbaum SE, Meng L, Bilotta F. Recent trends in the anesthetic management of craniotomy for supratentorial tumor resection. Curr Opin Anaesthesiol. 2016;29(5):552–7.
4. Wang L, Shen J, Ge L, et al. Dexmedetomidine for craniotomy under general anesthesia: A systematic review and meta-analysis of randomized clinical trials. J Clin Anesth. 2019;54:114–25.
5. Vacas S, Van de Wiele B. Designing a pain management protocol for craniotomy: A narrative review and consideration of promising practices. Surg Neurol Int. 2017;8:291.
6. Vadivelu N, Kai AM, Tran D, et al. Options for perioperative pain management in neurosurgery. J Pain Res. 2016;9:37–47.
7. Badenes R, Gruenbaum SE, Bilotta F. Cerebral protection during neurosurgery and stroke. Curr Opin Anaesthesiol. 2015;28(5):532–6.
8. Sandhu K, Gupta N. Anesthesia for posterior fossa surgery - ScienceDirect. Essentials of Neuroanesthesia. 2017;14:255–76.
9. Gheorghita E, Ciruea J, Balanescu B. Considerations on anesthesia for posterior fossa-surgery. Anesthesia for posterior fossa-surgery. Romanian. Neurosurgery. 2012;XIX 3:183–92.
10. Ho S, Hambidge O, John R. Anaesthesia for neurosurgery - ScienceDirect. Anaesthesia & intensive care medicine. 2020;21(1):33–8.

9 Surgical Evacuation of Brainstem Hematoma Via Subtemporal Approach

Hongtian Zhang and Haiquan Tao

9.1 Overview

The subtemporal approach provides an effective and direct exposure of the brainstem. By lifting the temporal lobe and opening the tentorium, the lateral aspect of the pons can be accessed easily, facilitating rapid hematoma evacuation. This area constitutes a relatively safe zone in proximity to the brainstem, resulting in minimal secondary damage to this vital structure. Additionally, opening the tentorium can effectively alleviate any compression exerted by the swollen brainstem. For brainstem hemorrhage, this approach is regarded as a simple, direct, and effective entry point that is easy to learn and master.

9.2 Indications and Contraindications

9.2.1 Indications

Currently, there is no unified surgical standard for brainstem hemorrhage. However, the following conditions are generally considered suitable for surgical treatment:

1. Patients under the age of 60 years old.
2. Hematoma located in the upper portion of the pons and certain areas of the midbrain.
3. Hematoma volume > 5 mL or maximum hemorrhage cross-sectional area occupying >50% of the same level of the brainstem.
4. Patients with a GCS score < 8, indicating moderate to severe coma.
5. Stable circulation without a history of cardiac arrest and cardiopulmonary resuscitation.
6. Normal coagulation function.
7. Strong willingness for surgery expressed by the patient's family after being fully informed of the surgical risks and potential economic and family burdens.

9.2.2 Contraindications

1. Hematoma volume < 5 mL.
2. Patients without significant impairment of consciousness.
3. Unstable circulation and inability to maintain basic vital signs.
4. Coagulation disorders or multi-organ dysfunction.
5. Patient's family refusal of surgery.

9.3 Preoperative Preparation and Surgical Instruments

9.3.1 Preoperative Preparation

Thorough preoperative preparation is a crucial measure for improving the efficacy of brainstem hemorrhage surgery. Maintaining clear airways, early tracheal intubation, and actively controlling blood pressure are indispensable. For patients with significant hydrocephalus, external ventricular drainage should be conducted first. When conditions and time permit, the combination of image-guided navigation and microsurgery can notably enhance the efficiency and safety of the surgery. Various imaging workstations can currently simulate surgical approaches, greatly improving surgical efficacy and safety.

Supplementary Information The online version contains supplementary material available at https://doi.org/10.1007/978-981-95-8942-5_9.

H. Zhang (✉)
Department of Neurosurgery, Chinese PLA General Hospital, Beijing, China

H. Tao
Department of Cerebrovascular Diseases, Zhuhai People's Hospital (The Affiliated Hospital of Beijing Institute of Technology, Zhuhai Clinical Medical College of Jinan University), Zhuhai, China

G. Chen, C. You (eds.), *Surgical Treatment of Primary Brainstem Hemorrhage*, https://doi.org/10.1007/978-981-95-8942-5_9

9.3.2 Surgical Instruments

The requirements of surgical equipment include a dedicated electric operating table, neurosurgical operating microscope, head frame and automatic retractor, electric craniotomy drill, bipolar coagulation and monopolar electrocautery, microsurgical instruments, etc.

9.4 Surgical Methods, Precautions, and Techniques

9.4.1 Surgical Methods

1. Positioning and head placement

   The patient is positioned in a supine position with a cushion beneath the ipsilateral shoulder to aid in head tilting. A Mayfield head frame, equipped with three pins for secure fixation, is utilized, with one pin positioned at the forehead to enhance intraoperative maneuverability. Initially, the head is elevated above the chest to facilitate venous return and alleviate pressure on the cervical region and airway. Subsequently, the head is rotated 60° to 100° toward the contralateral side, with the angle of rotation depending on the location of the lesion. For hematomas located in the anterior region of upper pontine, the zygomatic arch should be positioned nearly horizontally, with the head rotated approximately 90°; for hematomas in the upper cerebellopontine angle, a rotation of approximately 75° is recommended. Following this, the head is laterally flexed 15° to 20° to compensate for the steep upward angle of the medial aspect of the middle cranial fossa to provide an efficient working position for the surgeon. Additionally, lateral flexion allows the temporal lobe to retract under the influence of gravity, preventing potential injury to the base of the temporal lobe due to mechanical retraction. Finally, the head is slightly extended by approximately 10° to prevent compression of airway, pharyngeal, and major neck vessel (Fig. 9.1). Lateral decubitus positioning is also an alternative approach.
2. Incision

   The standard incision for the procedure is characterized by a slightly arched linear incision, which is commonly employed. The lower margin of this incision is positioned at the root of the zygomatic arch or just superior to it, while the curvature of the incision arches superiorly, with the upper margin situated anterior to the parietal tubercle. Furthermore, alternative incisions, such as a horseshoe-shaped or a small question mark-shaped incision, are less frequently utilized but may also be employed in specific clinical contexts (Fig. 9.2).
3. Dissection of subcutaneous tissue and muscles

   The scalp is incised in full thickness. When employing the keyhole surgical approach, the use of scalp clips may be unnecessary. The temporal muscle fascia is incised in a "Y" configuration, and a periosteal elevator is subsequently used to dissect the temporalis muscle from the supramastoid crest and the upper temporal line, flipping it toward the external auditory meatus direction and securing it with a retractor (Fig. 9.3).
4. Bone Window

   The bone window is approximately 3 cm × 4 cm in size. The anterior portion of the window exposes the root of the zygomatic arch, while the posterior aspect reveals parietomastoid suture and upper crest of the mastoid process. The posterior edge is located at the confluence of parietomastoid suture and scaly suture, just anterior to the transition between the transverse and sigmoid sinuses, with the superior edge being the temporal squamous suture. Three holes are drilled: one at the upper part of the zygomatic arch, another at the suprameatal spine, and a third at the temporal squamous suture (Fig. 9.4). The inner margin of the bone window is ground down to flatten it, facilitating the elevation of the temporal lobe.
5. Dural opening

   The dural membrane should be carefully suspended around the perimeter of the bone window. The dura is then incised in a crescent-shaped manner, with the opened flap being reflected toward the zygomatic arch. This flap is subsequently secured with two sutures to maintain the exposure (Fig. 9.5).

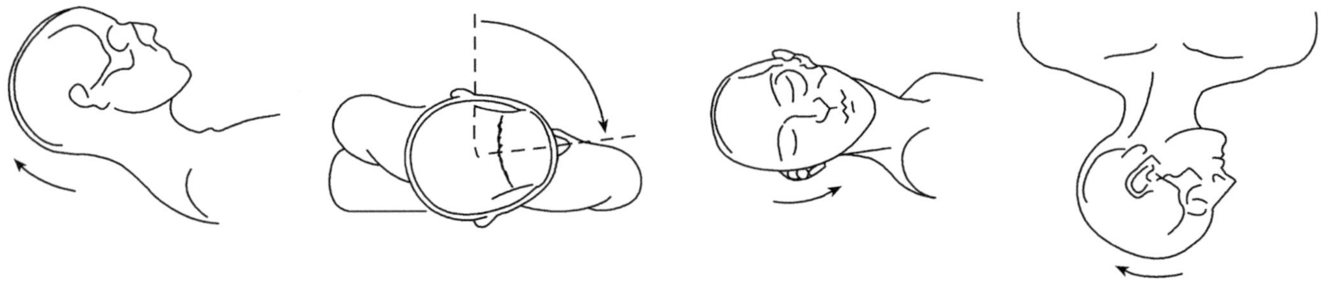

Fig. 9.1 Position

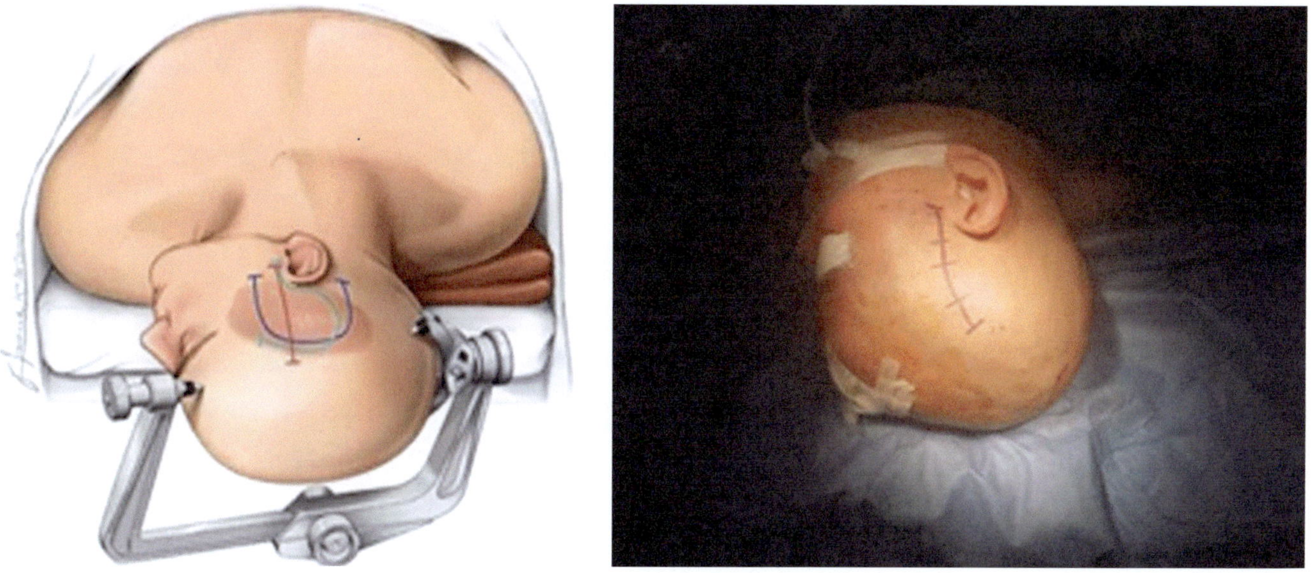

Fig. 9.2 Incision pattern diagram and actual incision

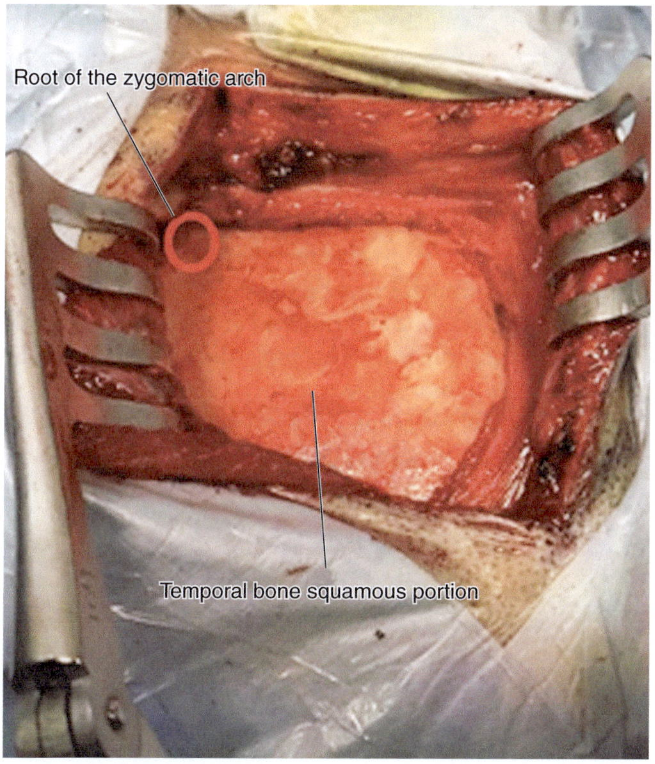

Fig. 9.3 Dissection of subcutaneous tissue and muscles. 1 root of the zygomatic arch 2 temporal bone squamous portion

6. Exposure of the tentorium

   Under microscopic visualization, gently elevate the base of the temporal lobe using a 0.5 cm brain spatula, releasing cerebrospinal fluid while continuously delving deeper, gradually exposing the superior petrosal sinus, and along the posterior aspect of the superior petrosal sinus to locate the edge of the tentorium (refer to Fig. 9.6).

7. Tentorial incision and exposure of the brainstem

   A 0.5–1 cm incision parallel to the posterior edge of the superior petrosal sinus is sufficient to access the upper lateral aspect of the pons (Fig. 9.7). By opening the ambient cistern, cerebrospinal fluid is further released, which serves to expand the surgical exposure range and fully reveal the lateral aspect of the brainstem. A 0.5 mL needle is used to puncture the brainstem to ascertain the precise location of the hematoma (Fig. 9.8).

8. Evacuation of hematoma

   To expose the hematoma cavity, a fine-tip bipolar coagulator is employed, while the contralateral hand operates a microsuction device to meticulously extract the hematoma with controlled suction. If the blood clot is firm, it can be fragmented with tumor forceps before removal. Once the evacuation is complete, a small amount of hemostatic sponge can be used to control bleeding in the surgical cavity (Fig. 9.9).

9. Dural suturing

   Upon the conclusion of the intracranial procedure, the subdural space should be filled with warm saline solution to maintain optimal conditions within the surgical field. The dural incision is sutured in a watertight manner. If there is high tension in the dural plane, it may be necessary to implant a small piece of temporal muscle or artificial material.

10. Skull closure

    Position gelatin foam extradurally and secure the skull with titanium plates. Once hemostasis is achieved, intermittently suture the muscle layer and subcutaneous tissue, and close the skin. Generally, no drainage tube is placed in the subcutaneous area (Video 9.1).

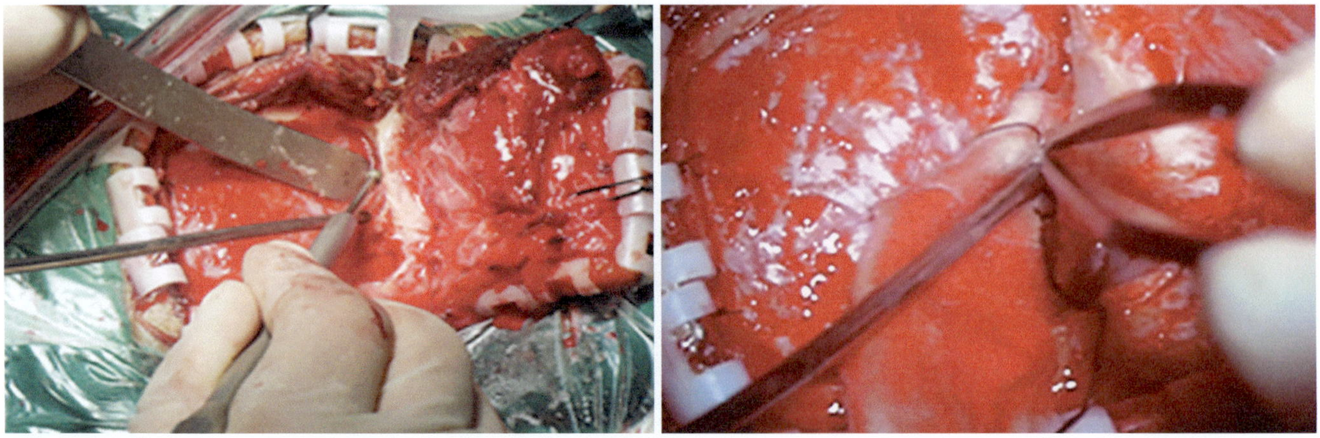

Fig. 9.4 Grinding of the inner edge of the bone window

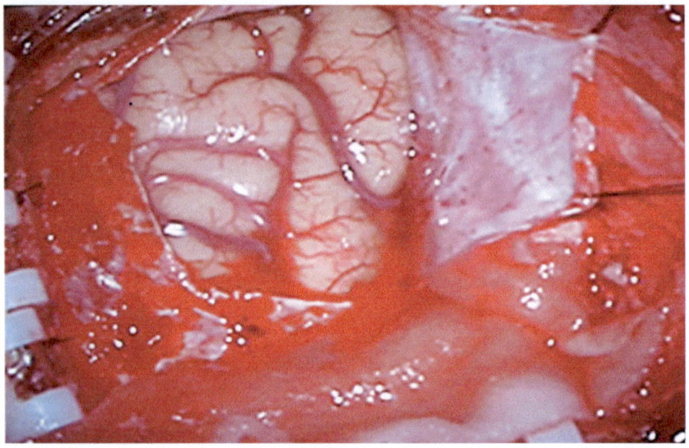

Fig. 9.5 Opening of the dura

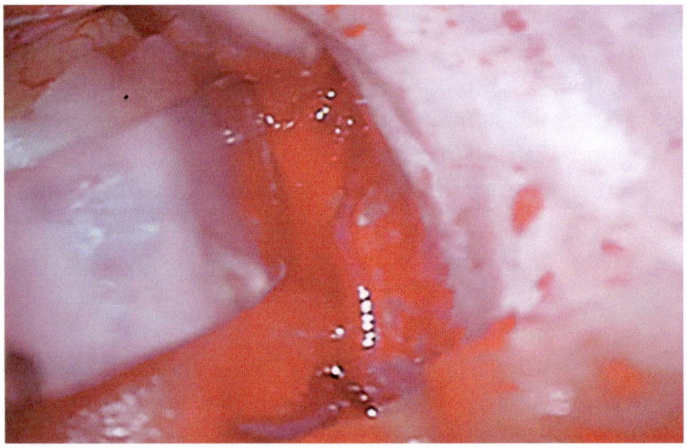

Fig. 9.6 Elevation of the temporal lobe, release of cerebrospinal fluid

9.4.2 Surgical Techniques and Considerations

1. Craniotomy phase
   (a) During the incision, particular care should be taken to avoid damage to the superficial neurovascular structures in the preauricular temporal region, such as the superficial temporal artery, auriculotemporal nerve, and temporal branch of the facial nerve.
   (b) Prevent postoperative masticatory dysfunction and temporalis muscle atrophy by avoiding traumatic separation and excessive traction on the muscle.
   (c) When performing bone flap milling, be cautious to avoid damage to the sigmoid and transverse sinuses in the posterior edge. After shaping the bone flap, seal the temporal bone mastoid air cells with bone wax.
   (d) After removing the bone flap, grinding the inner edge of the bone is crucial for observing and operating within the dura. During grinding, the assistant should use a brain spatula positioned above the dura to prevent the drill from slipping, which could result in damage to brain tissue.
   (e) Completely seal the temporal bone and mastoid air cells with bone wax to prevent cerebrospinal fluid leakage.
2. Intracranial operation phase
   (a) Thoroughly control extracranial bleeding in the epidural space to prevent blood from infiltrating the intracranial space.
   (b) It is essential to fully release cerebrospinal fluid gradually using a brain spatula to elevate the temporal lobe, thereby preventing iatrogenic trauma. Additionally, proper positioning, minimal dura incision, and careful surgical dissection are crucial factors in averting temporal lobe contusion.
   (c) When incising the tentorium, take care to protect the trochlear nerve.
3. Hematoma evacuation phase
   (a) Select the point where the hematoma ruptures into the brainstem or the bluish area beneath the brainstem as the entry point. If the hematoma is within the brainstem, it is critical to choose an incision site with minimal damage to vital neural nuclei for consciousness and motor function. Use a small suction device

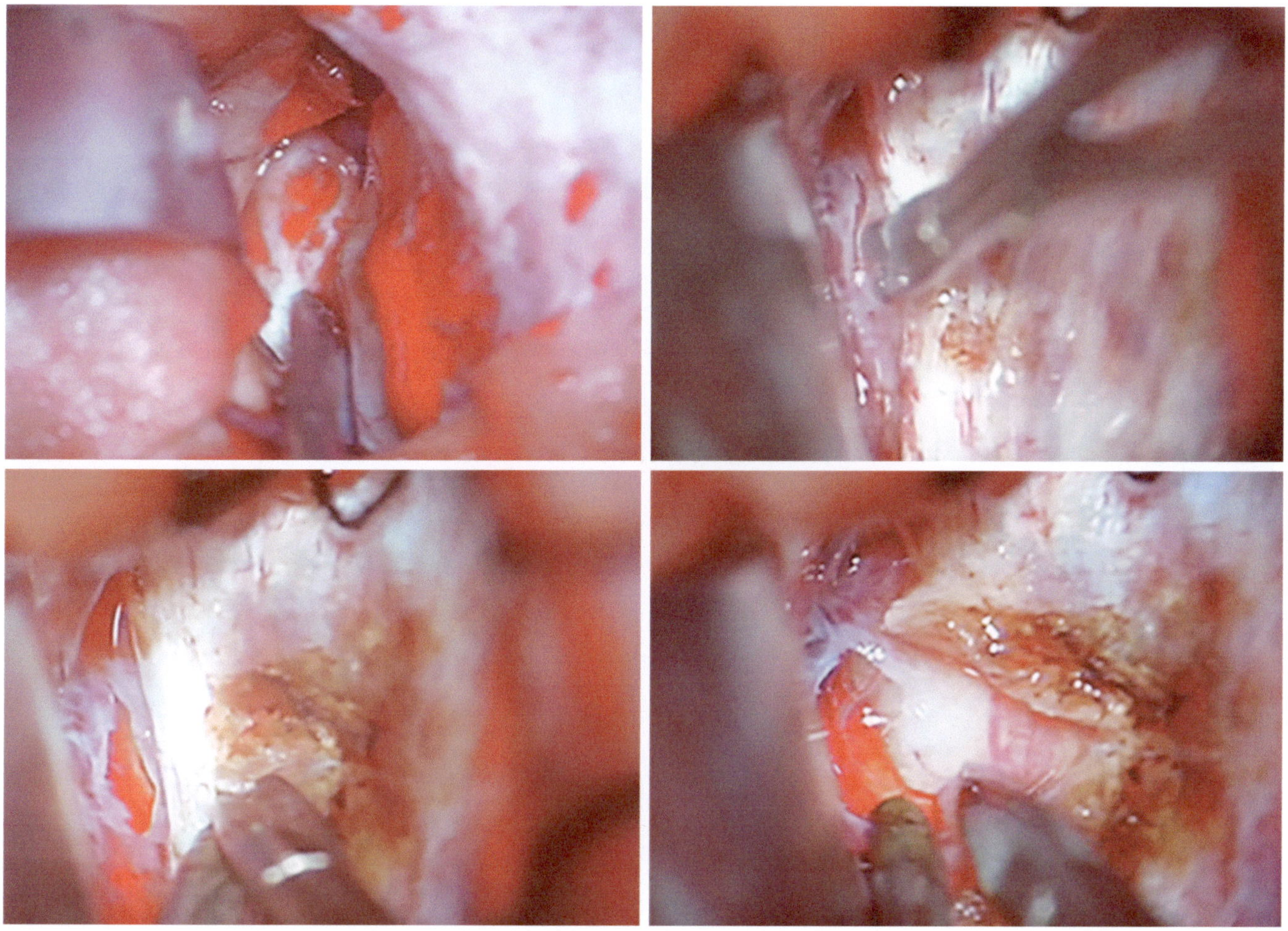

Fig. 9.7 Opening of the tentorium, process of exposing the brainstem

to remove the hematoma, preferably confined within the hematoma cavity, taking care to avoid damage to surrounding tissues beyond the hematoma edge. Use irrigation to loosen blood clots.

(b) Conduct the surgery primarily within the hematoma cavity to minimize damage to brainstem tissue and ensuing bleeding. In case of significant bleeding, the application of cotton pads or hemostatic gauze with gentle pressure can be effective. Utilize bipolar coagulation judiciously, reserving it for active bleeding sites. If active bleeding occurs, consider using bipolar coagulation after identifying and securing the bleeding vessel. Set the bipolar coagulator power to 5 to prevent heat transfer and avoid contact with brainstem tissue.

4. Skull closure phase
   (a) Ensure a tight closure of the dura, especially if the mastoid antrum was opened during surgery, as it may lead to cerebrospinal fluid rhinorrhea. Temporal muscle or artificial implant materials can be used for watertight dural suturing.
   (b) Insufficient control of bleeding in the soft tissue may lead to intracranial or soft tissue hematoma postoperatively.

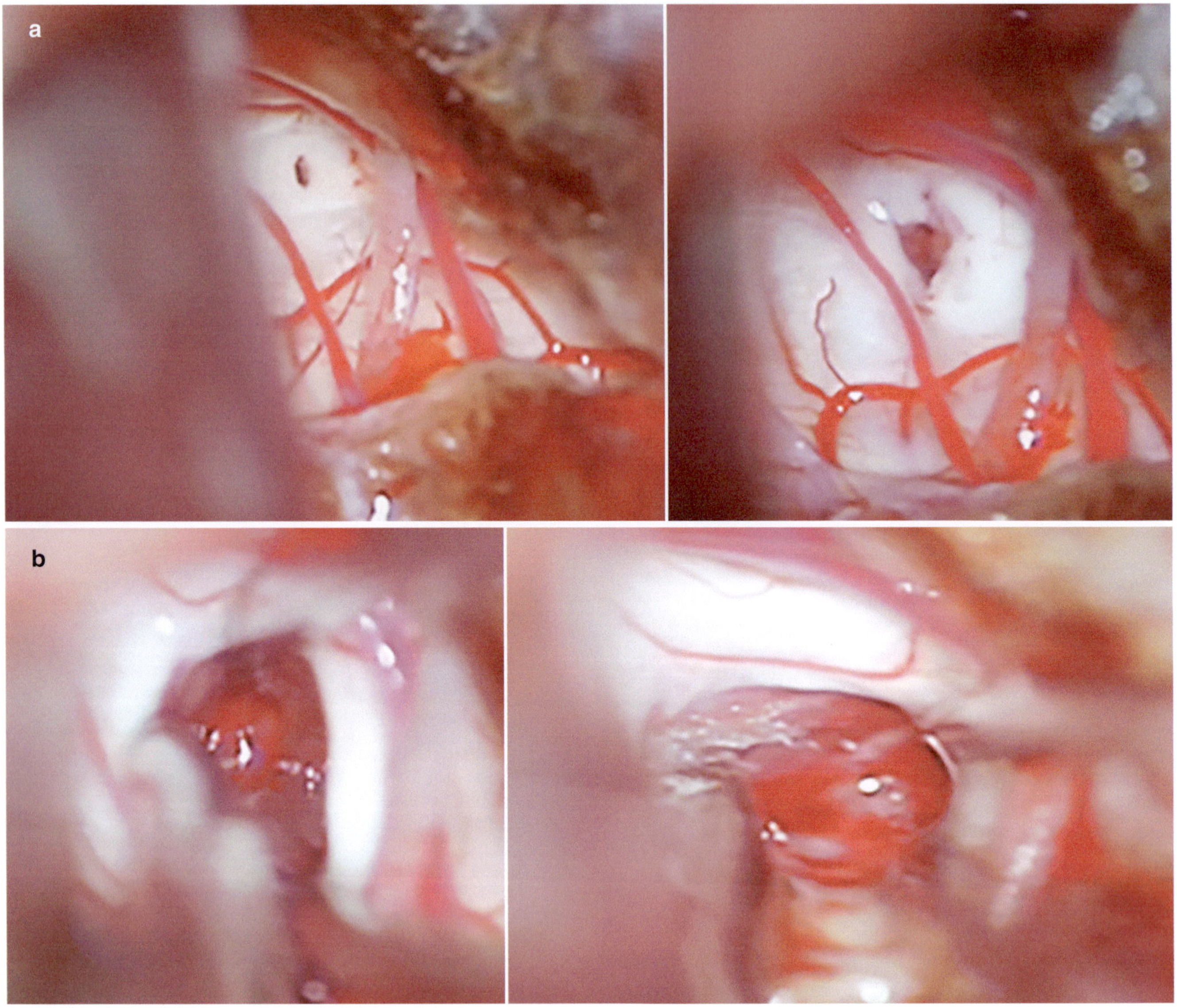

Fig. 9.8 Locating the hematoma, determining the hematoma's position

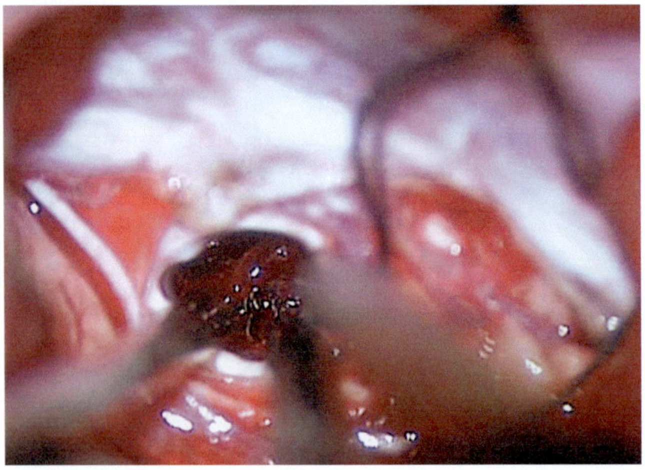

Fig. 9.9 Evacuation of hematoma

9.5 Postoperative Care and Complication Prevention

1. Pulmonary infection

   In comatose patients, postoperative expectoration may be compromised, consequently increasing the risk of pulmonary infection. Early tracheostomy facilitates sputum removal, reduces airway resistance, diminishes dead space ventilation, enhances effective gas exchange in the alveoli, and improves cerebral oxygenation. For instances characterized by hypoxemia or respiratory failure, early ventilator assistance is recommended. After the onset of pulmonary infection, the selection of targeted antibiotics, informed by the outcomes of sensitivity testing, is imperative.

2. Stress ulcer bleeding in the upper gastrointestinal tract

   In the postoperative period, the administration of acid suppressants is instrumental in preventing alleviating stress-induced acute gastric mucosal lesions. Patients unable to ingest food for 24 hours necessitate the placement of a gastric tube for nasogastric fluid feeding and the provision of mucosal protection. For patients with gastrointestinal bleeding, intragastric injection with ice saline plus coagulation enzyme or 0.02% epinephrine can effectively control bleeding.
3. Central hyperthermia

   Brainstem hemorrhage-induced central hyperthermia is a severe manifestation of significant brain injury, characterized by noninfectious hyperthermia with temperatures often reaching around 40 °C. Prolonged hyperthermia exacerbates brain damage and is associated with increased short-term mortality in patients. In the postoperative setting, the application of physical cooling modalities, such as ice blankets and caps, can effectively reduce cerebral oxygen consumption and metabolic rates, alleviate brain edema, lower intracranial pressure, mitigate neuronal damage, and promote functional recovery. Caution should be exercised in using pharmacological cooling due to the potential to induce stress ulcers, and it is imperative to limit the use of such cooling methods.
4. Postoperative rebleeding

   Elevated blood pressure is a predominant factor contributing to postoperative rebleeding. Postoperative care should prioritize the stabilization of blood pressure, targeting a systolic/diastolic range of 140/90 mmHg as a general guideline, though this may be tailored to align with the individual patient's baseline measurements. The judicious application of sedation and analgesia is also recommended to facilitate blood pressure control.
5. Fluid and electrolyte disturbance

   Routine surveillance of serum electrolytes and renal function is crucial for the preservation of fluid and electrolyte equilibrium. Upon the patient's return to consciousness, it is imperative to promptly institute neurorehabilitation interventions, including hyperbaric oxygen therapy, to enhance the quality of life and promote functional recovery.

9.6 Advantages, Disadvantages, and Lessons Learned

The subtemporal approach is recognized for its efficiency and directness in exposing the brainstem from the lateral aspect. By elevating the temporal lobe and opening the tentorium, the brainstem's lateral aspect becomes quickly accessible, allowing rapid access to hematomas. This region is a relatively safe zone for the brainstem surgery, as it significantly reduces the risk of secondary damage. The use of a surgical microscope equipped with direct illumination enhances procedural precision and ensures deft manipulation of delicate neural structures. Additionally, opening the tentorium effectively alleviates compression on the swollen brainstem. Opening the ambient cistern releases hemorrhagic cerebrospinal fluid, reducing irritation to the brainstem effectively. Hematomas often manifest as localized elevations or changes in color. In the event of a hematoma rupture, the presence of blood within the ambient cistern becomes readily apparent. During the surgery procedure, longitudinal incisions are made on the side of the localized elevation in the brainstem tissue, and a micro-aspirator is used under the microscope to remove the hematoma. This approach is minimally invasive, accurate, easy to perform, and associated with minimal bleeding. If the mastoid air cells are opened, proper closure with bone wax is essential. Care must be exercised to avoid injury to Labbé's vein during the exposure. Preserving the integrity of this vein is essential to prevent exacerbation of brainstem edema and to avoid compressive effects on the brainstem tissue, which could lead to irreversible neural function impairments. The subtemporal approach also has limitations, such as a confined operating space, limited exposure, and a narrow field, making surgical procedures challenging. Exerting improper traction on brain tissue poses a significant risk of severe brain injury and should be avoided. The most effective method is to open the cistern to release cerebrospinal fluid, facilitating the natural retraction of brain tissue. Preoperative external ventricular drainage, in conjunction with intraoperative cerebrospinal fluid release, is a critical strategy to reduce intracranial pressure. Unlike in supratentorial bleeding, caution is advised against sacrificing surrounding brainstem tissue for the sake of achieving radiological perfection, especially when dealing with heavily adhered blood clots.

9.7 Procedure Evaluation and Prospects

The subtemporal approach is recognized for its rapidity and efficiency in addressing brainstem hemorrhages from the lateral aspect. It has a short learning curve, making it easy to master. Effectively opening the tentorium cerebelli alleviates the compressive impact of the cerebellar tentorial incisura on the brainstem. Opening the ambient cistern releases hemorrhagic cerebrospinal fluid, reducing irritation to the brainstem. As experience in microsurgery accumulates, microsurgical techniques are refined, microsurgical instruments advance, and neuroimaging technology progresses, the subtemporal approach for clearing brainstem hemorrhages holds promise as an effective method to enhance both patient survival rates and quality of life.

9.8 Typical Case

9.8.1 Brief Medical History and Imaging Data

1. Patient: 52-year-old male presented with sudden consciousness disturbance for 6 hours upon admission. History of uncontrolled hypertension for 5 years without regular antihypertensive medication. Smoking history of 23 years, consuming one pack per day, and alcohol intake of 500 g per day.
2. Physical examination: Blood pressure 220/90 mmHg, respiratory rate 19 breaths/min, heart rate 102 beats/min, and temperature 39 °C. Deep coma status, GCS: 5. Both pupils were constricted and of equal size, approximately 1 mm in diameter, with sluggish light reflex and nystagmus. Slight flexion movements were observed in bilateral limbs after stimulation, with positive pyramidal tract signs.
3. Auxiliary examination: Head CT revealed a high-density mass in the dorsolateral aspect of the pons, suggestive of brainstem hematoma, measuring up to 3.5 cm in maximum diameter, resulting in compression of the fourth ventricle and mild bilateral ventricular dilation (Fig. 9.10).
4. Admission diagnosis: Spontaneous brainstem (dorsolateral upper pons) hemorrhage (approximately 14 mL); Grade 3 hypertension (extremely high-risk group); diabetes; and old cerebral infarction.

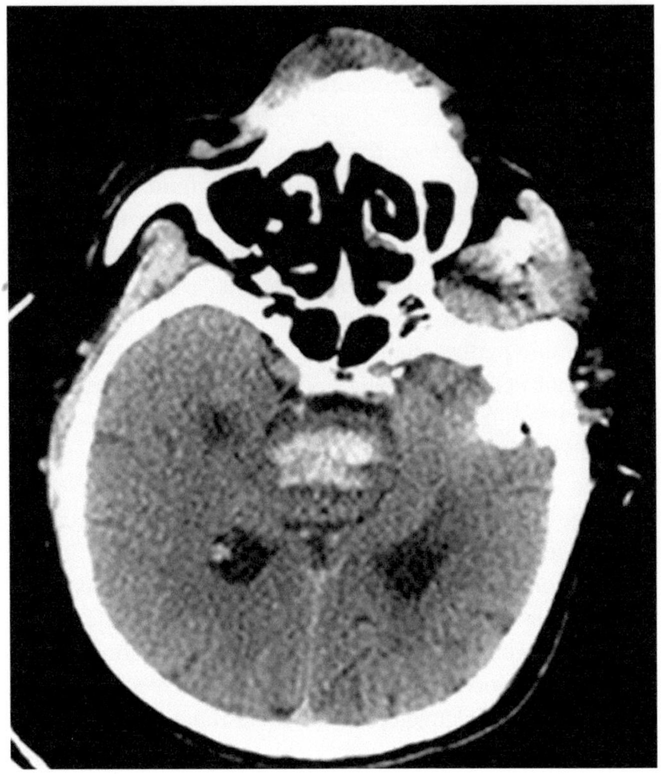

Fig. 9.10 Preoperative head CT scan

9.8.2 Surgical Procedure and Key Points

Under general anesthesia, the patient was positioned on the left lateral decubitus. After routine disinfection and draping, a straight incision of approximately 4 cm was made above the right subtemporal zygomatic arch. The scalp and muscles were incised and then turned forward. Two burr holes were created at the root of the zygomatic arch and the upper edge of the temporal squamous suture, followed by the formation of a 3 cm x 2 cm bone flap. The dura mater was incised in an arc and turned toward the bottom of the middle cranial fossa. After lifting the temporal lobe, the ambient cistern was slowly opened to release cerebrospinal fluid. Following the satisfactory reduction of intracranial pressure, the temporal lobe was further retracted to expose the tentorium. The trochlear nerve within the ambient cistern was visible. The tentorium was incised behind the trochlear nerve to expose the pons. A 3 mm incision was made at the point nearest to the brainstem hematoma, and the hematoma was exposed. A 1–1.5 mm diameter aspirator was used to gently and slowly remove the hematoma. Adequate hemostasis was achieved, and the dura mater was watertightly sutured. The bone flap was repositioned, and the scalp was closed in layers with sterile dressings applied (refer to the surgical video for details).

9.8.3 Postoperative Imaging and Recovery

A follow-up examination on the first day postoperatively revealed satisfactory clearance of the hematoma (Fig. 9.11), with improved pain response compared to preoperatively. Three weeks after the surgery, the patient regained consciousness and was able to respond appropriately. Central facial palsy was observed on the left side, with muscle strength at level II in the left limb and level III in the right lower limb, and level III in the right upper limb. By 6 weeks postoperatively, the patient was able to self-feed using hand. By 10 weeks postoperatively, the patient could sit and stand independently and could walk unassisted (Fig. 9.12).

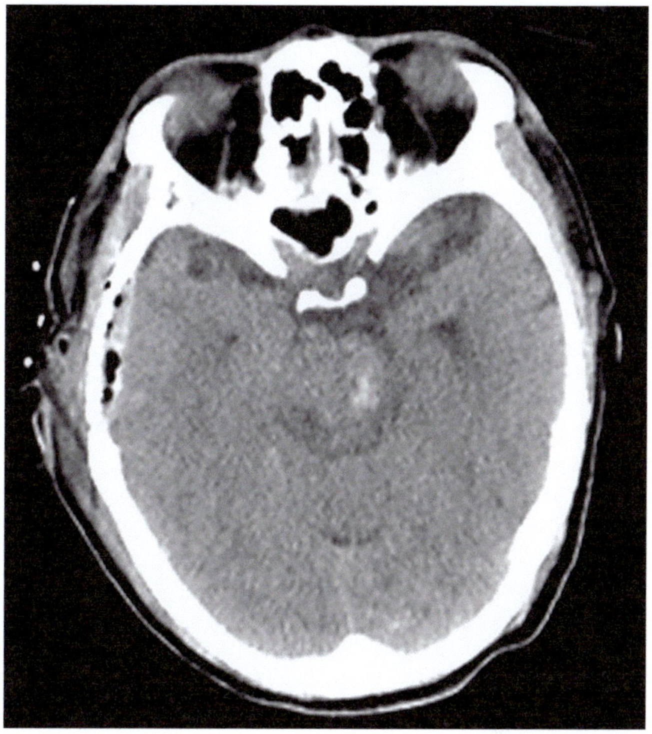

Fig. 9.11 Postoperative head CT scan

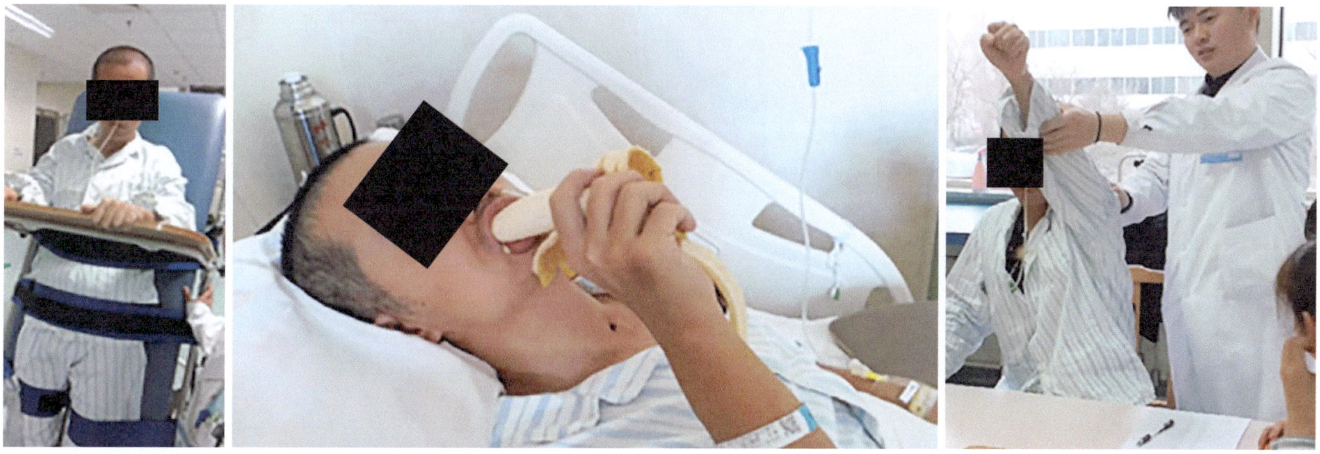

Fig. 9.12 Patient's recovery progress

Surgical Evacuation of Brainstem Hematoma Via Suboccipital Retrosigmoid Approach

10

Gang Chen, Yan Qu, Quan Zhou, Chao Sun, and Minfeng Sheng

10.1 Overview

The suboccipital retrosigmoid approach is a classic surgical entry route for lesions in the cerebellopontine angle region. The pons is the most common site of brainstem hemorrhage. The retrosigmoid approach facilitates expeditious access to the lateral aspect of the pons, allowing for a safer longitudinal incision along the lateral aspect of the pons. Therefore, this approach is most suitable for brainstem hemorrhages that are in close proximity to or have breached the brainstem's surface [1, 2].

10.2 Indications and Contradictions

10.2.1 Indications

There is no unified standard for the surgical indications of brainstem hemorrhage. Generally, the following conditions may be considered for surgical treatment:

1. The main part of the hematoma is situated within the pons, predominantly affecting one side, relatively concentrated, and close to or penetrating the surface of the brainstem.
2. Hematoma volume exceeds 5mL.
3. The maximum bleeding cross-sectional area occupies >50% of the same level of brainstem cross-sectional area.
4. Patients exhibit a range from mild to moderate coma, as indicated by a Glasgow Coma Scale (GCS) score below 8, and may present with severe vital sign disturbances.
5. The patient's family has expressed a strong preference for surgical intervention and has confirmed that their financial resources are sufficient to cover the costs associated with extended postoperative care [3, 4].

10.2.2 Contraindications

1. Patients with a small amount of brainstem hemorrhage (≤3mL) without obvious obstruction of the ventricular system or consciousness disturbances.
2. Patients with a significantly large hemorrhage that severely damages the vital centers of the brainstem, leading to bilateral dilated pupils and extreme instability of vital signs (lack of spontaneous breathing for more than 2 hours, occurrence of cardiac arrest, or low blood pressure requiring vasopressors for maintenance) are generally not suitable for surgery.
3. Diffuse brainstem hemorrhage, where it is difficult to achieve sufficient decompression through various surgical approaches.
4. Other surgical contraindications, such as severe coagulation disorders, or inability of the cardiopulmonary system to withstand anesthesia [5].

Supplementary Information The online version contains supplementary material available at https://doi.org/10.1007/978-981-95-8942-5_10.

G. Chen (✉) · M. Sheng
Department of Neurosurgery, Zhuhai People's Hospital (The Affiliated Hospital of Beijing Institute of Technology, Zhuhai Clinical Medical College of Jinan University), Zhuhai, China

Y. Qu
Department of Neurosurgery, The Second Affiliated Hospital of Air Force Military Medical University, Chinese People's Liberation Army, XiAn, China

Q. Zhou
Department of Neurosurgery, The Fiist Affiliated Hospital of Guangxi Medical Universityy, NanNing, China

C. Sun
Department of Neurosurgery, The Second Affiliated Hospital of Soochow Universityy, SuZhou, China

G. Chen, C. You (eds.), *Surgical Treatment of Primary Brainstem Hemorrhage*, https://doi.org/10.1007/978-981-95-8942-5_10

10.3 Preoperative Preparation and Surgical Instruments

Before surgery, it is essential to engage in thorough and comprehensive discussions with the patient's family. The patient's family members should make a definitive decision to proceed with the surgery only after fully understanding the surgical risk, possible prognosis, long-term prognosis, and high treatment cost.

10.3.1 Preoperative Preparation

Thorough preoperative preparation is an important measure to improve the effectiveness of brainstem hemorrhage surgery. This preparation encompasses several key elements: ensuring airway patency, early endotracheal intubation, active blood pressure control, and, in cases of significant hydrocephalus, performing preoperative ventriculostomy drainage [6]. If the condition and time permit, the combination of image-guided navigation, intraoperative neuroelectrophysiological monitoring, and microsurgery can greatly enhance both the efficiency and safety of the surgery [7]. Modern imaging workstations can simulate surgical approaches, significantly improving surgical effectiveness and safety.

10.3.2 Surgical Instruments

The surgical equipment required includes a specialized dedicated electric operating table, neurosurgical operating microscope, navigation system, intraoperative neuroelectrophysiological monitoring device, head frame and automatic retractor, electric cranial drill, fine bipolar coagulation, monopolar electrocautery, and a set of fine microsurgical instruments.

10.4 Surgical Techniques and Precautions

10.4.1 Surgical Techniques

1. Positioning and Head Position

   The patient is typically positioned in a lateral decubitus or lateral prone position, with the affected side facing upward. The head should be flexed forward as much as possible and rotated 20° to 30° toward the opposite side based on the lateral position, so that the plane of the mastoid process is at the highest point in the surgical field [8]. The head is fixed with a pin-type head frame (Fig. 10.1).

2. Incision and Bone Window

   The superficial projection of the transverse sinus and sigmoid sinus is preliminarily determined. A linear incision, approximately 6 cm in length, is made downward from about 1.5–2 cm behind the root of the mastoid process. The incision's superior limit is positioned 1 cm above the junction line between the external occipital protuberance and the root of the mastoid process. The skin and subcutaneous tissues are sequentially incised, followed by the dissection of the deep muscular layers using an electric knife. Care should be taken as the occipital artery emerges from the origin of the trapezius to the termination point of the sternocleidomastoid muscle and passes through the subcutaneous tissue. After exploration, it should be thoroughly electrocoagulated and cut. A periosteal raspatory is used for subperiosteal dissection, and a mastoid retractor is used to expand the mastoid, exposing the local bony landmarks. A burr hole is drilled at the junction of the transverse sinus and sigmoid sinus. After the dura mater is dissected, a milling cutter is used to mill inward and downward in an arc shape, creating a bone window with a diameter of approximately 3 cm. The upper edge is horizontal to the lower margin of the transverse sinus, and the outer edge is posterior to the posterior margin of the sigmoid sinus.

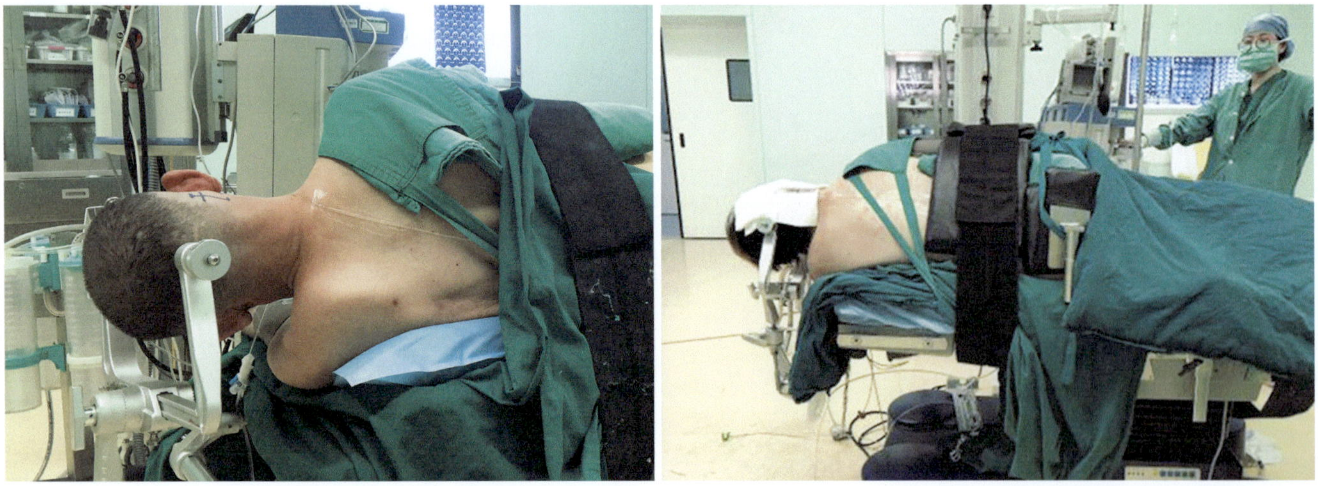

Fig. 10.1 Surgical positioning. Demonstrating the surgical incision, lateral decubitus position, and placement of the head frame

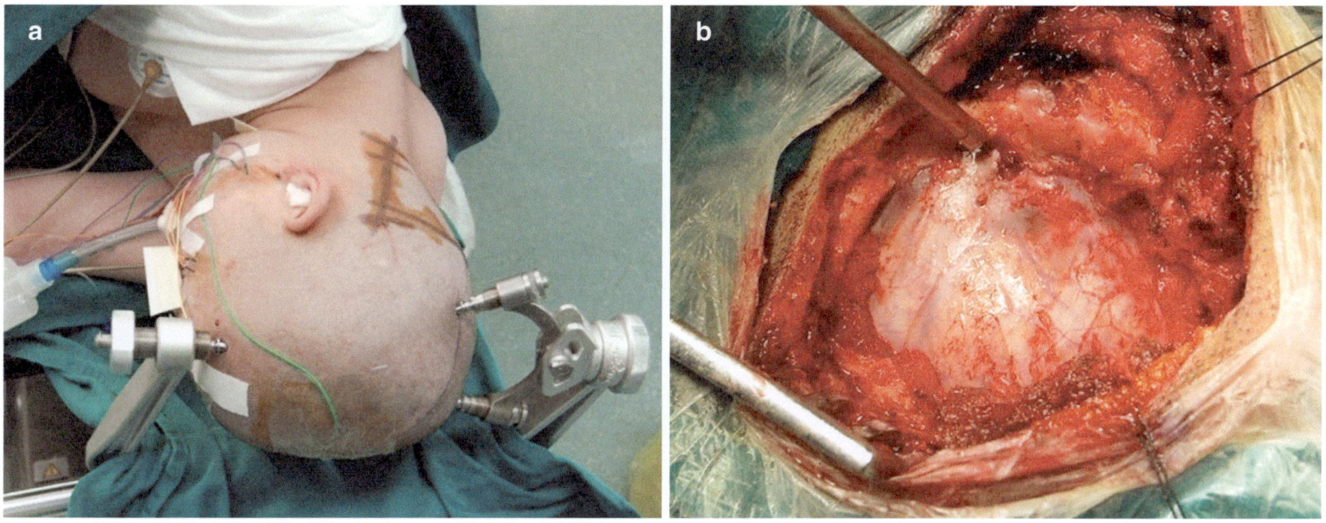

Fig. 10.2 Incision and bone window. (**a**). Illustration of the surgical incision location. (**b**) The bone window exposed to the junction of the transverse sinus and sigmoid sinus

Should the mastoid air cells be inadvertently opened during the procedure, they are sealed with bone wax to prevent complications. If necessary, the surrounding skull inner lamina on the edge of the bone window can be grounded away to expand the surgical field of view (Fig. 10.2).

3. Dural Incision

   The dura mater is incised in a flap-like manner to release cerebrospinal fluid. The base is located on the side of the sigmoid sinus. Under the microscope, the lateral aspect of the cerebellum is gently pulled inward, gradually deepening the dissection. This maneuver opens the lateral recess of the cerebellomedullary cistern, which facilitates the release of cerebrospinal fluid and consequently reduces intracranial pressure. The cerebellar hemisphere is gently pulled inward, gradually exposing the arachnoid membrane of the cerebellomedullary cistern and separating it. Further medial retraction of the cerebellar hemisphere is performed to enhance the exposure of the cerebellopontine angle, providing an expanded surgical field (Fig. 10.3).

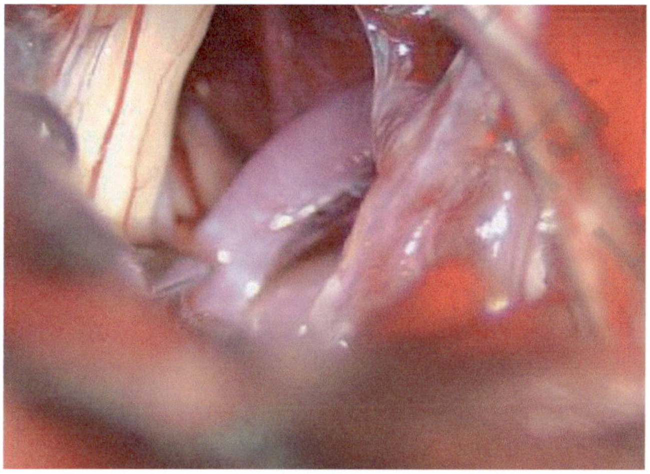

Fig. 10.3 Entry and exposure of the cerebellomedullary cistern. The dura mater is incised in a flap-like manner and suspended. The lateral recess of the cerebellomedullary cistern is opened, releasing cerebrospinal fluid to reduce intracranial pressure

4. Microscopic removal of Hematoma and Hemostasis in the Surgical Area

   After the brain pressure decreases, the cerebellar hemisphere is further pulled inward to expose the posterior group of cranial nerves. Using the posterior group of cranial nerves as a reference, the surgical field is systematically explored to gradually reveal the facial and auditory nerves, the anteroinferior cerebellar artery, the superior petrosal vein, and the trigeminal nerve. With the facial and auditory nerve as a reference, the surgical dissection is directed medially toward the lateral aspect of the pons. The hematoma that has entered the subarachnoid space can be seen as it passes through the interval between the trigeminal nerve and the facial nerve. The brainstem hematoma is extracted in segments through this interstitial space. Electrocoagulation is used judiciously within the hematoma bed, and the surgical site is covered with hemostatic gauze and gelatin sponge, followed by the placement of appropriate-sized cotton pads or cotton balls. An aspirator is used for compression and suction assistance, which generally achieves satisfactory hemostasis (Fig. 10.4).

5. Closure of the Cranium

   After confirming that there is no active bleeding in the hematoma cavity and achieving satisfactory hemostasis in the surgical area, the dura mater or artificial dura is sutured without leakage. The bone flap is repositioned and fixed with connecting plates. The muscle layers are intermittently sutured, and the tendon membrane layer is tightly sutured with high tension, with a recommended stitch interval of 5 mm. The scalp is closed using conventional sutures to complete the procedure (Fig. 10.5, Video 10.1).

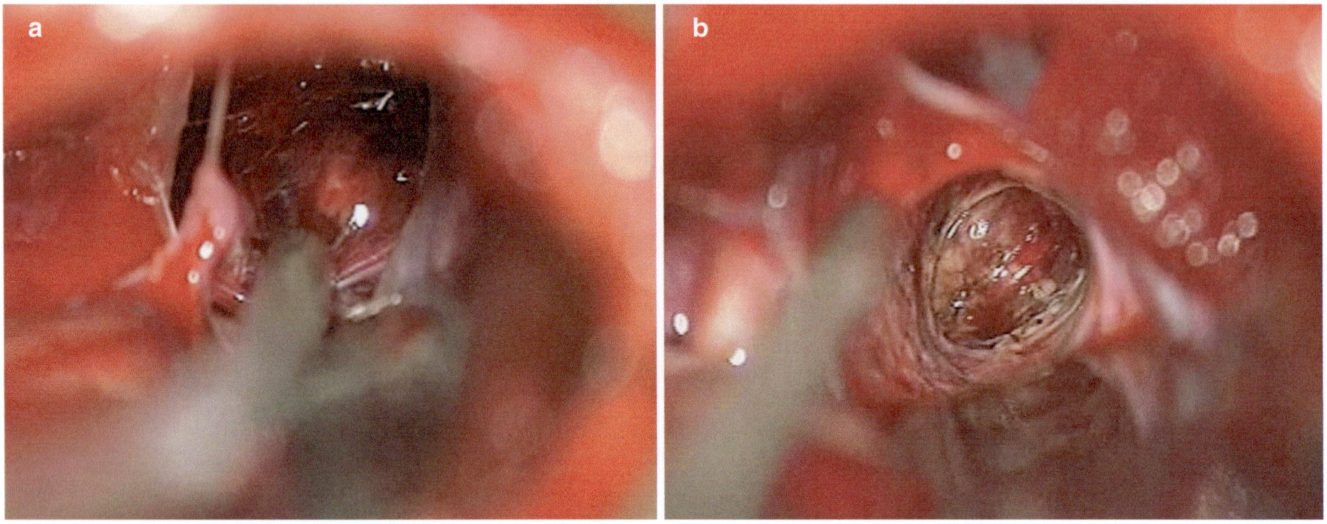

Fig. 10.4 Evacuation of brainstem hematoma. (**a**) The cerebellar petrosal surface is pulled open, and the lateral aspect of the brainstem is most exposed during the surgery (between the trigeminal nerve and the facial nerve). The hematoma ruptured through the brainstem cortex, and the hematoma is sucked out and cleared through the breakthrough point along the brainstem cortex. The black area below the suction device is the hematoma. (**b**) Satisfactory hemostasis in the residual cavity

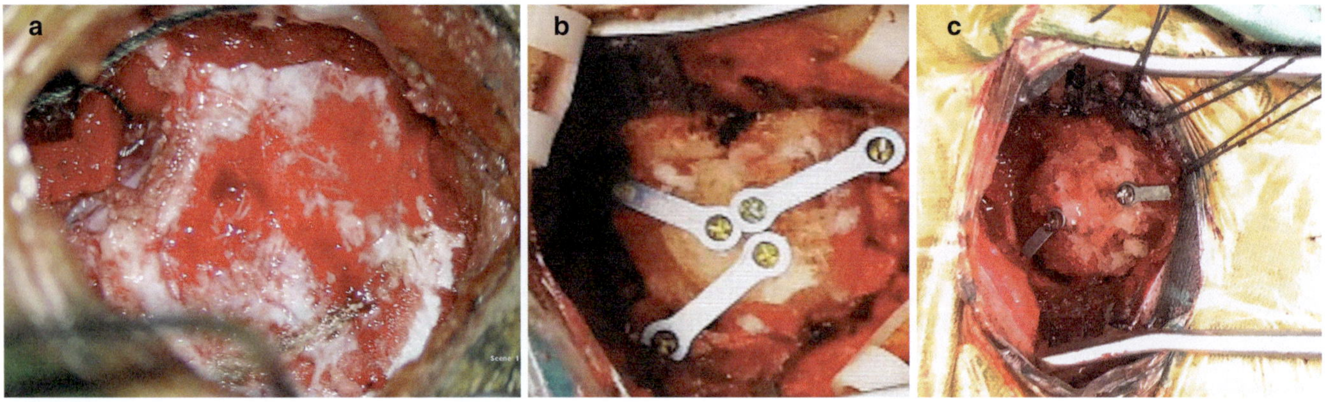

Fig. 10.5 Cranium closure. (**a**) Dura mater tightly sutured. (**b** and **c**) Bone flap repositioned and fixed with cranial connecting plates

10.4.2 Surgical Techniques and Precautions

1. The timing of the surgery should be carefully determined. Around 6 hours after post-brainstem hemorrhage (PBSH), edema and necrosis begin to appear around the hematoma. The surgical outcome is more favorable when the surgery is performed in the early stages of hemorrhage rather than 24 hours after the event.
2. Before the surgery, a lumbar drainage tube should be placed. Initially, it should be temporarily clamped, and once the bone flap is formed, the drain tube should be released to drain 30–50 mL of cerebrospinal fluid, which can reduce traction on the cerebellum.
3. During the craniotomy, it is important to prevent injury the venous sinuses, especially the sigmoid sinus. In patients with severe adhesions between the dura mater and the inner surface of the skull, a bone window with a diameter of approximately 2 cm can be created using a burr drill to prevent inadvertent penetration of the venous sinuses during craniotomy. The bone above the sigmoid sinus can be carefully polished with a burr drill, and the remaining thin bone can be removed with bone forceps.
4. After cutting the dura mater, gently retract the petrous surface of the cerebellum to release cerebrospinal fluid from the cerebellomedullary cistern. Once the intracranial pressure has significantly decreased, the arachnoid membrane in the cerebellopontine angle can be carefully dissected to expose the middle cerebellar peduncle and the lateral aspect of the pons.
5. During the surgery, the preferred approach is to access the brainstem through the site of hematoma rupture. Should this not be feasible, the safe zone of the brainstem can be used as an alternative option. Intraoperative navigation systems can be used to accurately locate the hematoma and the brainstem cortical fistula site.

6. During the clearance of the hematoma, fluctuations in evoked potentials provide accurate and sensitive electrophysiological indicators of brainstem functional activity, objectively reflecting the functional status of the brainstem and avoiding iatrogenic injury to the brainstem around the hematoma.
7. Whenever possible, suction should be involved within the hematoma cavity during the surgical procedure. This technique, when combined with irrigation, facilitates the loosening and piecemeal removal of blood clots. It is imperative to avoid penetrating the hematoma wall to prevent additional damage to the brainstem.
8. Microscopes have attenuation and blind spots in deep illumination. The use of neuroendoscopy in conjunction with a microscope enables clear deep illumination, eliminates surgical blind spots, allows close observation, improves hematoma clearance, and reduces secondary damage to the brainstem. It also facilitates thorough hemostasis and reduces the risk of postoperative rebleeding.
9. Efforts should be made to thoroughly remove the hematoma and relieve obstructive hydrocephalus.
10. Surgeons must proficiently employ hemostasis techniques to manage bleeding effectively. For active bleeding, fine bipolar electrocoagulation with low power is indicated. In cases of oozing from the wound, the wound can be covered with a water-moistened gelatin sponge or hemostatic gauze, followed by the application of gentle pressure using cotton pads to control hemorrhage.
11. Take measures to protect the draining veins to prevent postoperative exacerbation of brainstem edema and compression of neural tissues, which can lead to neurological deficits [7–9].

10.5 Postoperative Management and Prevention of Complications

1. Postoperative Rebleeding

   The primary cause of postoperative rebleeding is elevated blood pressure. Therefore, blood pressure should be stabilized and maintained within a target range of 130–140/70–90 mmHg in the postoperative period. Sedation and analgesia, as appropriate for the patient's condition, can assist in maintaining stable blood pressure.
2. Pulmonary Infection

   In comatose patients, postoperative sputum clearance may be compromised, leading to a high incidence of pulmonary infections. Early tracheostomy not only facilitates sputum removal but also reduces airway resistance, decreases dead space ventilation, enhances effective gas exchange in the alveoli, and improves cerebral oxygenation. Early ventilator support is recommended in cases of hypoxemia or respiratory failure. Following the diagnosis of pulmonary infection, appropriate antibiotics should be selected based on the results of sensitivity testing.
3. Stress Ulcer Bleeding

   Postoperative administration of proton pump inhibitors (PPIs) is indicated to prevent and mitigate the occurrence of acute gastric mucosal lesions induced by stress. Patients who are unable to eat for 24 h should be given a nasogastric tube for liquid feeding to protect the gastric mucosa. For patients with gastrointestinal bleeding, the administration of an intragastric infusion comprising an ice-saline solution with thrombin or a 0.02% epinephrine solution has been demonstrated to effectively manage hemorrhage.
4. Central Fever

   Central fever resulting from brainstem hemorrhage is a severe manifestation of brain injury and is characterized by noninfectious high fever, often reaching around 40 °C, which exacerbates brain damage and can lead to short-term mortality. In the postoperative period, physical cooling using ice blankets and caps can effectively reduce cerebral oxygen consumption and metabolic rates, alleviate brain edema, lower intracranial pressure, reduce neuronal damage, and promote functional recovery. However, caution should be exercised with the use of pharmacological cooling, as it may induce stress ulcers and should be employed judiciously to minimize such risks.
5. Internal Environment Monitoring and Rehabilitation

   Regular monitoring of electrolytes, liver and kidney function, and maintaining water and electrolyte balance are crucial for nutritional support therapy. If the patient regains consciousness, early neurorehabilitation and measures such as hyperbaric oxygen therapy should be initiated to improve the quality of survival.

10.6 Advantages, Disadvantages, and Lessons Learned

The suboccipital retrosigmoid approach is a classic surgical approach for lesions in the cerebellopontine angle region. The pons, located in the cerebellopontine angle region, is recognized as the most frequent site for brainstem hemorrhage. The approach allows for rapid access to the lateral aspect of the pons. The hematoma site often presents as a local bulge or discoloration. In cases where the hematoma ruptures, it becomes readily apparent within the surrounding ambient cistern. Longitudinal incision of the brain stem on one side at the site of the local bulge and the use of a micro-suction device under the microscope for hematoma clearance is minimally invasive, precise, and easy to perform, with minimal bleeding. During craniotomy, care should be taken to avoid damaging the transverse sinus and sigmoid sinus. If the mastoid air cells are opened, they must be properly sealed with bone wax. During exposure, care should be taken to avoid damaging the petrous vein, and every effort should be made to protect the draining veins to prevent postoperative exacerbation of brainstem edema and compression of neural tissues, which can lead to neurological deficits. The retrosigmoid approach has limited operating space and narrow exposure, making surgical procedures difficult. Inappropriate traction of brain tissue can cause more severe brain damage and should be avoided. The most effective method is to release cerebrospinal fluid by opening the cistern and allowing brain tissue to retract on its own. For some patients with high intracranial pressure, if diuretics are ineffective, ventricular puncture to release cerebrospinal fluid can be performed before surgery. Alternatively, a lumbar puncture to place a catheter in the subarachnoid space can be done before surgery to release cerebrospinal fluid and reduce intracranial pressure.

10.7 Evaluation and Perspective of Techniques

Suboccipital retrosigmoid approach for the treatment of PBSH exhibits a clear surgical field and a relatively short operation time. It is a proactive, straightforward, and effective surgical method, particularly suitable for cases of lateral pontine hemorrhage and unilateral occurrences. With the accumulation of microsurgical experience, improvement in microsurgical techniques, advancements in microsurgical instruments, and progress in neuroimaging technology, early clearance of brainstem hematoma via the suboccipital retrosigmoid approach significantly enhances the survival rate and quality of life for severe PBSH patients.

10.8 Typical Cases

10.8.1 Brief Medical History and Radiological Data

1. The patient, a male, 38 years old, presented with sudden consciousness disturbance and was admitted 3 hours after onset. He had a 5-year history of hypertension and was regularly taking antihypertensive medication.
2. Physical examination blood pressure of 151/78 mmHg, weak respiration at 16 times/min, a heart rate of 102 times/min, and a body temperature of 39 °C. The patient was in a shallow coma with a GCS score of 6. His pupils were equal and round bilaterally, approximately 2.0 mm in diameter, with a sensitive light reflex. There was no response to painful stimuli on the left side, but a localized response on the right side, and positive Babinski sign bilaterally.
3. Auxiliary examination: Head CT revealed a pontine hemorrhage, estimated at about 8mL (Fig. 10.6).
4. Admission diagnosis: Brainstem hemorrhage (anterolateral pontine); Grade 3 hypertension (extremely high-risk group).

10.8.2 Surgical Procedure and Key Points

Under general anesthesia, the patient was positioned on the right lateral decubitus postition. After routine disinfection and draping, a 6 cm straight incision was made behind the

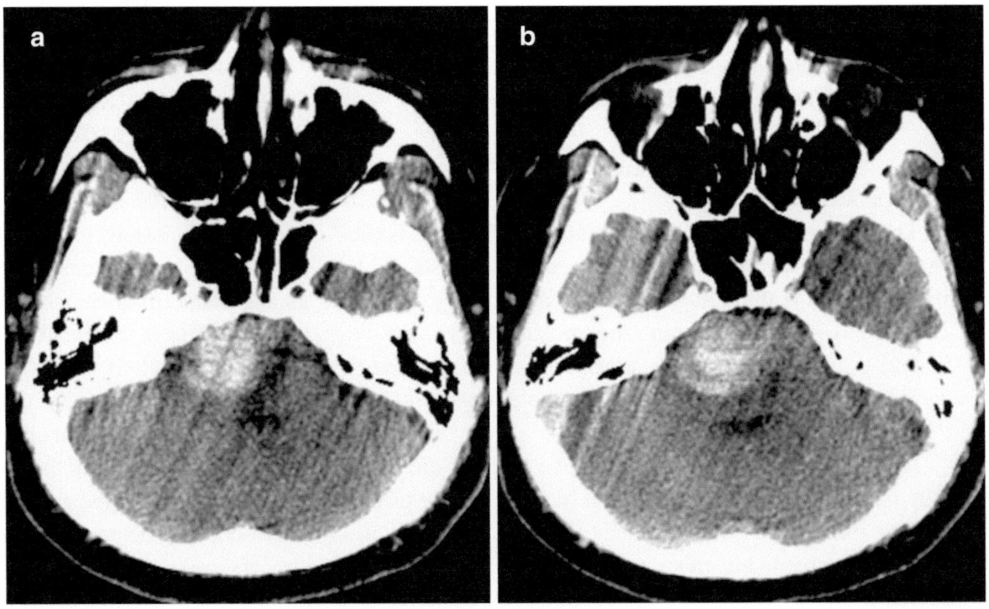

Fig. 10.6 (**a**) Emergency CT scan for patient with pontine hemorrhage. (**b**) Emergency CT showing acute pontine hematoma, approximately 8mL in volume

left mastoid process. The scalp and muscles were incised to expose the apex of the digastric groove. A keyhole was created using a drill, and a 3 cm bone flap was formed. The dura mater was opened in an arc shape and suspended. Cerebrospinal fluid was slowly released from the cerebellomedullary cistern until a satisfactory reduction of intracranial pressure was achieved. The cerebellar hemisphere was retracted, and the hematoma was visualized between the entry and exit of the facial and auditory nerves and trigeminal nerves in the brainstem. A 1–1.5 mm diameter suction device was used to gently and slowly evacuate the hematoma along the site of rupture. Hemostasis was achieved satisfactorily within the residual cavity. The dura mater was meticulously sutured, the bone flap was replaced, and the scalp was closed in layers with sterile dressings applied.

10.8.3 Postoperative Imaging and Recovery

1. On the first day after surgery, the patient remained in a shallow coma. His pupils were equal and round bilaterally, measuring 1.5 mm in diameter, with a sensitive light reflex. There was a localized response to painful stimuli on the left side but no response on the right side (Fig. 10.7).
2. Three months postoperatively, a follow-up CT scan revealed a small softening lesion in the pons in the absence of hydrocephalus (Figs. 10.8).
3. Neurological examination 3 months after the operation showed the patient to be conscious with equal and reactive pupils. Muscle strength in the left lower limb was at Grade IV, while the right upper limb was at Grade IV-, and the right lower limb was at Grade V. Bilateral Babinski signs were negative (Fig. 10.9).

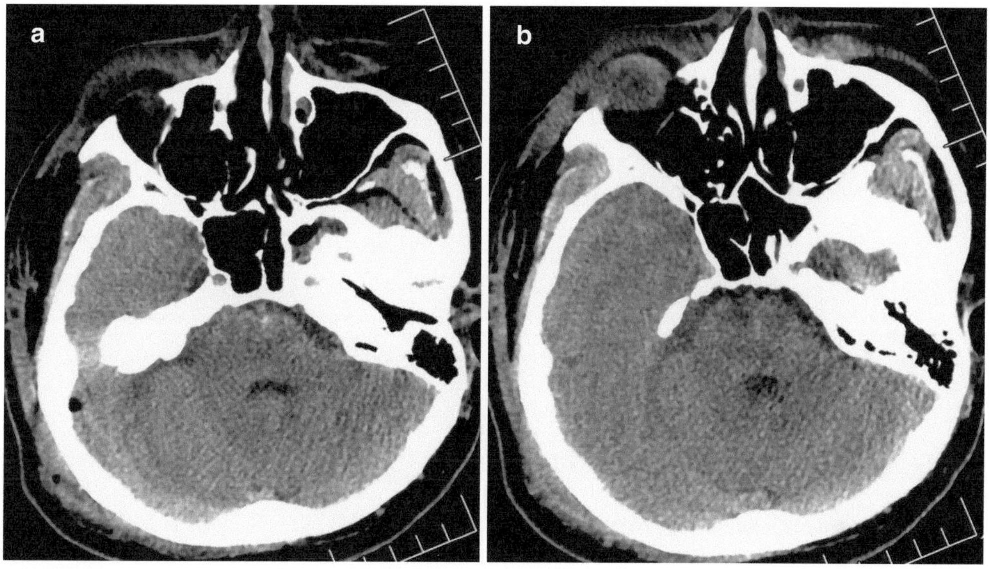

Fig. 10.7 (**a**) Postoperative CT on the first day. (**b**) Postoperative CT on the first day showing complete clearance of the intracranial hematoma

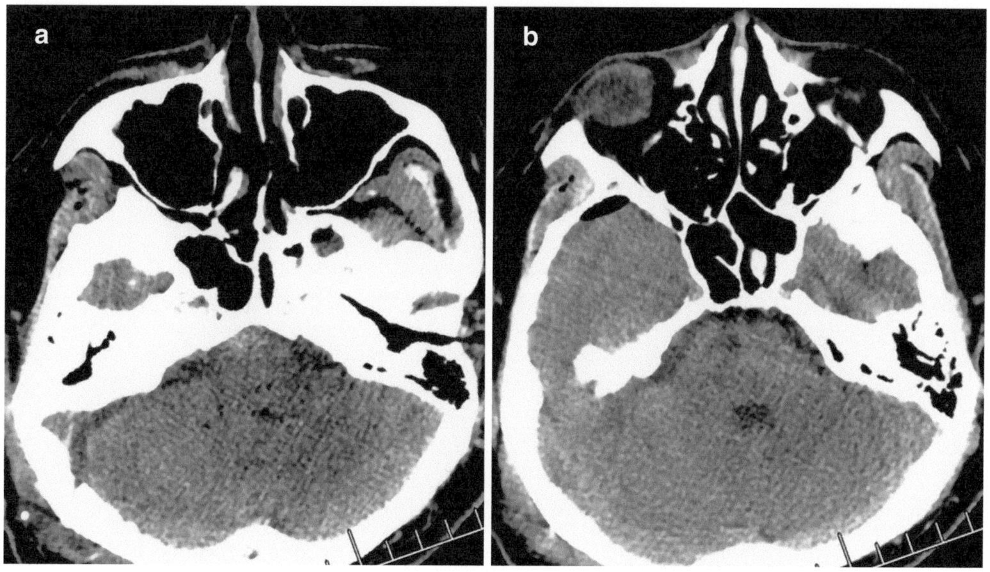

Fig. 10.8 (**a**) Postoperative head CT at 3 months. (**b**) Postoperative head CT at 3 months showing a small softening lesion in the pons and normal ventricular size

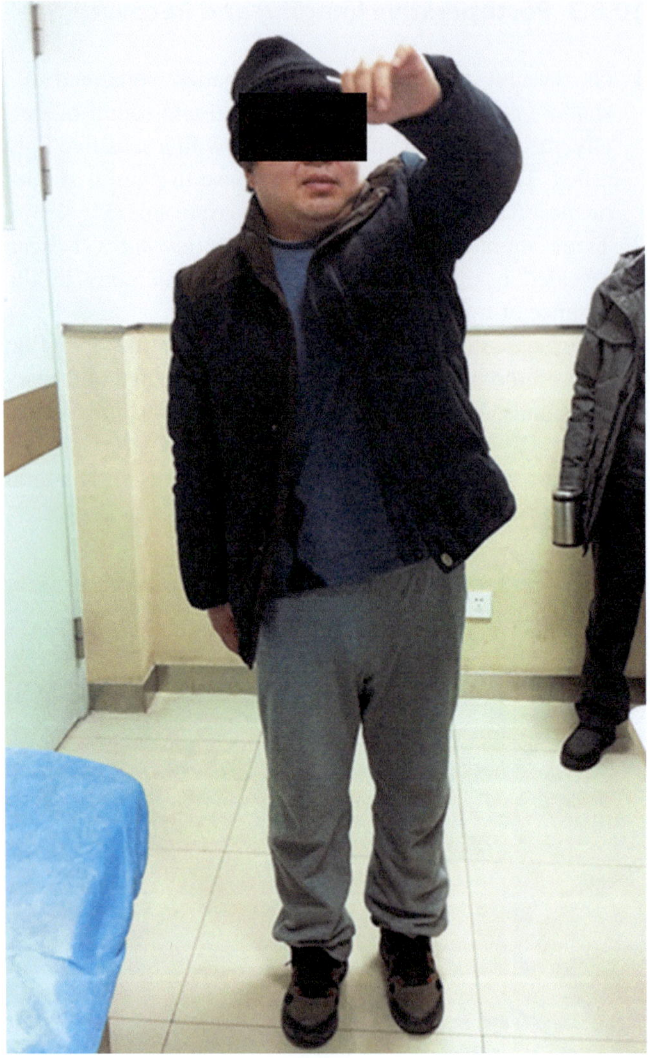

Fig. 10.9 Patient's condition at 3 months postoperatively. Patient's condition at 3 months postoperatively, demonstrating clear consciousness, equal and reactive pupils, and specific muscle strength assessment

References

1. Chen LH, Wei Q, Xu RX, et al. Minimally invasive surgical treatment of primary brainstem hemorrhage. J Clin Neurosurg. 2015;12(5):349–53.
2. Hao L, Li GP, You C, et al. Microsurgical treatment of PBSH: clinical analysis of 21 cases. Chinese J Neurosurg. 2007;23:944.
3. Chen LH, Xu RX. Minimally invasive treatment of primary brainstem hemorrhage. Chinese J Electron Trauma Neurosurg. 2016;2(4):252–4.
4. Liu X, Li H, Hu X, et al. Discussion on the treatment of spontaneous brainstem hemorrhage. J Clin Neurosurg. 2013;10:287.
5. Shi H, Zhou H, Wang FY, et al. Surgery via the tela choroidea sail route for hypertensive pontine hemorrhage. J Clin Neurosurg. 2017;14(1):49–51.
6. Zhang YF, He SM, Lv WH, et al. Observation of the efffcacy of microsurgical treatment for primary brainstem hemorrhage. Chinese J Clin Neurosurg. 2014;19(4):200–2.
7. Li H, Liu WK, Lin S, et al. Discussion on the treatment of primary brainstem hemorrhage. Chinese J Neurosurg. 2013;29(4):339–41.
8. Liang JG, Dong J, Qu MQ, et al. Neuroendoscopic-assisted surgical treatment of brainstem hemorrhage penetrating the fourth ventricle. Chinese J Neurol. 2013;12:197.
9. Li J, Zheng J. Insights into microsurgical treatment of primary brainstem hemorrhage. Chinese J Neurosurg. 2017;33(2):184–5.

11 Surgical Evacuation of Brainstem Hematoma Via the Posterior Median Approach

Gang Chen, Linsen Mu, Junfeng Huo, Xin Gao, and Zong Dai

11.1 Overview

In the surgical evacuation of brainstem hematoma via the posterior median approach, the "telovelar approach" and the "transvermian approach" are the two most commonly used approaches. The "transvermian approach" requires an incision of the vermis structure to reach the midline portion of the fourth ventricle, which often leads to nystagmus, dysarthria, ataxic gait, trunk ataxia, and balance disturbances [1, 2]. In contrast, the "telovelar approach" allows for a natural cleavage to access the fourth ventricle, eliminating the risk of neurological deficits associated with the approach [3]. Consequently, an increasing number of neurosurgeons are inclined to choose the "telovelar approach" as the preferred approach for exposing the floor of the fourth ventricle. This chapter primarily discusses the relevant technical points of this approach.

11.2 Indications and Contraindications

11.2.1 Indications

1. Hematoma extends beyond the maximal level of the brainstem by more than 50%, resulting in brainstem displacement or significant mass effect, particularly when located in the middle and lower portion of the pons and the dorsolateral medulla, in close proximity to the floor of the fourth ventricle.
2. GCS < 8, severe neurological impairment, or progressive deterioration, with an anticipated better outcome from surgical intervention compared to conservative treatment.
3. Brainstem hemorrhage >5 mL, with bleeding penetrating into the ventricle or causing obstructive hydrocephalus.
4. Hematoma located at the dorsolateral medulla and middle-lower pons, with penetration toward the floor of the fourth ventricle or a tendency to approach it closely.
5. Strong desire for resuscitation from the patient's family, actively seeking surgery despite being informed of poor prognosis [4–6].

11.2.2 Contraindications

1. Hematoma shows no increase after conservative treatment, and brainstem edema is controllable.
2. Hematoma volume is less than 5 mL, or the maximal level does not extend beyond 50% of the maximal level of the brainstem, without a significant mass effect.
3. GCS ≥ 8, with good consciousness and no apparent neurological deficits.
4. Deep coma, irreversible brainstem dysfunction, brain herniation, bilateral fixed and dilated pupils, loss of spontaneous respiration, circulatory failure, extremely unstable vital signs, and a GCS score of 5 or lower, resulting in a high expected mortality and severe disability post-surgery, serving as a relative contraindication for surgery.
5. The presence of other surgical contraindications, such as severe coagulation disorders, inability to tolerate general anesthesia due to cardiopulmonary dysfunction, etc.

Supplementary Information The online version contains supplementary material available at https://doi.org/10.1007/978-981-95-8942-5_11.

G. Chen (✉)
Department of Neurosurgery, Zhuhai People's Hospital (The Affiliated Hospital of Beijing Institute of Technology, Zhuhai Clinical Medical College of Jinan University), Zhuhai, China

L. Mu · X. Gao · Z. Dai
Department of Neurosurgery, Guangdong Sanjiu Brain Hospital, Guangzhou, China

J. Huo
Department of Neurosurgery, Shanghai Donglei Brain Hospital, Shanghai, China

G. Chen, C. You (eds.), *Surgical Treatment of Primary Brainstem Hemorrhage*, https://doi.org/10.1007/978-981-95-8942-5_11

6. Diffuse bleeding, making it difficult to achieve sufficient decompression through surgery.
7. Refusal by the patient's family [4–8].

11.3 Preoperative Preparation and Surgical Instruments

11.3.1 Preoperative Preparation

1. Preoperative CT examination is necessary to determine the axial and sagittal positions of the hematoma and assess the condition of the atlantooccipital region and cervical spine joints [9, 10].
2. Complete biochemical tests and evaluate circulatory function to rule out common surgical contraindications.
3. Prepare the occipital area for skin preparation, and arrange for intraoperative administration of steroid medications and blood preparation.
4. Engage in thorough communication with the patient's family regarding surgical risks and unfavorable prognosis, ensuring their understanding.

11.3.2 Surgical Instruments

Microscope, head fixation device, brain spatula, intraoperative electrophysiological monitoring equipment, and neurosurgical microinstruments. Neuroendoscope, serving as an observational tool, provides additional perspectives and clearer imaging during the surgery [11].

11.4 Surgical Techniques, Considerations, and Tips

11.4.1 Surgical Techniques

The fundamental principle of the surgery is to protect brainstem function to the greatest extent possible while effectively evacuating the hematoma and alleviating mass effects and irritation on brain cells caused by the hematoma. Intraoperative electrophysiological monitoring and neuronavigation devices can be utilized as adjuncts to achieve a safe, minimally invasive, and expedient surgical approach.

1. Positioning: The "park bench position" and the "prone position" with the Mayfield head fixation device are the commonly used surgical positions (Fig. 11.1).

   (a) Park Bench Position (also Known as "Lateral Decubitus Position")

   Advantages: The positioning is convenient and easily achievable, allowing the surgeon to operate in a seated position. The "surgical field" is roughly parallel to the ground, facilitating drainage of blood and cerebrospinal fluid from the surgical area. There is minimal interference with the patient's vital sign monitoring during the procedure.

   Disadvantages: In this position, the handle of the microscope and the patient's back tissue often come into contact, sometimes obstructing the microscope's light from reaching the position of the opening of the mesencephalic aqueduct, thus hindering better exposure of the structures in the rostral direction of the floor of the fourth ventricle. Muscles and ligaments in the neck and shoulder area are prone to strain, and there is a higher likelihood of twisting and damaging the vertebral artery. Additionally, this position places the surgeon's arms in a constantly extended and tense state during the operation, leading to potential fatigue [12].

   (b) Prone Position

   Advantages: The positioning is simple, making it easy to identify the midline position. The surgeon's "top" and "side" microsurgical operation positions are more comfortable and less fatiguing. There is a high degree of freedom for microscope observation, allowing for easy exposure of the floor of the fourth ventricle and the mesencephalic aqueduct opening.

   Disadvantages: The surgeon often needs to adopt a "standing" position for the operation. Tracheal intubation is prone to distortion, and with pressure on the chest, it increases airway pressure, leading to potential interference with intraoperative vital sign monitoring. Without a head fixation device, there is a risk of pressure-related injury to the eyes and nose.

   In both of the above positioning methods, the patient's head should be positioned above the level of the heart to alleviate venous congestion in the head and reduce intracranial pressure.

2. Scalp, Soft Tissue, and Skull Handling

   The posterior midline incision starts from 2.0 cm above the external occipital protuberance and extends down to the level of C3–C4. After incising the scalp, the fatty connective tissue is dissected along the midline using an electric scalpel, exposing the external occipital protuberance, posterior arch of the atlas, and spinous process of the axis. The suboccipital muscles are dissected (a large piece of periosteum can be preserved for repairing the dura mater if needed), revealing the occipital bone, foramen magnum, and the vertebral arch of the atlas. Due

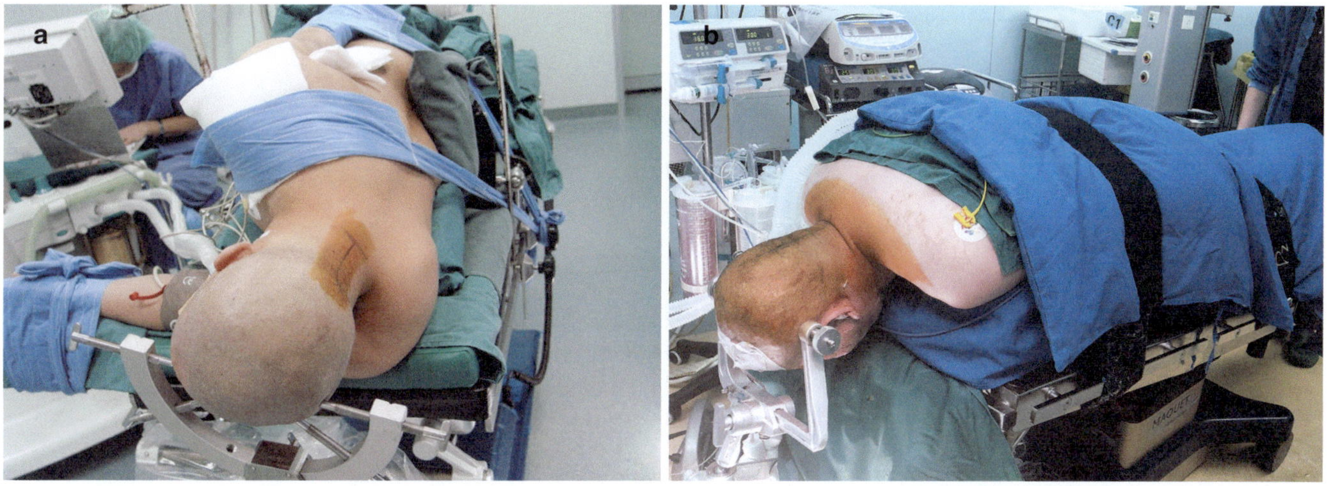

Fig. 11.1 Positions. (**a**) Park bench position, tilting the patient's head downward at a 45° angle and securing it with the head fixation device. (**b**) Prone position with the head elevated above the heart level to facilitate venous return and reduce intracranial pressure

to the lack of bony structures between the foramen magnum and the atlas, the electric scalpel should be used with reduced current to avoid damaging the dura mater and vertebral artery. Blunt dissection in the area of the vertebral plate of the atlas is recommended.

Two burr holes are drilled on both sides of the midline below the external occipital protuberance, and then a milling cutter is used to assist in freeing the occipital bone flap, which is the common practice for most surgeons. Personally, I prefer to directly drill a burr hole on the midline below the external occipital protuberance and use a burr to detach the cristae occipitalis interna within the hole. Then, a milling cutter is used to free the bone flap from the hole, and the edge of the foramen magnum is carefully removed using a powered cranial drill. Subsequently, the bone flap is pried open, and the cut end of the bone in the foramen magnum is further refined using a burr, ultimately forming a bone flap approximately 4 cm x 4 cm in size. The opening of the vertebral plate of the atlas is necessary to achieve an unobstructed optical pathway for the microscope toward the rostral of the floor of the fourth ventricle.

3. The Management of the Dura Mater and Arachnoid

   "Y"-shaped incision of the dura mater is a natural and reasonable selection. This design allows for the maximum exposure of the "target surgical area" with minimal incision distance. The incised occipital sinus is sutured, and the dural flap is flipped and secured to the skin, avoiding the use of electrocoagulation for dural hemostasis to ensure the final watetight suture closure. The arachnoid membrane of the cisterna magna is incised in midline and is suspended under the dura mater with sutures, exposing the cerebellar tonsils, inner side of lobulus biventer, the vermis, the pyramis vermis, the junction of the medulla and the cervical medulla, the foramen of Magendie, and the posterior inferior cerebellar artery (PICA).

4. Exposure of the Fourth Ventricle

   A brain spatula is used to pull the tonsils outward and upward, thus exposing the lower part of the cerebellomedullary space. After achieving better exposure of the vermis, the brain spatula is used to pull the vermis inward and upward, subsequently revealing the choroid and the inferior medullary velum. Electrocoagulation of the microvessels on the choroid and inferior medullary velum, followed by microscopically cutting these membranous structures, can thoroughly expose the floor of the fourth ventricle, the opening of the aqueduct, and the lateral recess of the same side. Throughout the dissection of these structures, every effort is made to prudently preserve each branch of the PICA (Fig. 11.2).

5. Evacuation of Hematoma and Hemostasis in the Surgical Area

   In cases of brainstem hemorrhage rupturing into the fourth ventricle, the hematoma is initially evacuated. Subsequently, the floor of the fourth ventricle is exposed, and the location of the hematoma can be accurately determined through the ruptured site on the surface of the brain stem. If the hematoma is entirely within the brain stem, its location can be determined by observing the slightly bulge, bluish-gray area on the dorsal aspect of the pons, just above the medullary striae. A 5–10 mm incision is made at this site to access the hematoma cavity. Before incising the brain stem, superficial small blood vessels are preferably coagulated using low-flow electrocautery to minimize damage to the brain stem by bipolar coagulation. The micro-forceps enter the orificium fistulae with a closed position and then bluntly expand the incision. A suction device with a diameter smaller than 2.0 mm is used whenever possible. The suction pressure is adjusted, and gentle manipulation with the micro-dissector is performed at the center of the hematoma to "fragmentally

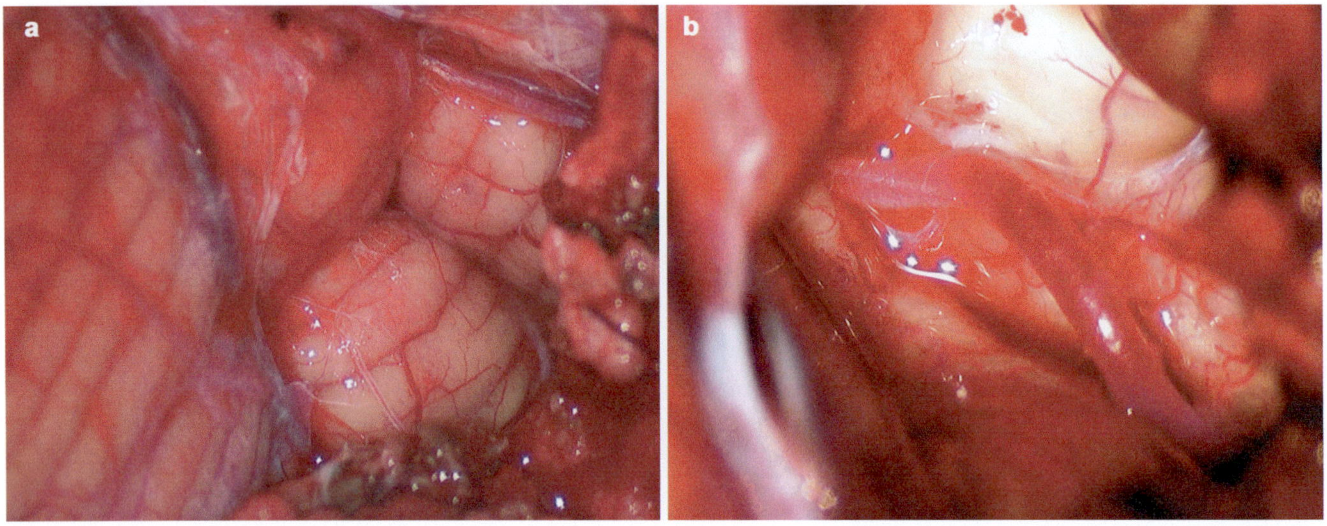

Fig. 11.2 Exposure of the fourth ventricle during craniotomy. Revealing the dural sinus after removing the occipital bone. (**a**) Surface anatomy of the cerebellum. (**b**) exposure of the inferior medullary velum and choroid after retracting the tonsils, the fourth ventricle was then exposed

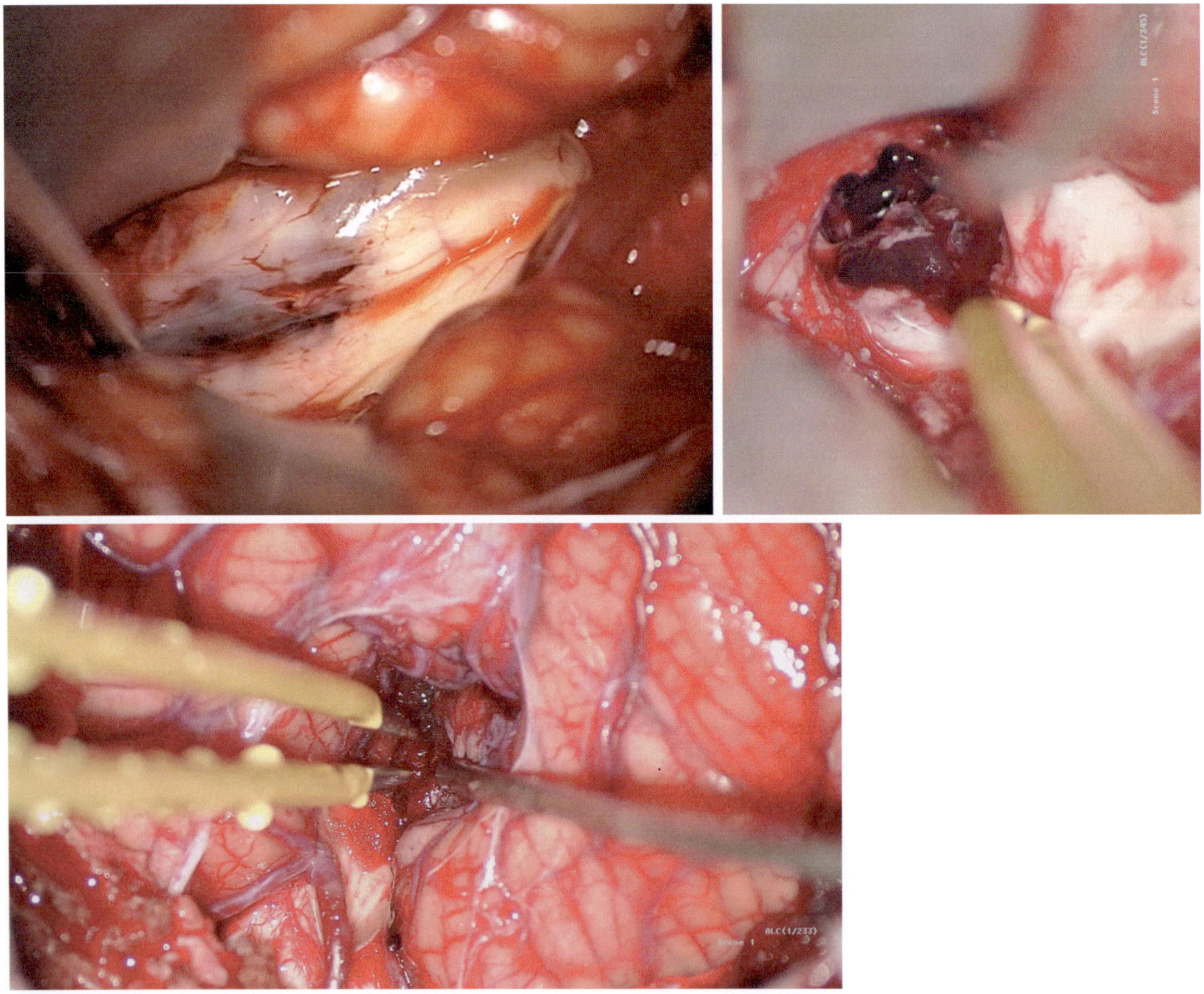

Fig. 11.3 Hematoma evacuation. After dissecting the tonsils, separating the inferior medullary velum and choroid, the location of the hematoma protruding from the brainstem surface can be accurately identified and evacuated, achieving satisfactory hemostasis in the surgical area

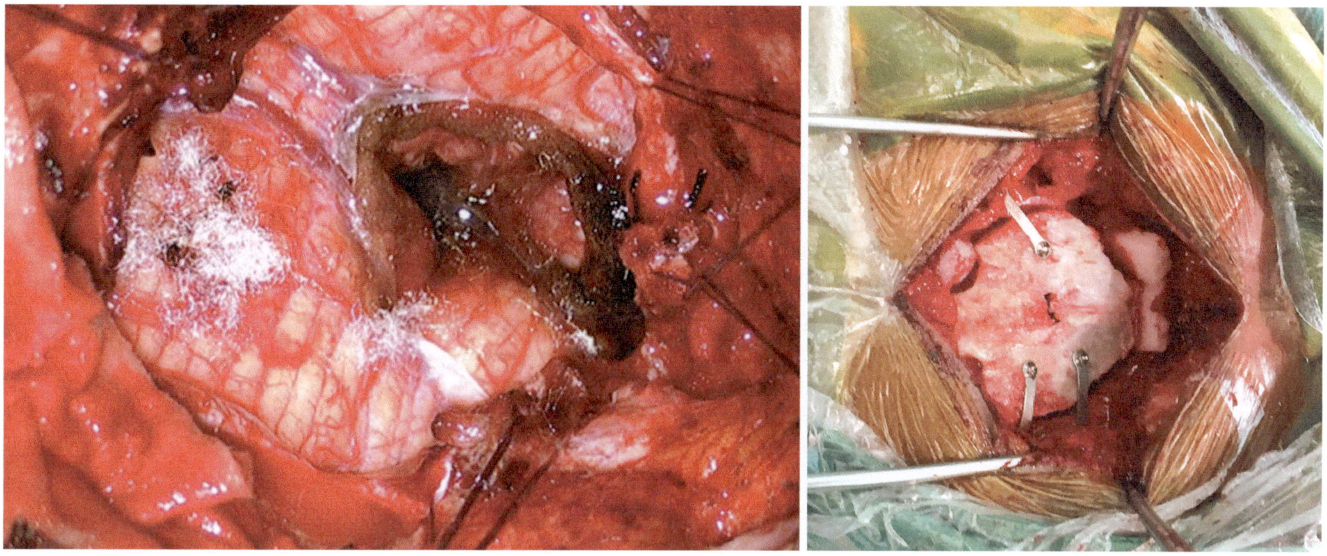

Fig. 11.4 Closure. Using cervical fascia or artificial dura mater for watertight suturing of the dura mater, followed by replacement and fixation of the bone flap

aspirate" and remove the hematoma while minimizing disruption of the normal brainstem interface within the hematoma cavity. Frequent use of electrocoagulation for hemostasis is avoided at the hematoma bed. Hemostatic sponges are placed over the wound, followed by appropriate-sized cotton pads or balls, and hemostasis is generally achieved with the assistance of a suction device (Fig. 11.3).

6. Closure

After achieving hemostasis within the hematoma cavity, further exploration under the microscope is necessary to ensure the patency of the aqueduct opening, preventing postoperative obstructive hydrocephalus due to hematoma blockage. The cervical fascia or artificial dura mater is taken, and the dura mater is sutured watertightly. The bone flap replacement and fixation are performed using a connecting plate. The material of the connecting plate should be chosen to avoid interference with magnetic resonance imaging. The muscles in the midline of the neck are gently sutured, as excessive tension in muscle closure may lead to postoperative muscle necrosis and neck pain, while the tendon membrane layer requires meticulous, high-tension suturing (Fig. 11.4, Video 11.1).

11.5 Postoperative Management and Prevention of Complications

Damage to the nuclei caused by brainstem hematoma can lead to long-term coma in patients as well as induce a series of complications such as muscle spasms, respiratory failure, hoarseness, coughing, digestive ulcers, aspiration pneumonia, and deep vein thrombosis in the lower limbs. Postoperatively, strict control of blood pressure stability, hemostasis, antiacid treatment, anti-inflammatory medication, prevention of pressure sores, and measures to prevent lower limb thrombosis are necessary. For patients expected to be in a prolonged coma, early tracheostomy is recommended for airway management. Short-term use of corticosteroids can alleviate brain edema and secondary brainstem injury. The use of nimodipine can improve local circulation, prevent cerebral vasospasm, and other ischemic-related secondary damage. In some patients, deep occipital subcutaneous effusions and cerebrospinal fluid leakage may be seen after surgery. In addition to the emphasized "watertight dural closure" mentioned earlier, the "external drainage of the lumbar cistern" method can be employed to address these complications.

11.6 Advantages, Disadvantages, and Lessons Learned

1. This surgical technique utilizes natural anatomical spaces to access the hematoma area, obviating the need to open the vermis of the cerebellum, thereby achieving the goal of removing brainstem hematoma with minimal secondary damage and a lower probability of neurological complications. Simultaneously, hematomas in the fourth ventricle and at the aqueduct opening can be evacuated, restoring the cerebrospinal fluid circulation pathway and resolving obstructive hydrocephalus in patients.
2. During the surgery, it is crucial to focus on protecting the PICA and its branches. In some cases, when PICA branches obstruct the inferior medullary velum, after cauterization and disconnection, postoperative cerebellar edema has been observed in some patients. This may also be related to brain contusion caused by traction during

the surgery and vascular spasm induced by vascular involvement. Therefore, gentle handling and minimizing vascular disconnection are key factors in reducing postoperative brain edema [13]. If there is concomitant obstructive hydrocephalus before the surgery, prioritize external ventricular drainage during the procedure to reduce posterior fossa pressure, minimize secondary damage caused by brain spatula, and facilitate exposure of deep structures of the fourth ventricle.

3. In cases of cerebellar hemorrhage, the size of the bone flap opening can be determined based on the volume and location of the intracerebral hemorrhage. In some cases, postoperative posterior fossa pressure increases, disappearance of the ambient cistern, and continued compression of the brainstem causing circulation failure due to factors such as traction on the cerebellum, cerebellar lobe hematoma, and preoperative ischemia and hypoxia. For such cases, it is recommended to simultaneously perform intracranial and/or extracranial decompression of the posterior fossa while removing the brainstem hematoma [6, 14].

11.7 Surgical Evaluation and Prospects

The telovelar approach utilizes natural anatomical interspaces around the fourth ventricle, without damaging the vermis of the cerebellum, to expose various aspects of the fourth ventricle, providing the optimal surgical pathway for clearing pons hematomas adjacent to the floor of the fourth ventricle. As this approach gradually gains wider acceptance and with the continuous improvement in microscopic surgical training for neurosurgeons at all levels of hospitals, this minimally invasive surgical approach will undoubtedly benefit more patients meeting the surgical indications.

However, as we proceed with the clearance of brainstem hematomas using this approach, there are issues worth further exploration, such as whether the range of occipital bone flaps can be further reduced, whether the resection of the posterior arch of the atlas is necessary, and how this approach compares to the current "stereotactic introcerebellar brainstem hematoma aspiration" in terms of minimally invasive nature and potential for wider application.

In recent years, with the widespread application of neuroendoscopy techniques, the surgical removal of intracranial hematomas has been performed entirely under endoscopy. Choosing the appropriate endoscopic endoport or using neuroendoscopy as an observation tool will provide the "telovelar approach" with a more unique surgical perspective, and the design of incisions, muscles, and bone flaps may become even more minimally invasive as a result [14, 15].

11.8 Typical Cases

11.8.1 Case One

11.8.1.1 Brief Medical History and Imaging Data

The patient is a 46-year-old male who was admitted with a chief complaint of "sudden onset of unconsciousness for 2 hours." Physical examination: heart rate 101 beats/min, respiratory rate 26 breaths/min, and blood pressure 185/110 mmHg. The patient presented with light coma, posterior tongue falling, bilateral pupils equal round and approximately 2.5 mm in diameter, light reflex disappeared, and bilateral Babinski signs were positive; head CT scan showed a brainstem hematoma, approximately 5 mL in volume (Fig. 11.5). Admission diagnosis: brainstem hemorrhage (anterolateral pontine region), grade 3 hypertension (extremely high-risk group).

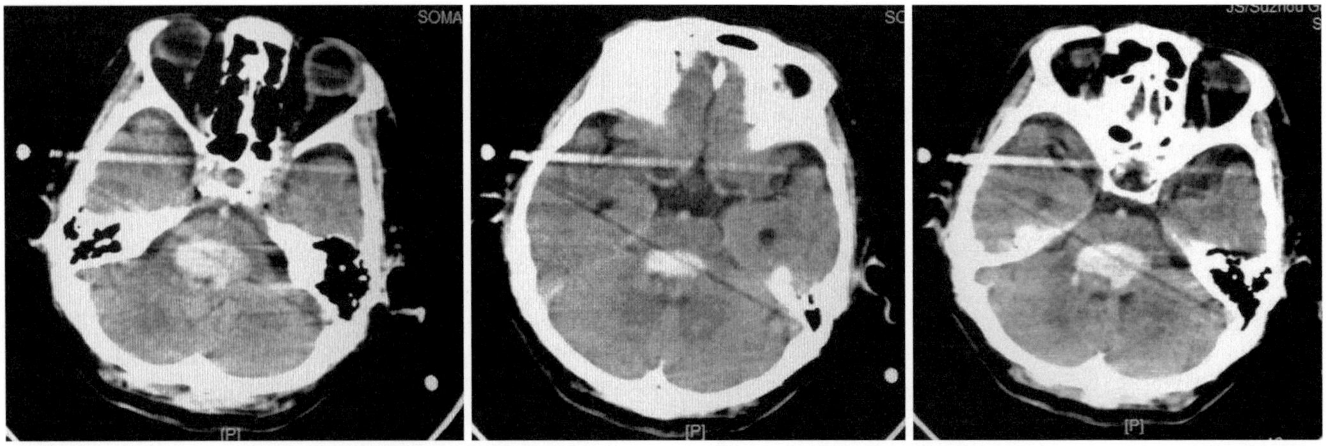

Fig. 11.5 Typical case one. Preoperative CT: hematoma located in pons, adjust to the floor of the fourth ventricle

11.8.1.2 Surgical Procedure and Key Points

The patient was placed in a prone position. The posterior median was marked for the incision site. The subcutaneous fat layer was incised along the midline, and the muscles of the posterior occipital and suboccipital region were divided to both sides, exposing the occipital bone, the inferior nuchal line, the foramen magnum, and the posterior arch of the atlas. A hole was drilled 0.5–1.0 cm below the external occipital protuberance, and the remaining cristae occipitalis interna was carefully ground away using a burr. Along the burr hole and downward, the milling cutter was used to create an arc-shaped opening in the occipital bone, reaching the edges of the foramen magnum on both sides. The thickened edges of the foramen magnum were further smoothed ground away with a 3 mm diameter burr until a thin "internal edge plate of the foramen magnum" was retained. The bone flap was lifted using a periosteal dissector, revealing the close adhesion between the occipital internal plate of the foramen magnum and the atlantooccipital fascia. At this point, a No. 11 blade was used to sharply free the attachment between the atlantooccipital fascia and occipital bone, or monopolar electrocoagulation was used for separation. After the bone flap was freed, a circular bone window with a diameter of approximately 4–6 cm was created.

The dura mater was incised in a "Y" shape, with attention paid to protecting the subdural cortical tissue. Simultaneous attention was given to protecting the occipital sinus. The severed occipital sinus was sutured for hemostasis, and the dura mater was suspended to expose the bilateral cerebellar tonsils, the vermis, and the "cortical segment" of the posterior inferior cerebellar artery (in this case, the left cerebellar tonsil shifted to the contralateral side). The bilateral cerebellar tonsils were retracted to fully expose the cerebellar vallecula, revealing the lower part of the floor of the fourth ventricle, the obex, the area postrema, and the opening of the central canal.

With the assistance of a brain spatula, the vermis was pulled to the right, and the left cerebellar tonsil was pulled laterally, revealing the choroid structure, which was cauterized and then incised. After incising the choroid, further exposure toward the lateral recess revealed the slightly thickened "inferior medullary velum" structure. Incising the "inferior medullary velum" provided a broader space at the floor of the fourth ventricle. As the hematoma appeared dark brown, under the cover of thin white matter, a "gray-blue" shadow could be seen on the floor of the fourth ventricle, which was the site of the fistula. Creating a fistula in this area revealed a dark hematoma. Micro-forceps and a suction device were used in combination to carefully flip and remove the blood clot. In the case of bridging vessels, electrocoagulation was used for cauterization and disconnection. After removing all clots, low-current bipolar electrocoagulation was used to achieve hemostasis within the hematoma cavity. To protect more brainstem tissue and reduce the secondary damage from electrocoagulation, a thin layer of gelatin sponge was placed between the bipolar forceps and the brainstem to allow for gentle heat transfer. Slow bleeding from the hematoma cavity was managed by applying hemostatic gauze and cotton, which generally achieved effective hemostasis. It is recommended that during this step, a combined "irrigation-suction" operation be performed to observe the hematoma cavity for at least 5 minutes, ensuring more thorough and appropriate hemostasis (Figs. 11.6 and 11.7).

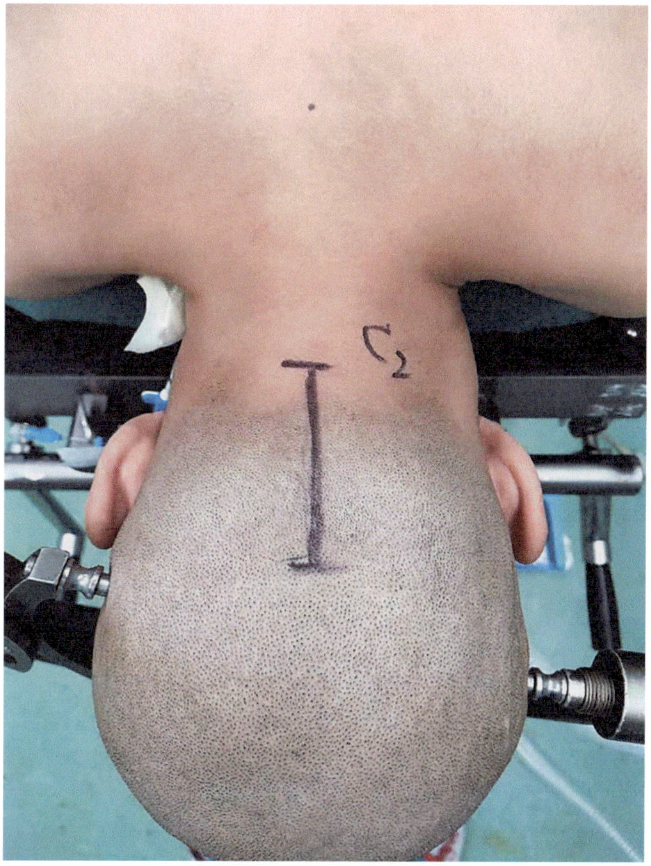

Fig. 11.6 Posterior median incision. A midline incision was made to free the bone flap and expose the dura mater

11.8.1.3 Comparison of Preoperative and Postoperative Imaging (Fig. 11.8).

11.8.2 Case Two

11.8.2.1 Brief Medical History and Imaging Data

The patient, a 36-year-old male, was admitted with a chief complaint of "sudden onset of altered consciousness with vomiting for 10 hours." Upon admission, his vital signs were as follows: heart rate 95 beats/min, respiratory rate 29 breaths/min, and blood pressure 195/110 mmHg. He presented with deep coma, GCS 4 (E1V1M2), bilaterally equal and irregularly shaped pupils, approximately 4 mm in diameter, with absent light reflex. His extremities exhibited decer-

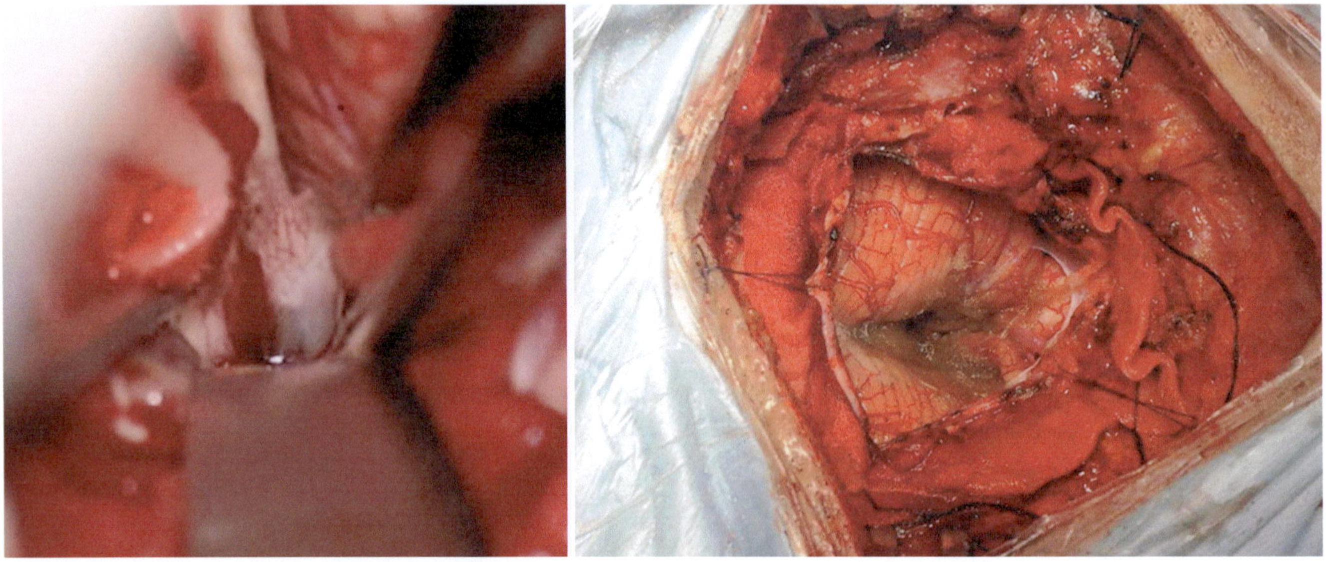

Fig. 11.7 Hematoma evacuation process. The bilateral cerebellar tonsils were separated and retracted, revealing a gray-blue area on the surface of the floor of the fourth ventricle, indicating the location of the hematoma. A brainstem fistula was created in this area, allowing for the careful and gentle removal of the hematoma, followed by the application of hemostatic gauze and cotton to achieve effective hemostasis. Minimizing the secondary damage caused by electrocoagulation was emphasized

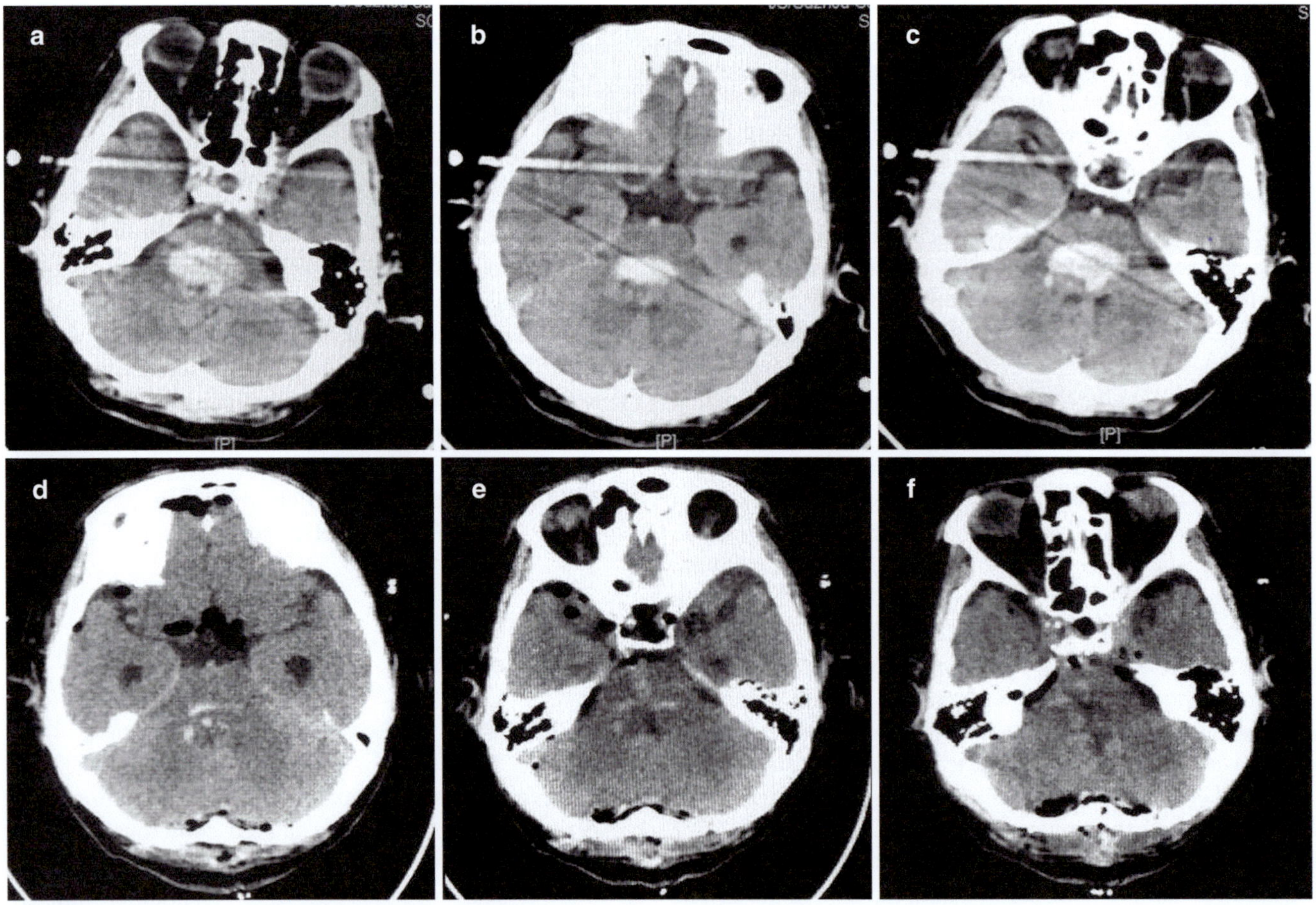

Fig. 11.8 Preoperative and postoperative CT. (**a–c**). Preoperative CT. (**d–f**) postoperative CT showing satisfactory evacuation of the hematoma

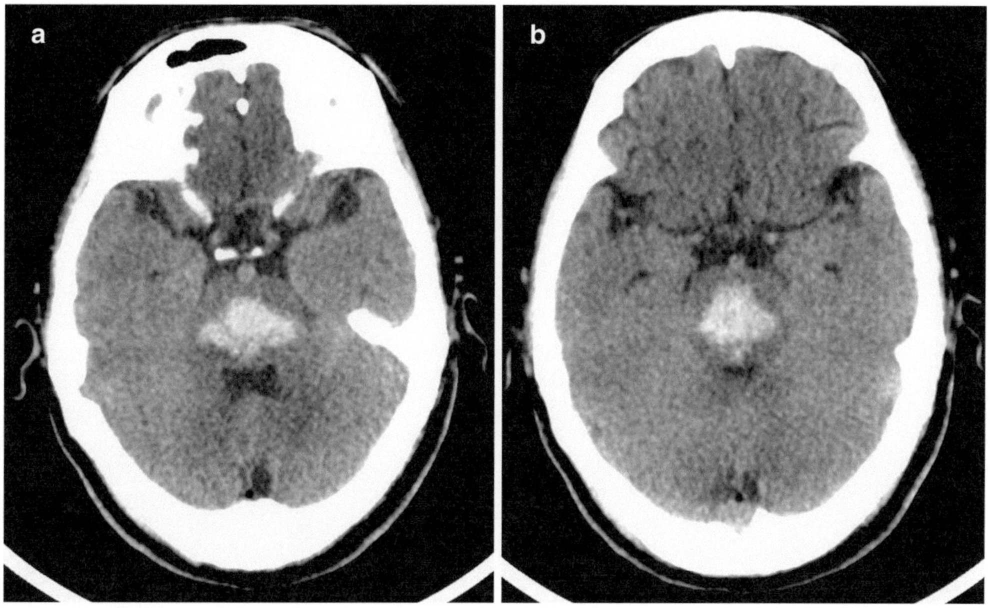

Fig. 11.9 (**a**) Preoperative head CT. (**b**) Preoperative head CT showing an 8 mL intrapontine hematoma

ebrate posturing when were stimulated, and bilateral pathological signs were positive. Head CT revealed an intrapontine hematoma, approximately 8 mL in volume (Fig. 11.9). The admission diagnosis was pontine hemorrhage (anterolateral pontine region) and grade 3 hypertension (extremely high-risk group).

11.8.2.2 Surgical Procedure

The patient was placed in a prone position. The scalp was incised 1.5 cm above the external occipital protuberance to the level of the second cervical vertebra, strictly along the nuchal ligament, using an electric scalpel. The rhomboid muscle was preserved at the external occipital protuberance. A hole was drilled at the external occipital protuberance, and the occipital bone was milled down from the external occipital protuberance to the foramen magnum and opening a 5 cm × 4 cm bone window.

Under the guidance of neuro-navigation and intraoperative electroneurophysiological monitoring, the lower one-third of the cerebellar vermis was incised to enter the fourth ventricle. After exposing the floor of the fourth ventricle and identifying the location of the hematoma, a suction device with low-to-medium negative pressure was used, under high magnification, to slowly and gently aspirate small amounts of the hematoma from the fourth ventricle. The hematoma cavity was entered through the ruptured site of the hematoma in the pons, and the entire hematoma was aspirated. After confirming the absence of active bleeding, the exit foramina of the aqueduct, the median aperture, and the lateral apertures of the fourth ventricle were opened, confirmed the patency of the cerebrospinal fluid circulation, placed a drainage tube in the surgical cavity. The dura mater was watertightly sutured with tension suture, the occipital bone was fixed, and the occipital muscles and scalp were sutured layer by layer (Fig. 11.10).

11.8.2.3 Comparison of Preoperative and Postoperative Imaging](Fig. 11.11)

11.8.2.4 Surgical Key Points

1. Accurately identify the incision site for brainstem entry, cutting along the prominent bulging edema band.
2. If the hematoma ruptures into the ventricle, entry into the hematoma cavity should be through the original channel.
3. The use of neuro-navigation and intraoperative electrophysiological monitoring can reduce postoperative complications and protect important functional areas.
4. During surgery, attention should be paid to protecting the drainage veins to avoid postoperative brain swelling.
5. Emphasize the use of compression hemostasis, minimizing or avoiding electrocoagulation for hemostasis. If necessary, use low-power, rapid, and precise electrocoagulation for hemostasis.
6. Ensure the patency of the cerebrospinal fluid circulation pathway, and strive to completely remove intraventricular hematomas.
7. If a significant amount of bleeding and high intracranial pressure is suspected preoperatively, external ventricular drainage may be performed first to facilitate the separation and protection of the brainstem during surgery.
8. Postoperatively, a lumbar cistern drainage may be left in place to promote the renewal of cerebrospinal fluid circulation.
9. Based on the author's experience, the prognosis of patients with brainstem hemorrhage rupturing into the ventricle is better than that of those with the hematoma not rupturing into the ventricle. For such patients, even

Fig. 11.10 Surgical procedure. (**a**) Showing the incision site. (**b**) exposing the floor of the fourth ventricle and the inferior medullary velum, identifying the location of the hematoma. (**c**) revealing the breach of the hematoma cavity

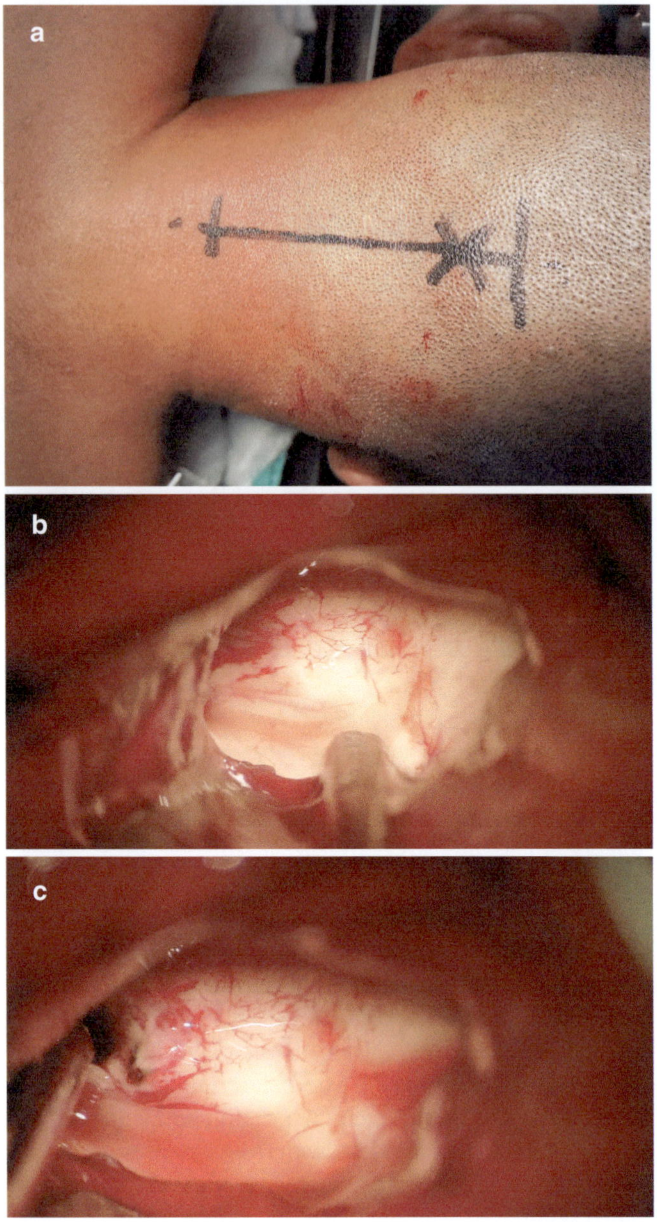

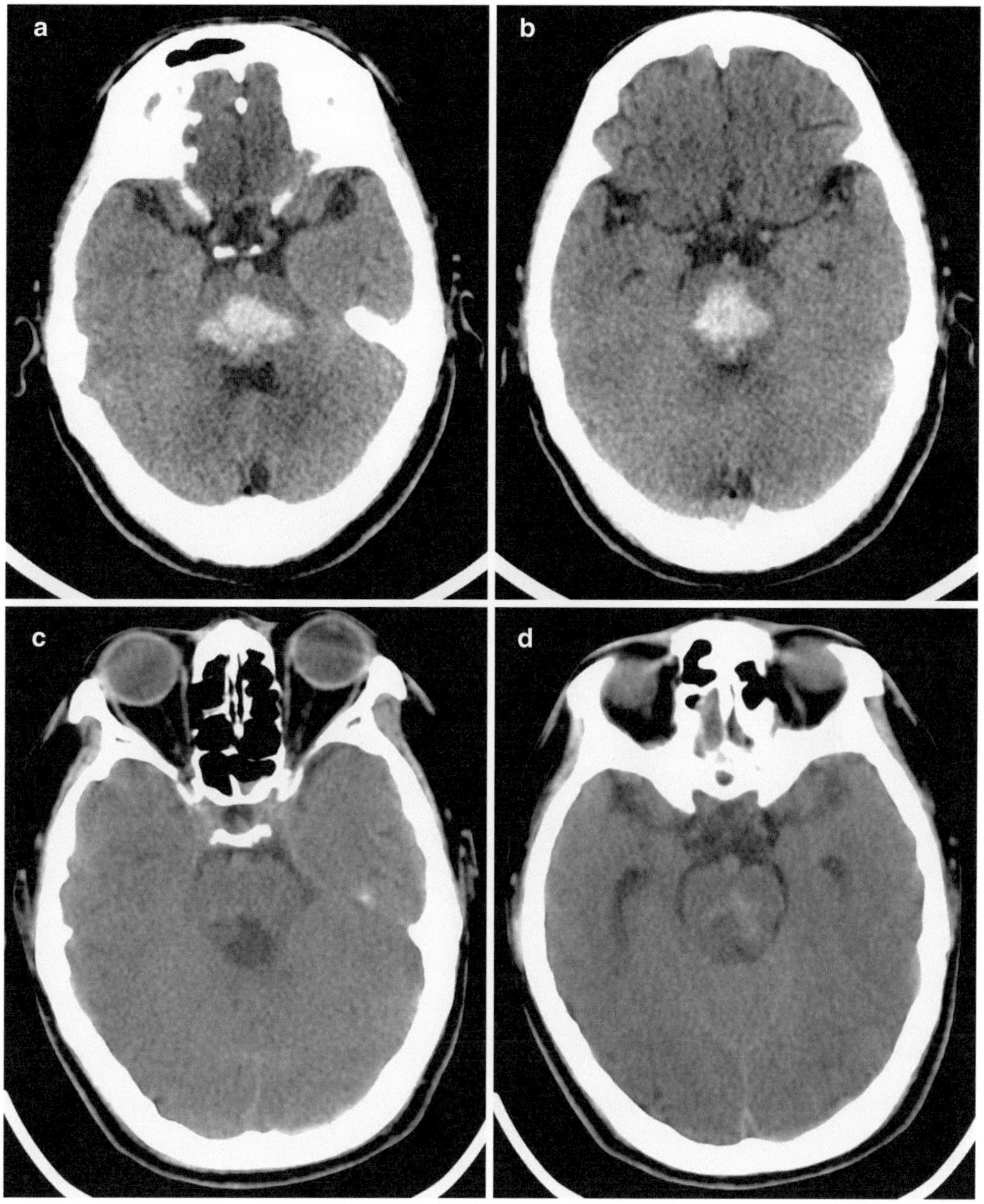

Fig. 11.11 Preoperative and postoperative CT. (**a** and **b**). Preoperative CT. (**c** and **d**) postoperative CT

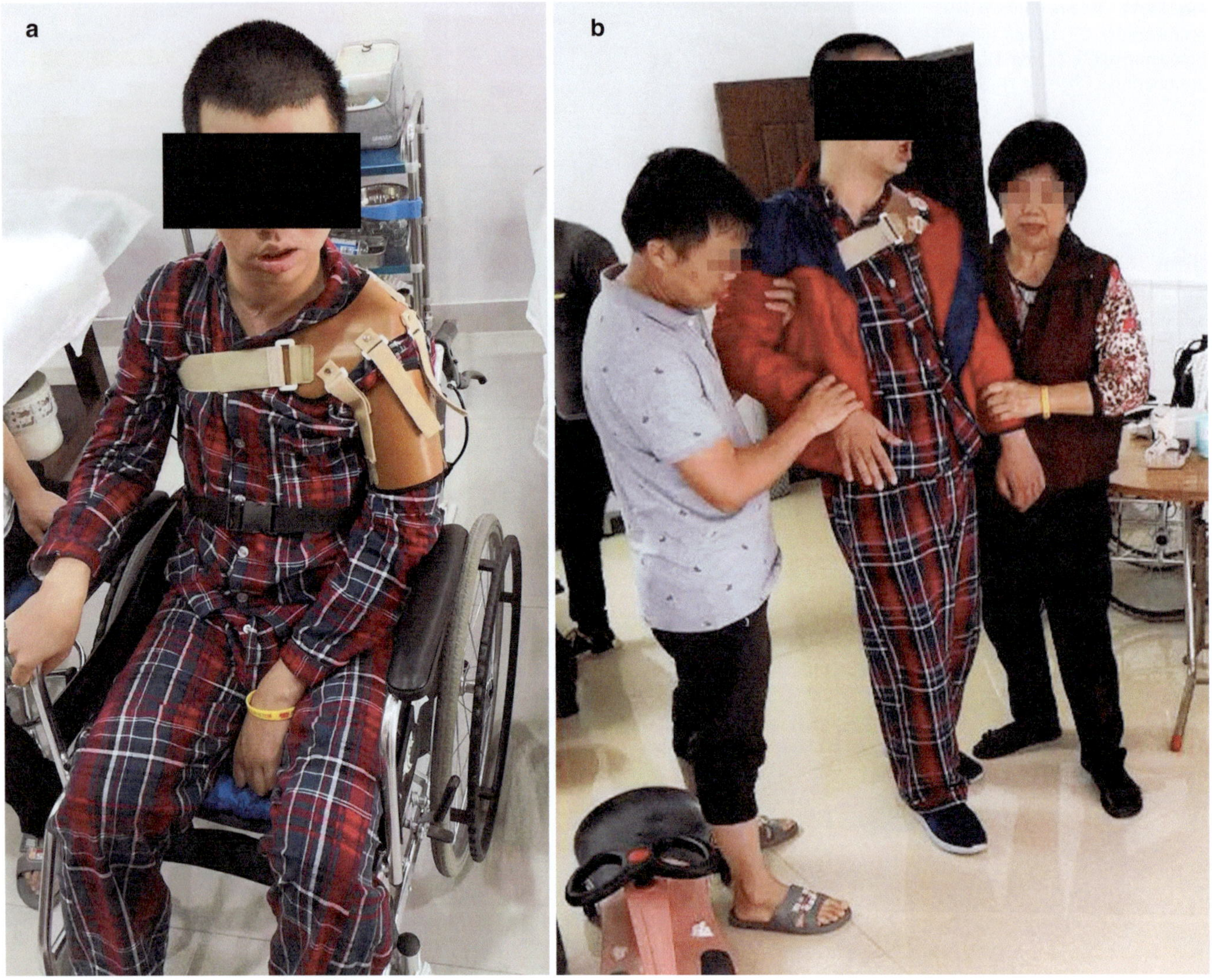

Fig. 11.12 Patient's condition at discharge

if the preoperative GCS score is low, active surgical treatment may be considered under appropriate conditions.

11.8.2.5 Postoperative Patient Condition (Fig. 11.12)

References

1. Gudrunardottir T, Sehested A, Juhler M, et al. Cerebellar mutism: review of the literature. Childs Nervous Syst. 2011;27(6):867–8.
2. Tanriover N, Ulm AJ, Rhoton AL, et al. Comparison of the transvermian and telovelar approaches to the fourth ventricle. J Neurosurg. 2004;101(3):484–98.
3. Mussi ACM, Rhoton AL. Telovelar approach to the fourth ventricle: microsurgical anatomy. J Neurosurg. 2000;92(5):812–23.
4. Chen LH, Wei Q, Xu RX, et al. Minimally invasive surgical treatment of primary primary brainstem hemorrhage. J Clin Neurosurg. 2015;5:349–53.
5. Liu X, Li H, Hu X, et al. Discussion on the treatment of spontaneous brainstem hemorrhage. J Clin Neurosurg. 2013;10(5):287–8.
6. Ichimura S, Bertalanffy H, Nakaya M, et al. Surgical treatment for primary brainstem hemorrhage to improve post-operative functional outcomes. World Neurosurg. 2018;120:1289–94.
7. Zhou H, Wang FY, Sun WY, et al. Resection of dorsal pontine cavernous malformations via the telovelar approach: report of 12 cases. Chinese J Neurol. 2016;15:1059.
8. Chen LH, Xu RX. Minimally invasive treatment of primary brainstem hemorrhage. Chinese J Neurotrauma Neurosurg. 2016;2(04):252–4.
9. Greenberg (US). Neurosurgery Manual. Zhao JZ, Trans, vol. 8. 8th ed. Nanjing: Phoenix Science and Technology Publishing House; 2017. p. 1811–20.

10. Liu QL. Anatomical and clinical aspects of neurosurgical approaches. Beijing: Science Press; 2007. p. 79–84.
11. Liu Y, Zou YJ, Liu HY, et al. Microsurgical resection of fourth ventricle tumors via the telovelar approach. Chinese J Neurosurg. 2017;33:1147.
12. Rhoton. Rhoton's Cranial anatomy and surgical approaches. Liu QL, Trans. Beijing: Science Press, 2010: 439–59.
13. Matsumoto K, Yagmur K, Kohno M, et al. Anatomy and approaches along the cerebellar-brainstem fissures. J Neurosurg. 2015:1–16.
14. Winkler EA, Birk H, Safaee M, et al. Erratum to: Surgical resection of fourth ventricular ependymomas: case series and technical nuances. J Neuro-Oncol. 2017;131(2):423.
15. Tomasello F, Conti A, Cardali S, et al. Telovelar approach to fourth ventricle tumors: highlights and limitations. World Neurosurg. 2015;83(6):1141–7.

12 Combined Microscopic and Endoscopic Surgical Treatment of Primary Brainstem Hemorrhage Via CPA Approach

Quan Zhou, Lihua Chen, and Zhiheng Jian

12.1 Overview

Historically, the brain stem has been considered a surgical no-go zone with extremely high risks, and clinical outcomes for primary brainstem hemorrhage have been very poor. According to domestic literature in 2013, the mortality rate for hemorrhages of 2–5 mL was 36%, 5–10 mL was 85.7%, and >10 mL was 100%. Over the past 5 years, advancements in micro-neurosurgical techniques, minimally invasive approaches, intraoperative neuronavigation, electroneurophysiological monitoring, and neuroendoscopy, combined with effective intensive care unit management, have significantly improved outcomes for brainstem hemorrhage and reduced mortality. Currently, there is increasing attention on the surgical treatment of primary brainstem hemorrhage. This chapter primarily elaborates on the combined use of microscopy and neuroendoscopy in the treatment of primary brainstem hemorrhage.

12.2 Surgical Indications and Contraindications

Currently, there is no unified standard for surgical indications and contraindications for primary brainstem hemorrhage in the guidelines. The following is a summary based on references:

12.2.1 Indications

1. Significant mass effect, with the largest dimension of the hemorrhage exceeding half of the brainstem, severe or progressively worsening neurological dysfunction.
2. Hemorrhage volume ≥5 mL.
3. Relatively concentrated hematoma, close to the brain cortex surface or ruptured into the fourth ventricle and subarachnoid space.
4. Poor response to conservative treatment, with a progressive deterioration of the condition.
5. GCS score of 3–8.
6. Strong family desire for surgery.

12.2.2 Contraindications

1. Deep coma with bilateral dilated and fixed pupils, absent light reflex.
2. The absence of spontaneous breathing for more than 2 h.
3. Unstable vital signs, experiencing cardiac arrest or hypotension requiring vasopressor support.
4. Disseminated brainstem hemorrhage, where various surgical approaches are difficult to achieve adequate decompression.
5. Other surgical contraindications, such as coagulation disorders, or inability of the cardiovascular and pulmonary systems to withstand anesthesia.

Supplementary Information The online version contains supplementary material available at https://doi.org/10.1007/978-981-95-8942-5_12.

Q. Zhou (✉) · L. Chen
Department of Neurosurgery, The First Affiliated Hospital of Guangxi University School of Medicine, Nanning, China

Z. Jian
Department of Neurosurgery, Zhuhai People's Hospital (The Affiliated Hospital of Beijing Institute of Technology, Zhuhai Clinical Medical College of Jinan University), Zhuhai, China

G. Chen, C. You (eds.), *Surgical Treatment of Primary Brainstem Hemorrhage*, https://doi.org/10.1007/978-981-95-8942-5_12

12.3 Preoperative Preparation and Surgical Instruments

12.3.1 Preoperative Preparation

1. Clear Diagnosis: Most patients have a clear history of hypertension. For patients with an uncertain history of hypertension, a CTA examination is performed to exclude aneurysms or arteriovenous malformations.
2. Maintain Airway Patency: Comatose patients are prone to vomiting, leading to aspiration or suffocation. For patients with breathing difficulties, prompt endotracheal intubation is performed to maintain airway patency, preventing an increase in intracranial pressure and worsening of cerebral tissue hypoxia.
3. Stable Blood Pressure Control: Effective blood pressure control can prevent rebleeding. Patients with an acute onset often experience significant blood pressure fluctuations, typically leading to blood pressure elevation, with severe cases reaching 200/110 mmHg, resulting in rebleeding and hematoma enlargement. Preoperatively, antihypertensive medications are used to maintain blood pressure within the range of 140–150/80–90 mmHg.
4. Coagulation Function Monitoring: For patients who were taking aspirin or other anticoagulants before the onset of the condition, intravenous administration of fresh platelets or intramuscular injection of vitamin K is necessary to correct coagulation function.
5. Determine the surgical indications: Based on the volume, location, and type of hemorrhage, as well as the patient's level of consciousness, pupil response, and respiratory condition, the decision for surgery is made.

12.3.2 Surgical Equipment and Instruments

The surgical equipment includes a specialized neurosurgical operating table, neurosurgical operating microscope, head frame with automatic retractor, electric cranial drill, specialized microsurgical instruments, neuroendoscope (length 18 cm, diameter 4 mm, angle 0°), etc. If a dedicated neuroendoscope is not available, an otolaryngology nasal endoscope can be used as a substitute.

12.4 Surgical Techniques and Considerations

12.4.1 Surgical Techniques

1. Surgical Principles: Adhere to the principles of minimally invasive surgery, aiming to achieve optimal surgical outcomes with minimal trauma.
2. Timing of Surgery: Generally, earlier surgery is believed to yield better therapeutic effects. Pathophysiologically, around 6 h following intracerebral hemorrhage, cerebral tissue edema and necrosis begin to appear around the hematoma and worsen over time. If the bleeding has persisted for over 3 days, the outcomes are notably poor, as evident brainstem edema has developed. Performing surgery at this stage may exacerbate brainstem edema, leading to suboptimal surgical outcomes. Therefore, early reduction of the hematoma to alleviate cerebral tissue compression and interrupt the malignant cycle of secondary changes following hemorrhage can improve survival rates and prognosis. According to Li Guoping, surgery within the ultra-early phase, within 6 h of bleeding, yields better outcomes, with superior neurological function recovery compared to mid to late-stage surgeries.
3. Common Surgical Approaches
   (a) Suboccipital posterior median transcerebellomedullary fissure approach: suitable for pontine hemorrhage rupturing posteriorly into the fourth ventricle.
   (b) Suboccipital retrosigmoid approach: For pontine hemorrhage approaching or rupturing the brainstem surface laterally.
   (c) Subtemporal transtentorial approach: Suitable for midbrain and pontine hemorrhage approaching or rupturing the brainstem surface laterally.
   (d) Pterion approach: suitable for midbrain hemorrhage.
   (e) Far lateral supracerebellar infratentorial approach: suitable for the hemorrhage on the junction of midbrain and pontine approaching or rupturing the brainstem surface lateral posteriorly (see Video 12.1).

12.4.2 Considerations

1. Preoperative volumetric CT scanning of the head provides a comprehensive understanding of the location and extent of the hematoma from axial, coronal, and sagittal perspectives, facilitating the accurate selection of the most suitable surgical approach.
2. The positioning for dual endoscopic and microscopic surgeries should accommodate the surgical requirements of both instruments, and adequate long microsurgical instruments should be prepared to facilitate deep operations.
3. Whenever possible, surgery should be performed within 24 h. If this time window is exceeded, the decision for surgery should be based on the patient's vital signs and GCS score.

12.4.3 Surgical Techniques

1. Enter the brainstem through the hematoma rupture site or through a safe zone in the brain stem. Initially, use the microscope to remove the superficial hematoma beneath the brainstem rupture, and then switch to the endoscope to remove the deeper hematoma, reducing traction on the brainstem rupture.
2. Perform a longitudinal incision of 3–5 mm in the brain stem to minimize traction on the brain stem.
3. During aspiration within the hematoma cavity, avoid damaging the surrounding normal brainstem tissue. For tougher hematomas, use suction devices, pistol-grip forceps, or tumor forceps to assist with removal.
4. Manage active bleeding by using a suction device to hold small blood vessels, and apply low-power bipolar coagulation. During coagulation, attention should be paid to irrigation to reduce temperature and prevent adhesion between the coagulation probe and blood vessels. For oozing, cover the wound with a thin gelatin sponge or hemostatic gauze, and apply light pressure with cotton pads.
5. Thoroughly remove the hematoma to relieve obstructive hydrocephalus.
6. Protect draining veins as much as possible to prevent exacerbation of brainstem edema and compression of neural tissues postoperatively, which may lead to neurological dysfunction.

12.5 Postoperative Management and Prevention of Complications

12.5.1 Prevention of Postoperative Complications

1. Postoperative bleeding in the hematoma cavity: Resulting from improper handling of bleeding vessels. For instance, inadequate compression using gelatin sponge for small arterial bleeding may lead to recurrent bleeding due to postoperative agitation and subsequent blood pressure elevation. Therefore, precise hemostasis using bipolar coagulation under endoscopic observation is essential to reduce the likelihood of secondary bleeding. If recurrent bleeding causing hematoma compression on the brainstem is detected, a secondary surgical evacuation may be necessary.
2. Postoperative intracranial air accumulation: Occurring due to the patient's lateral positioning, often leading to residual gas accumulation in the subdural space over the frontal and temporal lobes. Tension pneumocephalus resulting from excessive intracranial air can lead to increased intracranial pressure. Therefore, during the conclusion of the surgery and dural closure, thorough injection of saline into the subdural space should be performed to expel the air.
3. Postoperative exacerbation of cerebellum or brainstem edema: Resulting from surgical traction on cerebellar tissue, brain stem, or injury to major drainage veins, leading to postoperative brain edema. Excessive or prolonged traction on brain tissue can cause ischemic infarction, which is the primary cause of postoperative brain edema. Therefore, during surgery, draining cerebrospinal fluid to relieve pressure on the brain and employing gentle traction or intermittent traction on brain tissue without causing excessive pulling can alleviate the occurrence of postoperative brain edema.

12.5.2 Postoperative Management

1. Upon detecting rebleeding, it is essential to increase sedation and pain management, maintain stable blood pressure, and continue using hemostatic agents to prevent hematoma expansion. If the hematoma enlarges and compresses the brain stem, a secondary surgical evacuation may be necessary.
2. Minor postoperative intracranial air can be absorbed naturally and does not require specific intervention. However, in the case of excessive air accumulation leading to tension pneumocephalus and brain tissue displacement, external drainage through burr holes may be performed to release the trapped gas.
3. In the event of cerebellar or brainstem edema postoperatively, dehydration therapy can be intensified. If necessary, intravenous administration of human albumin can be considered to increase plasma colloid osmotic pressure and enhance the resolution of edema. If conservative treatment yields unsatisfactory results and cerebellar edema worsens, leading to brainstem compression, emergency decompressive craniectomy or further internal decompression surgery may be required.

12.6 Advantages, Disadvantages, and Lessons Learned

The advantages of microscopic combined with neuroendoscopic surgery for treating brainstem hemorrhage include a high rate of complete hematoma clearance and mild postoperative brainstem edema. Minimal traction on the brainstem allows for the clearance of deep hematomas under direct vision, ensuring good protection of surrounding normal brainstem tissue. Responsible bleeding vessels can be precisely coagulated, reducing the probability of postoperative rebleeding. However, the disadvantages include the limited widespread use of endoscopy and a longer learning curve, especially in adapting to the challenges of hand-eye separation during operations in the short term.

The progression of microscopic combined with neuroendoscopic surgery should be gradual. Initially, a thorough understanding of anatomy and anatomical training, mastery of various skull base approaches, and proficient clearance of brainstem hematomas under the microscope are essential. Simultaneously, training in hand-eye separation under endoscopy is crucial. Once the technique is mastered, the endoscope can be fixed using an arm, allowing for bimanual operation and clearance of deep brainstem hematomas.

During the initial stages of brainstem hemorrhage surgery, the following issues may be encountered:

1. Incomplete hematoma clearance, often related to incorrect approach selection or blind spots in the microscopic field of view.
2. Exacerbation of brainstem edema, often related to inadequate proficiency in endoscopic operations, leading to increased damage to normal tissue.

12.7 Evaluation and Prospects of the Procedure

Microscopic combined with neuroendoscopic surgery for clearing brainstem hemorrhage is an effective method that allows for the direct visualization and clearance of hematomas, ensuring excellent preservation of normal brainstem tissue. The initial clearance rate of hematomas is high, and under endoscopy, there are no blind spots or dark areas. This approach enables close observation and treatment of responsible bleeding vessels, thereby reducing the probability of postoperative rebleeding. Once surgical proficiency is achieved, complete endoscopic clearance of brainstem hematomas can be performed, resulting in reduced trauma, shorter surgical duration, and improved postoperative recovery for patients.

12.8 Typical Case

12.8.1 Brief Medical History and Imaging Data

1. Patient: Male, 64 years old, transferred from an external hospital due to "sudden consciousness disturbance for 7 days."
2. Physical examination: Weak spontaneous respiration, tracheostomy, assisted ventilation, moderate coma, GCS score of 5, bilateral pupils equal and round, with a diameter of 3 mm, the presence of light reflex, and flexion of both upper limbs to pain stimulation, with positive pathological signs on both sides.
3. Head CT scan revealed pontine hemorrhage extending into the fourth ventricle, approximately 6.8 mL in volume (Figure 12.1a, b).
4. Admission diagnosis: brainstem hemorrhage; grade 3 hypertension (extremely high-risk group).

12.8.2 Surgical Procedure and Key Points

1. Positioning and Incision: The patient is typically placed in a three-quarter prone position (Park-bench position) (Fig. 12.2). The head and upper body are elevated by 20°–30°, positioning the head higher than the level of the chest, facilitating venous return. A 45° forward flexion of the head aids the separation operation on the undersurface of the cerebellum and within the fourth ventricle. The surgical incision involves a posterior suboccipital

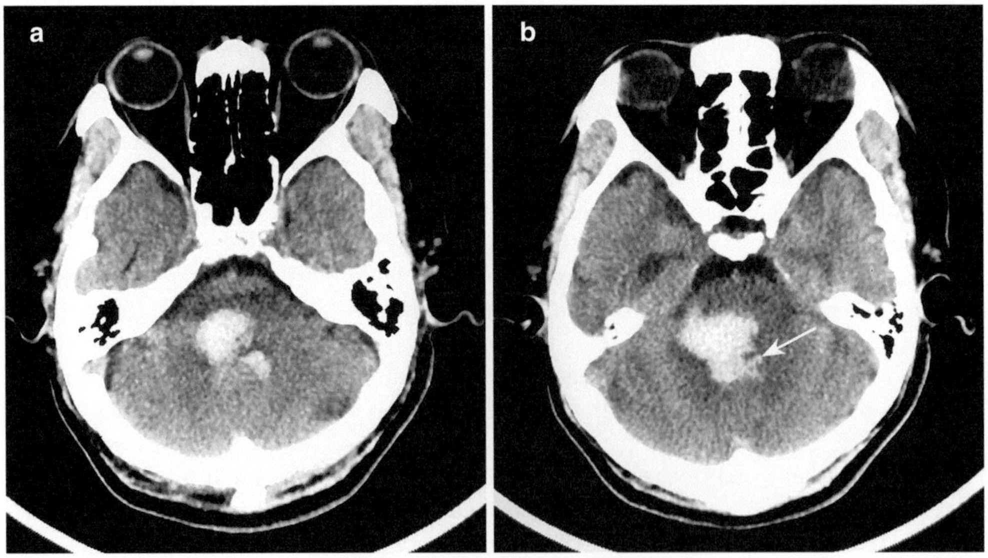

Fig. 12.1 Preoperative head CT scan. (**a**) Right-sided posterior pontine hemorrhage. (**b**) pontine hemorrhage extending into the fourth ventricle (indicated by the white arrow)

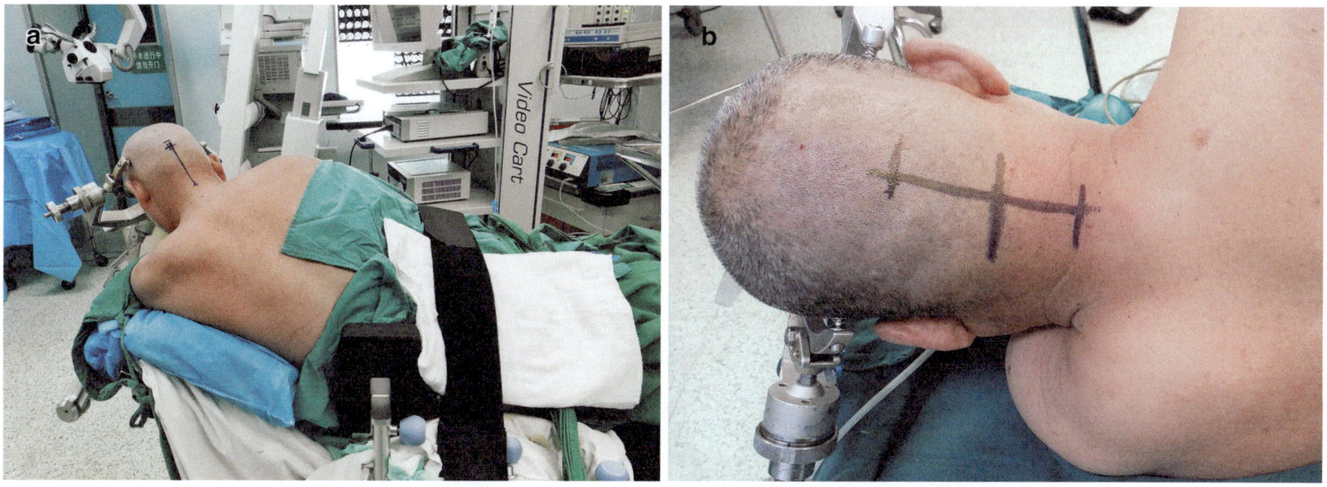

Fig. 12.2 Surgical positioning and incision. (**a**) The patient was placed in a left lateral decubitus position with the upper body elevated by 30° The head was secured with a three-pin head frame. (**b**) suboccipital posterior median vertical incision

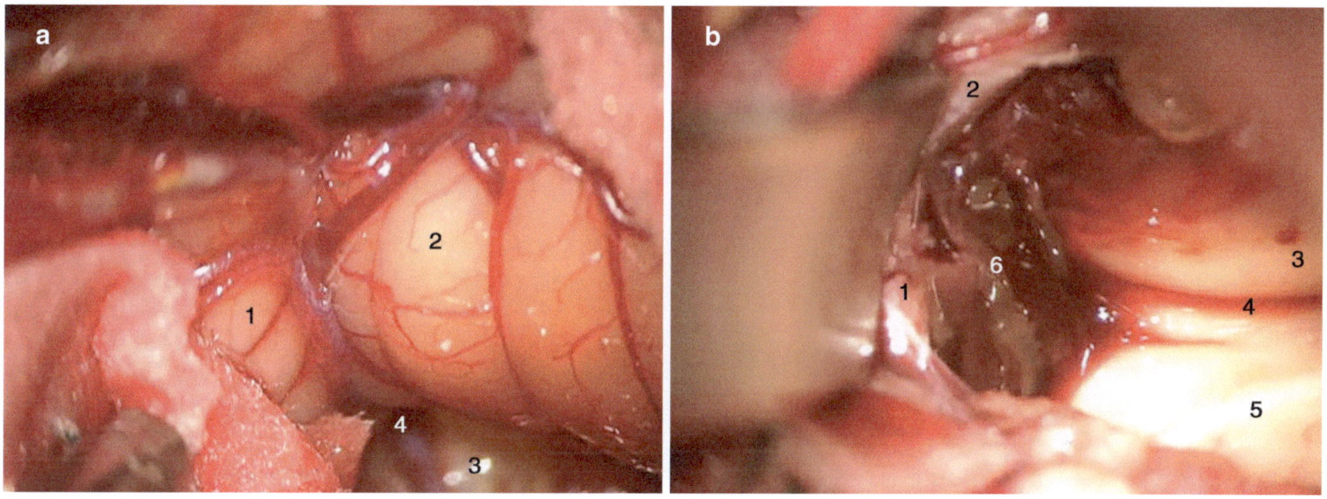

Fig. 12.3 Opening the cerebellomedullary fisture under the microscope. (**a**) The micrograph shows the separation of the cerebellar vermis and the right cerebellar tonsil, revealing the cerebellomedullary fissure. 1 Vermis. 2 right cerebellar tonsil. 3 medulla. 4 cerebellomedullary fissure. (**b**) separation of the cerebellomedullary fissure, revealing the hematoma entering into the fourth ventricle. 1 Choroid plexus. 2 inferior medullary velum. 3 floor of the fourth ventricle. 4 median sulcus. 5 medullary striae. 6 hematoma

median vertical incision, extending from the external occipital protuberance to the spinous process of the fourth cervical vertebra.

2. Skin and Muscle Layer Incision: Following the incision and retraction of the skin and subcutaneous tissues, the ligamentum nuchae is carefully identified, and a strict midline incision is made. The posterior rectus capitis muscle is dissected from the posterior arch tubercle of the atlas to expose the foramen magnum and the posterior arch of the atlas.
3. Bone Flap Craniotomy: A bone orifice is drilled below the external occipital protuberance, and the bone is milled bilaterally in an arc-shaped manner to the foramen magnum, creating a bone flap. In most cases, it is unnecessary to remove the majority of the posterior arch of the atlas. However, if the skull base is flat or severely depressed, and the hematoma is close to the medulla, removal of the posterior arch of the atlas is necessary to facilitate exposure and adequate decompression.
4. Dural Incision: After ligating the occipital and atlas sinuses, a "Y"-shaped incision is made in the dura mater, followed by traction and fixation.
5. Opening of the Cerebellomedullary Fissure (Figs. 12.3 and 12.4): Upon opening the arachnoid membrane, the cervical medulla, medulla, and the undersurface of the cerebellum are visible. The right cerebellar tonsil is retracted, and with microscissors, the cerebellomedullary fissure is sharply dissected. After opening the foramen of

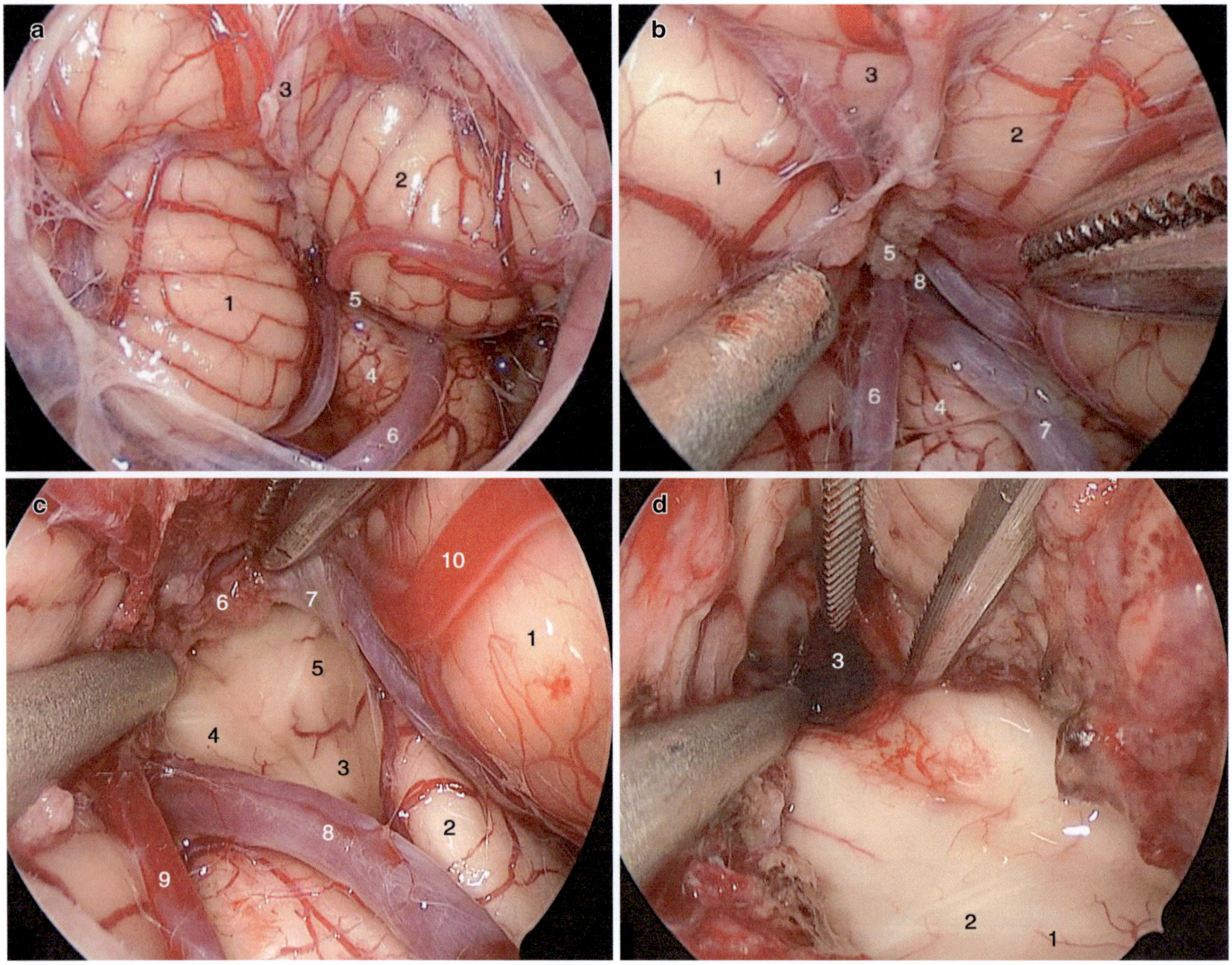

Fig. 12.4 Opening the cerebellomedullary fissure under the neuroendoscope providing a clearer anatomical structure than the microscope (another patient, used for comparison). (**a**) The neuroendoscope provides a clearer display of the anatomical structure. 1 Left cerebellar tonsil. 2 right cerebellar tonsil. 3 vermis. 4 medulla. 5 cerebellomedullary fissure. 6 posterior medulla segment of posterior inferior cerebellar artery on the left. (**b**) sharp incision of the cerebellomedullary fissure, exposing the choroid plexus. 1 Left cerebellar tonsil. 2 right cerebellar tonsil. 3 vermis. 4 medulla. 5 choroid plexus. 6 internal branch of posterior inferior cerebellar artery on the left. 7 posterior medulla segment of posterior inferior cerebellar artery on the right. 8 median aperture of the fourth ventricle. (**c**) exposing the rhomboid fossa of the floor of the fourth ventricle. 1 right cerebellar tonsil. 2 medulla. 3 floor of the fourth ventricle. 4 left medullary striae. 5 right medullary striae. 6 choroid plexus. 7 inferior medullary velum. 8 posterior medulla segment of posterior inferior cerebellar artery on the left. 9 lateral branch of the posterior inferior cerebellar artery on the left. 10 lateral branch of the posterior inferior cerebellar artery on the right. (**d**) revealing the hematoma rupture on the dorsal side of the brainstem. 1 Floor of the fourth ventricle. 2 left medullary striae. 3 protruding hematoma rupture of the brainstem

Magendie (the median aperture of the fourth ventricle) and the choroid plexus, the inferior medullary velum and cerebellar vermis are gently retracted, providing a broad view of the fourth ventricle. At the rostral end of the fourth ventricle, the hemorrhage ruptured on the posterior pontine can be observed.

6. Microscopic Hematoma Evacuation (Fig. 12.5): Under the microscope, the hematoma cavity is entered through the rupture, and the hematoma is carefully removed. The rupture is appropriately enlarged to 5 mm, and a 1.5 mm diameter micro-suction device is used to carefully aspirate the hematoma. Large, solid clots can be fragmented with micro-forceps and then aspirated in chunks. Care should be taken to work within the hematoma cavity and avoid damaging surrounding tissues beyond the edge of the hematoma cavity (Fig. 12.6).
7. Neuroendoscopic Hematoma Evacuation: Due to the small size of the brainstem rupture, the deep illumination under the microscope diminishes, resulting in areas of poor visibility. Without pulling the brainstem incision, it is difficult for the microscope to completely evacuate the hematoma. The advantage of the neuroendoscope lies in

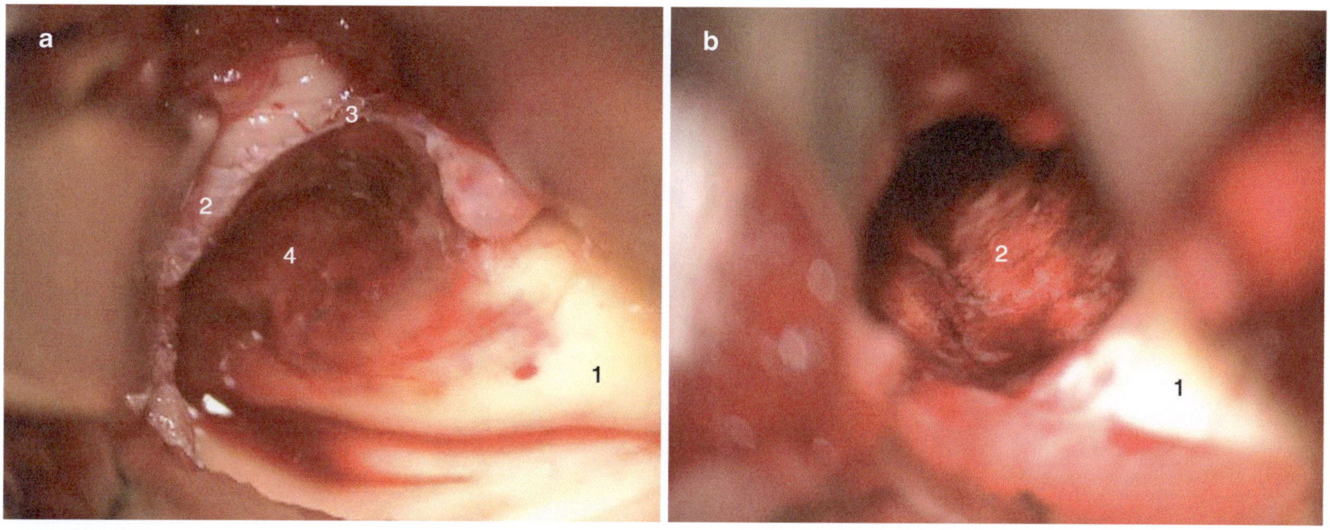

Fig. 12.5 Evacuation of the partial brainstem hematoma. Under the microscope. (**a**) Clearance of the superficial brainstem hematoma under the microscope. 1 Floor of the fourth ventricle. 2 choroid plexus. 3 inferior medullary velum. 4 hematoma. (**b**) under the microscope, there is a decrease in deep illumination, resulting in areas of poor visibility and blind spots. 1 Floor of the fourth ventricle. 2 wound after hematoma clearance

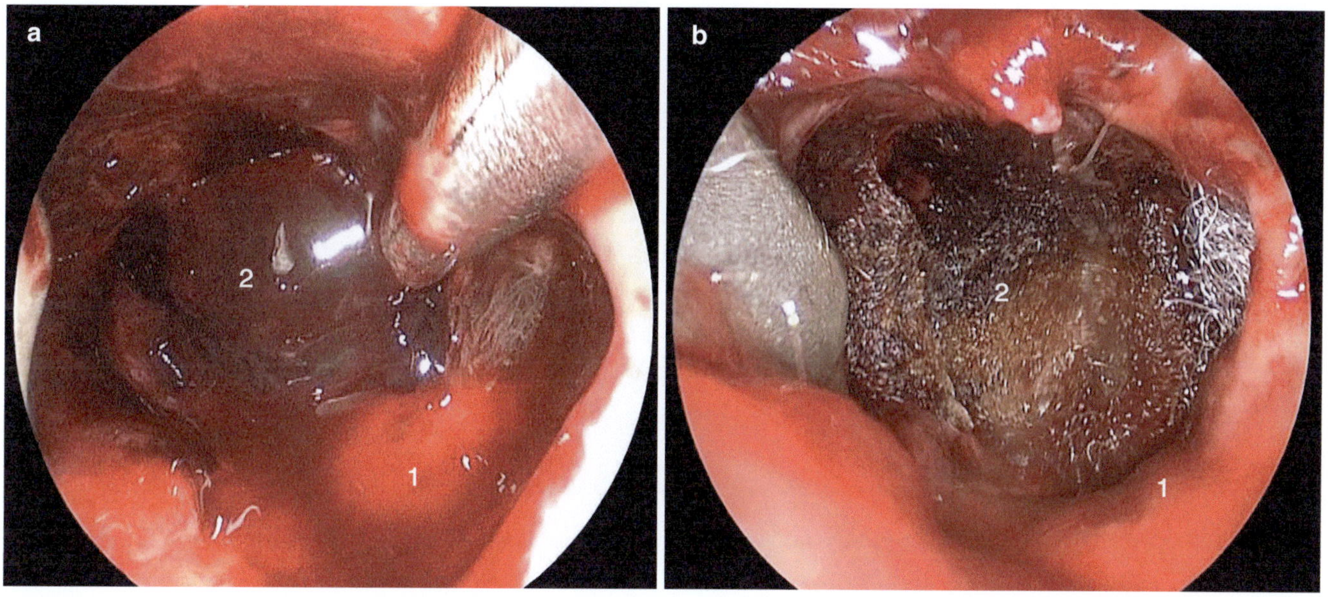

Fig. 12.6 Direct visualization and complete hemostasis of the residual deep brainstem hematoma under the endoscope. (**a**) Under the neuroendoscope, there are no dark areas or blind spots, allowing complete clearance of the hematoma. 1 Floor of the fourth ventricle. 2 hematoma. (**b**) complete hemostasis of the wound. 1 Floor of the fourth ventricle. 2 immediate application of gauze to cover the wound, achieving thorough hemostasis

its ability to clearly display deep-seated hematomas and evacuate them under direct vision without increasing traction on the brainstem. In cases of deep bleeding, a mechanical arm can be used to fix the endoscope, allowing precise manipulation with both hands to cauterize bleeding vessels, reducing the probability of postoperative rebleeding. The endoscope also allows for an enlarged field of view to confirm complete hematoma evacuation while avoiding secondary damage. The hematoma cavity is covered with hemostatic gauze to achieve thorough hemostasis, and the cavity is flushed until the fluid is clear. This approach preserves the integrity of the cerebellar vermis, preventing the occurrence of postoperative mutism and cerebellar ataxia.

12.8.3 Preoperative and Postoperative Imaging Comparison (Fig. 12.7)

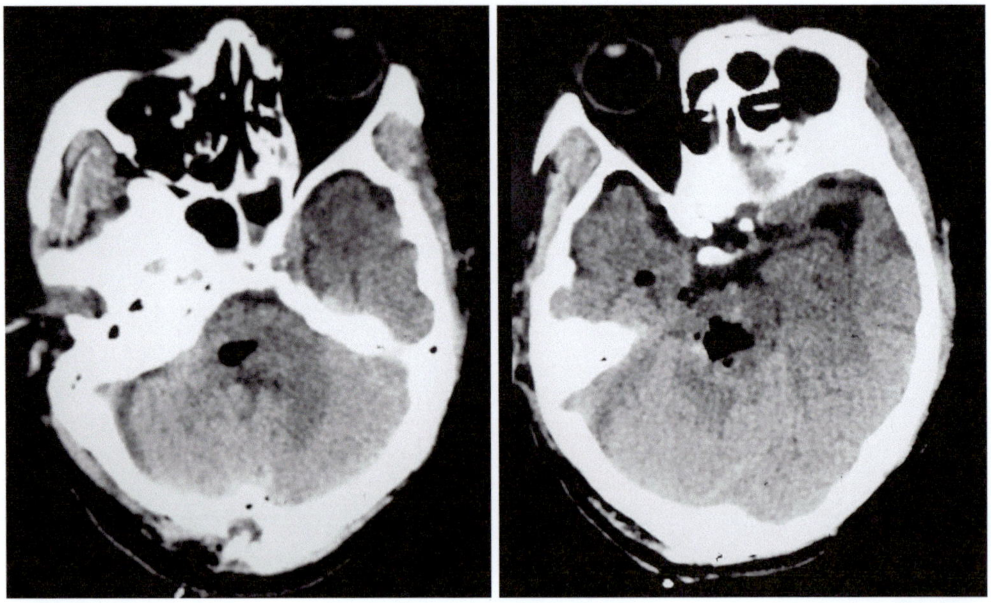

Fig. 12.7 Complete clearance of the hematoma in the postoperative cranial CT

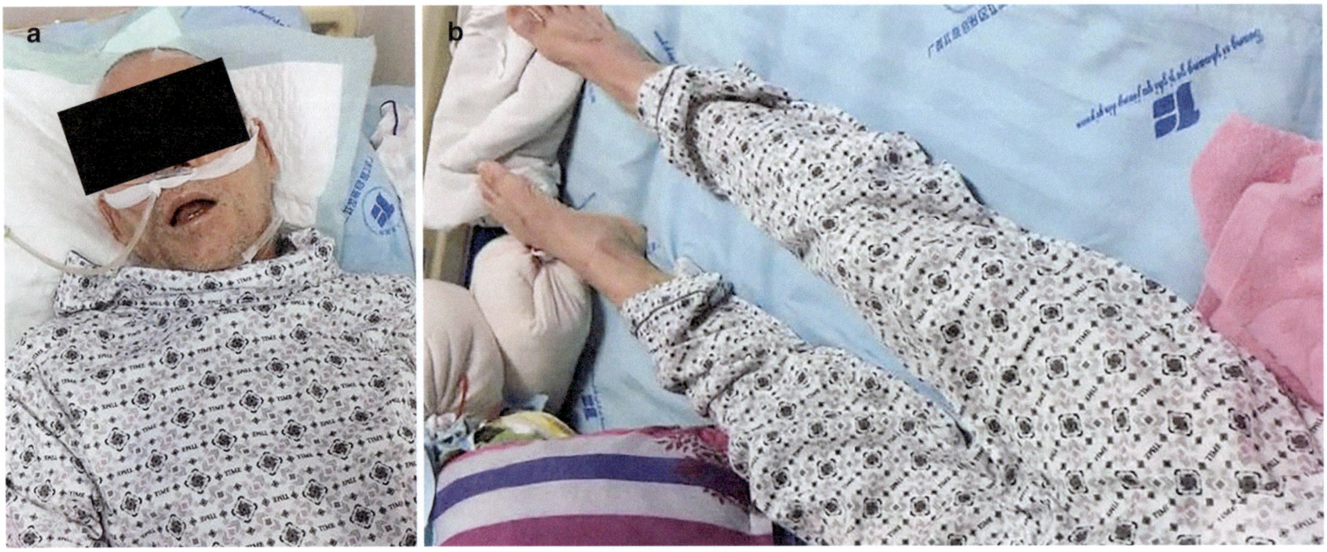

Fig. 12.8 Patient's condition 2 months postoperatively. (**a**) The patient regained consciousness. (**b**) both lower limbs can move

12.8.4 Imaging Data and Video of Postoperative Neurological Examination

At 2 months postoperatively, the patient regained consciousness (Fig. 12.8). They can independently blow their nose, move both lower limbs, and make a fist with both hands.

13 Surgical Treatment of Primary Brainstem Hemorrhage Via Keyhole Approach

Gang Chen, Chao Sun, and Junfeng Huo

13.1 Overview

The concept of keyhole surgery was introduced by Wilson in 1971. In 1991, Fukushima applied a 3 cm diameter bone window for clipping an anterior communicating artery aneurysm via the interhemispheric keyhole approach. The publication of the monograph on keyhole neurosurgery by Perneczky at the University of Mainz in Germany in 1999 marked the maturity of this technique. In 2000, Professor Lan Qing in China studied keyhole surgical techniques with Professor Perneczky and subsequently dedicated himself to the research and promotion of keyhole surgery [1]. The formulation of the "Chinese Expert Consensus on Neurosurgical Keyhole Microsurgery" in 2017 reflected the promotion and standardization of keyhole minimally invasive techniques in China. The publication of the "International Expert Consensus Statement about Methods and Indications for Keyhole Microneurosurgery from the International Society on Minimally Invasive Neurosurgery" in 2019 demonstrated China's efforts and achievements in the field of minimally invasive keyhole surgery to the global community [2].

Keyhole neurosurgery is a product of the combination of modern microsurgery technology, neuroimaging technology, and neuroendoscopic technology with the concept of modern minimally invasive surgery. It is not merely about the size of the surgical incision, and it represents a surgical concept where minimally invasive, precise, and personalized approaches are the essence of keyhole surgery. The primary goal of keyhole microsurgery is to design a surgical approach tailored to the location and nature of the lesion and make full use of limited space to remove unnecessary structural exposure or damage, ensuring the shortest and most accurate surgical path to reach the lesion. During the procedure, normal anatomical space in the brain tissue is utilized to minimize traction on the brain, enabling the complete removal of the lesion with minimal trauma to achieve the best surgical outcome [3].

Neurosurgical keyhole microsurgery relies on advanced microsurgical techniques and is based on local anatomy and lesion characteristics [4]. It utilizes the "keyhole" effect to develop a novel minimally invasive approach, enabling a rational reduction of the craniotomy bone window while ensuring optimal exposure and treatment of the lesion. The size of the keyhole approach incision and bone window is tailored to meet the principle of "sufficient exposure of the lesion with minimal craniotomy trauma." Although the location of brainstem hemorrhage is deep, it is relatively fixed. Through the magnification effect of the "keyhole," a large field of view can be obtained under the microscope through a small bone window, facilitating surgical procedures. Therefore, using the keyhole approach to evacuate brainstem hemorrhage is entirely feasible from a technical perspective [5].

The keyhole neurosurgical technique has been developed for over 20 years. Looking back at its development over the past two decades, keyhole microsurgery can meet the basic requirements of the majority of neurosurgical procedures. Under current technical conditions, for most deep-seated lesions, a bone window with a diameter of less than 3 cm is sufficient for microsurgical procedures, usually requiring a scalp incision of approximately 4 cm [6]. This minimally invasive approach not only maintains surgical quality and

Supplementary Information The online version contains supplementary material available at https://doi.org/10.1007/978-981-95-8942-5_13.

G. Chen (✉)
Department of Neurosurgery, Zhuhai People's Hospital (The Affiliated Hospital of Beijing Institute of Technology, Zhuhai Clinical Medical College of Jinan University), Zhuhai, China

C. Sun
Department of Neurosurgery, The Second Affiliated Hospital of Soochow University, Suzhou, China

J. Huo
Department of Neurosurgery, Shanghai Donglei Brain Hospital, Shanghai, China

G. Chen, C. You (eds.), *Surgical Treatment of Primary Brainstem Hemorrhage*, https://doi.org/10.1007/978-981-95-8942-5_13

efficacy but also reduces trauma and postoperative complications, such as infections. The straightforward approach not only reduces the duration of the craniotomy but also allows the surgeon to focus more on the treatment of the lesion, further enhancing surgical quality. Moreover, it can shorten the patient's recovery period, reduce the burden of nursing care, and save treatment costs [7].

13.2 Basic Requirements for Implementing Keyhole Surgery

It is essential to recognize that keyhole surgery is a development of microsurgical techniques and a natural result of the combination of excellent equipment and skilled techniques. Keyhole surgery must be based on microanatomy, professional techniques, extensive experience, and sophisticated instruments. Clinical implementation is a gradual process of adaptation and improvement and should not be pursued under inadequate conditions, which could lead to counterproductive results [8]. For surgeons new to keyhole surgery, meeting the necessary prerequisites and proceeding step by step is essential to ensure surgical safety.

1. Profound Understanding of Individual Diseases and Anatomy

   The keyhole approach does not allow changes to the surgical approach during the procedure. Therefore, precise preoperative design and individualized surgical management are prerequisites for successful keyhole microsurgery, requiring a profound understanding of individual diseases and anatomy. Training is necessary for the implementation of keyhole surgery, and anatomical training for the keyhole approach can enhance the surgeon's adaptability to instrument manipulation, familiarity with intracranial anatomical structures, and exposure ranges under various keyhole approaches, thereby increasing the surgeon's confidence in keyhole surgery (Fig. 13.1).
2. Thorough and Comprehensive Imaging and Other Auxiliary Examinations [9]

   The development of imaging technology is crucial for advancing modern neurosurgery and ensuring precise and minimally invasive procedures. Comprehensive imaging examinations play a vital role in preoperative planning, surgical navigation, and intraoperative guidance. Neuro-navigation enables efficient and safe preoperative planning of surgical approaches while providing real-time visualization of lesions and surgical sites in three-dimensional space. With the recent advancements in various 3D imaging workstations, navigation software, and mobile phone-assisted applications, preoperative thin-slice CT scans can now facilitate intraoperative neuro-navigation for critical conditions like brainstem hemorrhage, significantly enhancing surgical safety. Additionally, the application of mobile CT plays a significant role in ensuring surgical safety and improving the treatment of critical patients. Mobile CT enables the assessment of intraoperative hematoma clearance, detection of residual blood clots, and timely evaluation of hydrocephalus, providing substantial assistance (Fig. 13.2).
3. Sophisticated Surgical Instruments and Equipment

   (a) Neurosurgical Microscope: A microscope is a fundamental requirement for keyhole microsurgery, and a microscope with a considerable depth of field provides more precise visualization of deep structures. Due to the small surgical bone window, the microscope's viewing angle must be continuously adjusted. An electromagnetic lock-adjustable surgical microscope can better meet these requirements.

   (b) Headframe and Automatic Retractor: Keyhole surgery has high requirements on the patient's position, especially the position of the head. The use of a headframe system facilitates head placement and fixation. The Mayfield headframe system is most commonly used and offers simple and rapid installation. The automatic retractor helps secure the surgical field without requiring manual retraction, ensuring an unobstructed operative view. Due to the small bone window in keyhole surgery, retractors fixed on the bone window are unsuitable. Instead, bedside retractors are more convenient for operation, with their snake-like retracting arms providing easy adjustment. Generally, they are positioned approximately 15 cm below the surgical bone window, and the width of the brain spatula can range from 0.3 to 1.0 cm. A rod-shaped brain spatula with a width of 0.1 to 0.3 cm can also be used for deep-seated procedures.

   (c) Fine Microsurgical Instruments: Gun-type rod-shaped instruments effectively increase the visual space during surgery and minimize the interference caused by the surgeon or the instruments in the microscope's field of view [10]. In keyhole microsurgery, it is advisable to use rod-shaped or narrow-bladed micro-scissors, dissectors, or aneurysm clip retainers. As for suction devices, adjustable negative pressure suction with a distal diameter of 1–3 mm is commonly used.

   (d) Power System: During surgery, a drill can be used to create a burr hole with a diameter of approximately 3 mm, followed by a milling cutter to form a small bone flap and remove the inner lamina of the bone window to expand the field of view.

   (e) Navigation System: Neuro-navigation enables accurate lesion localization and selection of the surgical approach. In keyhole surgery for deep-seated brainstem hemorrhages, implementing navigation enhances surgical safety. Its capabilities in precise

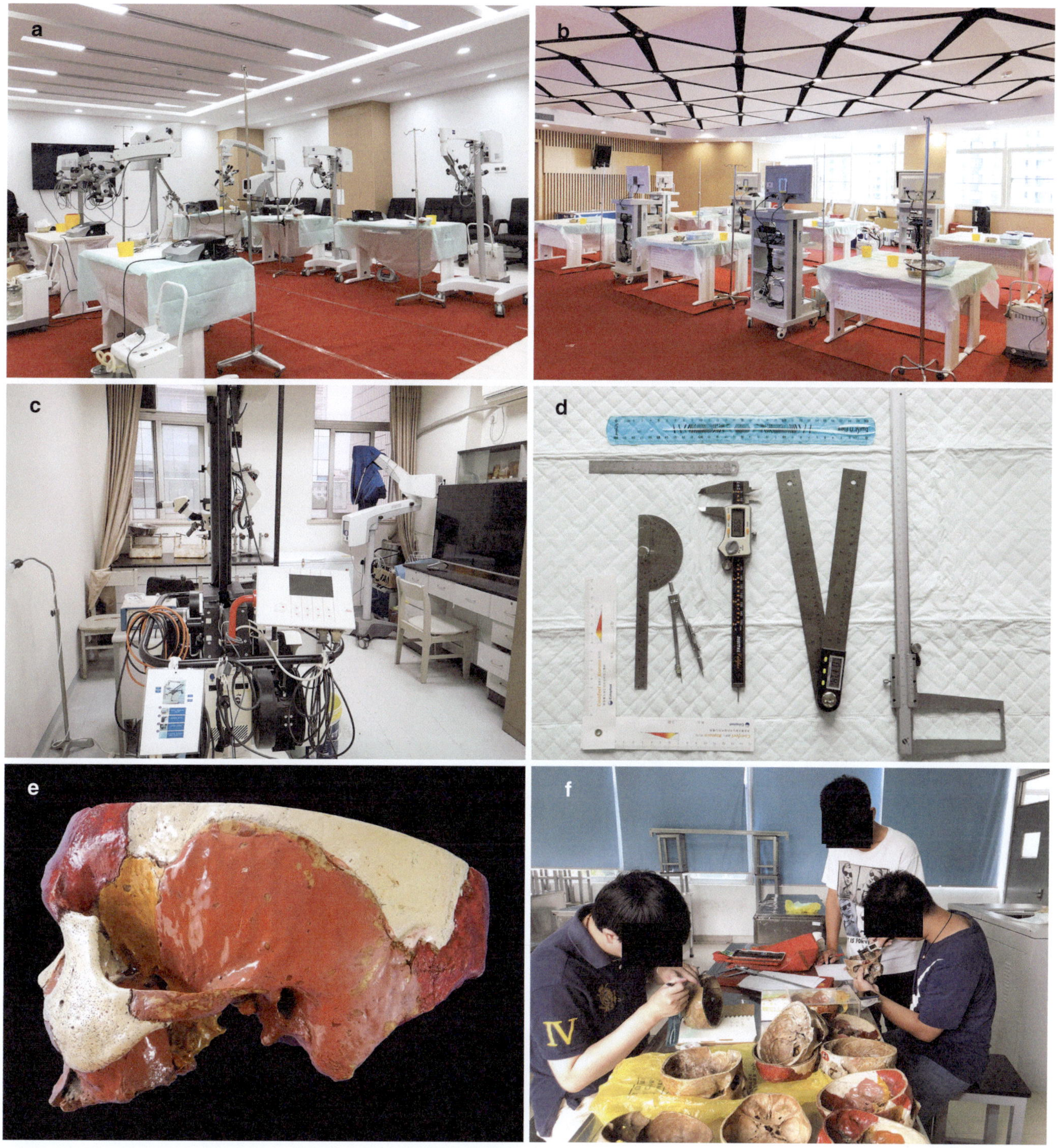

Fig. 13.1 Conditions and training content for cranial microscopic anatomy training. (**a**) Microsurgical technique training. (**b**) endoscopic technique training. (**c**) anatomy laboratory setup. (**d**) tools for measuring cadaveric head anatomy. (**e**) standard lateral view of dry skull bones. (**f**) measurement of anatomical data. (**g**, **h**) anatomy course on the application of the keyhole approach led by the author. (**i**) incision length of approximately 4 cm for the retromastoid keyhole approach on the right side. (**j**) incising the dura, retracting the cerebellar hemisphere laterally, and exposing the posterior cranial nerves to the caudal side. (**k**) exposing the trigeminal nerve and facial and auditory nerve. (**l**) exposing the lateral aspect of the brainstem

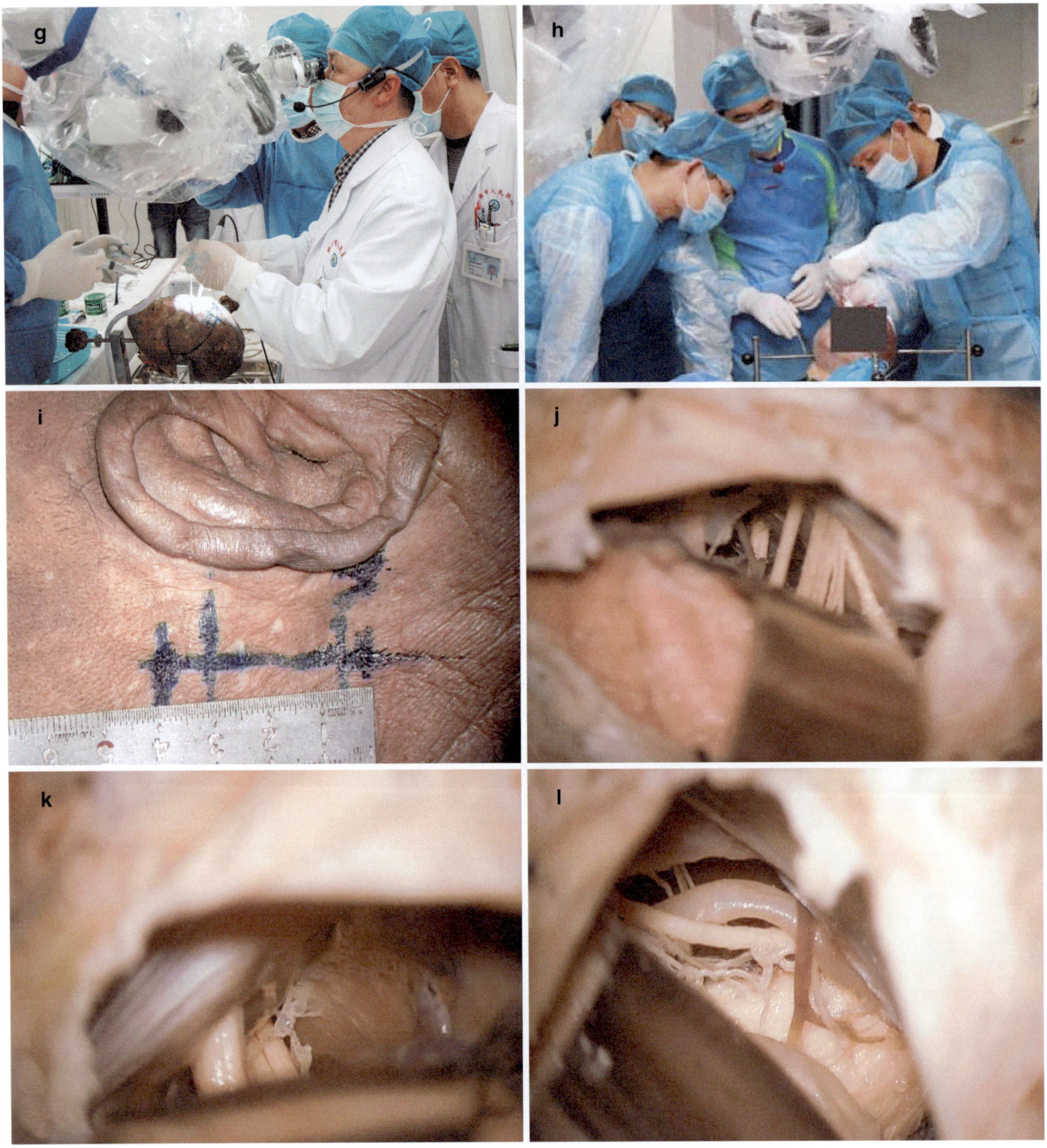

Fig. 13.1 (continued)

positioning, orientation, and real-time guidance provide reliable support for minimally invasive procedures. The main advantages of neuro-navigation include precise localization, optimal surgical approach, and real-time tracking and guidance during surgery. The navigation system provides surgeons with real-time feedback on intraoperative information, allowing for a better understanding of the relationship between anatomical structures and pathologies. Deep-seated lesions in functional areas like brainstem hemorrhages enable safer, faster, and more accurate identification of the lesion's location,

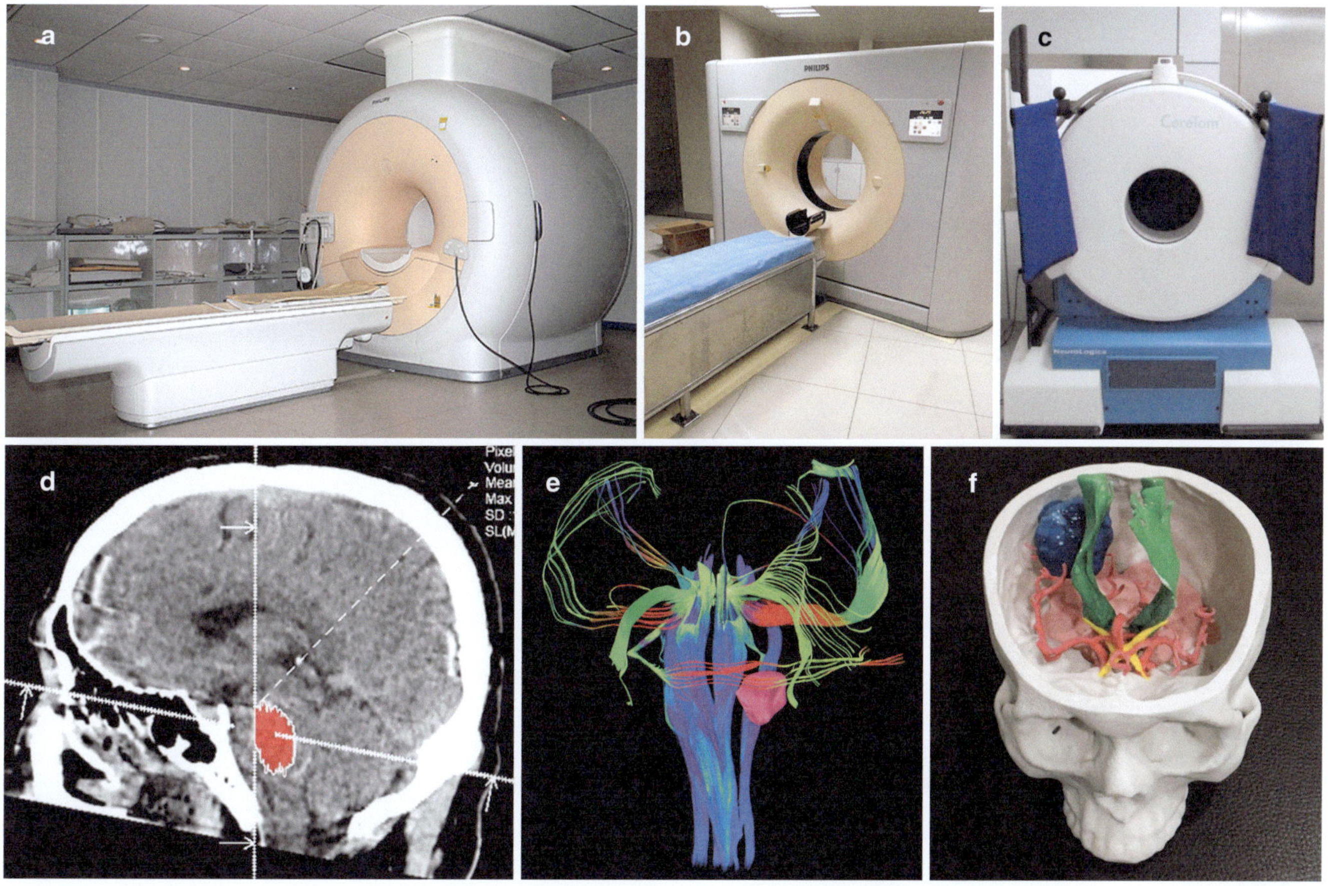

Fig. 13.2 Essential imaging equipment support for keyhole surgery. (**a**) 3.0 T MR. (**b**) 64-slice spiral CT. (**c**) bedside mobile CT. (**d**) displaying hematoma location using imaging software after CT scanning. (**e**) fiber bundle imaging F. 3D printing of hematoma models after three-dimensional reconstruction

effectively reducing intraoperative secondary damage, shortening surgical time, and improving surgical quality.

(f) Neuroendoscope: The development and improvement of neuroendoscopy have provided favorable conditions for keyhole microsurgery, allowing for their use as an adjunct in cases where the visual field is poor. Neuroendoscopes with a diameter of 2–4 mm can provide a bright and detailed image of deep-seated lesions, and the closer to the lesion, the better and more precise the image magnification effect. Angled endoscopes can reveal visual blind spots that are difficult to detect under the microscope, reducing traction and damage to normal tissues while enhancing surgical efficacy (Fig. 13.3).

(g) Intraoperative Neurophysiological Monitoring: Intraoperative neuroelectrophysiological monitoring has become an indispensable component of neurosurgical procedures for assessing the integrity of neural function, minimizing tissue disruption, and improving surgical quality. It allows for early detection and identification of nerve injuries caused by surgery, enabling prompt correction of the underlying cause and preventing permanent nerve damage.

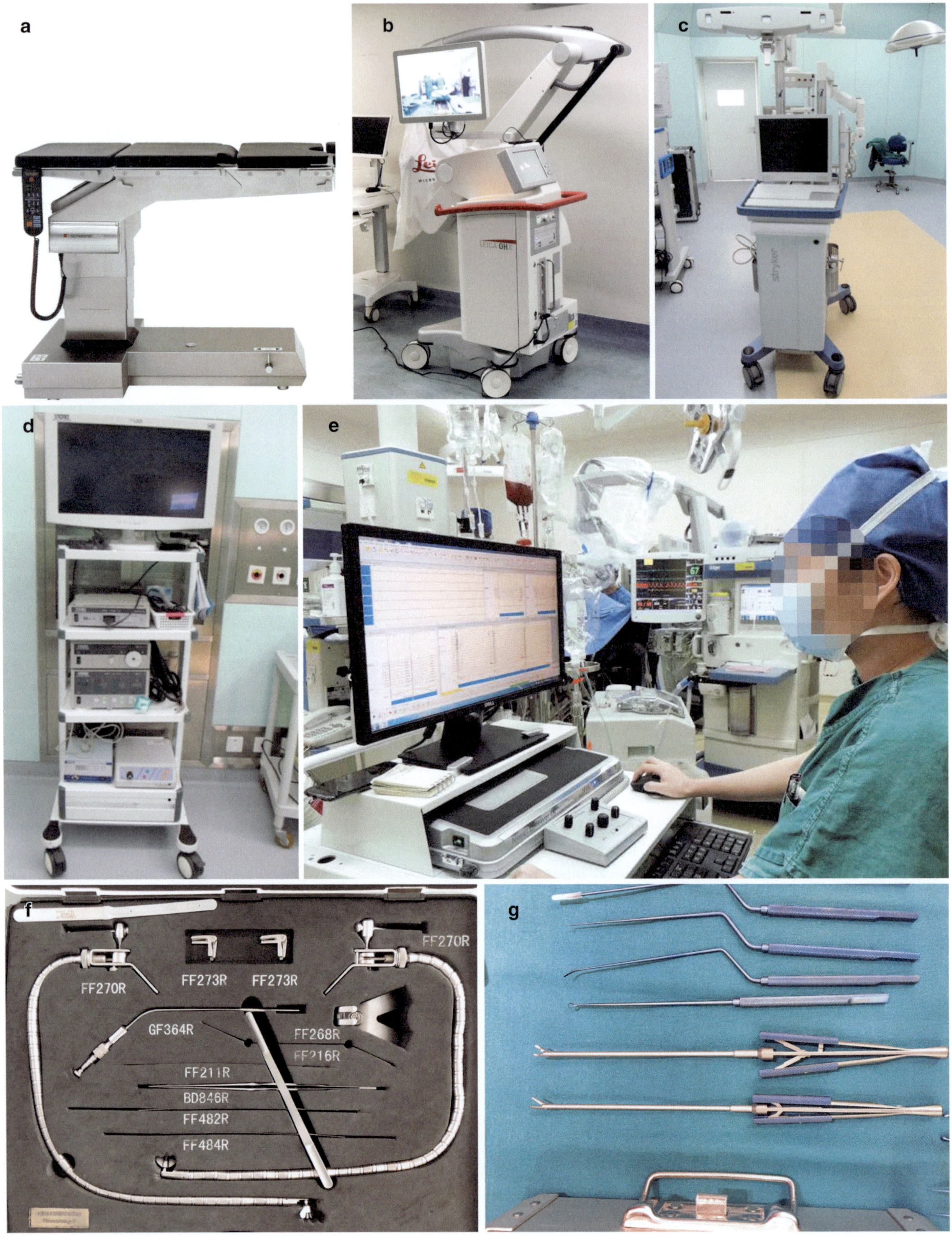

Fig. 13.3 Essential surgical equipment and instrumentation for keyhole surgery. (**a**) Fully automated operating table for convenient intraoperative adjustments. (**b**) Leica high-definition microscope. (**c**) navigation device. (**d**) neuroendoscopy. (**e**) neuroelectrophysiological monitoring equipment. (**f**) automatic retractors and suction devices. (**g**) microsurgical instruments

13.3 Subtemporal Keyhole Approach for Brainstem Hemorrhage Evacuation

13.3.1 Surgical Indications and Contraindications

1. Indications

   No unified surgical standard for brainstem hemorrhage. However, the following conditions are generally considered suitable for surgical intervention:

   (a) Hematoma located in the upper pons and the lower midbrain, especially when biased toward one side, relatively concentrated, and close to or protruding from the surface of the brainstem.
   (b) Hematoma volume > 5 mL or the maximum cross-sectional bleeding area > 50% of the corresponding brainstem section.
   (c) GCS score < 8, severe neurological impairment, or progressive deterioration of neurological function.
   (d) After fully informing the patient's family about the surgical risks and potential financial burdens, and consequences, the family strongly expresses the desire for surgery.

2. Contraindications
   (a) Hematoma volume < 5 mL.
   (b) No significant impairment of consciousness.
   (c) Unstable circulation, inability to maintain basic vital signs.
   (d) Severe coagulation dysfunction or multi-organ failure.
   (e) Patient or family refusal of surgery.

13.3.2 Preoperative Preparation and Surgical Instruments

1. Preoperative Preparation

   Maintain airway patency. Early endotracheal intubation is performed for patients with airway obstruction or inadequate airway. Control blood pressure, conduct comprehensive biochemical and coagulation function tests, and rule out contraindications. Prior to surgery, a lumbar puncture is performed to place a lumbar drain in the lumbar cistern and temporary clamp the drainage tube. In cases of significant hydrocephalus, external ventricular drainage should be prioritized.

2. Surgical Instruments

   The surgical equipment required includes a specialized electric operating table, neurosurgical microscope, headframe, automatic retractor, electric cranial drill, bipolar coagulation, and microsurgical instruments. Navigation systems and intraoperative neuroelectrophysiological monitoring equipment are recommended.

13.3.3 Surgical Techniques and Considerations

1. Surgical Techniques

   (a) Patient Positioning and Head Placement: Generally, a lateral decubitus position is sufficient, with the zygomatic arch in a horizontal position, tilted 15° posteriorly and 15° laterally toward the opposite side to compensate for the upward tilt of the middle cranial fossa.
   (b) Incision: The skin incision is located approximately 1 cm in front of the tragus of the ear, and a straight incision about 4 cm in length is made above the lower border of the zygomatic arch (Fig. 13.4).
   (c) Craniotomy: After the skin incision, the subcutaneous tissue is dissected to avoid injury to the facial nerve frontal branch and superficial temporal artery. The skin is retracted, and the temporal muscle fascia is incised in a "Y" shape. The fascial flap below the incision is flipped toward the zygomatic arch. The remaining fascia is pulled laterally along with the

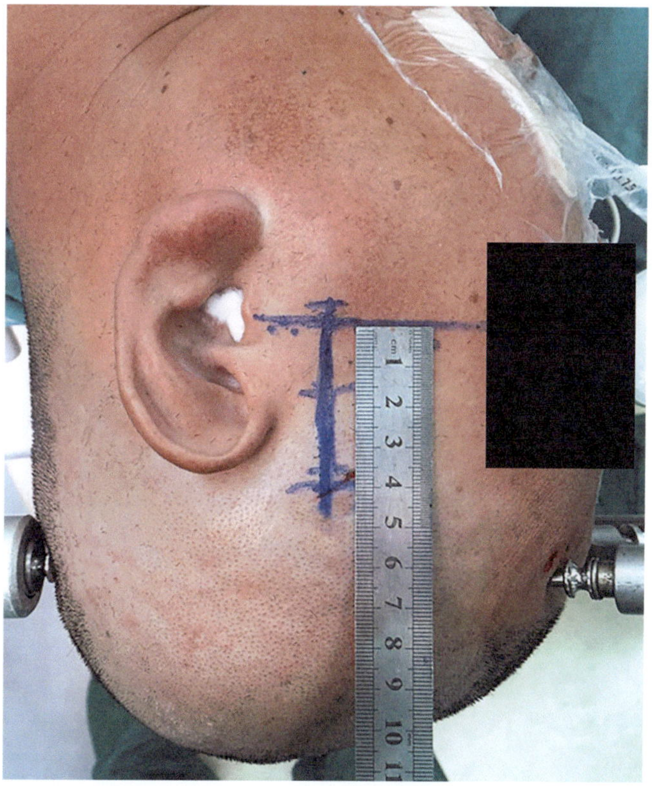

Fig. 13.4 The incision for the keyhole approach is located in front of the ear, starting from the lower border of the zygomatic arch, approximately 4 cm in length

skin. The temporal muscle is vertically incised and retracted bilaterally to expose the squamous part of the temporal bone. A hole is drilled at the root of the zygomatic arch, and the bone flap is shaped with a milling cutter, approximately 25 mm × 20 mm in size. The lower edge of the bone window should be in close contact with the zygomatic arch and its root. To achieve good exposure, the upper inner edge of the zygomatic arch root should be removed (Fig. 13.5).

(d) Dural Incision and Opening of the Tentorial Internal Edge: Open the lumbar cistern drainage tube to release approximately 30 mL of cerebrospinal fluid, and then clamp the drainage tube. Under the microscope, the dura mater is incised flap-like and suspended. Lift the base of the temporal lobe gently under the microscope, gradually releasing cerebrospinal fluid to reduce intracranial pressure. Proceed deeper and expose the tentorial edge, where the trochlear nerve runs parallel to it. Take care to avoid injury. The trochlear nerve enters the tentorial point approximately 1–1.5 cm behind it. Incise and suspend the tentorium's free edge and the tentorium's inner side by approximately 1 cm, exposing the lateral aspect of the mid-upper part of the pons and the lower part of the midbrain (Fig. 13.6).

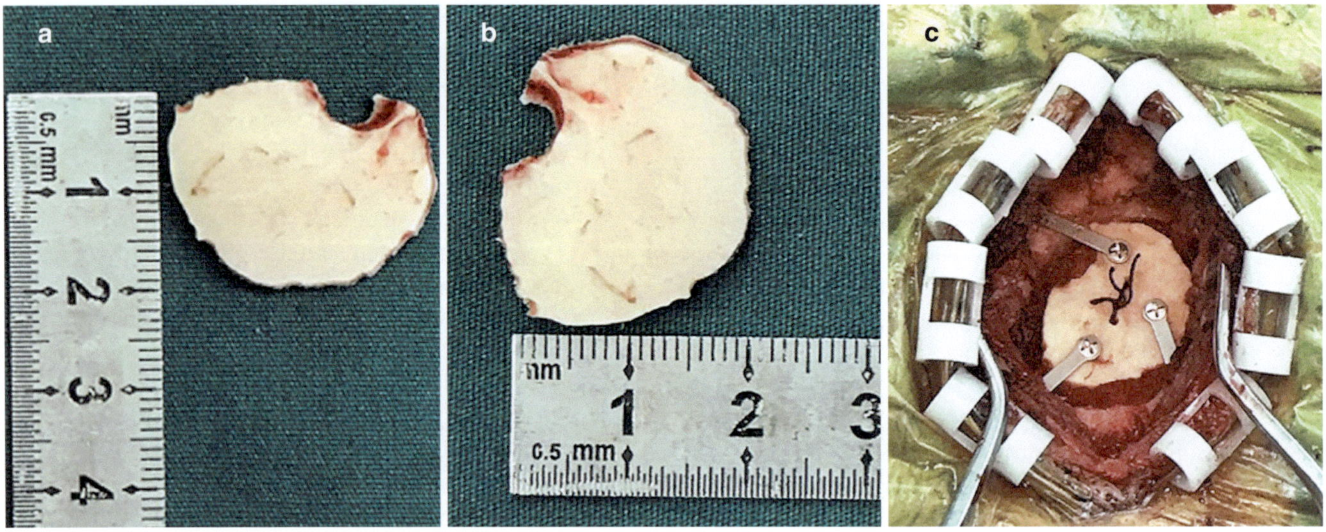

Fig. 13.5 Craniotomy. (**a**, **b**) The diameter of the bone window is approximately 2 cm C. The small bone flap is fixed with titanium connecting plates

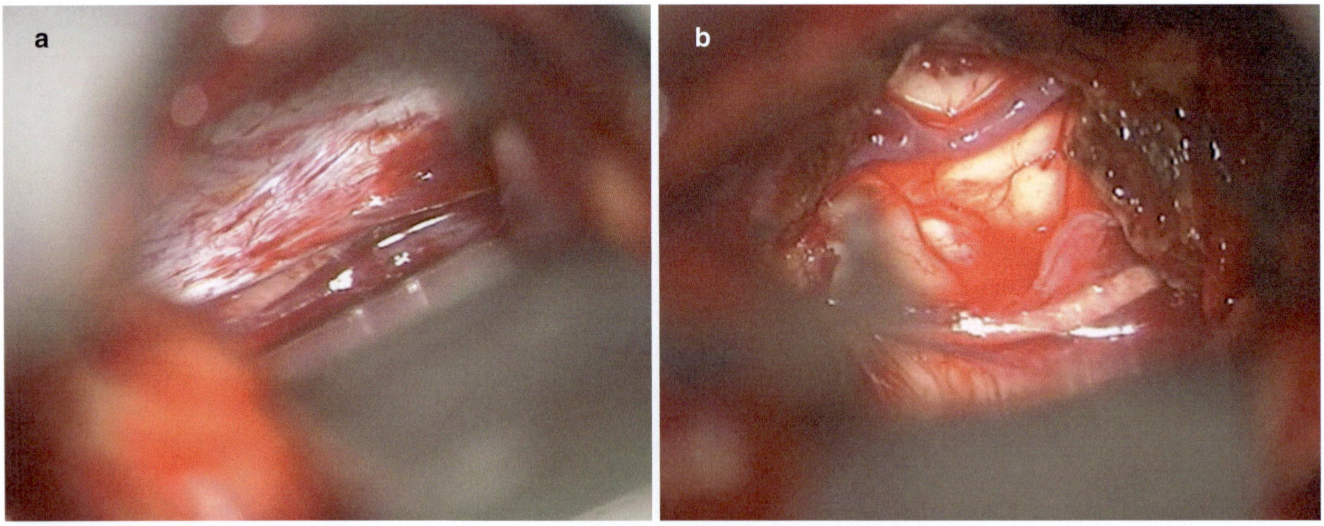

Fig. 13.6 Dural incision and opening of the tentorial internal edge. (**a**). Incision of the free edge of the tentorium and the inner side of the tentorium. (**b**) exposing the lateral aspect of the upper part of the pons and the lower part of the midbrain

(e) Hematoma Evacuation: Under the microscope, select the area of abnormal cortical coloration in the brainstem or above and below the superior cerebellar artery. Use a micro-dissector to separate the cortical tissue of the brainstem gradually, from superficial to deep, until reaching the hematoma cavity. Use a small suction device to operate within the hematoma cavity slowly and gently, ensuring gentle movements. The entire surgical procedure should be performed within the hematoma cavity without crossing the edema zone around the hematoma. For adherent small blood clots on the hematoma cavity wall, forceful removal is not necessary. For a small amount of bleeding, compression with Surgicel can be applied to achieve hemostasis. In the case of arterial bleeding, identify the bleeding artery, lower the bipolar power, and gently coagulate to achieve hemostasis (Fig. 13.7).

(f) Craniotomy Closure: After satisfactory hemostasis in the surgical area, suture the dura mater, reposition and fix the bone flap, and perform layered closure of the temporal muscle, its fascia, and the subcutaneous layers (Fig. 13.8, Video 13.1).

2. Surgical Considerations

(a) The small size of the keyhole bone flap limits the extent of traction on the temporal lobe. Prior to surgery, a lumbar drain tube can be placed, and after the bone flap is formed, the drainage tube can be opened to drain 30–50 mL of cerebrospinal fluid, which can reduce traction on the temporal lobe.

(b) The principle of the keyhole approach lies in the doorhole effect, so the skin flap and bone window should be as smooth as possible, and any bony protrusions on the lateral wall of the middle cranial fossa should be removed to ensure a radiating expansion of the intracranial target field of view. If the mastoid air cells are opened during the drilling process, they should be properly sealed with bone wax, and a final check should be performed during the closure of the skull to prevent cerebrospinal fluid leakage.

(c) The trochlear nerve runs below the tentorial edge. When cutting the tentorial free edge, it is essential to make the incision behind the point where the trochlear nerve enters the tentorium.

(d) During the procedure, the preferred entry point into the brainstem is through the site of hematoma rupture or abnormal cortical coloration near the brainstem or above and below the superior cerebellar arteries. The changes in evoked potentials during the hematoma evacuation process provide accurate and sensitive electrophysiological indicators of brainstem functional activity, objectively reflecting the functional status of the brainstem and avoiding damage to the brainstem around the hematoma wall.

(e) Whenever possible, suction should be performed within the hematoma cavity. Large clots should be fragmented and removed in sections, avoiding breaching the hematoma wall to prevent further damage to the brainstem.

(f) Pay attention to mastering hemostasis techniques. For active bleeding, low-power bipolar electrocoagulation can be used. In cases of bleeding from the surgical site, the wound can be covered with a water-moistened gelatin sponge or hemostatic gauze, and gentle pressure can be applied with a cotton pad to achieve hemostasis.

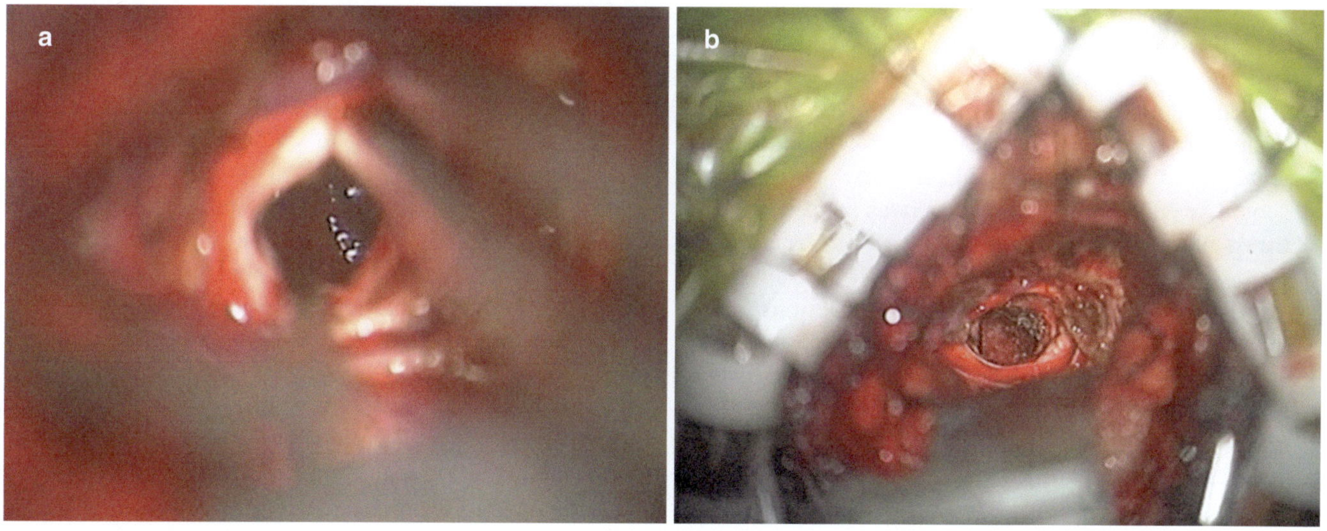

Fig. 13.7 Hematoma evacuation. (**a**) Slow and gentle removal of the hematoma with suction. (**b**) hemostasis is satisfactory in the surgical area after hematoma evacuatio

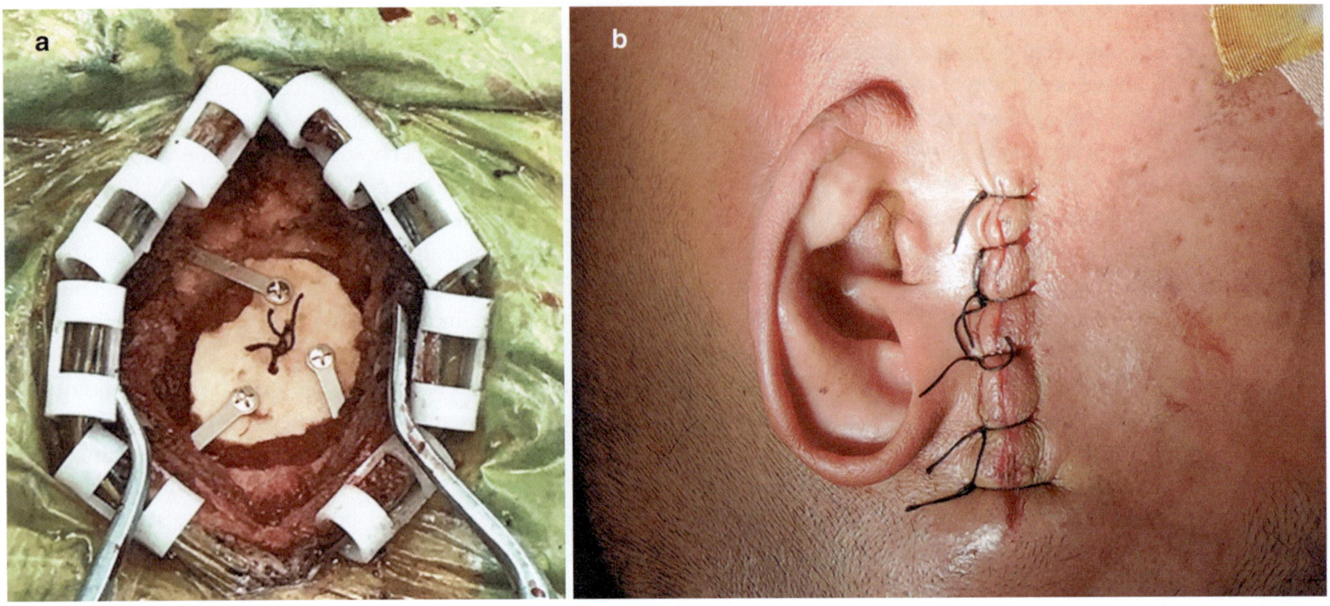

Fig. 13.8 Craniotomy closure. (**a**) Fixation of the bone flap. (**b**) layered closure of the scalp

13.3.4 Postoperative Management and Prevention of Complications

1. Postoperative rebleeding: Elevated blood pressure is the leading cause of rebleeding within the hematoma cavity. Therefore, blood pressure should be stabilized and maintained at a level of 140/90 mmHg postoperatively. Sedation and analgesia can be used appropriately based on the patient's condition to help maintain stable blood pressure. During the procedure, prolonged traction on the temporal lobe or injury to the basal temporal vein, especially the Labbé vein, can lead to temporal lobe contusion, delayed hematoma, and edema. Every effort should be made to avoid these complications. If significant brain swelling occurs postoperatively, decompression of the bone flap may be necessary.
2. Pulmonary infection: For patients expected to remain in a coma for a prolonged period, an early tracheostomy should be performed to facilitate airway management.
3. Stress ulcer bleeding in the upper gastrointestinal tract: Proton pump inhibitors can be used postoperatively to prevent and alleviate acute gastric mucosal lesions caused by stress.
4. Central fever: Central fever caused by brainstem hemorrhage is a severe manifestation of brain injury and belongs to the noninfectious fever category. Body temperature can reach around 40 °C, and sustained hyperthermia worsens brain damage, often leading to the patient's death within a short period. Postoperatively, physical cooling methods such as ice blankets and caps can lower the temperature.
5. Regular monitoring of electrolytes and renal function in patients to maintain water and electrolyte balance. If the patient's consciousness recovers, early neurorehabilitation and hyperbaric oxygen therapy should be initiated to improve the quality of life.

13.3.5 Advantages, Disadvantages, and Lessons Learned

1. Advantages

   (a) The subtemporal keyhole approach causes less damage, saves surgical time, and reduces intraoperative bleeding, leading to a lower incidence of complications.
   (b) The incision for the subtemporal keyhole approach starts 1 cm in front of the ear, and only a minimal vertical dissection and slight retraction of the temporal muscle are required to expose the surgical field. The limited dissection of the temporal muscle minimizes the risk of atrophy, with minimum injury to arteries and nerves.
   (c) Compared to the traditional subtemporal approach, the keyhole approach avoids excessive traction on the temporal lobe and damage to the Labbé vein due to the limitations of the bone window.

2. Disadvantages

   This approach has specific requirements for surgical instruments, and the surgeon needs to have a deep understanding of microanatomy, proficient microsurgical techniques, and extensive clinical surgical experience. Good illumination and more advanced surgical instruments are required for deep-seated operations. Careless manipulation can easily damage surrounding vital structures.

13.3.6 Evaluation and Prospects of the Approach

The subtemporal keyhole approach offers the advantages of shorter surgical and closure times, more minor trauma, and faster postoperative healing. It is not simply a "miniaturization" of the traditional subtemporal approach but rather a comprehensive application of minimally invasive principles in every detail of the surgical procedure. Therefore, it places significant demands on the surgeon's anatomical knowledge, microsurgical techniques, and ability to handle unexpected situations. Careless manipulation can easily lead to damage to surrounding vital structures. In clinical practice, the approach must be determined based on the location of the hematoma to ensure surgical quality.

13.3.7 Brief Introduction of a Typical Case

13.3.7.1 Brief Medical History and Radiographic Data

The patient, a male 36 years old, was admitted with the chief complaint of "sudden loss of consciousness accompanied by vomiting for 10 hours." On admission, physical examination revealed a heart rate of 95 beats/min, respiratory rate of 29 breaths/min, and blood pressure of 195/110 mmHg. The patient was in a moderate coma with a GCS 5. The pupils were equal and irregular, approximately 4 mm in diameter, with no light reflex. The limbs exhibited decerebrate posturing, and bilateral pathological signs were positive. Head CT showed brainstem hemorrhage, with an estimated volume of approximately 8 mL. The admission diagnosis was brainstem hemorrhage (the anterolateral aspect of the pons) and grade 3 hypertension (extremely high-risk group) (Fig. 13.9).

13.3.7.2 Surgical Procedure and Key Points

After anesthesia, a lumbar puncture was performed to place a catheter in the lumbar cistern. The patient was positioned in a proper lateral decubitus position, with the zygomatic arch in a horizontal position and tilted 15° backward and 15° toward the contralateral side to compensate for the upward tilt of the middle cranial fossa. A straight incision of approximately 1 cm in front of the ear and 4 cm above the lower edge of the zygomatic arch was made. The skin was dissected layer by layer. The temporal muscle fascia was incised in a "Y" shape, longitudinally incising the temporal muscle and pulling it to both sides to expose the squamous part of the temporal bone. A hole was drilled at the root of the zygomatic arch, and the bone flap was shaped with a milling cutter, measuring approximately 25 mm × 20 mm. The lower edge of the bone window should be closely attached to the zygomatic arch. To achieve good exposure, the upper inner edge of the zygomatic arch root should be ground away.

The lumbar cistern drainage tube was opened, and approximately 30 mL of cerebrospinal fluid was released.

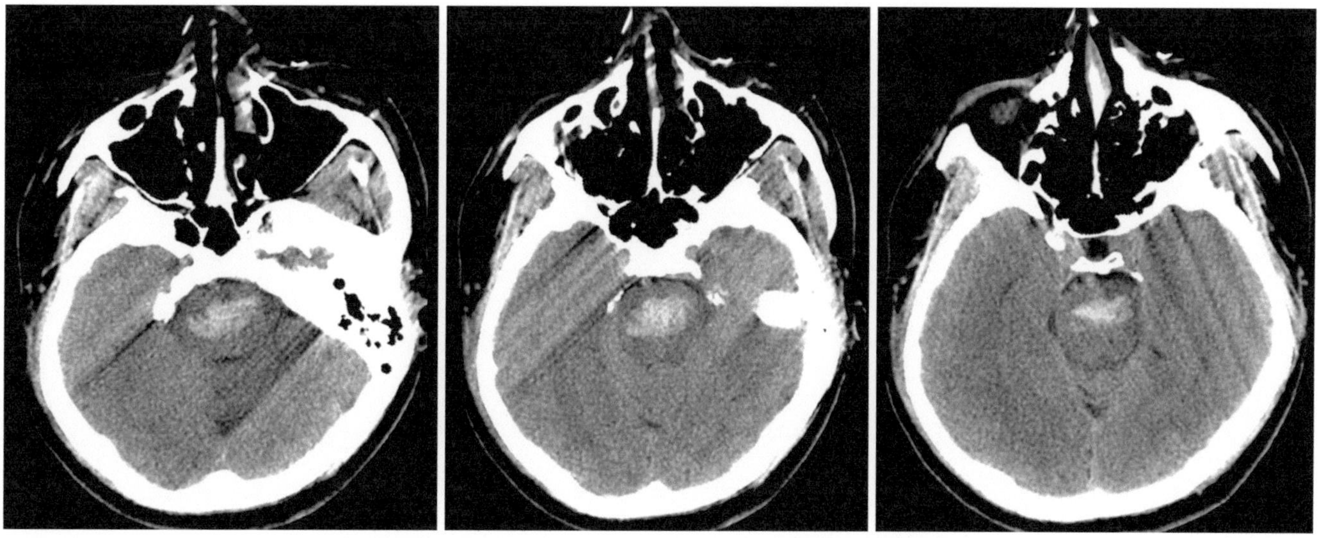

Fig. 13.9 Preoperative head CT of the patient

The dura mater was incised in a flap-like manner. Under the microscope, the base of the temporal lobe was gently lifted to gradually release cerebrospinal fluid, reduce intracranial pressure, and expose the free edge of the tentorium. At approximately 1–1.5 cm behind the entry of the trochlear nerve into the tentorium, the tentorium was incised for about 1 cm and suspended. The abnormal cortical area of the brainstem or the upper and lower aspects of the superior cerebellar artery were selected, and a microdissection instrument was used to separate the cortical tissue of the brainstem. Gradually, the hematoma cavity was reached, and a small suction device was used to remove the hematoma. After satisfactory hemostasis in the surgical area, the dura mater was sutured, the bone flap was repositioned and fixed, and the temporal muscle and scalp were sutured layer by layer (Fig. 13.10).

13.3.7.3 Preoperative and Postoperative Radiographic Comparison (Fig. 13.11)

13.3.7.4 Postoperative Neurological Examination Imaging Data

1. 1 week postoperatively: The patient had blurred consciousness, bilateral pupils were equal and round with a diameter of 1.5 mm, and the light reflex was sensitive. Muscle strength in the left limb was grade III, while in the right limb was grade I upon stimulation (Fig. 13.12).
2. (1 month postoperatively: The patient had clear consciousness and equal-sized pupils with a sensitive light reflex. Muscle strength in the left limb was grade IV-, while in the right limb was grade III. The bilateral Babinski sign was positive (Fig. 13.13).

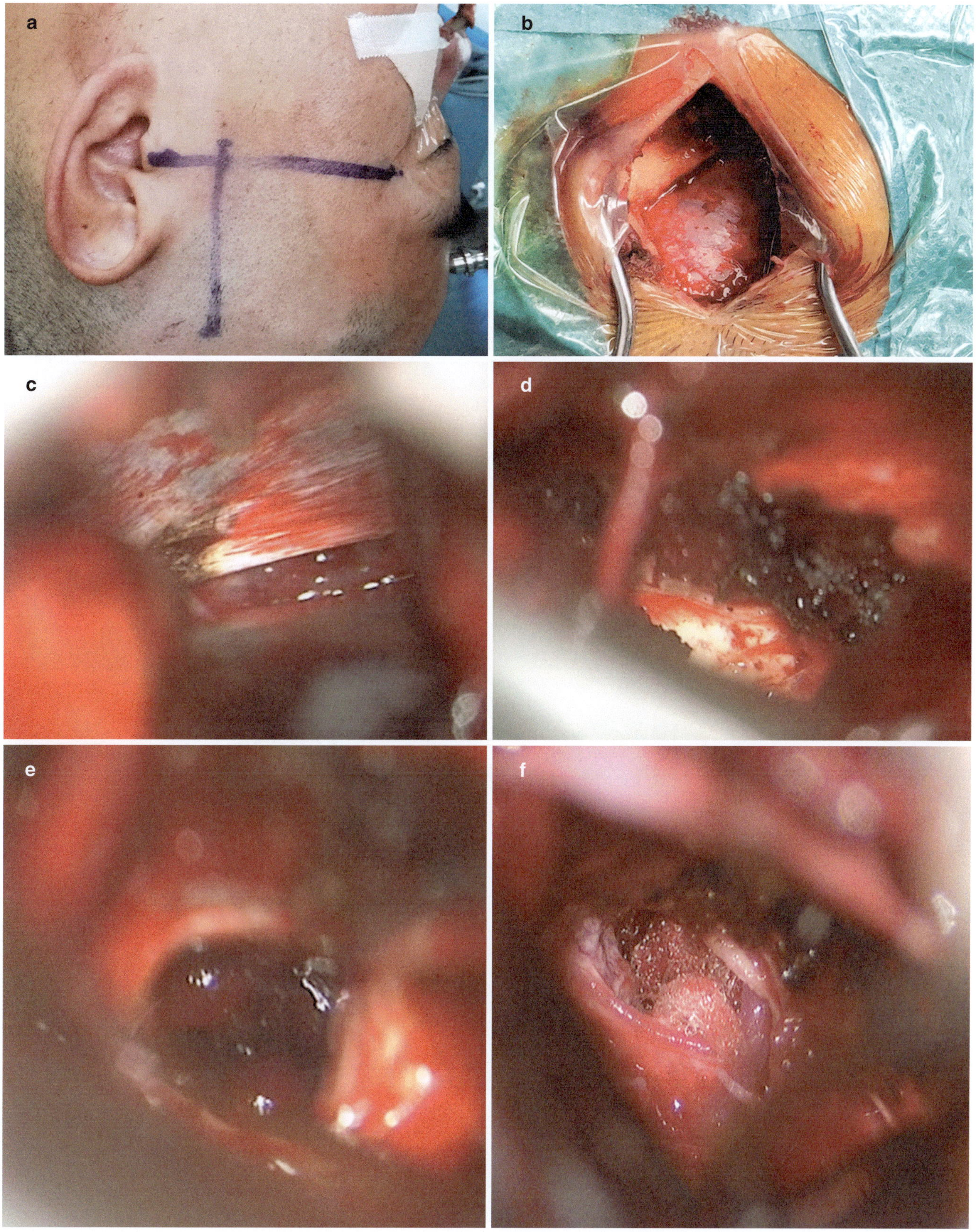

Fig. 13.10 Intraoperative process. (**a**) Straight incision in front of the left ear, starting from the lower edge of the zygomatic arch and about 4 cm long. (**b**) Mastoid retractor used to retract the skin flap and temporal muscle to both sides. Zygomatic arch root drilling and milling cutter used to mill a bone flap measuring approximately 25 mm × 20 mm. (**c**) Exposing the edge of the tentorium, incising the tentorium at a point approximately 1–1.5 cm behind the entry of the trochlear nerve into the tentorium. (**d**) Separating the cortical tissue of the brainstem from the abnormal color cortical area. (**e**) Gradually reaching the hematoma cavity from superficial to deep, removing the hematoma in blocks. (**f**) Satisfactory removal of the hematoma, minor oozing can be controlled by applying gelatin sponge compression

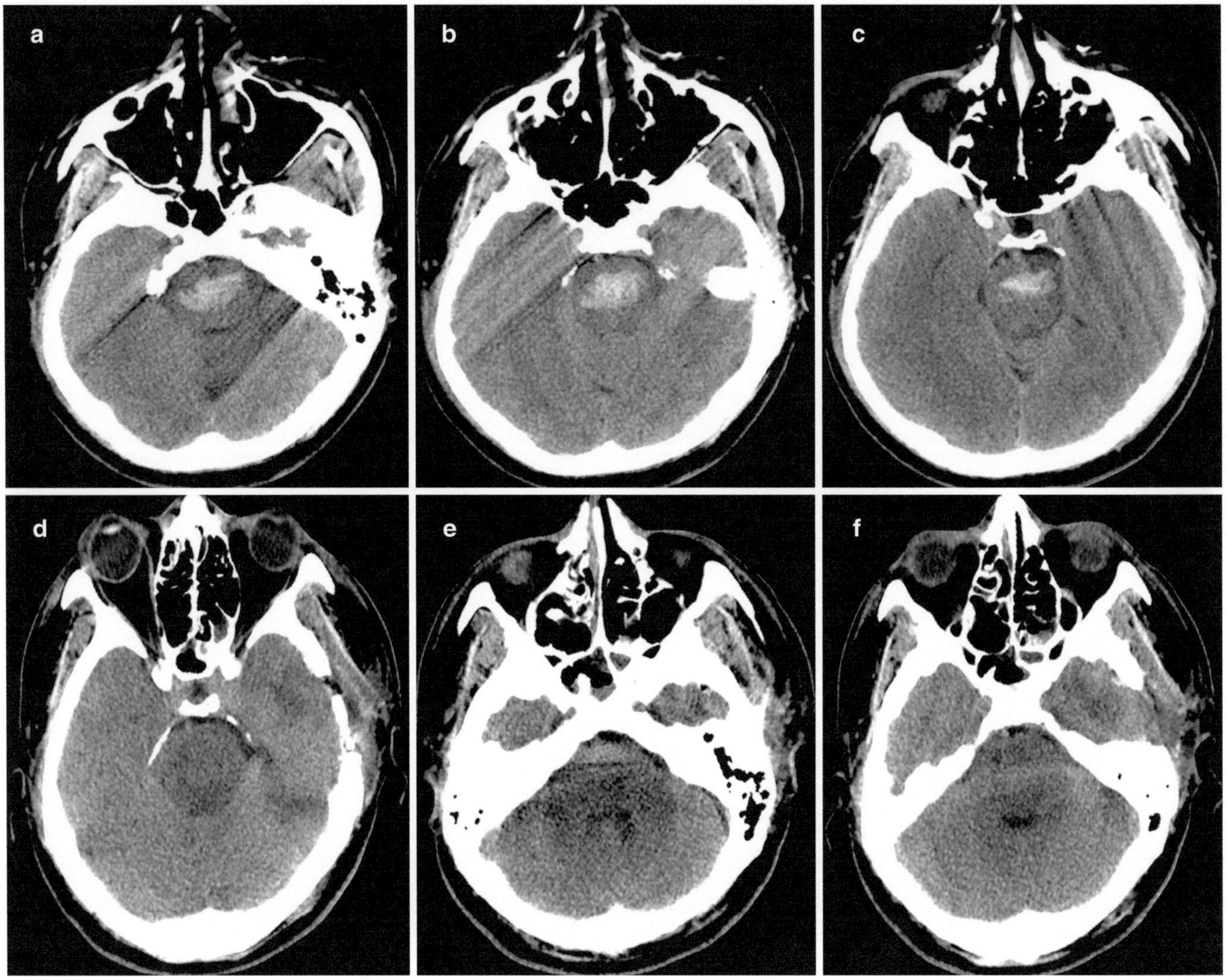

Fig. 13.11 Comparison of CT before and after surgery. (a–c) Preoperative CT. (d–f) Head CT 1 month after surgery

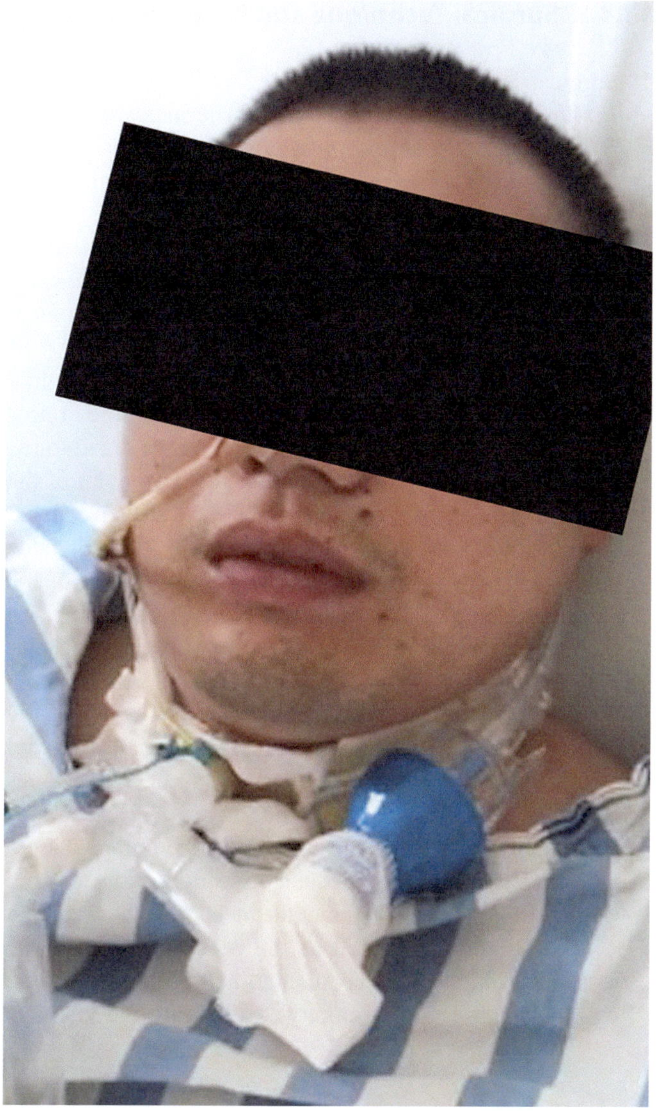

Fig. 13.12 Patient's condition 1 week postoperatively

13.4 Retrosigmoid Keyhole Approach for Brainstem Hematoma Evacuation

13.4.1 Indications and Contraindications

1. Indications

   There is no unified standard for the surgical indications of brainstem hematoma. Generally, the following conditions may be considered for surgical treatment.

   (a) The main part of the hematoma is located in the brainstem, predominantly on one side, relatively concentrated, and the hematoma is close to or breaks through the surface of the brainstem.

   (b) The hematoma volume is larger than 5 mL.

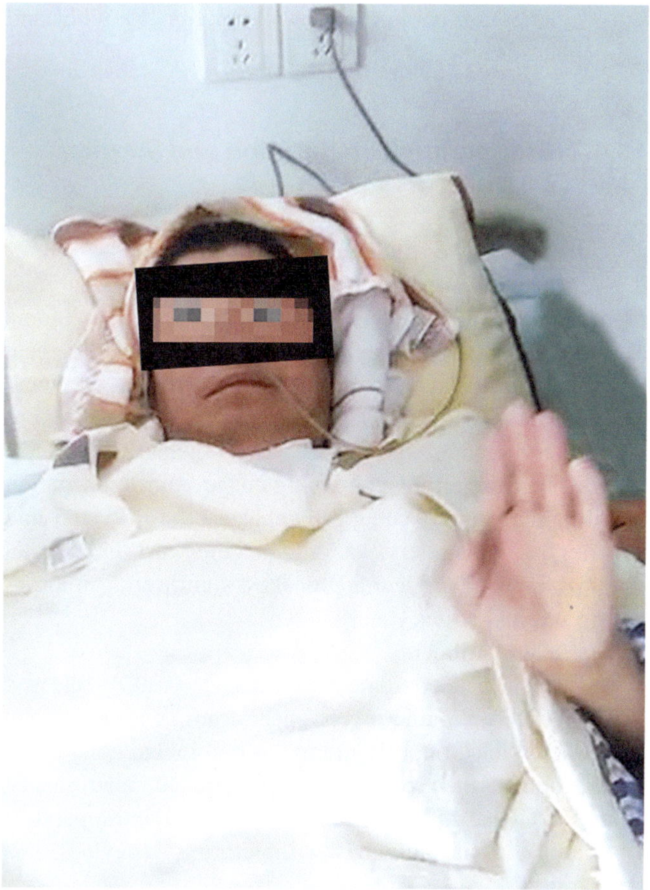

Fig. 13.13 Patient's condition 1 month postoperatively

   (c) The patient is in a state of light to moderate coma, with a GCS score of <8, accompanied or not accompanied by severe disturbances in vital signs.

   (d) The patient's family strongly desires surgery, and the family's financial situation can support long-term postoperative treatment.

2. Contraindications

   (a) Patients with small brainstem hematoma ($\leq$3 mL) without obvious obstruction of the ventricular system or unconsciousness.

   (b) For patients with an excessively large hematoma that severely damages the vital centers of the brainstem, leading to bilaterally dilated pupils and extreme instability of vital signs (no spontaneous breathing for more than 2 hours, occurrence of cardiac arrest or hypotension requiring vasopressors), surgery is generally not recommended.

   (c) Diffuse brainstem hemorrhage where it is difficult to achieve sufficient decompression through various surgical approaches.

   (d) The presence of other surgical contraindications, such as severe coagulation disorders or the insufficiency of cardiopulmonary function to withstand anesthesia.

13.4.2 Preoperative Preparation and Surgical Instruments

1. Preoperative Preparation

   Adequate preoperative preparation is an important measure to improve the efficacy of brainstem hematoma surgery. Maintaining airway patency, early endotracheal intubation, and active blood pressure control are crucial. For patients with significant hydrocephalus, external ventricular drainage is performed first. If the patient's condition and time permit, combining image-guided navigation with microsurgery can greatly enhance the efficiency and safety of the surgery. Various imaging workstations can now simulate surgical approaches, significantly improving surgical efficacy and safety.
2. Surgical Instruments

   The surgical equipment required a specialized electric operating table, microscope, head frame with automatic retractor, electric craniotomy drill, bipolar coagulator, monopolar electrocautery, microsurgical instruments, etc. The use of navigation systems and intraoperative neuroelectrophysiological monitoring devices is recommended.

13.4.3 Surgical Technique and Precautions

1. Surgical Technique
   (a) Positioning and Head Position: The standard position is lateral decubitus or lateral prone position. The head is rotated anteriorly by 15° to 30° from the lateral position, placing the mastoid plane at the highest point of the surgical field. The head is fixed using a three-pin head frame. In hospitals with the necessary facilities, intraoperative neuroelectrophysiological monitoring is recommended (Fig. 13.14).
   (b) Incision and Bone Window: The author's original "one point, two lines, two distances" modified retrosigmoid keyhole approach is used for the craniotomy. Mark the mastoid apex and the posterior point of the digastric groove, and determine the transverse sinus. A straight incision of approximately 4 cm is made about 1.5 cm posterior to the posterior point of the digastric groove. Cutting through the skin and subcutaneous tissue, followed by the deep muscles using an electric scalpel. Carefully exploring the occipital artery, which emerges from between the starting point of the trapezius muscle and terminal point of the sternocleidomastoid muscle and pierces through to the subcutaneous layer, and then thoroughly coagulated and cut. A bone membrane dissector is used for subperiosteal dissection, and a mastoid retractor is used to retract the incision, exposing local bony landmarks such as the posterior point of the digastric groove. The "one point, two lines, two distances" method is employed to locate the keyhole.

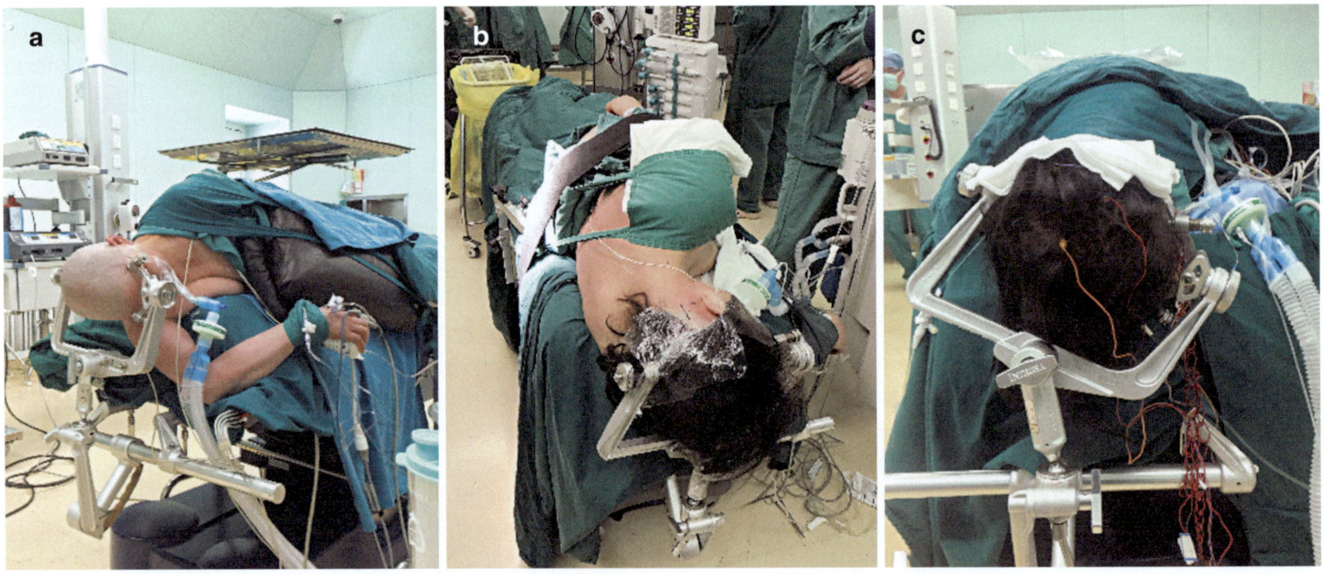

Fig. 13.14 Positioning and head position. (**a**) Lateral decubitus or lateral prone position with the head fixed in a head frame. (**b**) Anterior rotation of the head by 15°–30° from the lateral flexion position, placing the mastoid plane at the highest point of the surgical field. (**c**) Neuroelectrophysiological monitoring enhances the safety of the surgery

Drilling the keyhole with a diameter of 6 mm and creating a 2 cm × 2.5 cm bone flap with the milling cutter. The bone at the posterior edge of the sigmoid sinus is selectively removed depending on the individual variations. For the bone window, the upper boundary extends horizontally to the inferior margin of the transverse sinus, and the lateral boundary extends to the posterior edge of the sigmoid sinus. If the mastoid air cells are opened, seal them with bone wax. If necessary, the surrounding inner lamina of the cranial bone can be further removed to expand the surgical field (Fig. 13.15).

(c) Dural Incision: The lumbar cistern drainage tube is opened, and approximately 30 mL of cerebrospinal fluid is released. The dura is incised in a flap-like manner and suspended. Under the microscope, the lateral aspect of the cerebellum is gently pulled inward, gradually opening the cerebellomedullary

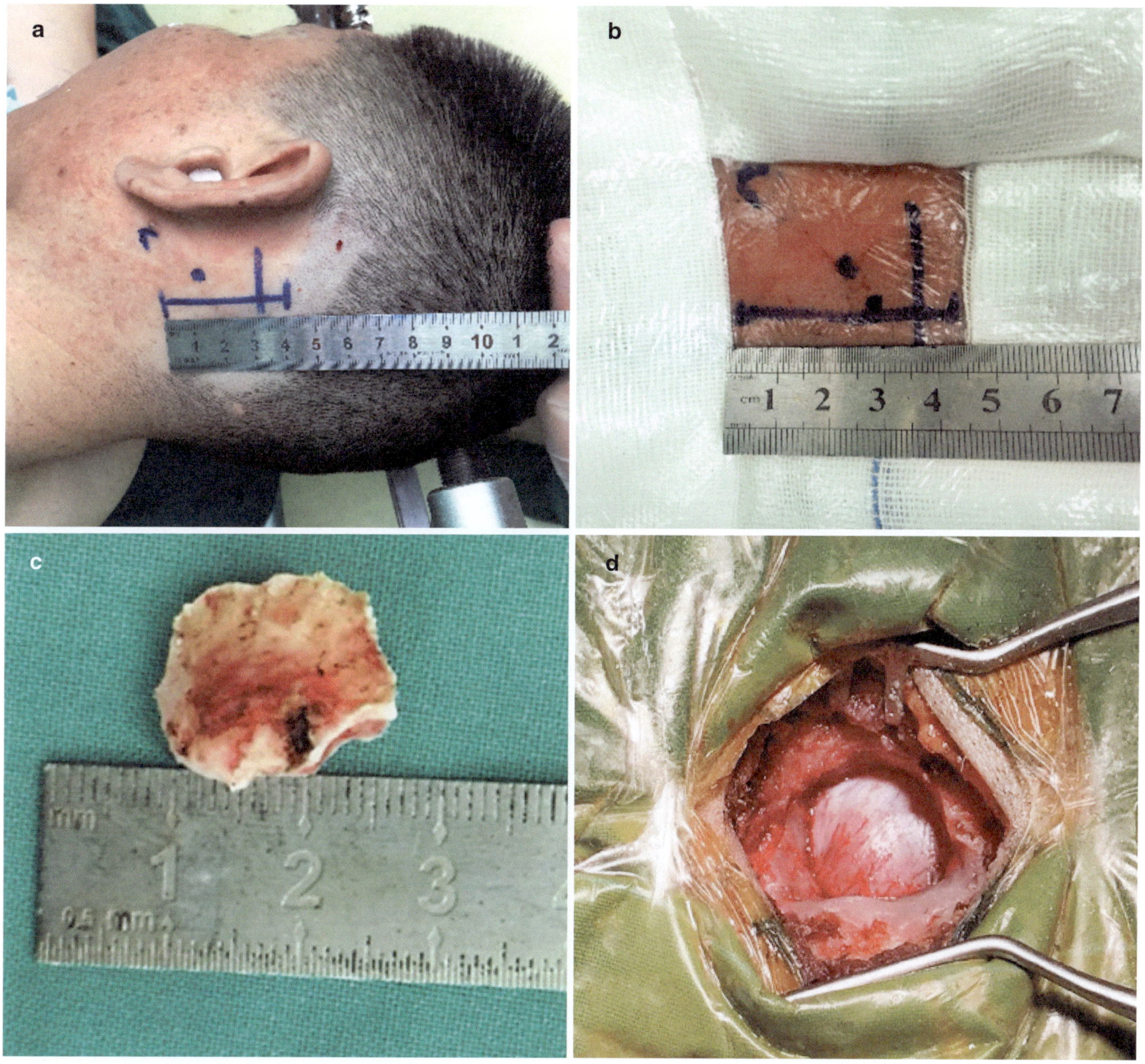

Fig. 13.15 Incision and bone flap. (**a**) Marking the mastoid apex and the posterior point of the digastric groove, determining the transverse line representing the inferior margin of the transverse sinus. Making an approximately 4 cm straight incision about 1.5 cm posterior to the posterior point of the digastric groove. (**b**) Removing the local hair behind the ear, covering the incision with sterile gauze, and securing it with a dressing film. The length of the incision is approximately 4 cm. (**c**) The diameter of the bone flap is approximately 1.5 cm. (**d**) After removing the bone flap, the bone window is exposed

cistern and releasing cerebrospinal fluid to reduce intracranial pressure. The hemisphere of the cerebellum is further pulled inward to increase the exposure space (Fig. 13.16).

(d) Hematoma Evacuation: After the intracranial pressure decreases, the hemisphere of the cerebellum is further pulled inward, and the superior petrosal vein, trigeminal nerve, facial nerve, and the blood clot that has entered the subarachnoid space through the lateral aspect of the pons are exposed under the microscope. The hematoma within the brainstem is cleared through a safe entry point in the paratrigeminal zone or at the site where the hematoma has reached the cortical surface of the brainstem. Hemostasis is achieved in the surgical area (Fig. 13.17).

(e) Closure: After observing the hematoma cavity for any inactive bleeding and achieving satisfactory hemostasis in the surgical area, the dura mater is watertight sutured. The bone flap is repositioned and fixed. The muscles are intermittently sutured in multiple layers, and the fascial layer is tightly and tensely sutured, with a recommended needle spacing of 5 mm. Subcutaneous and skin closure is performed routinely (Fig. 13.18, Video 13.2).

2. Surgical Techniques and Considerations

   (a) Use the author's original "one point, two lines, two distances" modified retrosigmoid keyhole craniotomy method. Mark the mastoid apex and the posterior point of the digastric groove, and determine the

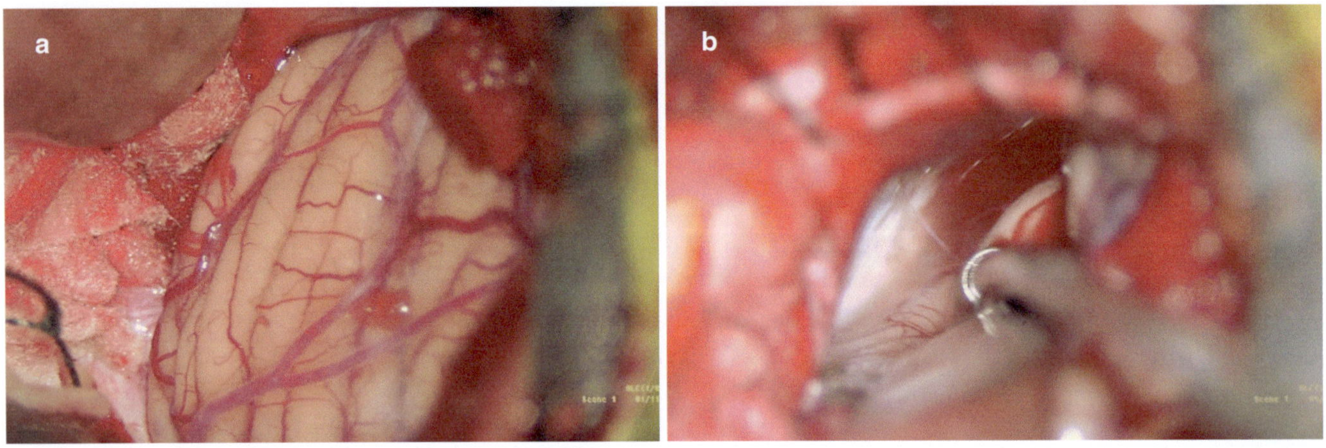

Fig. 13.16 Dural incision. (**a**) Incising the dura in a flap-like manner to expose the cerebellum. (**b**) Gradually opening the cerebellomedullary cistern, releasing cerebrospinal fluid to reduce intracranial pressure

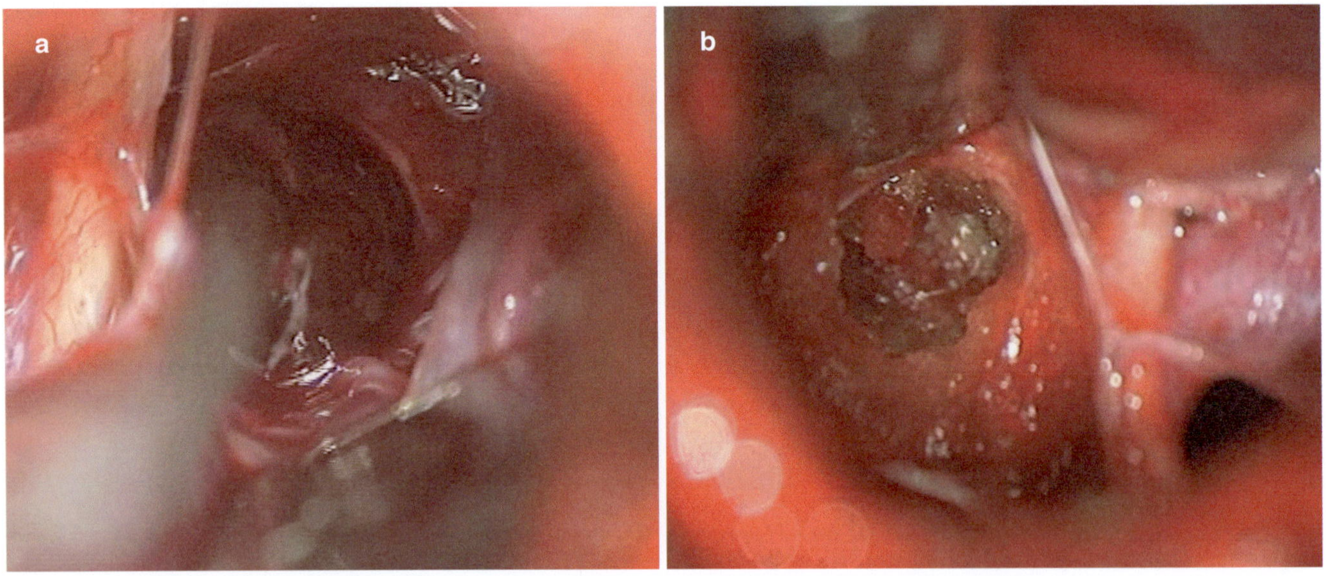

Fig. 13.17 Hematoma evacuation. (**a**) Suctioning and removing the hematoma through the cortical breakthrough site along the brainstem. The black area below the suction device represents the hematoma. (**b**) Hemostasis was achieved with the satisfactory removal of the hematoma, followed by filling the residual cavity with moist gelatin sponge or Surgicel

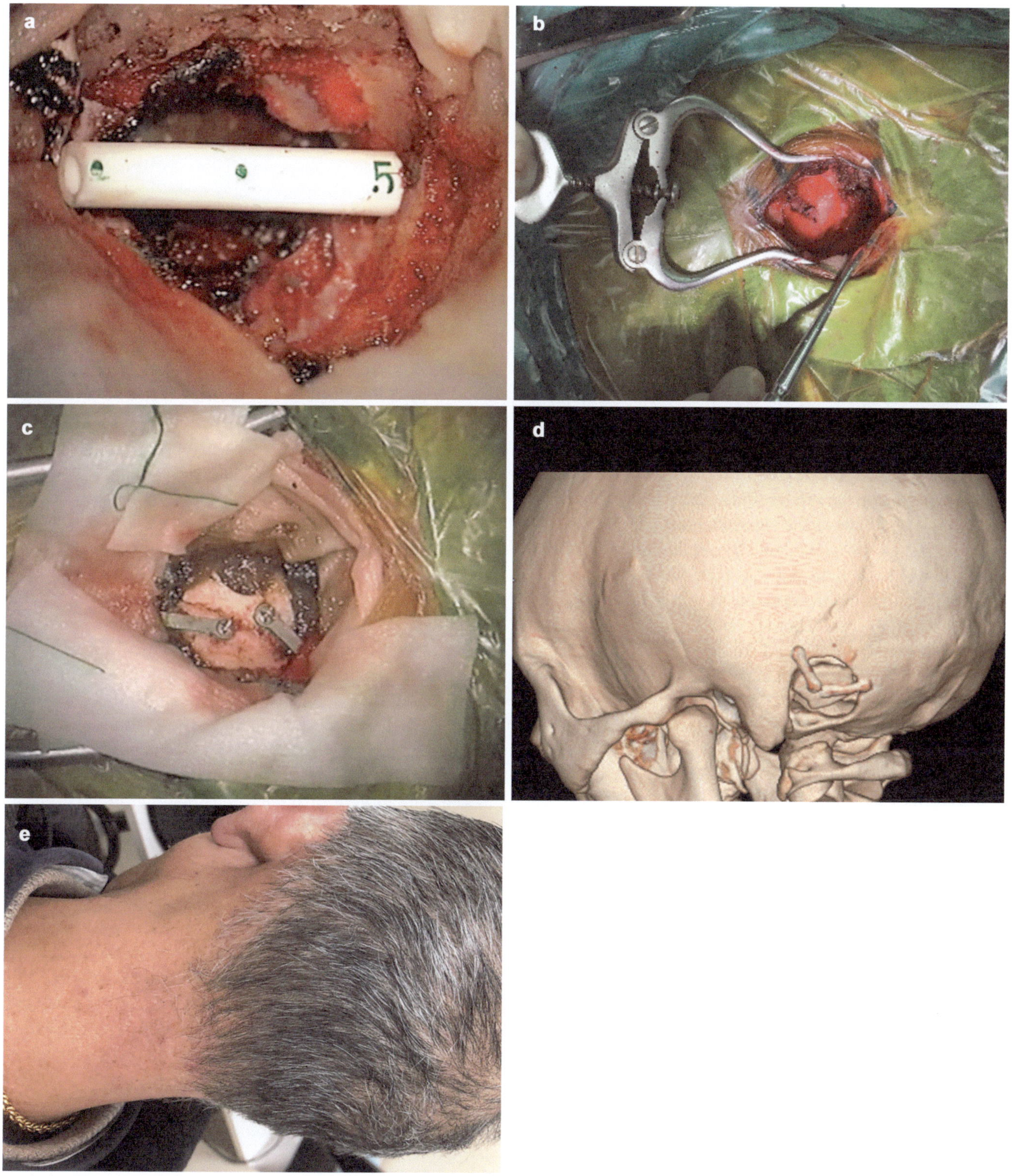

Fig. 13.18 Craniotomy closure. (**a**) Bone window with a diameter of less than 2 cm. (**b**) Dura mater tightly sutured. (**c**) Bone flap repositioned and fixed. (**d**) The three-dimensional reconstruction CT image showing the size of the bone window. (**e**) The surgical incision is not visible behind the mastoid when the patient is discharged

transverse sinus's surface projection. A straight incision of approximately 4 cm is made about 1.5 cm posterior to the posterior point of the digastric groove. Our original "one point, two lines, two distances" method is used to locate the keyhole. A burr hole with a diameter of 6 mm is created, and a bone flap of approximately 2 cm × 2.5 cm is formed using a milling cutter.

(b) Due to the small size of the bone window at the keyhole, a lumbar cistern drainage tube is placed preoperatively. It is temporarily clamped and then opened for drainage after the bone flap is formed, allowing slow drainage of 30–50 mL cerebrospinal fluid, which can reduce traction on the cerebellum.

(c) During the craniotomy, avoid damaging the venous sinuses, especially the sigmoid sinus. For patients with severe adhesions between the dura mater and the skull, a bone hole with a diameter of approximately 2 cm can be created using a burr to avoid milling through the venous sinuses during the craniotomy. The bone above the sigmoid sinus can be carefully polished with a burr, and the remaining eggshell-like bone can be removed with bone forceps.

(d) After incising the dura mater, the petrous bone surface of the cerebellum is pulled apart, further releasing cerebrospinal fluid from the cerebellomedullary cistern. Once the intracranial pressure significantly decreases, the arachnoid membrane in the cerebellopontine angle area is separated to expose the middle cerebellar peduncle and the lateral aspect of the pons. Special attention is paid to protecting the petrosal vein to avoid postoperative cerebellar swelling.

(e) Preferably, entry into the brainstem is through the site of hematoma rupture and, alternatively, through the safe zone of the brainstem. During hematoma evacuation, changes in evoked potentials provide accurate and sensitive electrophysiological indicators of brainstem functional activity, objectively reflecting the functional status of the brainstem and avoiding damage to the brainstem around the hematoma wall.

(f) Hematoma aspiration should be performed within the hematoma cavity. Combined with irrigation, it can loosen the blood clots. Large clots should be suctioned in fragments without breaching the hematoma wall to avoid increasing brainstem injury.

(g) Microscope illumination has attenuation and blind spots in deep areas. The combined use of neuroendoscopy allows clear illumination of deep areas, eliminates surgical blind spots, enables close observation, improves hematoma clearance rate, and reduces secondary damage to the brainstem. It also facilitates thorough hemostasis and reduces the probability of postoperative rebleeding.

(h) Pay attention to mastering hemostasis techniques. For active bleeding, low-power bipolar coagulation can be used. In cases of oozing, the wound can be covered with a gelatin sponge or hemostatic gauze, and gentle pressure with cotton pads can be applied to achieve hemostasis.

(i) Protecting the drainage veins as much as possible is important to prevent postoperative brainstem edema and compression of neural tissues, which can lead to neurological deficits.

13.4.4 Postoperative Management and Prevention of Complications

1. Postoperative rebleeding: The main cause of postoperative rebleeding is elevated blood pressure. Therefore, after surgery, blood pressure should be stabilized and maintained at a level of 140/90 mmHg. Sedation and analgesia may be used appropriately to help maintain stable blood pressure.
2. Pulmonary infection: Comatose patients often have poor sputum production after surgery and have a higher incidence of pulmonary infections. Early tracheostomy facilitates sputum clearance and reduces airway resistance, minimizing dead space ventilation and improving effective gas exchange in the alveoli, thus enhancing cerebral oxygen supply. Early mechanical ventilation assistance should be provided in cases of low blood oxygen saturation or respiratory dysfunction. In the event of pulmonary infection, appropriate antibiotics should be selected based on the sensitivity testing results.
3. Stress-related upper gastrointestinal bleeding: Proton pump inhibitors can be used postoperatively to prevent and alleviate acute gastric mucosal lesions caused by stress. Patients who cannot eat for 24 hours should receive gastric tube insertion and nasogastric feeding with a liquid diet to protect the gastric mucosa. For patients with gastrointestinal bleeding, gastric lavage with ice saline solution plus coagulation factors or intragastric injection of 0.02% norepinephrine can effectively control bleeding.
4. Central fever: Central fever caused by brainstem hemorrhage is a severe manifestation of brain injury and belongs to noninfectious fever. The body temperature can reach around 40 °C, and persistent high fever exacerbates brain damage, often leading to the patient's death within a short period. Postoperatively, physical cooling methods such as cooling blankets and ice caps can be used to lower cerebral oxygen consumption and metabolic rate, reduce cerebral edema, decrease intracranial pressure, alleviate

neuronal damage, and promote functional recovery. Drug-induced hypothermia may induce stress ulcers and should be minimized.

5. Regular electrolytes and renal function monitoring are necessary to maintain water and electrolyte balance. If the patient's consciousness improves, early neurorehabilitation and hyperbaric oxygen therapy should be implemented to improve the quality of life.

13.4.5 Advantages, Disadvantages, and Lessons Learned

1. The author's original "One Point, Two Lines, Two Distances" modified retrosigmoid keyhole craniotomy method is safe, accurate, simple, and minimally invasive, and worthy of clinical promotion.
2. The retrosigmoid keyhole approach allows for rapid access to the lateral aspect of the pons. The hematoma site often presents as a local bulge or color changes. If the hematoma ruptures, a local hematoma can be easily identified in the cisterna ambiens. During the surgery, a vertical incision is made in the brainstem cortex on one side of the bulge, and the hematoma is removed using a microsuction apparatus under microscope. This approach is minimally invasive, accurate, easy to perform, and results in less bleeding.
3. The retrosigmoid keyhole approach has limited operative space, limited exposure, and a narrow space, which can lead to difficulties in surgical manipulation. Inappropriate traction of brain tissue can cause more severe brain damage, which should be taken into consideration. The most effective method is to open the cistern and release cerebrospinal fluid, allowing the brain tissue to retract independently. For patients with high intracranial pressure, if dehydration therapy is ineffective, cerebrospinal fluid can be drained by ventricular puncture before the surgery. Alternatively, a lumbar cistern catheter drainage can be performed preoperatively to drain cerebrospinal fluid during the surgery and reduce intracranial pressure.

13.4.6 Evaluation and Prospects of the Surgical Technique

The retrosigmoid approach allows for rapid access to the lateral aspect of the pons, and a vertical incision on the lateral side is relatively safe [11]. The retrosigmoid keyhole approach for the treatment of severe primary brainstem hemorrhage provides a clear surgical field and shorter operation time, making it a simple and effective surgical method. The author's original "One Point, Two Lines, Two Distances" modified retrosigmoid keyhole approach craniotomy method has the advantages of accurate localization, safe and simple, and minimally invasive, which are worth promoting in clinical practice. With the accumulation of microsurgical experience, improvement of microsurgical techniques and instruments, and advancements in neuroimaging technology, the application of the modified retrosigmoid keyhole approach for early removal of brainstem hematoma can significantly improve the survival rate and quality of life of patients with severe primary brainstem hemorrhage [12].

13.4.7 Typical Case

13.4.7.1 Summary of Medical History and Radiographic Data

The patient, a 56-year-old male, was admitted due to "sudden unconsciousness for more than 2 hours." Physical examination: blood pressure 151/78 mmHg, weak respiration, moderate coma, GCS score of 5, equal and round pupils bilaterally with a diameter of approximately 2.0 mm, sensitive light reflex, flexion response of the left limbs to painful stimuli, no response of the right limbs to painful stimuli, and positive bilateral Babinski sign. Auxiliary examination: Head CT scan showed brainstem hemorrhage with a volume of approximately 9 mL. Admission diagnosis: brainstem hemorrhage and hypertensive disease (extremely critical type) (Fig. 13.19).

13.4.7.2 Surgical Procedure and Key Points

After general anesthesia, the patient was placed in a right lateral decubitus position. A lumbar puncture was performed preoperatively to place a catheter in the lumbar cistern, and the drainage tube was temporarily clamped. A 4 cm incision was made in the left posterior mastoid area. Standard disinfection and draping were performed, followed by incision of the scalp and muscles to expose the vertex of the digastric groove. The keyhole was located using the author's original "One Point, Two Lines, Two Distances" method, and a 6 mm diameter keyhole was created using a drill. A 2 cm × 2 cm bone flap was formed using a milling cutter.

The lumbar cistern drainage tube was opened, and approximately 30 mL of cerebrospinal fluid was released. The dura mater was incised in an arc shape and suspended. The brain tissue pressure obviously decreased and then was further released of cerebrospinal fluid from the cerebellomedullary cistern by retracting the petrous surface of the cerebellum. After the satisfactory reduction in brain pressure, the cerebellar hemisphere was retracted, and the hematoma was found to rupture the brainstem surface between the facial and auditory nerve and the trigeminal nerve [13]. Using a 1–1.5 mm diameter suction device along the site of hematoma rupture, the hematoma was gently and slowly removed in small fragments. Hemostasis of the residual cav-

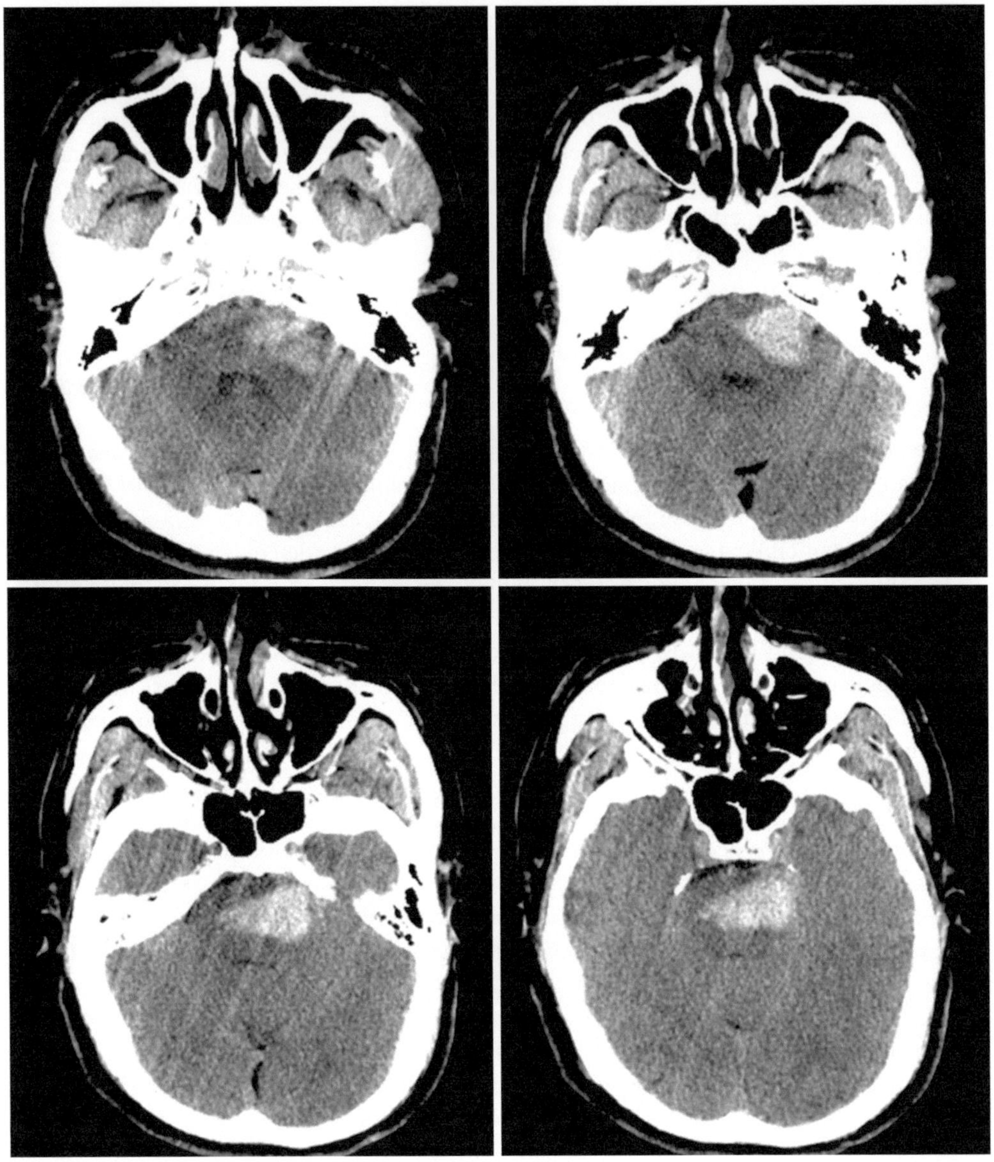

Fig. 13.19 Preoperative head CT scan

ity was satisfactory, and the dura mater was tightly sutured. The bone flap was repositioned, and the scalp was sutured layer by layer. Sterile dressings were applied (Fig. 13.20).

13.4.7.3 Preoperative and Postoperative Imaging Comparison

1. Postoperative Day 1: The patient was in a light coma with both pupils equal and round, measuring 1.5 mm in diameter. The pupillary light reflex was sensitive. The left-sided limb showed localized pain response, while there was no response to painful stimuli on the right side (Fig. 13.21).
2. Postoperative Day 5: The patient exhibited confusion with unequal pupils. The left pupil measured 2.5 mm, while the right pupil measured 3.0 mm. The pupillary light reflex was sensitive. The left-sided limb had muscle strength at grade III, whereas the right-sided limb had muscle strength at grade II. Both sides showed positive Babinski signs (Fig. 13.22).
3. Postoperative Week 5: The patient continued to experience confusion with unequal pupils. The left pupil measured 2.5 mm, and the right pupil measured 3.0 mm. The pupillary light reflex was sensitive. The left-sided limb had muscle strength at grade IV, while the right lower limb had muscle strength at grade III, and the right upper limb had muscle strength at grade II. Both sides exhibited positive Babinski signs (Figs. 13.23 and 13.24).
4. Postoperative Month 5: The patient regained clear consciousness, with equal-sized pupils measuring 2.5 mm. The pupillary light reflex was sensitive. The left-sided limb had muscle strength at grade V, while the right lower limb had muscle strength at grade III to IV, and the right upper limb had muscle strength at grade II (Figs. 13.25 and 13.26).

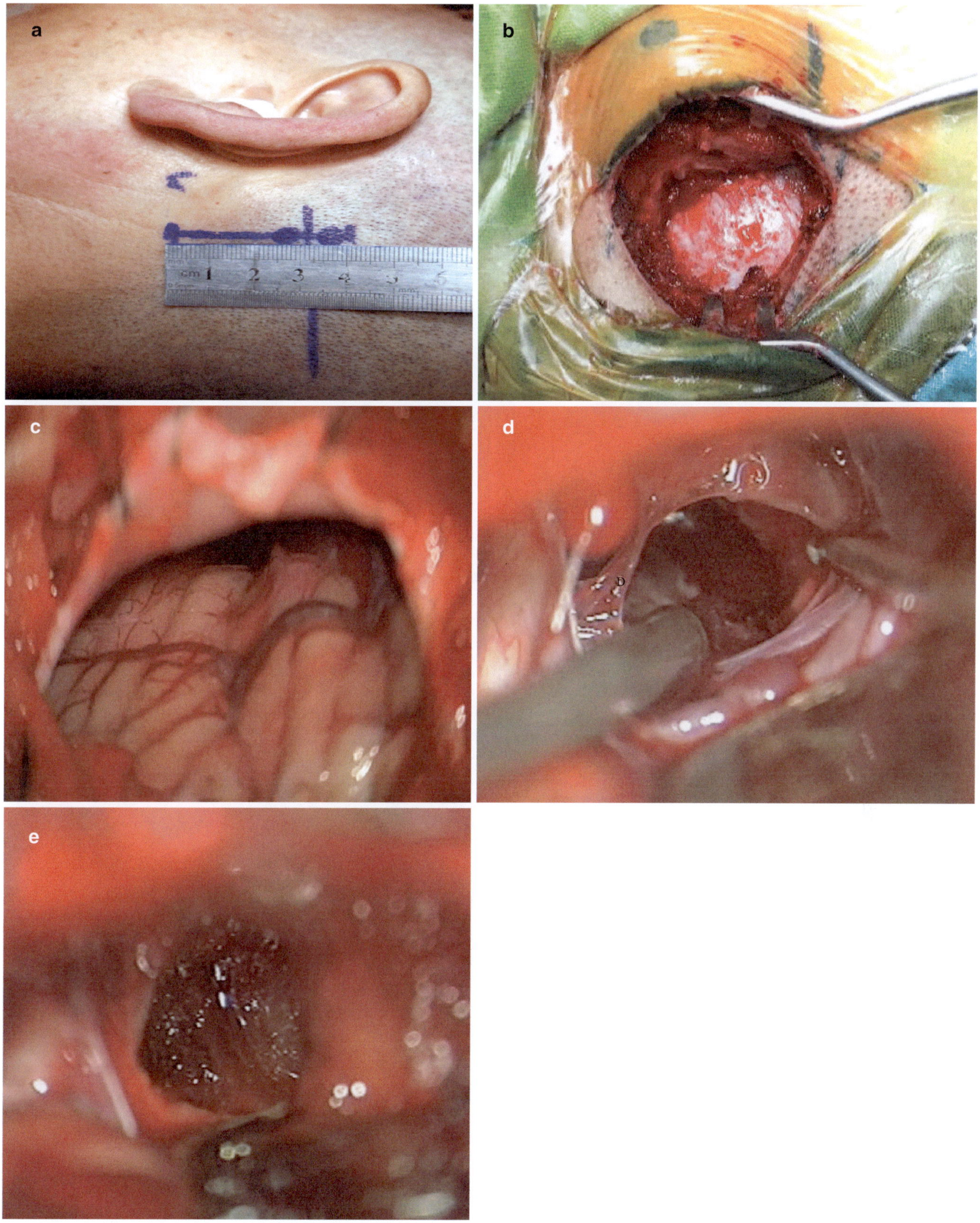

Fig. 13.20 Surgical procedure. (**a**) Mark the retromastoid straight incision. (**b**) Retraction of the posterior neck muscles, milling of the bone flap. (**c**) The dural flap was opened in a flap-like manner and turned toward the sigmoid sinus side, releasing cerebrospinal fluid. Satisfactory collapse of the cerebellum was observed, with minimal traction required. (**d**) Entry into the hematoma cavity along the surface of the brainstem where the hematoma ruptured. (**e**) Adequate hemostasis after hematoma removal

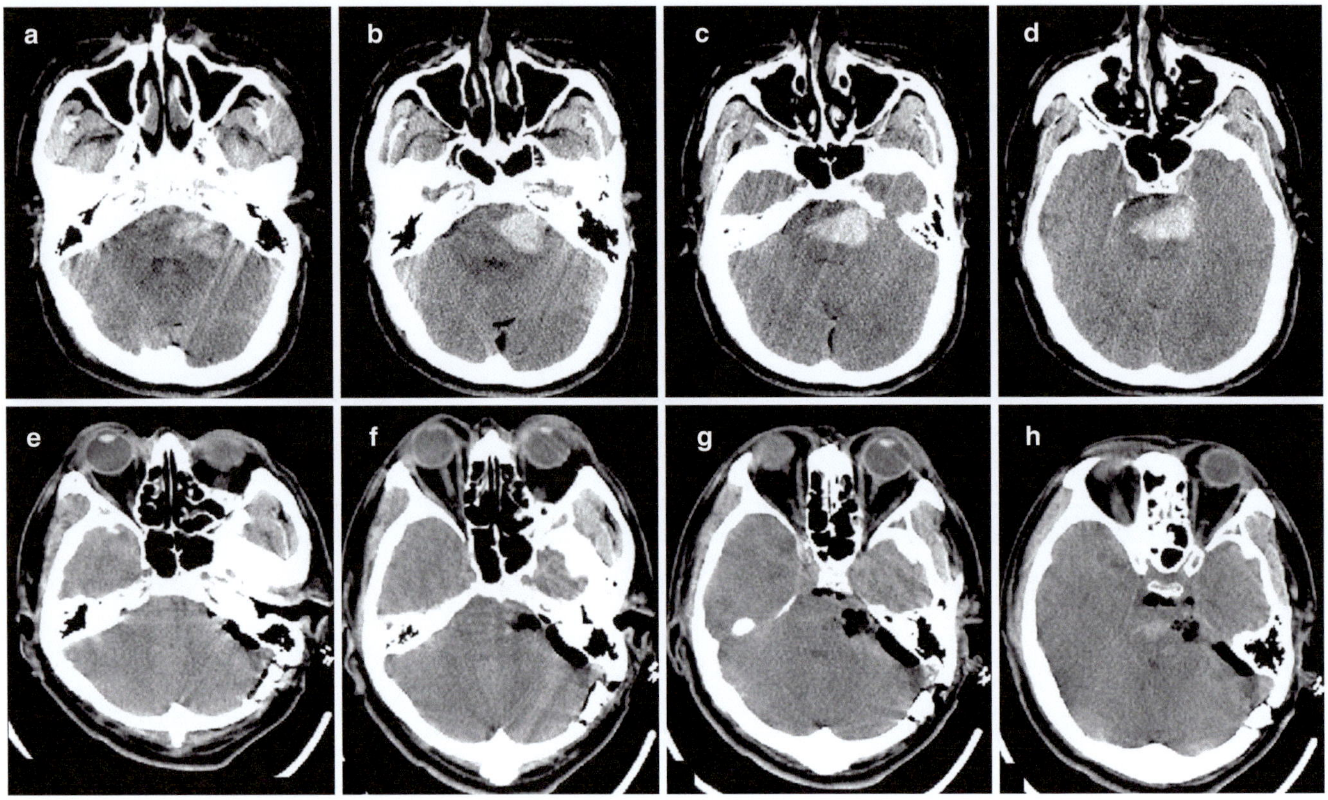

Fig. 13.21 Preoperative and postoperative day 1 head CT comparison (**a**–**d**) Preoperative head CT; (**e**–**h**) Follow-up head CT on postoperative day 1

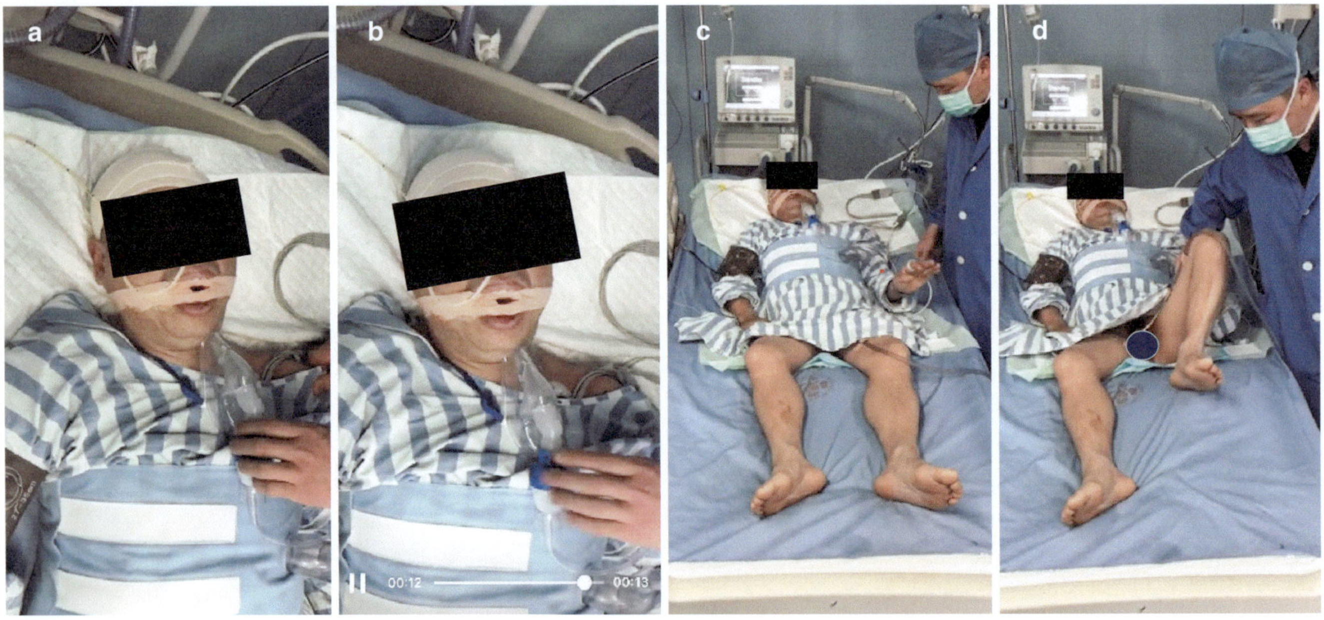

Fig. 13.22 Postoperative Day 5. (**a**, **b**) The patient exhibited confusion on postoperative day 5, with oropharyngeal airway maintained, and was able to follow commands to close and open eyes; (**c**, **d**) muscle strength at grade III in the left limb, grade II in the right limb

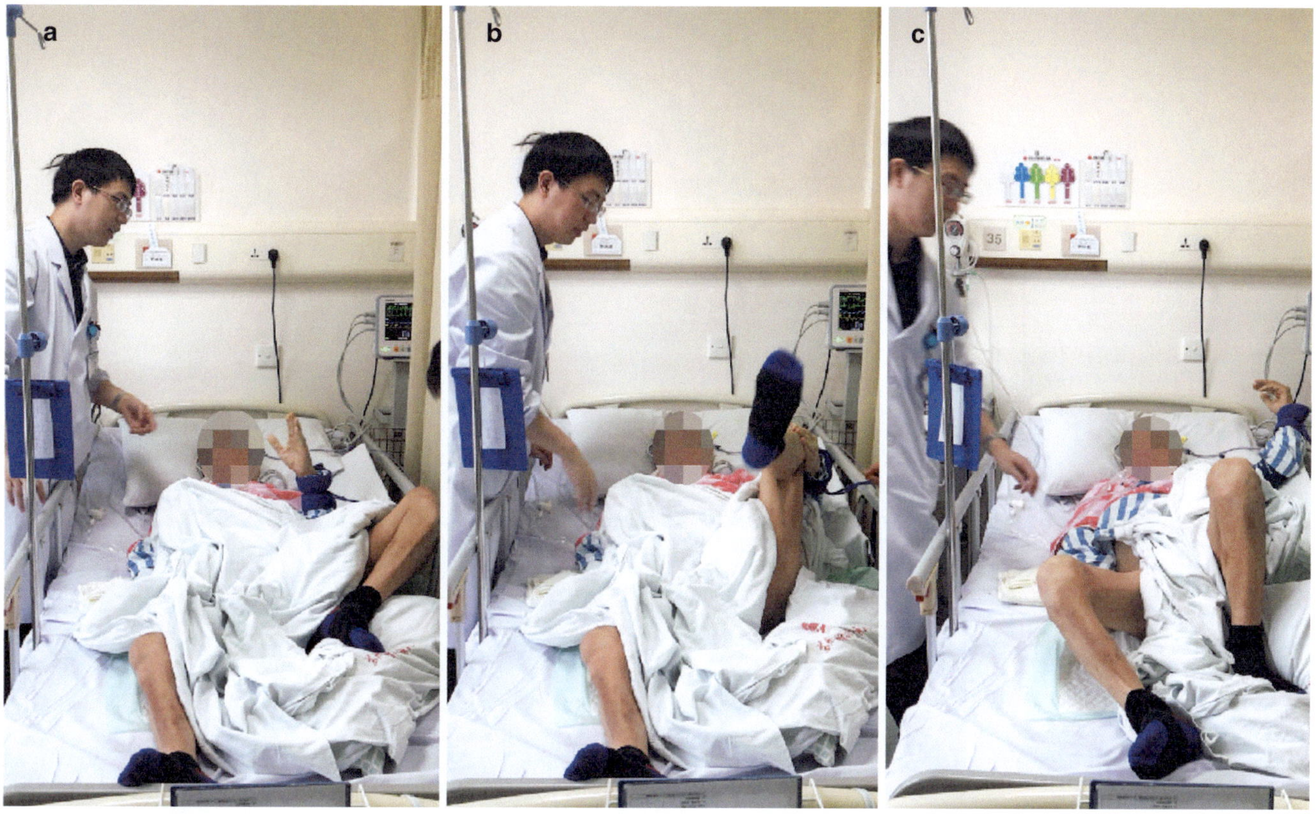

Fig. 13.23 Postoperative week 5. (**a**) The patient remained slightly confused on postoperative week 5 but was able to respond appropriately. (**b**) muscle strength at grade IV in the left limb. (**c**) muscle strength at grade III in the right lower limb and at grade II in the right upper limb

5. Postoperative Month 12: The patient achieved clear consciousness and significant improvement in cognitive function. Both pupils were equal in size, measuring 2.5 mm. The pupillary light reflex was sensitive. The muscle strength of the right upper limb was at grade III, while the remaining muscle strength was nearly normal. The patient demonstrated the ability to perform basic self-care tasks (Figs. 13.27 and 13.28).

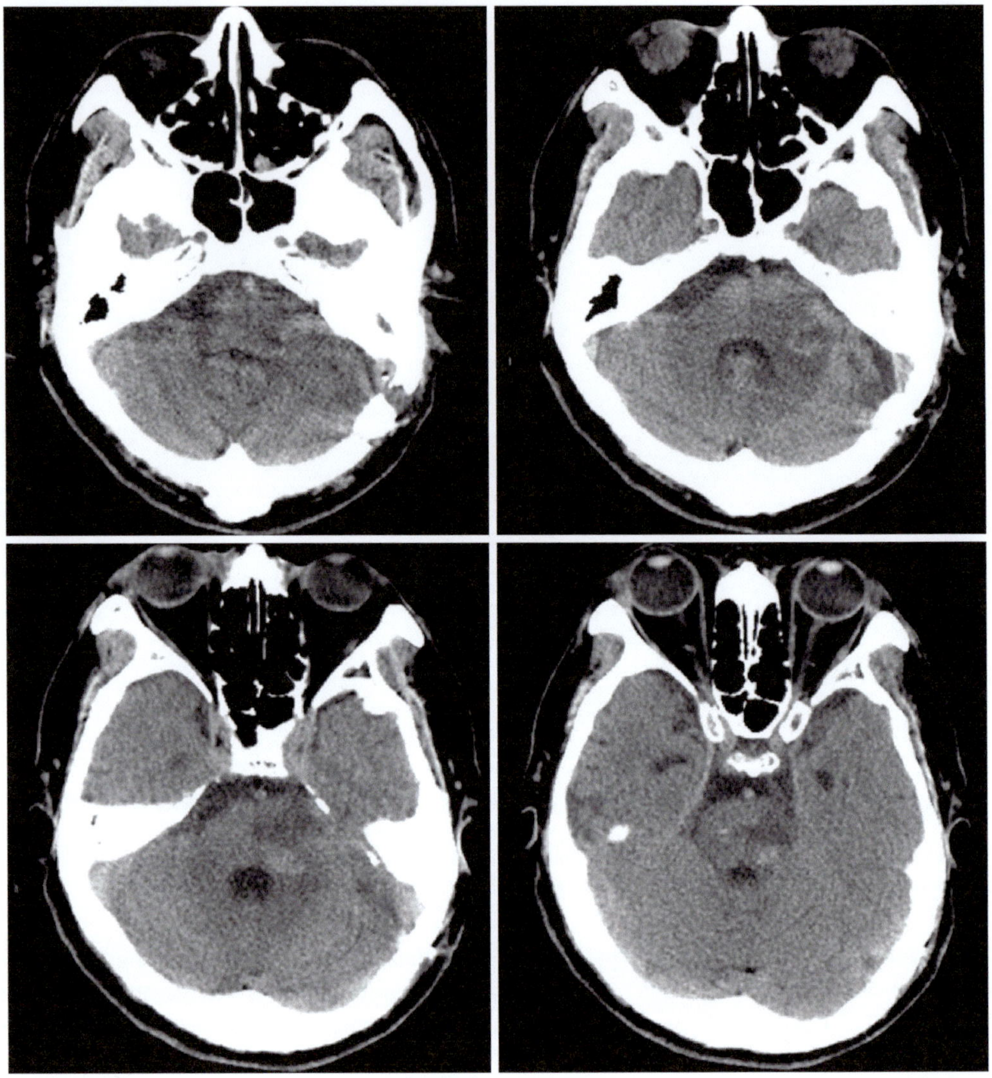

Fig. 13.24 Postoperative week 5 head CT

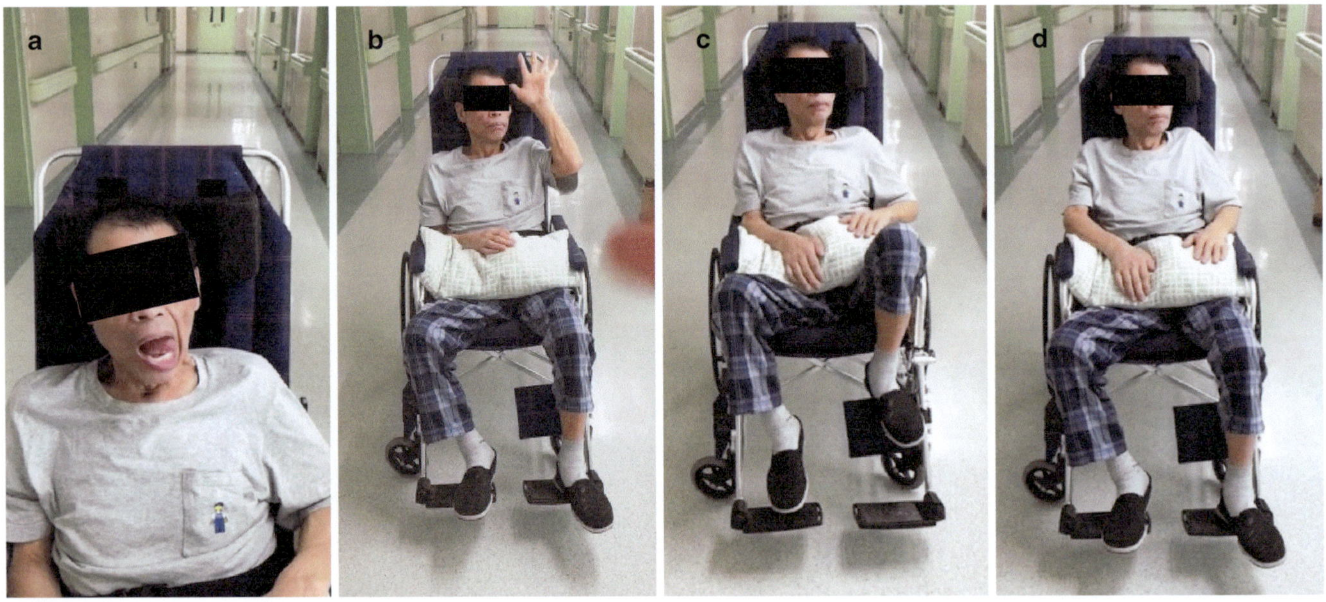

Fig. 13.25 Postoperative month 5. (**a**) The patient was alert and responsive, with improved cognitive abilities. (**b–d**) normal muscle strength in the left limb; muscle strength at grade III to IV in the right lower limb, at grade II in the right upper limb

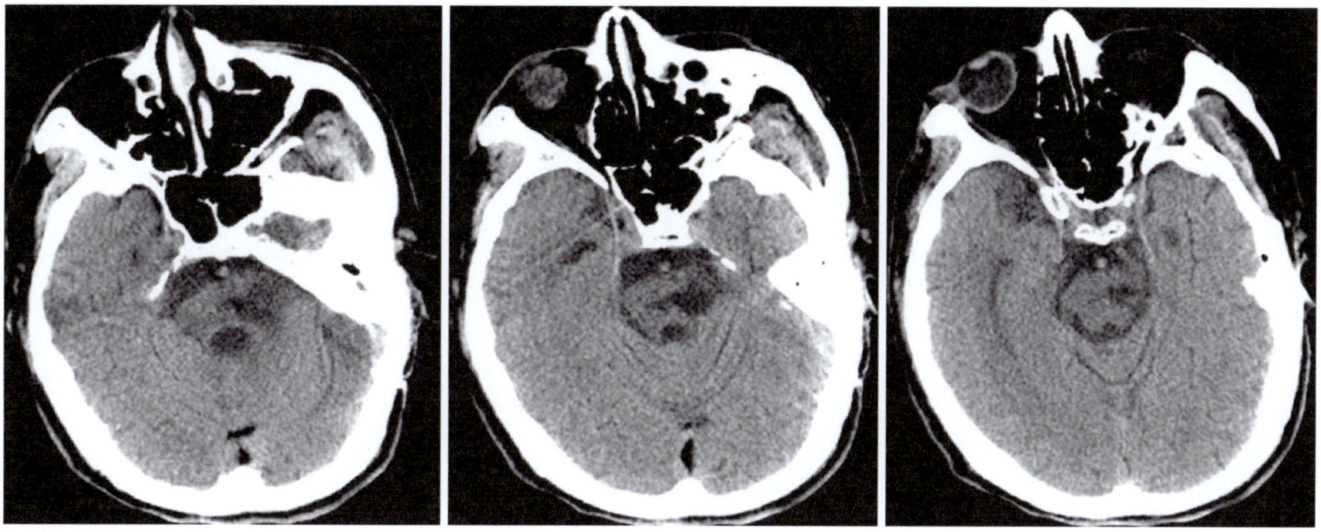

Fig. 13.26 Postoperative month 5 head CT

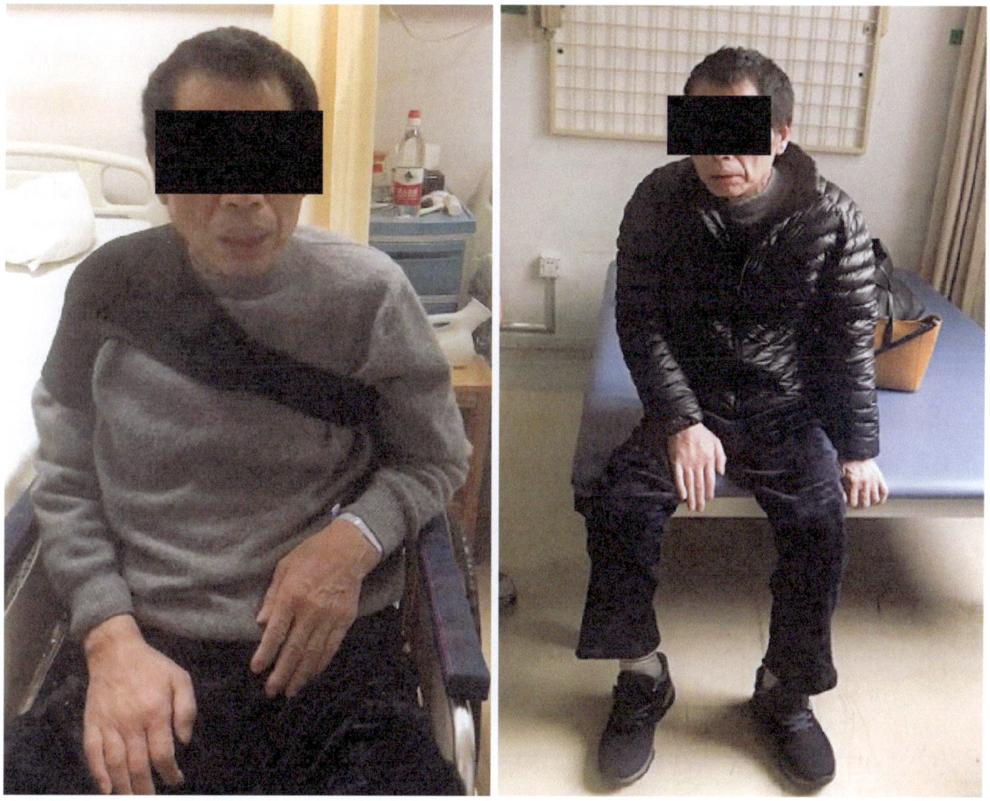

Fig. 13.27 Postoperative month 12. (a) The patient demonstrated further improvement in cognitive abilities, with appropriate responses; muscle strength at grade III in the right upper limb, nearly normal muscle strength in the remaining limbs, performing basic self-care abilities

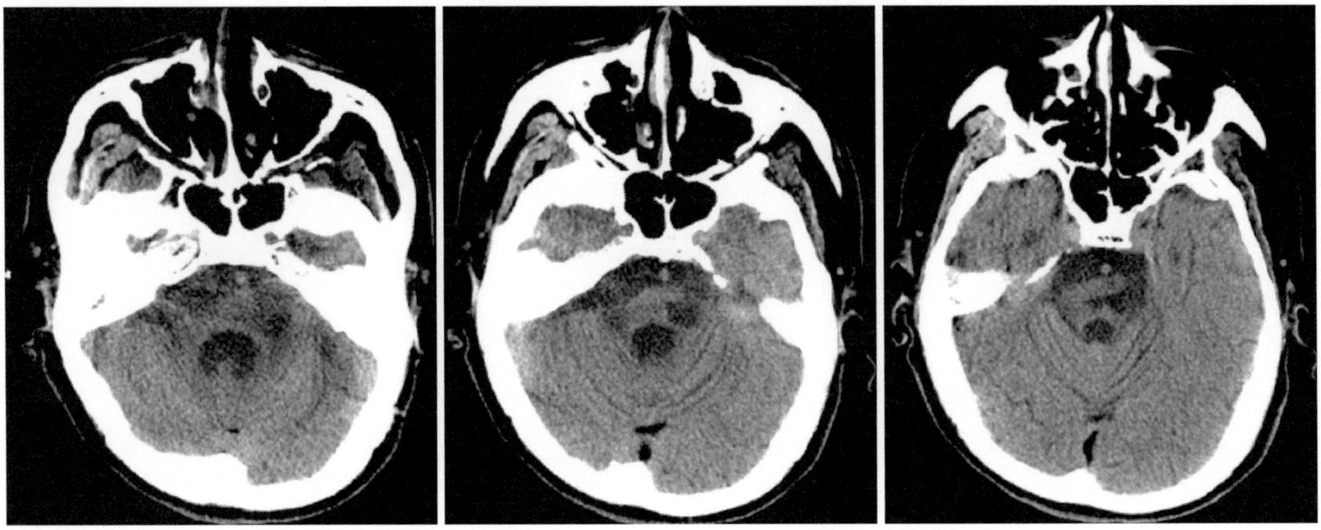

Fig. 13.28 Postoperative month 12 head CT

13.5 Posterior Median Keyhole Approach for Brainstem Hematoma Evacuation

13.5.1 Indications and Contraindications

1. Indications

   There is no unified surgical standard for brainstem hemorrhage. However, the following conditions are generally considered suitable for surgical treatment [14].

   (a) Hematoma located on the lateral aspect of the medulla oblongata or in the middle and lower portions of the pons, with rupturing through the fourth ventricle floor or a tendency to approach the fourth ventricle floor.
   (b) Hematoma volume exceeding 5 mL.
   (c) GCS <8, severe neurological dysfunction, or progressive deterioration.
   (d) Strong willingness expressed by the patient's family after being fully informed about the surgical risks and potential economic and family burdens.
2. Contraindications
   (a) Minimal hemorrhage volume (<5 mL).
   (b) The absence of significant impairment of consciousness.
   (c) Circulation unstable or inability to maintain basic vital signs.
   (d) Severe coagulation disorders or multi-organ dysfunction.
   (e) Patient or family refusal of surgery.

13.5.2 Preoperative Preparation and Surgical Instruments

1. Preoperative Preparation
   (a) Maintain airway patency. Early endotracheal intubation is performed in patients with airway obstruction or compromised airway. Blood pressure is controlled. For patients with significant hydrocephalus, external ventricular drainage is performed prior to surgery [15].
   (b) Complete biochemical and coagulation function tests to rule out common surgical contraindications.
2. Surgical Instruments

   The surgical equipment requirements include a specialized electric operating table, microscope, head frame with automatic retraction, electric cranial drill, bipolar coagulation, and preferably equipped with a navigation system and intraoperative neuroelectrophysiological monitoring device.

13.5.3 Surgical Techniques, Precautions, and Tips

1. Surgical Techniques
   (a) Positioning and Incision

   Positioning: The patient is placed in the prone position with fixation using the Mayfield head frame. The entire body is elevated at an angle of 20°–30°, ensuring that the head is higher than the chest to facilitate

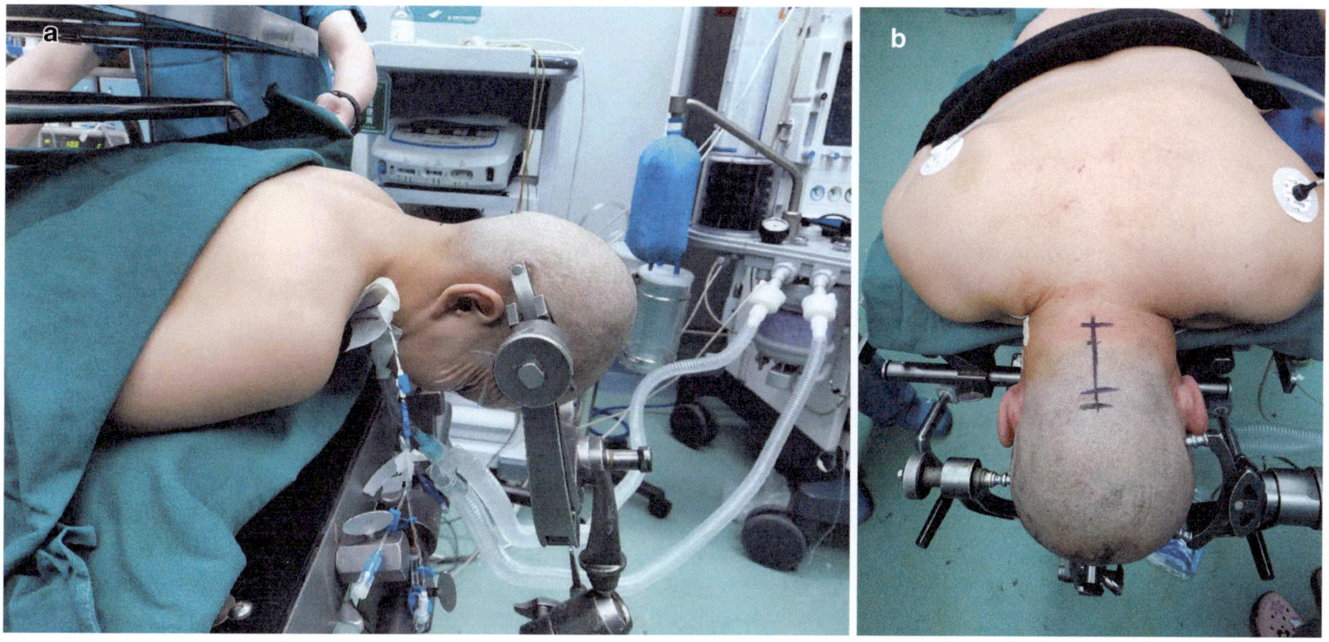

Fig. 13.29 Positioning and incision. (**a**) Patient in prone position with Mayfield head fixation. (**b**) Posterior median surgical incision

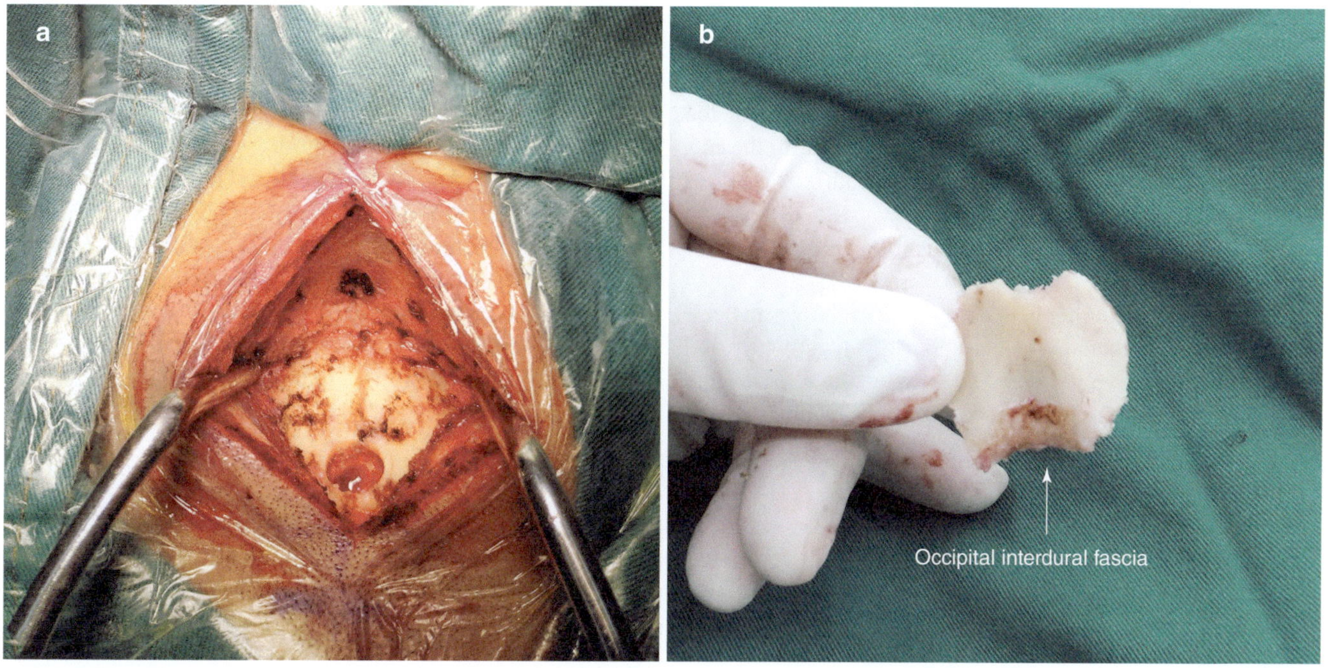

Fig. 13.30 Drilling and removal of bone flap. (**a**) Incision of the scalp, opening with retractor, and drilling a burr hole along the midline. (**b**) removal of the bone flap through the burr hole. 1 Occipital Interdural Fascia

venous drainage. The head is flexed approximately 30° forward, allowing for sufficient extension at the craniovertebral junction (Fig. 13.29a).

A median incision of approximately 6–8 cm (Fig. 13.29b).

(b) Craniotomy

The scalp is incised along the midline and sharply dissected. A retractor is used to hold the incision open. The dissection continues along the white line until reaching the skull. The muscles attached to the inferior nuchal line and the inferior border of the occipital bone are detached along with the bone surface, with the skin flap retracted using a retractor, exposing the occipital bone, foramen magnum, and the atlas plate (Fig. 13.30a).

A burr hole is drilled along the midline, and then a small bone flap is milled. Alternatively, a bone window with a diameter of approximately 2.5–3 cm can be created by grinding from the posterior edge of the foramen magnum upward (Fig. 13.30b).

(c) Dural Incision

Make a "Y"-shaped incision in the dura mater. Use a sharp scalpel to open the dura on both sides of the occipital sinus. Use tissue scissors to cut the dura toward anterolaterally on both sides. Cauterize or suture the occipital sinus, and then cut it and continue the incision inferolaterally on both sides creating four dural flaps. The dura remains suspended around the bone window (Fig. 13.31).

(d) Subdural Manipulation

Open the cisterna magna, where the tonsils of the cerebellum, biventral lobule, uvula of vermis, and cerebellomedullary fissure, the posterior inferior cerebellar artery (PICA) can be seen (Fig. 13.32a).

Pull the bilateral cerebellar tonsils apart to reveal the floor of the cerebellomedullary fissure, whose medial part is the roof of the fourth ventricle, composed of the medullary velum and choroid. The posterior aspect of the brainstem lies laterally. The bilateral choroid converges to form the foramen of Magendie, and the third and fourth segments of the posterior inferior cerebellar artery run within the cerebellomedullary fissure. A brain spatula is used to pull the tonsils outward and upward to expose the lower part of the cerebellomedullary fissure (Fig. 13.32b).

After obtaining better exposure of the vermis, use the brain spatula to pull the vermis inward and upward, revealing the structures of the choroid and inferior medullary velum. Further opening of the inferior medullary velum exposes the upper part of the fourth ventricle, including the superior medullary velum, the opening of the aqueduct, the medial eminence, and the superior cerebellar peduncles. When the bilateral inferior medullary velum is opened, lifting the cerebellar vermis allows for a panoramic view of the floor of the fourth ventricle (Fig. 13.32c).

(e) Hematoma Evacuation

First, remove the hematoma that has entered the fourth ventricle. Then, expose the floor of the fourth ventricle. The location of the hematoma can be accurately determined by examining the ruptured surface of the brain stem. Suppose the hematoma is entirely within the brain stem. In that case, it can be identified by observing a gray-bluish, slightly bulging area on the surface of the brainstem, located above the medullary stria. Make an incision within a range of 5 to 10 mm in the brainstem to access the hematoma cavity for manipulation (Fig. 13.33).

(f) Closure of the Cranium

Irrigate the subarachnoid space with saline, and inspect the patency of the aqueduct. Intermittently watertightly suture the dura mater. If the dura mater is under high tension, a small piece of muscle can be used for repair. Additionally, artificial dura mater can be used for repair (placing the gelatin sponge outside the dura mater). Reposition and fix the bone flap, and then perform layered suturing of the posterior cervical muscles, subcutaneous tissues, and skin (Fig. 13.34, Vid eo 13.3).

2. Surgical Precautions and Relevant Operative Techniques
   (a) Understand the surgical indications thoroughly, master the procedural steps and have a solid knowledge of the relevant anatomy.
   (b) Perform strict aseptic techniques to prevent intracranial infections.

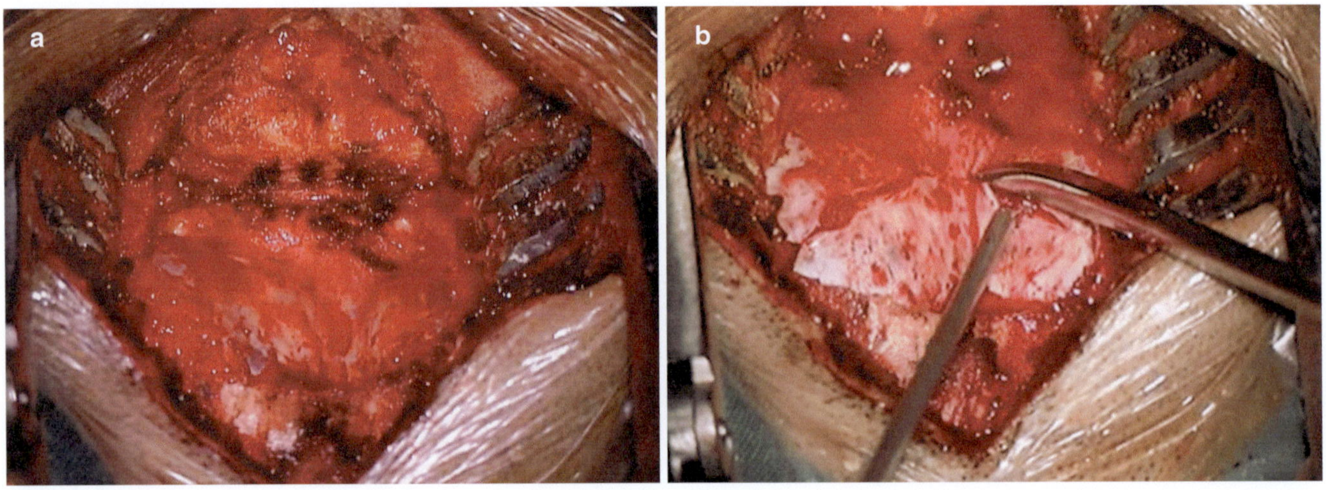

Fig. 13.31 Exposure and incision of the dura mater. (**a**) Exposure of the dura mater. (**b**) "Y"-shaped incision of the dura mater

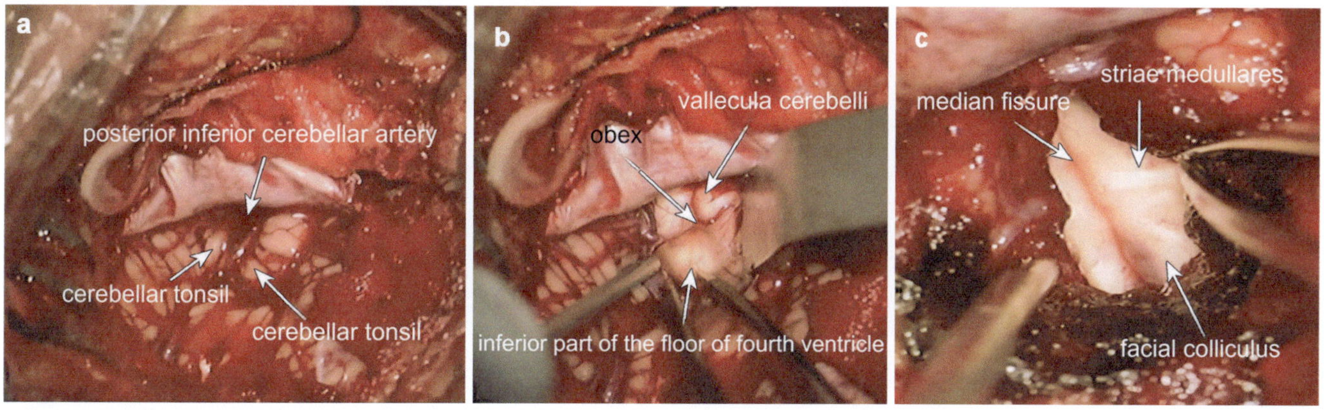

Fig. 13.32 Exposure of the floor of the fourth ventricle. (**a**) Open cistern magna, tonsils, vermis, and PICA are exposed. (**b**) retracting tonsils, the lower part of the fourth ventricle is exposed. (**c**) further exposing the upper part of the fourth ventricle. 1 PICA 2. Tonsils. 3 Vermis. 4 Obex. 5 Cerebellar Vallecular. 6 Lower Part of the Floor of the Fourth Ventricle. 7 Median Fissure. 8 Medullary Striae. 9 Facial Colliculus

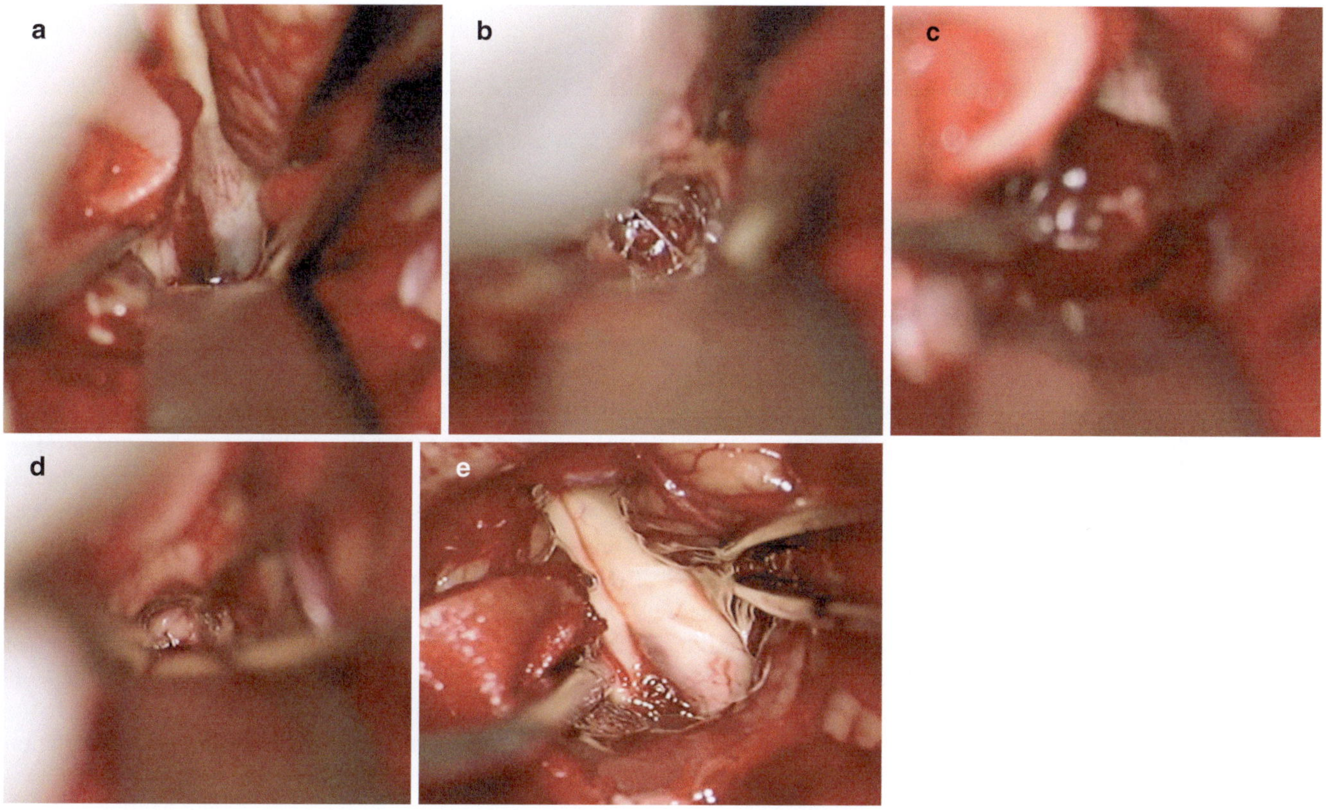

Fig. 13.33 Evacuation of hematoma. (**a**) Identification of the gray-bluish bulging hematoma on the floor of the fourth ventricle. (**b**) Hematoma location confirmed by creating a fistula in the gray-bluish area. (**c**) Removal of blood clots. (**d**) Coagulation of the inner wall of the hematoma cavity after evacuation. (**e**) Placement of hemostatic cotton in the hematoma cavity

(c) During the detachment of the bone flap, the occipital bone's inner lamina and the atlantooccipital membrane are tightly adhered at the foramen magnum. To preserve the integrity of the dura mater, a sharp No. 11 blade can be used to detach the attachment between the atlantooccipital membrane and the occipital bone. Monopolar electrocoagulation can also be employed to separate the adhesions.

(d) In some patients with obstructive hydrocephalus, increased intracranial pressure would cause surgical

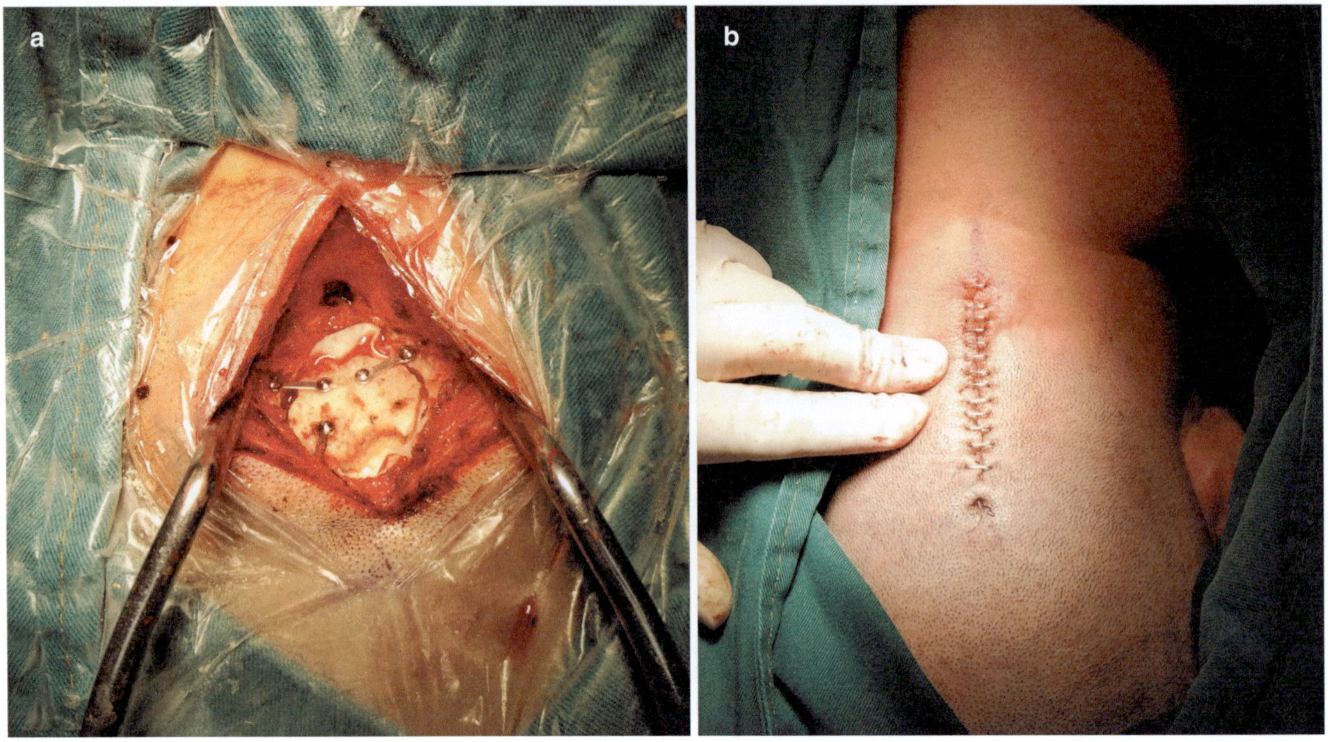

Fig. 13.34 Closure of the craniotomy. (**a**) Reposition the bone flap and fix it with cranial connecting plates. (**b**) suture the incision. Posterior midline incision 7.0 cm incision

difficulties. In such cases, external drainage through the posterior horn of the lateral ventricle can be performed before craniotomy to reduce intracranial pressure.

(e) The arachnoid membrane and the inferior medullary velum should be sharply cut to avoid excessive traction that may cause secondary damage to vessels or brain tissue [16].

(f) During the process of separating and exposing the inferior medullary velum, it is crucial to preserve the various branches of PICA encountered to avoid vermian ischemic injury and cerebellar infarction with subsequent edema, which would undermine the significance of this approach.

(g) To minimize secondary damage, low-power bipolar electrocoagulation is employed for bleeding within the hematoma cavity. Additionally, a thin layer of gelatin sponge can be placed between the bipolar forceps and the brainstem to facilitate gentle heat transfer.

(h) Ensure watertight dural closure, and secure repositioning of the bone flap to prevent subcutaneous fluid accumulation in the occipital region, cerebrospinal fluid leakage, and poor wound healing.

13.5.4 Postoperative Management and Complication Prevention

1. Compared to other types of brainstem hemorrhage, brainstem hematoma treated through this approach often breaks through the bottom of the fourth ventricle or is in close proximity to the floor of the fourth ventricle [17], making it more prone to causing hydrocephalus. Therefore, it is essential to explore the aqueduct's opening during surgery to ensure its patency.
2. Compared to other approaches, the suboccipital median approach may encounter complications such as suboccipital subcutaneous fluid accumulation, cerebrospinal fluid leakage, and poor wound healing [18]. During surgery, watertight dural closure should be performed. In the event of postoperative subcutaneous fluid accumulation or cerebrospinal fluid leakage, continuous lumbar drainage can be employed to facilitate wound healing.

13.5.5 Advantages, Disadvantages, and Lessons Learned

1. The incision is significantly smaller than the traditional suboccipital median approach, saving surgical time and reducing intraoperative bleeding. The incision avoids the

external occipital protuberance, preventing poor wound healing and reducing the occurrence of cerebrospinal fluid leakage [19].
2. The bone window does not extend beyond the inferior nuchal line, eliminating the need to remove the posterior arch of the atlas. This approach minimizes damage to the muscles in the occipital region and reduces the impact on craniovertebral stability.
3. The small bone window in the keyhole approach avoids unnecessary exposure of brain tissue and limits the extent of brain retraction, thus reducing the risk of brain injury caused by traction.
4. The application of neuronavigation and intraoperative neuroelectrophysiological monitoring can reduce postoperative complications and protect critical functional areas.

13.5.6 Evaluation and Prospects of the Surgical Technique

The suboccipital median keyhole approach shares similar anatomical pathways with the traditional approach. Due to the deep location and relative localization of brainstem hemorrhage [20], this approach effectively utilizes the "keyhole effect" to expose anatomical structures. After opening the cisterna magna and adequately releasing cerebrospinal fluid, sufficient surgical working space can be achieved. The smaller incision and bone window compared to the traditional approach not only shortens the surgical time and allows rapid access to the hematoma but also reduces unnecessary exposure and tissue damage.

13.5.7 Typical Cases

13.5.7.1 Typical Case One

13.5.7.1.1 Summary of Medical History and Radiological Data

The patient, a 55-year-old male, was admitted due to "sudden onset of unconsciousness for more than 2 hours." Physical examination revealed a blood pressure of 151/78 mmHg, weak respiration, light coma, GCS 5, bilateral equal and round pupils with a diameter of approximately 2.0 mm, sensitive light reflex, both limbs flexion to painful stimuli, and positive bilateral Babinski sign. Auxiliary examinations showed a brainstem hemorrhage of approximately 8 mL on the head CT scan (Fig. 13.35). Admission diagnosis: brainstem hemorrhage and hypertensive disease (extremely critical type).

13.5.7.1.2 Surgical Procedure and Key Points

The patient was placed in the prone position, and a midline incision of approximately 6–8 cm was made. The scalp and muscle layers were dissected layer by layer along the nuchal ligament (Fig. 13.36a, b).

Two burr holes were made on both sides of the external occipital protuberance, and a bone flap was freed using a milling cutter. The dura mater was opened in a "Y" shape. The tonsils were pulled outward and upward using a brain spatula, exposing the floor of the fourth ventricle. Under the guidance of neuro-navigation and neuroelectrophysiological monitoring, the hematoma location was identified, and a suction device with low to moderate negative pressure was used to slowly and gradually remove the hematoma under direct visualization through the microscope. After satisfactory hemostasis in the residual cavity, the dura mater was watertight sutured with relaxation suture, the bone flap was repositioned and fixed, and the occipital muscle and scalp were sutured layer by layer (Fig. 13.36c, d).

13.5.7.1.3 [Postoperative Imaging]

A postoperative cranial CT scan reveals complete hematoma clearance with minimal intracranial gas and a small bone window (Fig. 13.37).

13.5.7.1.4 Comparison of Postoperative and Discharge Condition

The patient underwent tracheostomy in the early postoperative period and was given nasal feeding. At the time of discharge, the patient was able to walk with the assistance of family members (Fig. 13.38).

13.5.7.2 Typical Case Two

13.5.7.2.1 Brief Medical History and Imaging Data

A 50-year-old male patient was admitted due to "sudden unconsciousness for more than 4 hours." Physical examination revealed blood pressure of 163/90 mmHg, weak respiration, moderate coma (GCS 5), bilaterally equal and round pupils with a diameter of approximately 2.0 mm, sensitive pupillary light reflex, unresponsive left limbs to painful stimuli, and flexion response of the right limbs, positive bilateral Babinski sign. Auxiliary examination showed head CT findings of brainstem hemorrhage with a volume of approximately 10 mL (Fig. 13.39). The admission diagnosis was brainstem hemorrhage and hypertensive disease (extremely critical type).

13.5.7.2.2 Surgical Procedure and Key Points

1. The patient was placed in the prone position, and a midline incision of approximately 6–8 cm was made. The scalp and muscle layers were dissected along the nuchal ligament. Two burr holes were drilled on both sides of the external occipital protuberance, and a bone flap was freed using a milling cutter. The dura was opened in a "Y" shape.

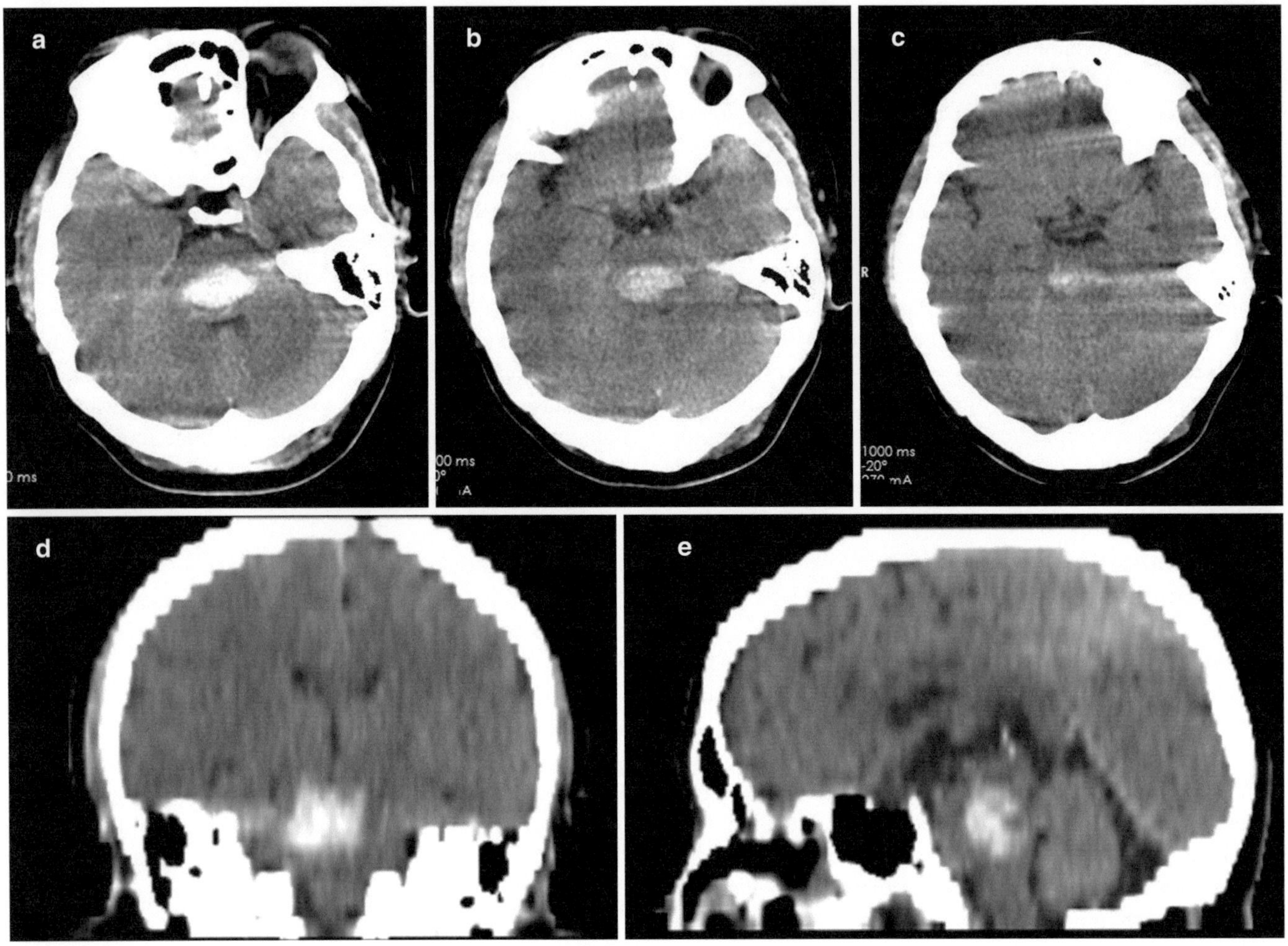

Fig. 13.35 Preoperative CT scan: hematoma located in the pons, close to the floor of the fourth ventricle. (**a–c**) Axial CT images in the acute phase showing a high-density hematoma located in the pons tegmentum, close to the floor of the fourth ventricle. (**d**, **e**) coronal and sagittal CT images in the acute phase, respectively, showing a high-density hematoma completely within the pons and close to the floor of the fourth ventricle

2. The tonsils were retracted outward and upward using a brain spatula, and the bilateral choroid inferior medullary velum was exposed to elevate the vermis of the cerebellum, exposing the floor of the fourth ventricle. The hematoma location was determined under the guidance of neuro-navigation and neuroelectrophysiological monitoring. A suction device with low to moderate negative pressure was used to slowly remove the hematoma in blocks under high magnification through a microscope. After achieving satisfactory hemostasis in the residual cavity, the dura mater was watertight sutured with relaxation suture, the bone flap was repositioned and fixed, and the occipital muscle and scalp were sutured layer by layer (Fig. 13.40).

13.5.7.2.3 Preoperative and Postoperative Imaging Comparison

Comparison of preoperative and postoperative head CT scans demonstrates complete clearance of the pontine hematoma after surgery (Fig. 13.41).

13.5.7.2.4 Neurological Examination Findings Postoperatively

Three weeks postoperatively, the patient remained in a state of drowsiness to light coma. The muscle strength in the left limbs was grade I–II, while the right limbs had a muscle strength of grade III (Fig. 13.42).

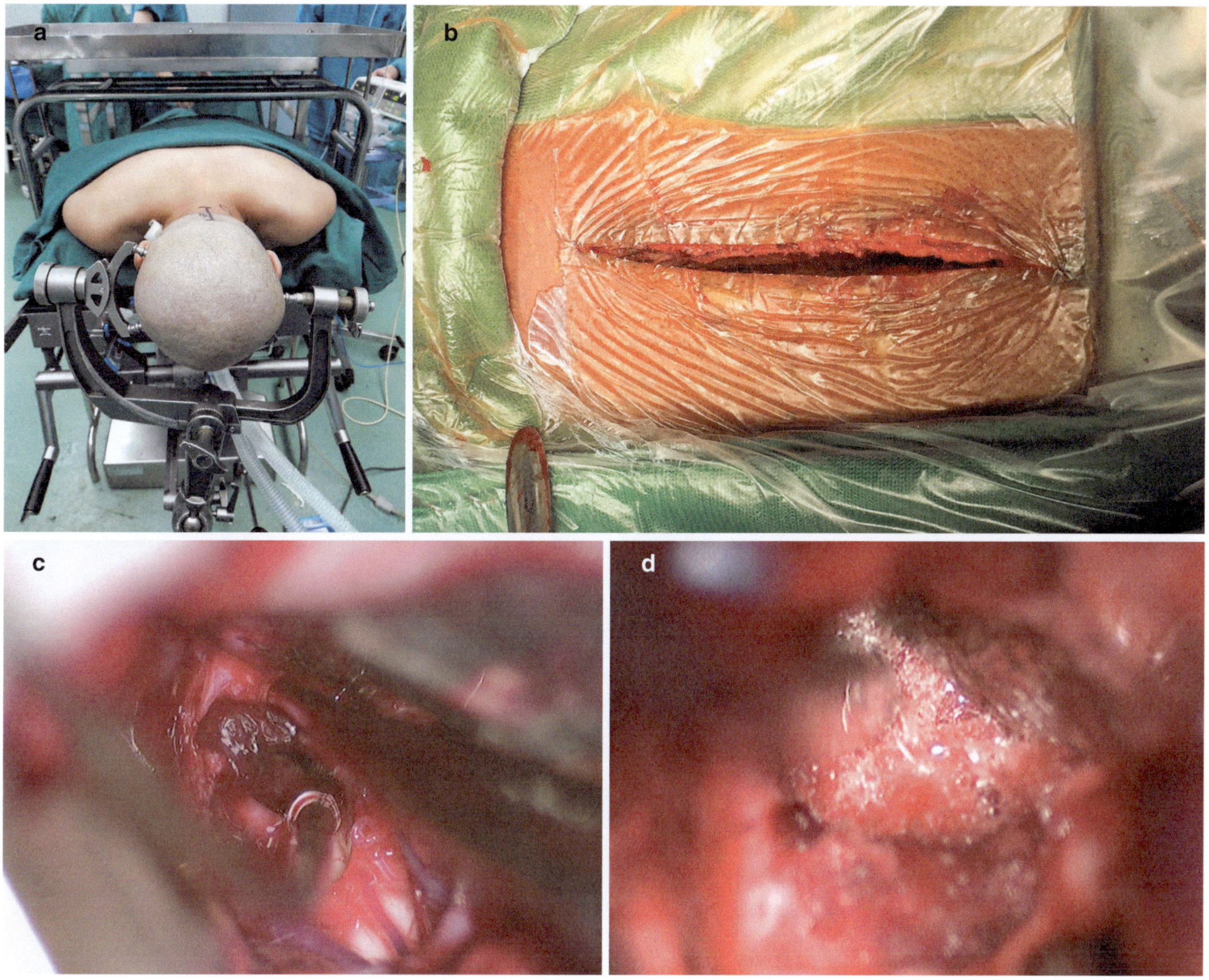

Fig. 13.36 Surgical procedure. (**a**) The patient is positioned prone with the head fixed using a three-pin head frame. (**b**) posterior median incision. (**c**) Accessing the hematoma cavity and removing the blood clots. (**d**) Thoroughly evacuating the hematoma and achieving satisfactory hemostasis, followed by the application of hemostatic gauze

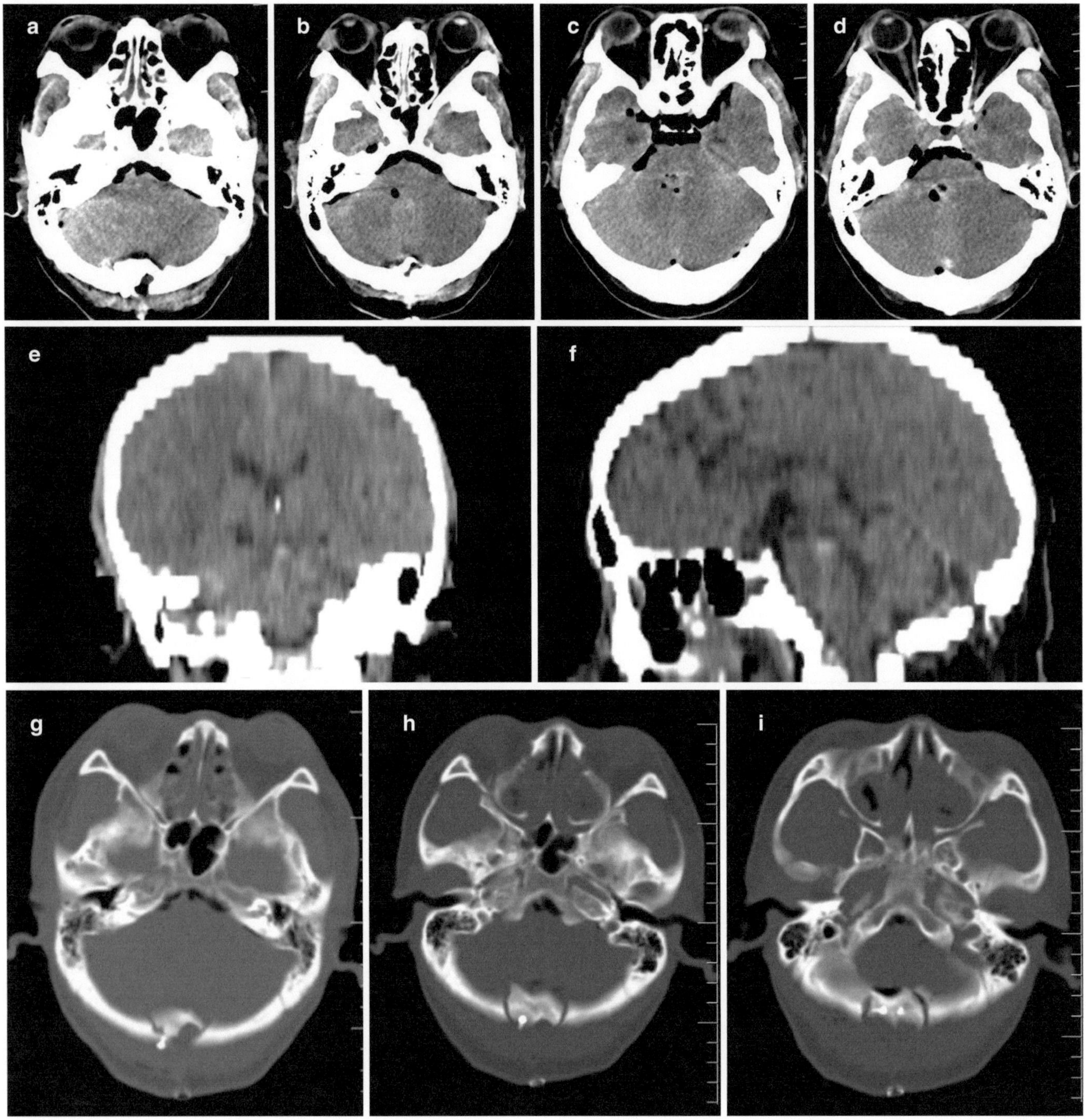

Fig. 13.37 Postoperative cranial CT scan. (**a–d**) Axial CT images demonstrate satisfactory clearance of the pontine hematoma with minimal residual intracranial gas. (**e**, **f**) coronal and sagittal CT images, respectively, confirm complete removal of the pontine hematoma. (**g–i**) bone window images display a small bone window

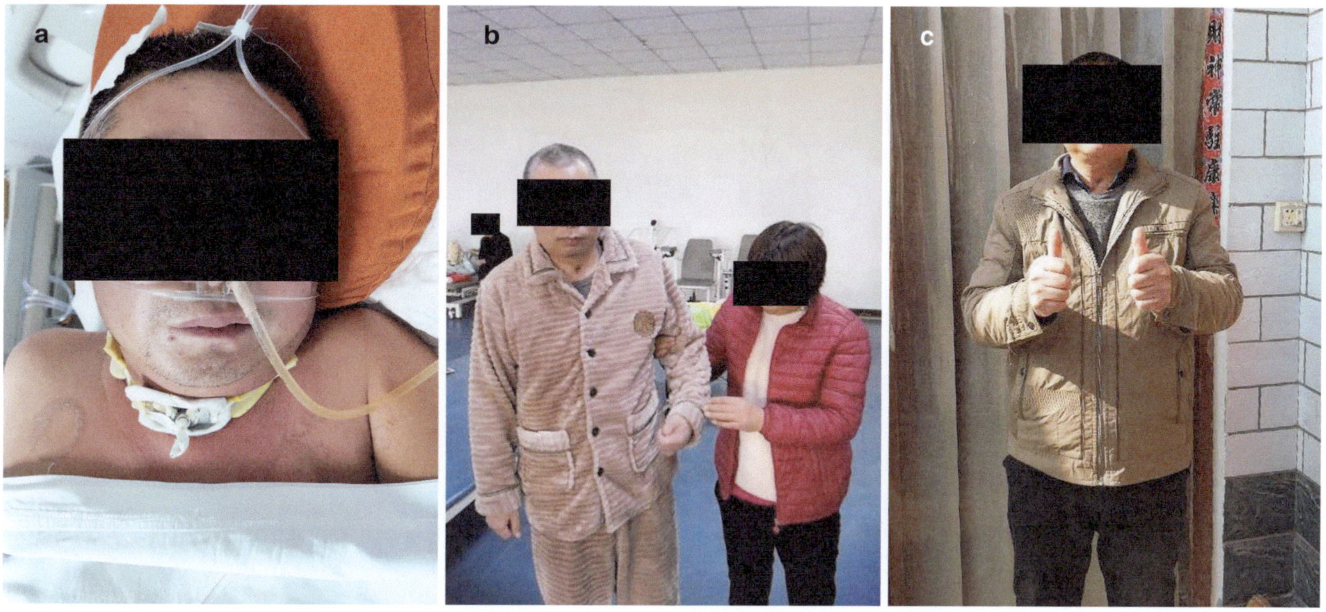

Fig. 13.38 Postoperative and discharge condition. (**a**) Early postoperative nasal feeding and tracheostomy. (**b**, **c**) At the time of discharge, the patient was able to walk with the assistance of family members and could raise thumbs with both hands

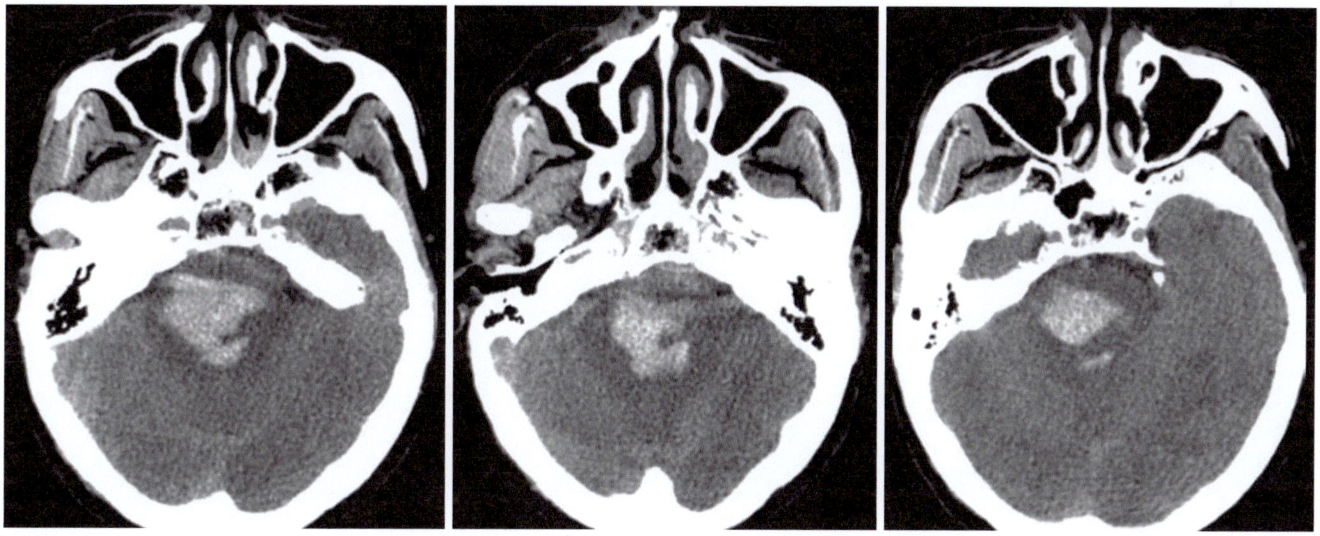

Fig. 13.39 Preoperative CT scan. Axial CT images in the acute phase show the hematoma located in the pons, extending into the fourth ventricle

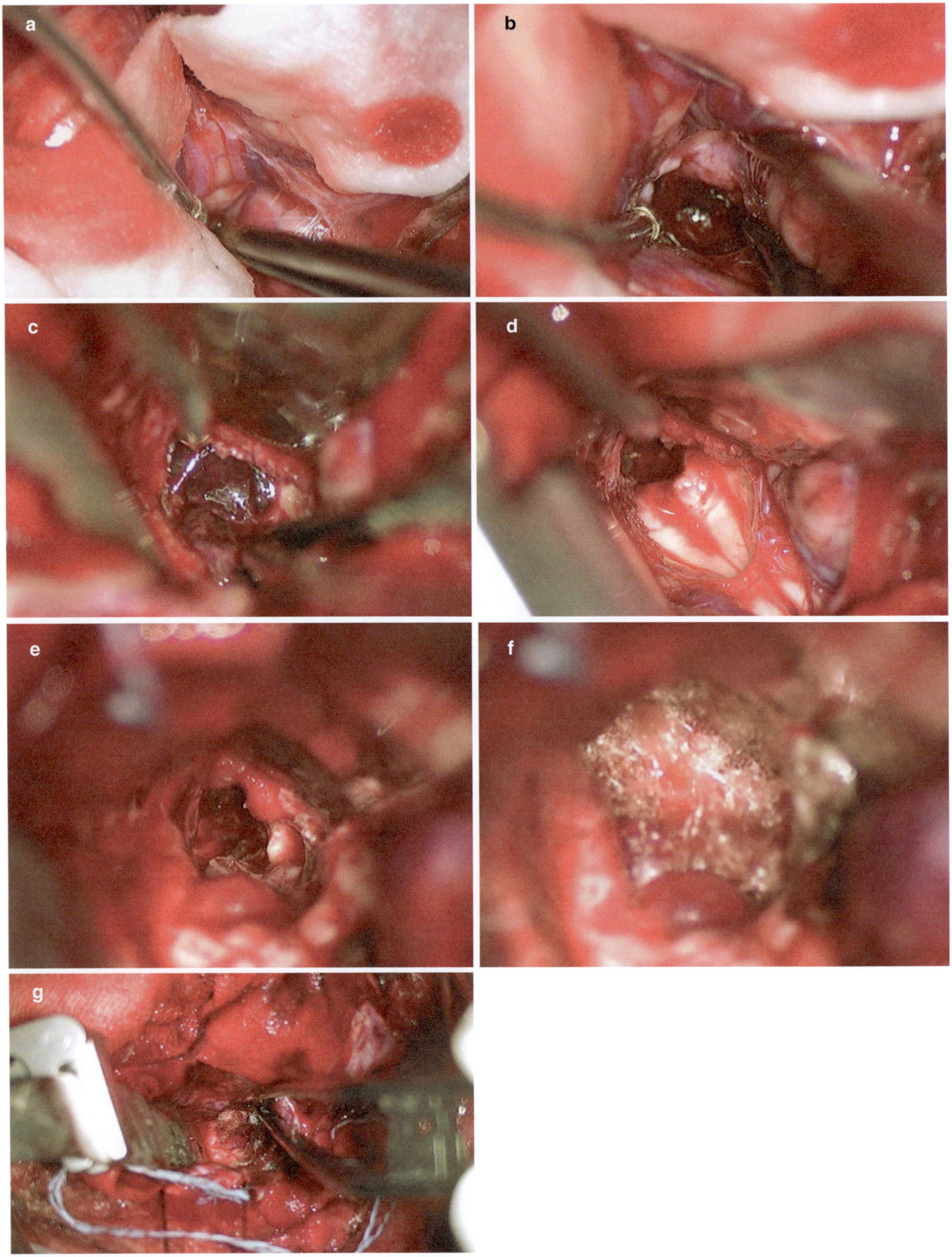

Fig. 13.40 Hematoma evacuation and hemostasis during surgery. (**a**) Tonsils retracted laterally to expose the fourth ventricle. (**b**) Fistula created at the floor of the fourth ventricle to access the hematoma cavity. (**c**, **d**) Blood clots within the hematoma cavity were removed. (**e**) The hematoma cavity was exposed after evacuation. (f, **g**) Thorough hemostasis achieved in the residual cavity and application of hemostatic cotton

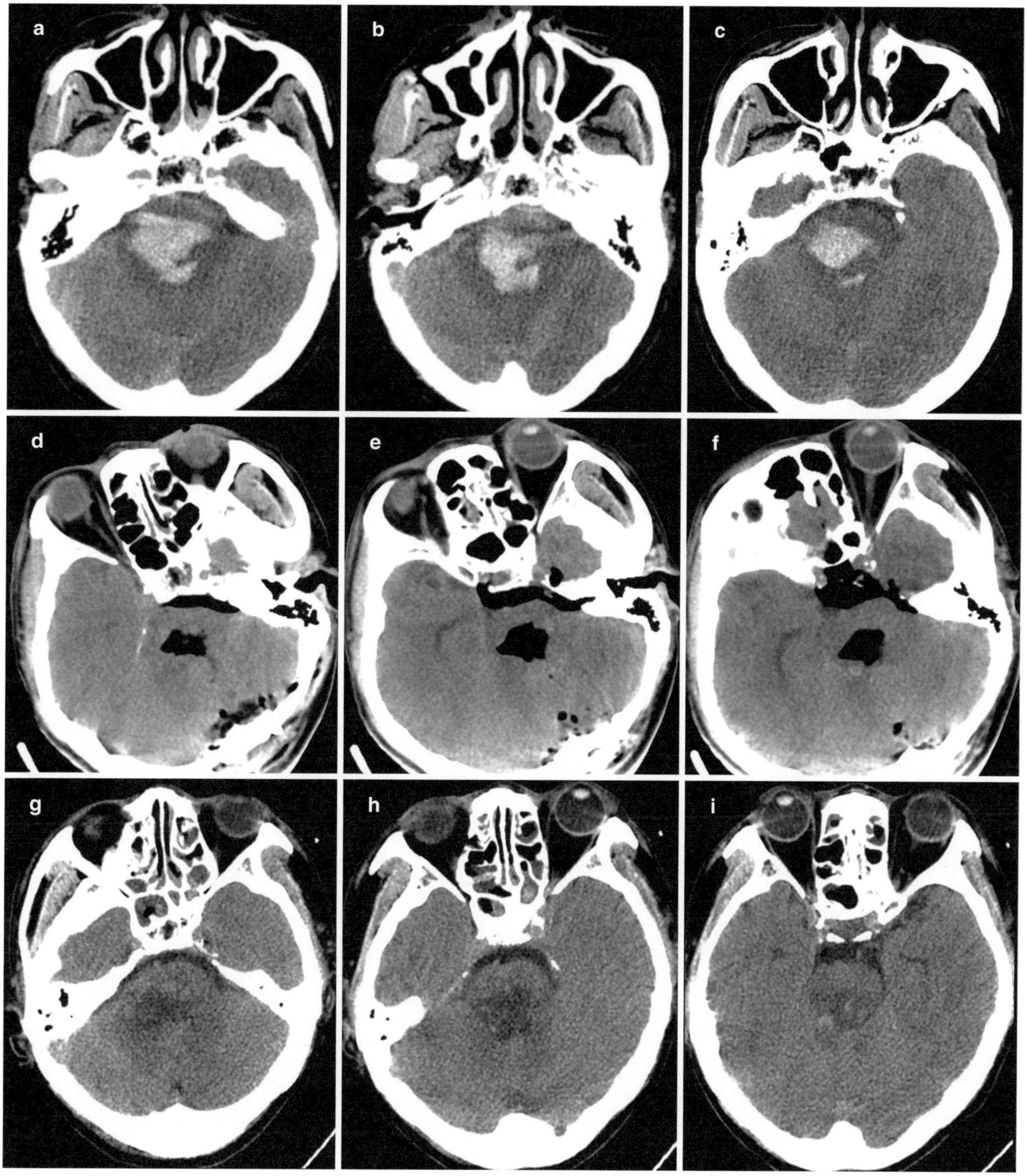

Fig. 13.41 Preoperative and postoperative cranial CT comparison (**a–c**) Preoperative axial CT images showing the hematoma located in the pons. (**d–f**) Axial CT images taken 6 h postoperatively demonstrating complete clearance of the pontine hematoma. (**g–i**) Three weeks postoperatively, axial CT images showing an intrapontine softening lesion

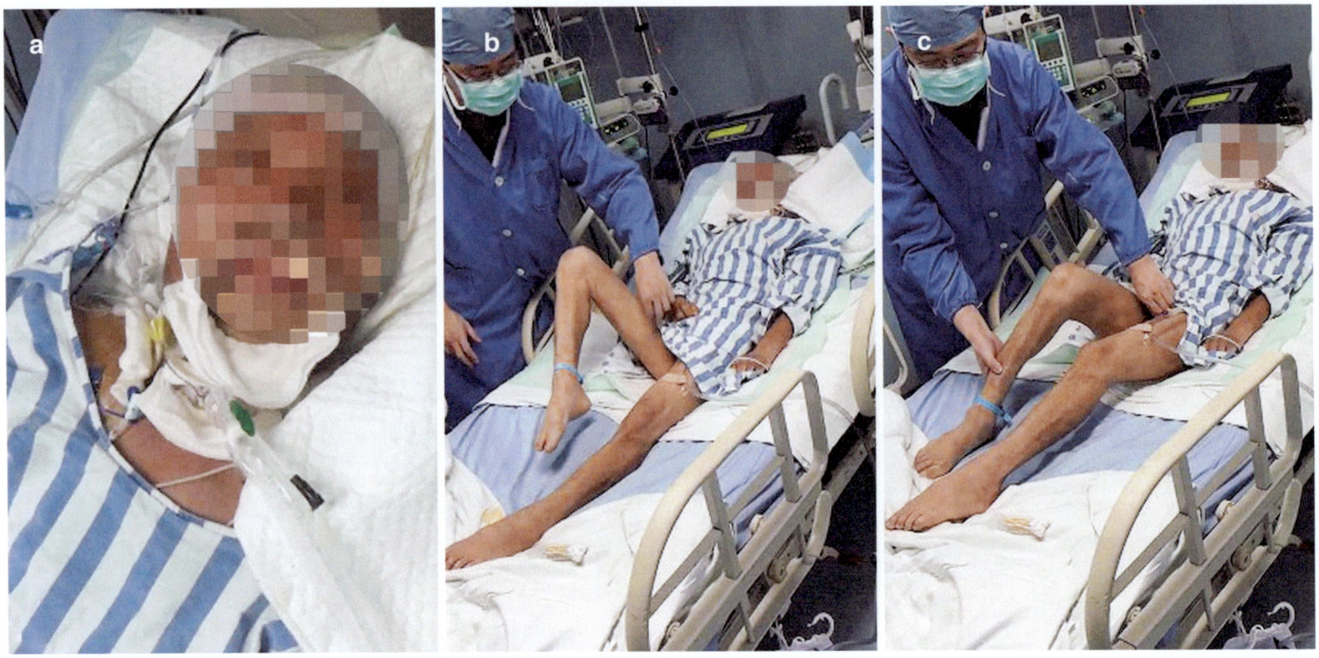

Fig. 13.42 Patient's Condition 3 Weeks Postoperatively. Neurological examination performed 3 weeks postoperatively shows muscle strength at grade III in the right lower limb

References

1. Lan Q. Actively carrying out minimally invasive neurosurgery through the keyhole approach. Chinese J Minimal Invasive Neurosurg. 2005;10(3):97–9.
2. Qin J, Qin SZ, Xu GZ, et al. Microscopic anatomical study of the subtemporal keyhole approach. Chinese J Clin Neurosurg. 2010;04:33–6.
3. Dong JJ, Lan Q. Study on the subfrontal keyhole approach. J Clinical Neurosurg. 2005;2(2):93–5.
4. Lan Q. Expert consensus on microscopic keyhole neurosurgery in China. Chinese J Neurosurg. 2017;33(6):548–53.
5. Qian ZY, Lan Q, Huang Q. Microsurgical keyhole surgery for brainstem and surrounding lesions. Chinese J Minimal Invasive Neurosurg. 2003;04:15–7.
6. Li ZQ, Lan Q. Microsurgical anatomy and quantitative evaluation of the suboccipital median keyhole approach via cerebellomedullary fissure. Chinese Medical J. 2009;89(39):2754–8.
7. Chen LH, Wei Q, Xu RX, et al. Minimally invasive surgical treatment of primary brainstem hemorrhage. Journal of Clin Neurosurg. 2015;12(5):349–53.
8. Li H, Li GP, You C, et al. Clinical analysis of microsurgical treatment of primary brainstem hemorrhage in 21 cases. Chinese J Neurosurg. 2007;23:944.
9. Brown AP, Thompson BG, Spetzler RF. The two-point method for evaluating brainstem lesions. BNI Quart. 1996;12:20.
10. Chen LH, Xu RX. Minimally invasive treatment of primary brainstem hemorrhage. Chinese J Neurotrauma Neurosurg. 2016;2(4):252–4.
11. Hao JM, Xue ZS. Preliminary exploration of the suboccipital retrosigmoid approach for the surgical treatment of severe primary brainstem hemorrhage. Chinese J Physic Edu. 2011;34(35):46–8.
12. Zhou Y, Ao XS, Huang X, et al. Microsurgical treatment of brainstem hemorrhage. Chinese J Clin Neurosurg. 2010;15(12):721–2.
13. Cavalcanti DD, Preul MC, Kalani MYS, et al. Microsurgical anatomy of safe entry zones to the brainstem. Journal of Neurosurgery. 2015:1–18.
14. Shi H, Zhou H, Wang FY, et al. Surgical treatment of hypertensive pontine hemorrhage related to brainstem through the transmembrane myelin approach. J Clin Neurosurg. 2017;14(1):49–51.
15. Liu X, Li H, Hu X, et al. Discussion on the treatment of spontaneous brainstem hemorrhage. J Clin Neurosurg. 2013;10:287.
16. You C, Liu M, Li H. Issues worthy of discussion in the diagnosis and treatment of diagnosing and treating cerebral hemorrhage. Chinese J Neurosurg. 2013;29:328.
17. Winkler EA, Birk H, Safaee M, et al. Erratum: Surgical resection of fourth ventricular ependymomas: case series and technical nuances. J Neuro-Oncol. 2017;131(2):423.
18. Matshushima K, Yagmurlu K, Kohno M, et al. Anatomy and approaches along the cerebellar-brainstem fissures. J Neurosurg. 2015:1–16.
19. Li H, Liu WK, Lin S, et al. Discussion on the treatment of primary brainstem hemorrhage. Chinese J Neurosurg. 2013;29(4):339–41.
20. Li J, Zheng J. Experience in microsurgical treatment of primary brainstem hemorrhage. Chinese J Neurosurg. 2017;33(2):184–5.

Puncture Evacuation for Brainstem Hemorrhage Via Stereotactic Frame-Assisted Positioning

14

Fengqiang Liu and Chi Gu

14.1 Overview

Primary brainstem hemorrhage is a severe neurological condition predominantly occurring in the pons, which has garnered limited interest among researchers due to its poor prognosis and challenging nature. In 2017, the "Expert Consensus on Monitoring and Treatment of Spontaneous Large Volume Intracerebral Hemorrhage in China" defined a hematoma volume of 5 mL or more in the brainstem as "large volume hematoma," indicating an unfavorable prognosis [1].

Upon admission, the GCS and hematoma volume are considered to be correlated with the 30-day mortality rate. Patients with a GCS below 7 and a hematoma volume of 5 mL or more have a 30-day mortality rate of at least 42.7%. For patients with a GCS score of 3–4 and a hematoma volume exceeding 10 mL, the mortality rate reaches 100%. Despite advancements in critical care medicine, which have extended the survival time of conservative patients, the prognosis remains unchanged. This not only consumes more medical resources but also necessitates the consideration of cost-effectiveness as one of the factors in medical decision-making.

Primary injuries resulting from brainstem hemorrhage are severe and extensive, with significant variations in the location, expansion, and extent of the hematoma among patients. The design of the surgical approach must adhere to personalized principles. However, imprecise puncture or a non-optimized precise operation may lead to inadvertent damage to the densely interconnected and complex structures surrounding the hematoma, such as important conduction tracts, neural clusters, blood vessels, and cranial nerves. Such iatrogenic injuries can easily cause secondary damage to already compromised neural functions, negating the potential benefits of the surgery and even resulting in worse outcomes.

The selection of surgical techniques should be carefully weighed against the iatrogenic injury-to-benefit ratio with utmost caution. Despite reported cases of surgical benefits, numerous factors, including case selection, surgical approach, technical proficiency, and perioperative management, influence the prognosis. Like spontaneous hemorrhages in other locations, there is also considerable controversy surrounding conservative versus surgical treatments [2, 3].

Stereotactic precise puncture and aspiration, with a sufficient and optimized preoperative plan, could be precisely conducted with minor trauma and short surgical time. It has gained increasing attention in the surgical treatment of brainstem hemorrhage. This chapter primarily focuses on the utilization of stereotactic frame-assisted surgery in treating brainstem hemorrhage [4, 5].

14.1.1 Primary Brainstem Hemorrhage Zhe-Er Classification and Its Surgical Value

Pontine hemorrhage accounts for 90% of primary brainstem hemorrhages. In the CT axial scan sequence, the largest cross-section of the hematoma is selected, and the midline and the boundary between the brainstem and the cerebellum on both sides are marked. Subsequently, the lines dividing the left and right sides, with midline, are designated as 1, 2, and 3. Hematomas located in the fourth ventricle or peripontine cistern, compressing the brainstem or blocking the cerebrospinal fluid circulation, belong to Type 0. Hematomas involving lines 1 or 3 but not crossing line 2 are classified as Type 1. Hematomas involving lines 1 and 2 or 2 and 3 are classified as Type 2. Hematomas involving lines 1, 2, and 3 are classified as Type 3. Among Type 2 and Type 3 hematomas, line 2 is divided into anterior, central, and posterior segments. Based on the range of hematoma involvement

Supplementary Information The online version contains supplementary material available at https://doi.org/10.1007/978-981-95-8942-5_14.

F. Liu (✉) · C. Gu
Department of Neurosurgery, The Second Affiliated Hospital of Zhejiang University School of Medicine, Hangzhou, China

G. Chen, C. You (eds.), *Surgical Treatment of Primary Brainstem Hemorrhage*, https://doi.org/10.1007/978-981-95-8942-5_14

across line 2, these are further categorized into subtypes A (ventral), C (central), and B (dorsal).

14.1.2 Surgical Value

Type 0 hematoma: The brainstem is not directly damaged by the hematoma. Following the principles of brain herniation management, urgent treatment often leads to a good prognosis.
Type 1 hematoma: The primary damage to the brainstem is relatively small, and significant benefits can be obtained by removing the hematoma.
Type 2 hematoma: The damage to one side of the brainstem is relatively mild, and removing the hematoma may be beneficial.
Type 3 hematoma: Both sides of the brainstem are damaged, and removing the hematoma can benefit some patients.

Among the three subtypes, different consequences are often observed due to the involvement of different brainstem structures.

Type A: Relatively distant from the reticular structures of the brainstem, with a higher probability of postoperative awakening. However, it is prone to affecting the corticospinal tract, leading to severe motor impairment. There are relatively more options for hematoma removal.
Type B: Proximity to the brainstem reticular structure and dorsal nuclei results in more pronounced damage to vegetative survival and posterior cranial nerves. It is essential to fully utilize the natural channels formed by hematoma expansion, and to precisely plan the surgical path to enhance the protection of residual function.
Type C: Involving the central area of the brainstem, when the hematoma volume is small (<5 mL), the damage to important functional areas is less than that of Type B. Evacuation of the hematoma is more likely to be beneficial. When the hematoma volume is large (>10 mL), benefits are difficult to achieve regardless of the method used.

14.2 Indications and Contraindications for Surgery

Surgical Indications: Existence of severe neurological deficits related to the hematoma, the absence of surgical contraindications, and the need for stereotactic surgery to salvage function and life. Specific criteria include:

1. Confirmation through imaging diagnosis, using CT quantitative measurement or "stereotactic surgical planning system" software to calculate the hematoma volume, and establishing the patient as having primary brainstem hemorrhage with a hematoma volume $\geq$ 3 mL.
2. GCS score $\leq$ 8; however, for patients with a score of 5–7, surgery may be more beneficial.
3. Stable vital signs at the onset of the condition, with no circulatory disturbances within 6 h.
4. Concomitant acute hydrocephalus requiring urgent surgical intervention.
5. Choice of surgical timing.

Personalized selection of the surgical timing based on GCS score, hematoma volume, disease progression, and family wishes.

1. Hematoma volume $\geq$ 5 mL, surgery is recommended within 72 h of the onset; in the presence of obstructive hydrocephalus, emergency evacuation of the hematoma is necessary, and depending on the extent of evacuation, external ventricular drainage may be considered.
2. Hematoma volume 3–5 mL, without obstructive hydrocephalus, observation for 2–3 days after the onset. If there is an improving trend in consciousness impairment, conservative management may be continued. Otherwise, surgery can be performed within 3–5 days after the onset.
3. Slow absorption of the hematoma, unresolved local mass effect, but good liquefaction, surgery can be delayed up to 3 weeks at the latest.

14.2.1 Contraindications

Radiologically confirmed secondary hemorrhage to the cerebral vascular abnormalities, such as cavernous malformation, ruptured aneurysm, arteriovenous malformation (AVM), or suspected tumor hemorrhage. Additionally, the following conditions apply:

1. Any irreversible coagulation disorders or known coagulation system diseases. Caution should be exercised when choosing surgery for individuals with a platelet count <100,000 or an INR >1.4.
2. Cautions should be exercised when choosing surgery for patients with circulatory failure who are unable to maintain blood pressure or have unstable heart rate despite the use of vasopressor medications.

14.3 Preoperative Preparation and Surgical Instruments

Preoperative preparation:

1. Installation of stereotactic frame in the supine position, with the expected puncture of the middle cerebellar peduncle through the lateral side, using the "3-nail method" to fix the frame, and selecting a disposable low- or no-artifact head nail as much as possible, with the upper edge of the base ring positioned below the level of the earlobe.
2. CT localization scan: the field of view (FOV) should be set at around 280, with the axial scan range including from the upper edge of the base ring to the scalp; The layer thickness should be <3 mm and continuous without gaps. CT data is transmitted to the navigation software for fine path planning, and the target point, entry point, and spin angle of the puncture needle are finely adjusted based on the path cutting plane and path vertical plane, and the surrounding structures of the path are fully evaluated.
3. Choose the appropriate position according to the planned surgical path, commonly used positions include: prone and lateral positions.

Surgical instruments: Use a frame stereotactic device, a 4 and 3 mm suction needle, and a lateral opening hematoma suction needle. In addition to general functions such as target point coordinate calculation, the surgical planning system should have at least basic 3D reconstruction functions such as displaying the puncture path sectional view and puncture path vertical plane.

14.4 Surgical Methods, Precautions, and Techniques

Standardized procedure for stereotactic precise aspiration surgery:

1. Surgical planning: The principles are as follows: (1) The surgical path should make full use of the natural channel formed by hematoma expansion as much as possible; (2) If the hematoma ruptures into the fourth ventricle, the route may pass through the fourth ventricle, but care must be taken to avoid the dorsal nuclei of the brainstem; (3) The route should be as consistent as possible with the long axis of the hematoma; (4) When additional external ventricular drainage is necessary, a single-target multi-channel scheme may be used. (5) Design the surgical position using three-dimensional images to make the puncture path tend toward vertical alignment with the ground.

Operational steps:

1. Arrange and fix the position according to the surgical plan.
2. Adhere to the standardized operation of disinfecting and draping, exposing only the scalp around the incision and the earpiece of the stereotactic instrument.
3. When setting the earpiece of the stereotactic instrument, the Y and Z values must be double-checked by two individuals.
4. It is recommended to drill under direct vision, strictly achieving hemostasis before puncture, and incising the pia mater.
5. According to the preoperative plan, precisely aspirate the hematoma until over 90% of the total volume is removed, or when fragmented brain tissue is observed. Then, stop aspiration, infuse the hematoma cavity with physiological saline to maintain a static water pressure level of 20–25 cm, and repeatedly irrigate the hematoma cavity with 3–5 mL of physiological saline until the effluent becomes noticeably diluted.
6. Maintain normal blood pressure throughout the perioperative period. After hematoma clearance, it is recommended to maintain systolic blood pressure at 120–130 mmHg.
7. Management of active bleeding: If fresh blood or effluent remains bright red after repeated irrigation and does not show a trend toward dilution, active bleeding within the hematoma cavity is diagnosed. Measures for management include controlled hypotension, targeting a sustained systolic blood pressure of 110 ± 10 mmHg; using cold saline or infusing the hematoma cavity with 0.5–2 mg of adrenaline in 100 mL of physiological saline and maintaining a static water pressure of over 20 cm of water.
8. When the hematoma cavity communicates with the fourth ventricle or in the absence of non-obstructive hydrocephalus preoperatively, additional lateral ventricular drainage may not be necessary.

14.5 Postoperative Complications, Prevention, and Postoperative Care

Unless there is severe intracranial hypertension, blood pressure should be strictly controlled within the normal range while maintaining normal cerebral perfusion pressure. Specialized external ventricular drainage products should be selected, and the drainage height should be set at 20–25 cm, following the management method for external ventricular drainage.

Perform a CT scan on the day of surgery or the following day to determine the timing of catheter removal based on the residual hematoma volume. If the residual volume is less than 3 mL and there is no hydrocephalus, the drainage tube can be removed within 24 h after surgery.

Major complications mainly include re-bleeding in the puncture tract or hematoma cavity. Attention should be paid to blood pressure management during the anesthesia recovery stage and the transfer process to the ICU. Blood pressure should be strictly controlled (below 140/90 mmHg, with a recommended systolic blood pressure control of 130 ± 10 mmHg), and drastic fluctuations should be avoided.

Assess consciousness and spontaneous breathing daily, enhance airway management, and initiate early weaning trials. If there is no expected short-term recovery or severe pulmonary infection, early tracheostomy and awakening-promoting therapy should be considered.

14.6 Advantages, Disadvantages, Experience, and Lessons Learned

14.6.1 Advantages

1. Stereotactic brainstem hematoma evacuation surgery is precise in positioning, with a high hematoma clearance rate and few complications. It allows for the visualization and design of the puncture path. Additionally, by evaluating the maximum deviation angle in the path planning (the lateral hole rotation angle), irregular hematomas in various orientations can be accurately removed.
2. It helps achieve the goal of "maximizing hematoma clearance with minimal surgical trauma."
3. The technical threshold is not high, and after systematic training, standardization can be easily achieved in the short term. It is predictable and has good reproducibility.

14.6.2 Disadvantages

1. It involves multidisciplinary collaboration, including radiology, anesthesia, and intensive care. Some clinical centers face difficulties in standardizing localization scanning, data acquisition, perioperative blood pressure control, and drainage management.
2. The procedure involves many detailed issues and requires systematic training; otherwise, smooth implementation is challenging.
3. There is a lack of entry requirements, leading to uneven technical proficiency.

14.6.3 Experience and Lessons Learned

1. Proper installation of the frame is crucial. Improper positioning can easily cause inconvenience for subsequent work, affecting localization scanning, anesthesia intubation, and even hindering puncture.
2. The planned path should adhere to rational principles; an irregular puncture path may cause accidental injury.
3. Gentle force should be used during aspiration, and blind increase in negative pressure should be avoided.
4. Blood pressure should be strictly controlled throughout the perioperative period, especially during the anesthesia recovery stage, with attention to treatment continuity during interdepartmental handovers.
5. Aspirating the hematoma as much as possible during surgery can relieve obstruction in the ventricular system and reduce the risk of obstructive hydrocephalus.
6. Prior to surgery, a comprehensive CTA examination should be performed to exclude the possibility of secondary bleeding, such as aneurysms and arteriovenous malformations.

14.7 Evaluation and Prospects of the Surgical Technique

Stereotactic surgery, due to its precise positioning and meticulous planning, minimizes iatrogenic damage by avoiding sensitive structures to the greatest extent possible. The procedure is brief, with minimal complications, and achieves a hematoma clearance rate of approximately 80–100%. Its advantages over other surgical methods are increasingly evident.

With the gradual popularization of stereotactic brain hemorrhage surgery and the development of clinical multicenter randomized controlled studies, this procedure is expected to bring more confidence to patients with brainstem hemorrhage. At the same time, the primary damage of brainstem hemorrhage is severe, and any improvement in surgical techniques is difficult to fundamentally change the poor prognosis. With the significant reduction in mortality rate, it is particularly urgent to improve the quality of life of surviving patients. In addition to improving surgical techniques, it is necessary to accelerate the development of related technologies such as neural functional reconstruction and rehabilitation.

14.8 Typical Case

14.8.1 Case 1

14.8.1.1 Summary of Medical History and Imaging Data

Patient: Male, 62 years old, admitted with a chief complaint of "sudden loss of consciousness for 10 h." The patient has a history of hypertension, managed with amlodipine, but the control status is unknown. Physical examination: BP 176/107 mmHg; the patient is in a comatose state with GCS 2 + T + 4. The heart rate is stable, bilateral pupils are 3 mm with sluggish light reflex, and there is flexion of limbs in response to painful stimuli. Muscle strength is 2/5 on the left side and 0/5 on the right side. Preoperative CT scan reveals a central hematoma in the left pons, partially extending into the fourth ventricle. The calculated volume of the hematoma is approximately 6.2 mL (Fig. 14.1).

14.8.1.2 Operative Procedure and Key Points

1. Preoperative planning: The hematoma is classified as Type I—lateral type. The target point is set at the center of the hematoma, considering both the brainstem and fourth ventricle hematomas. The angulation of the arc is maximized to avoid the transverse sinus. The coordinates are set as follows: X 110, Y 77, Z 128; arc angulation 198°; and Ring Arc 70°. The superficial and deep points of the hematoma are 15 mm above and 5 mm below the target, respectively. A catheter is placed 5 mm above the target (Fig. 14.2).
2. Intraoperative findings: A 0° needle is used to aspirate approximately 2–3 mL of blood from 5 mm above the target. Then, a 90° needle is inserted into the target, and approximately 1–2 mL of blood is aspirated. The cavity is washed until clear, and the pressure in the hematoma cavity is set at 25 cmH_2O (Fig. 14.3a, b).

14.8.1.3 Pre- and Postoperative Imaging Comparison

A postoperative CT scan on the first day shows that the hematoma has been largely cleared, and the drainage tube is appropriately positioned. A CT scan on the third day reveals that the fourth ventricle hemorrhage has been largely cleared, and there is no acute hydrocephalus (Fig. 14.3c–e).

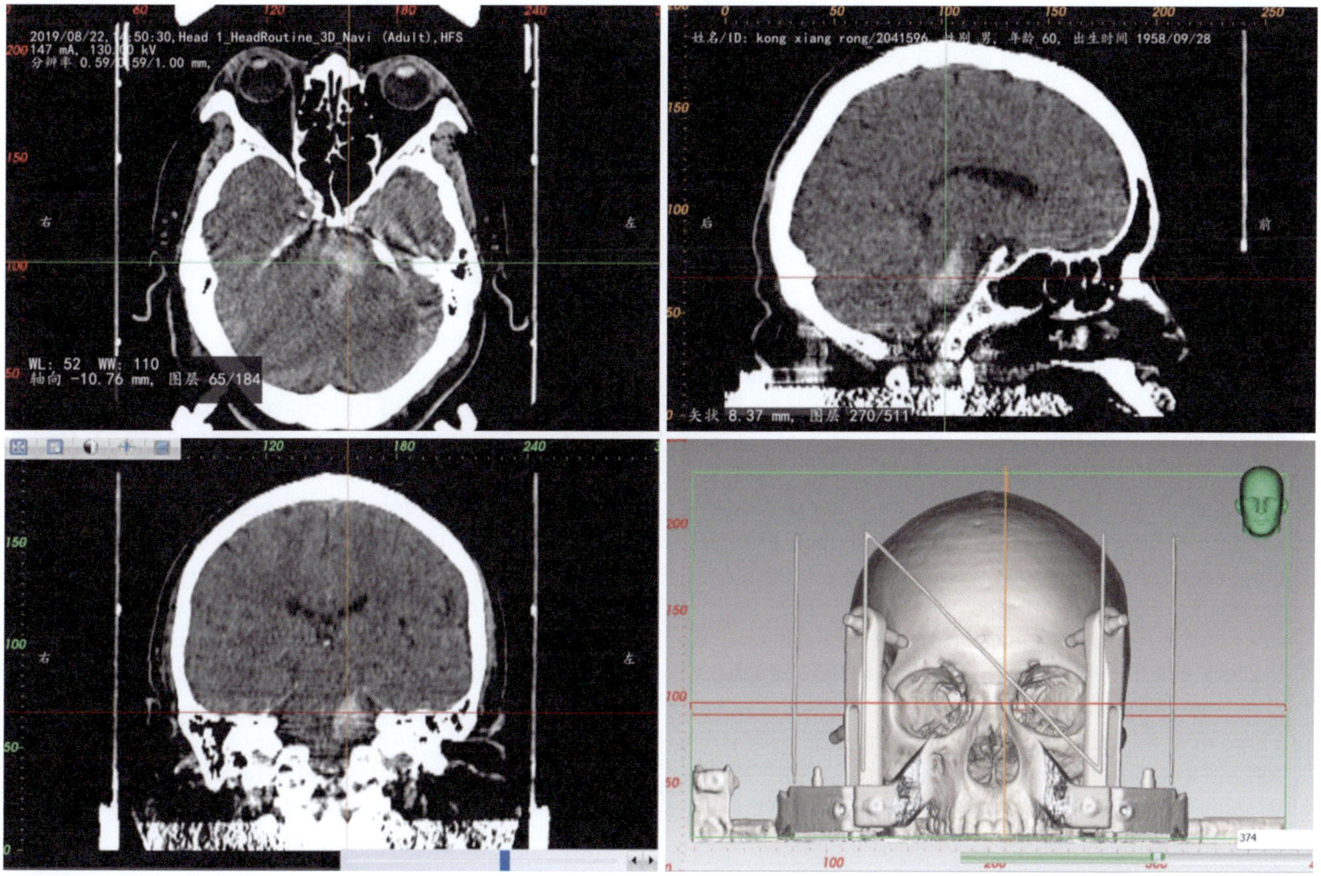

Fig. 14.1 Preoperative CT scan shows that the hematoma is relatively scattered, with the largest cross-section located above the pontomedullary sulcus, and the hematoma is elongated, with some entering the fourth ventricle

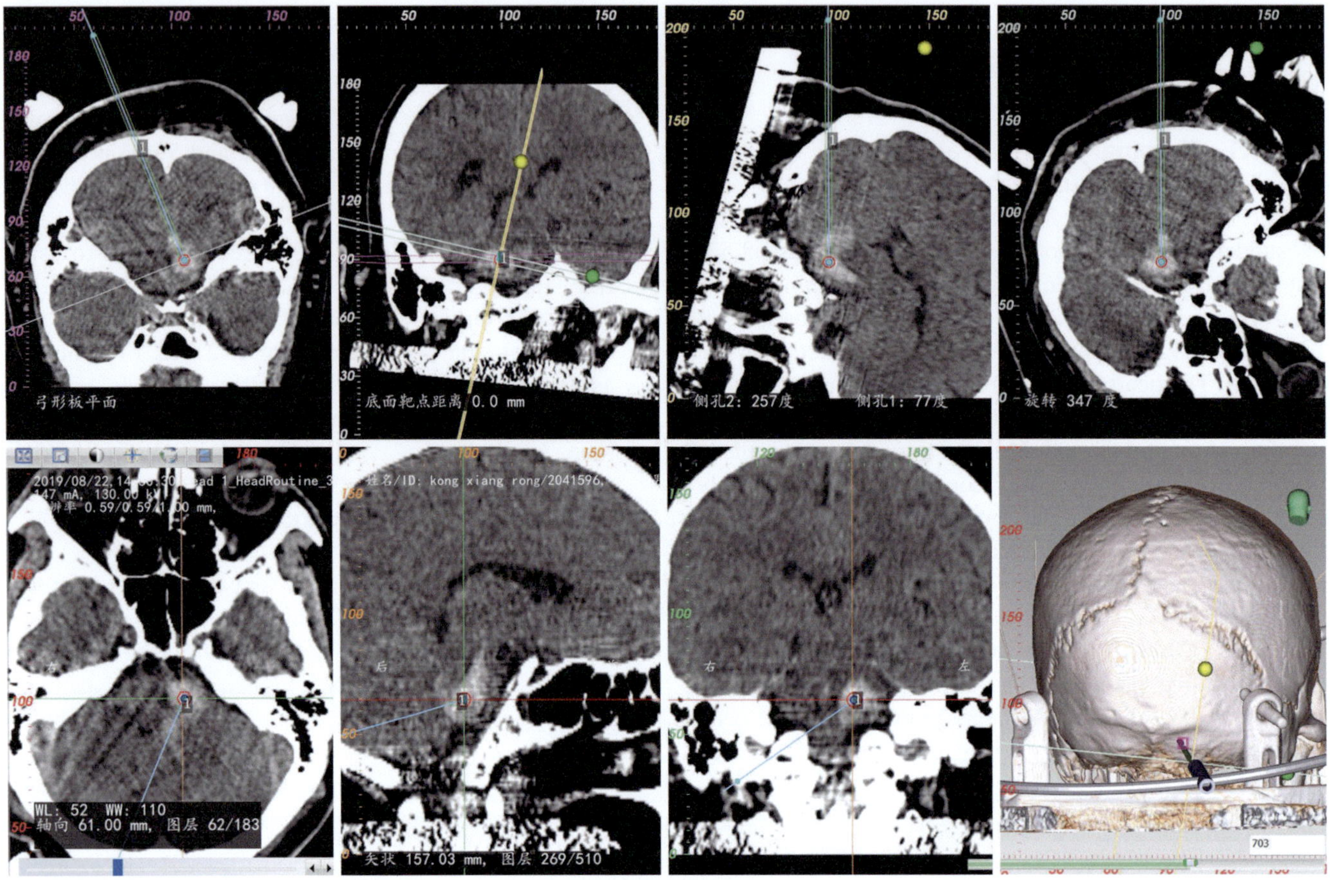

Fig. 14.2 Preoperative planning showing the puncture path from the contralateral cerebellum, traversing the entire length of the hematoma. By rotating the side hole of the puncture needle, aspirate the hematoma that extends deep into the brainstem

14.8.1.4 Postoperative Neurological Examination Imaging Data

1. The patient is transferred to the intensive care unit, and the systolic blood pressure is maintained between 120 and 140 mmHg. The patient regains consciousness on the third day, and undergoes tracheotomy, GCS 4 + T + 5. On the sixth day after surgery, the patient is transferred back to the general ward. On the tenth day after surgery, the patient is discharged with GCS 4 + T + 5 and muscle strength of 3/5 on the left side and 0/5 on the right side.
2. One month after surgery: The tracheostomy is not closed, and GCS 13 (4 + 4 + 5). The patient can follow instructions and perform movements. Muscle strength is 4/5 on the left side and 1/5 on the right side, GOS grade 3 (Fig. 14.4, Video 14.1).
3. Three months after surgery: GCS 14, and the patient can follow instructions and perform movements. Muscle strength is 4/5 on the left side and 1/5 on the right side. GOS grade 3.

14.8.2 Case 2

14.8.2.1 Summary of Medical History and Imaging Data

Patient: A 62-year-old male was admitted due to sudden headache, vomiting, and subsequent coma for 7 days. The patient has a history of hypertension, and the control status is unknown. Prior to admission, the patient underwent a tracheotomy at a local hospital. Physical examination: BP 168/105 mmHg; GCS = 1 + 1 + 4 = 6, comatose state, bilateral pupils measuring 2.5 mm with sluggish light reflex; slight withdrawal of the right limbs in response to painful stimuli. Preoperative CT scan revealed two hematomas, with one located in the right thalamus, estimated to be approximately 6 mL in volume. The other was located in the pons, slightly to the right side, with a more scattered hematoma measuring approximately 6.9 mL. Having been 7 days from the disease onset, the hematoma density was slightly higher, and the edges were not well-defined (Fig. 14.5).

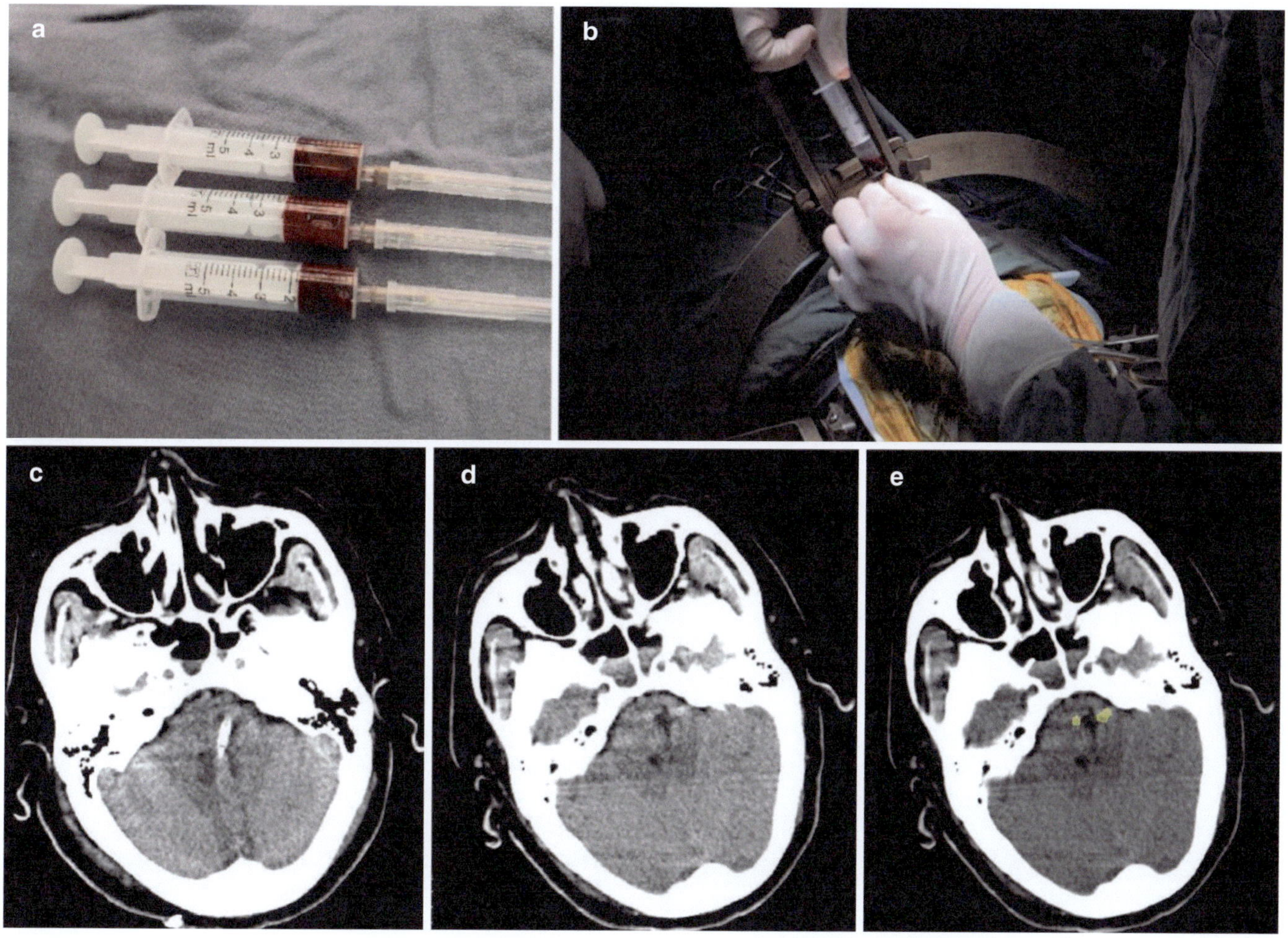

Fig. 14.3 (**a**, **b**) Approximately 5 mL of old blood-tinged fluid was aspirated during the surgery. (**c**) Complete clearance of brainstem hematoma was observed on the first postoperative day. (**d**, **e**) A CT scan on the third postoperative day indicated complete clearance of the hematoma in the ventricles and brainstem, with a residual hematoma volume of 0.26 mL after software modeling, achieving a satisfactory clearance rate

14.8.2.2 Operative Procedure and Key Points

Preoperative Planning: Given the considerable distance between the two hematoma locations and the need to adhere to aseptic requirements during surgery while minimizing frame adjustments, the target was set at the center of the brainstem hematoma, and two puncture paths were utilized.

Localization: Target setting: X 87 Y 71 Z 117.

Approach 1: Puncture of the thalamic hematoma, with the entry point positioned as far forward as possible to avoid the motor area, and the puncture path avoiding the lateral ventricle. Direction: Arc frame deviation angle 85°, arc plate deviation angle 56°.The superficial and deep points of the hematoma were 40 and 20 mm above the target, respectively, with the catheter placed 20 mm above the target upon completion (Fig. 14.6a).

Approach 2: Puncture of the brainstem hematoma, entering from the right side, with the arc frame deviation angle at 190° and the arc plate deviation angle at 56°. The catheter was placed at the target point upon completion (Fig. 14.6b).

Intraoperative Findings: Under general anesthesia and in the prone position, punctures were performed according to the preoperative planned paths: (1) Frontal approach: Approximately 3 mL of thalamic hematoma was aspirated. The catheter was placed 20 mm above the target. (2) Cerebellar approach: Approximately 7 mL of brainstem hematoma was aspirated, with fluid ingress (saline used for thalamic irrigation), and the catheter was placed at the target point. After the placement of two catheters, continuous irrigation was performed until the effluent was clear, ensuring unobstructed flow through both catheters. The hematoma cavity pressure was set at 20–30 cm in the supine position (Fig. 14.7).

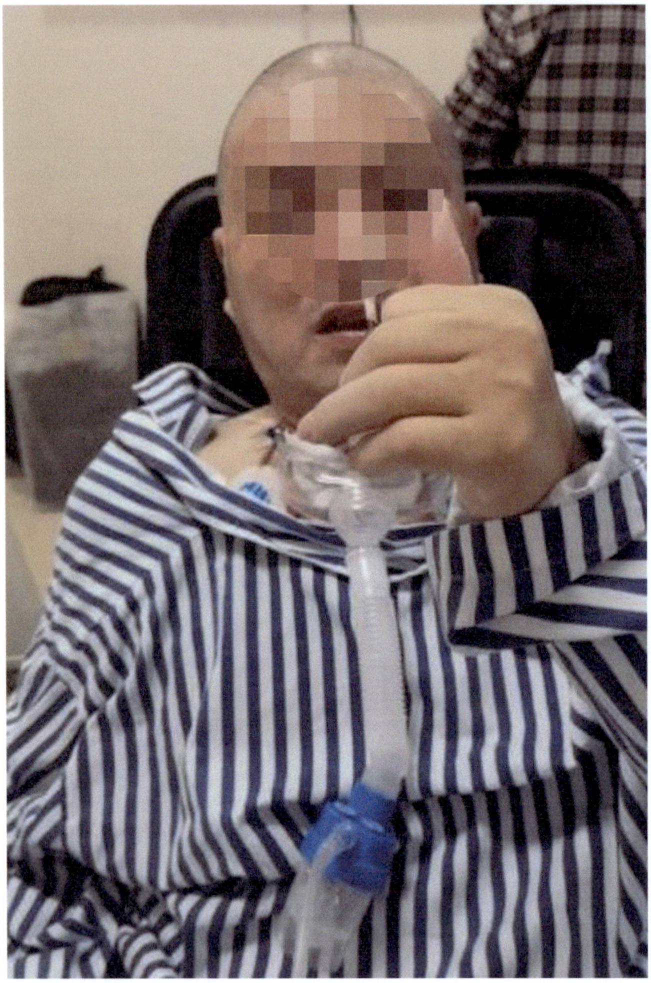

Fig. 14.4 Illustrating the patient's recovery 1 month postoperatively

14.8.2.3 Postoperative Neurological Examination

Postoperative Progress: The patient was transferred to the intensive care unit postoperatively, with systolic blood pressure maintained at 120–140 mmHg. On the fourth postoperative day, the patient's consciousness level was assessed at GCS 2 + T + 4, and a tracheostomy was performed, the ventilator was weaned. The patient was transferred to a rehabilitation hospital on the sixth postoperative day.

On the first postoperative day, a CT scan confirmed the presence of drainage tubes, with satisfactory clearance rates for both thalamic and pontine hematomas (Fig. 14.8).

One month postoperatively: GCS 3 + T + 5, partial compliance with instructions, ability to perform simple command-driven movements, right-sided limb muscle strength at level 4, left-sided limb muscle strength at levels 1–2. GOS score of 3.

14.8.3 Case 3

14.8.3.1 Brief Medical History and Imaging Data

Admission Information: A female patient, 62 years old, was admitted due to "sudden onset of altered consciousness for 2 days." History of hypertension, managed with amlodipine, with unclear control status. GCS improved from 3 to 5 after conservative treatment at a local hospital for 1 day, prompting transfer to our hospital.

Examination: BP 176/107 mmHg; GCS = 1 + 1 + 3 = 5, Pupils: left 4 mm, right 2 mm, both without light reflex, weak spontaneous breathing, no response to left-sided pain stimulation, flexion response to right-sided limb pain stimulation.

Preoperative CT revealed a pontine and medullary central hemorrhage, classified as type III in brainstem hemorrhage, with partial extension into the fourth ventricle. The calculated hematoma volume was approximately 14.8 mL (Fig. 14.9).

14.8.3.2 Operative Procedure and Key Points

Preoperative Planning: The target was set at the center of the hematoma, with the puncture path directed to the right to avoid important nuclei behind the brainstem.

Localization: Target setting: X 95 Y 73 Z 108, Direction: Arc frame deviation angle 190°, arc plate deviation angle 40°. The superficial and deep points of the hematoma were 20 mm above and 13 mm below the target, respectively; the catheter was placed at the target point upon completion (Fig. 14.10).

Intraoperative findings: Under general anesthesia and in the prone position, punctures were performed according to the preoperatively planned paths: gradual aspiration from the target point to 20 mm above the target, with hematoma liquefaction resulting in the aspiration of a total of 10 mL of blood and 10 mL of bloody cerebrospinal fluid. Subsequently, saline irrigation was performed repeatedly until the effluent was clear, and a drainage tube was placed at the target point. The hematoma cavity pressure was set at 20–30 cm in the supine position (Fig. 14.10a).

14.8.3.3 Postoperative Neurological Examination and Imaging Data

On the first postoperative day, a CT scan confirmed the presence of the drainage tube, with satisfactory clearance rates at the target point and above, and a small residual hematoma below the target. A CT scan on the third postoperative day revealed a further reduction in the residual hematoma volume, approximately 1.5 mL, with a hematoma clearance rate exceeding 90% (Fig. 14.11).

The patient received postoperative care in the intensive care unit, with systolic blood pressure maintained at

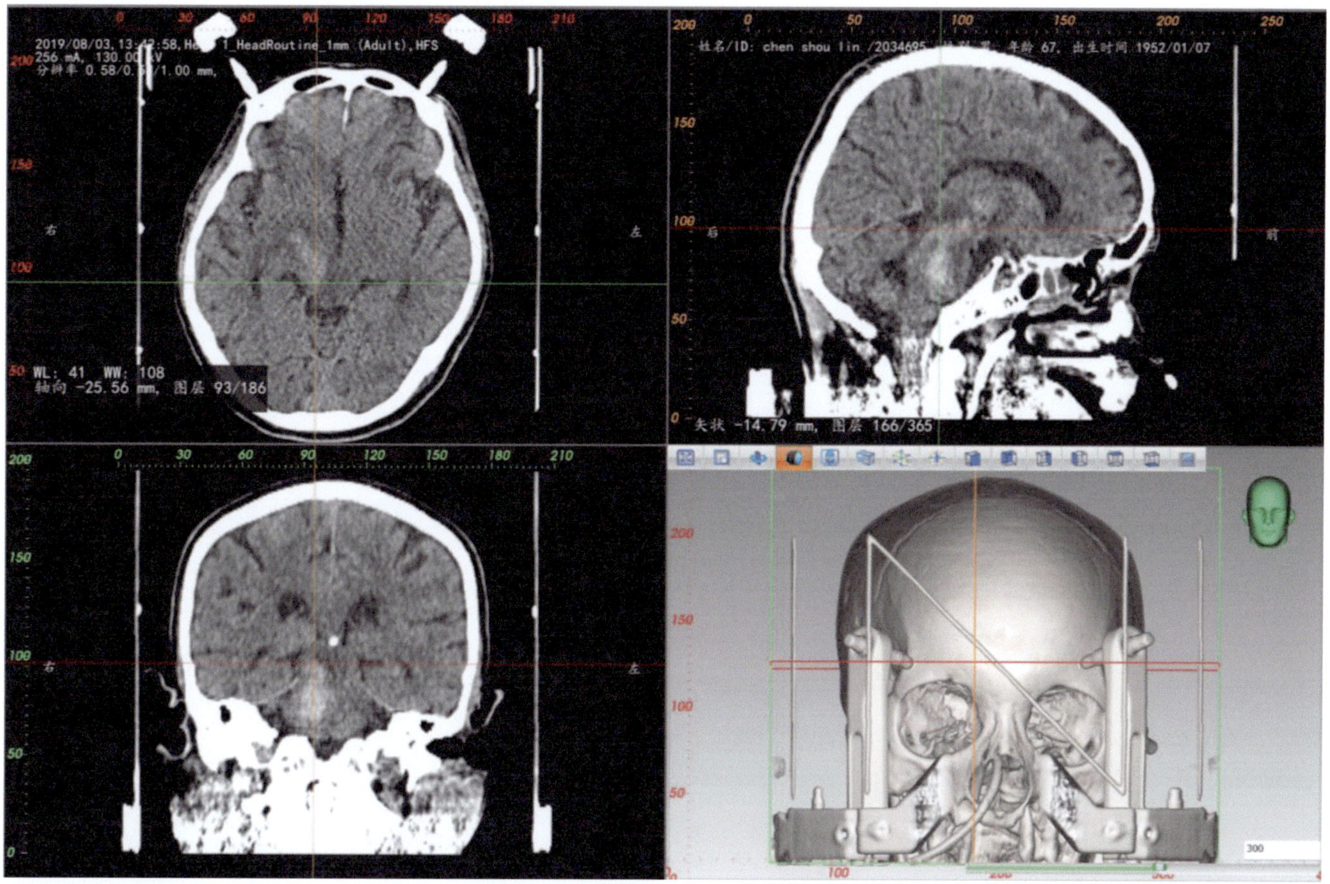

Fig. 14.5 Preoperative CT scans reveal a hematoma affecting the thalamus, midbrain, and pons, with slight compression of the ventricles and the posterior limb of the internal capsule, while the midline structures remain centrally positioned

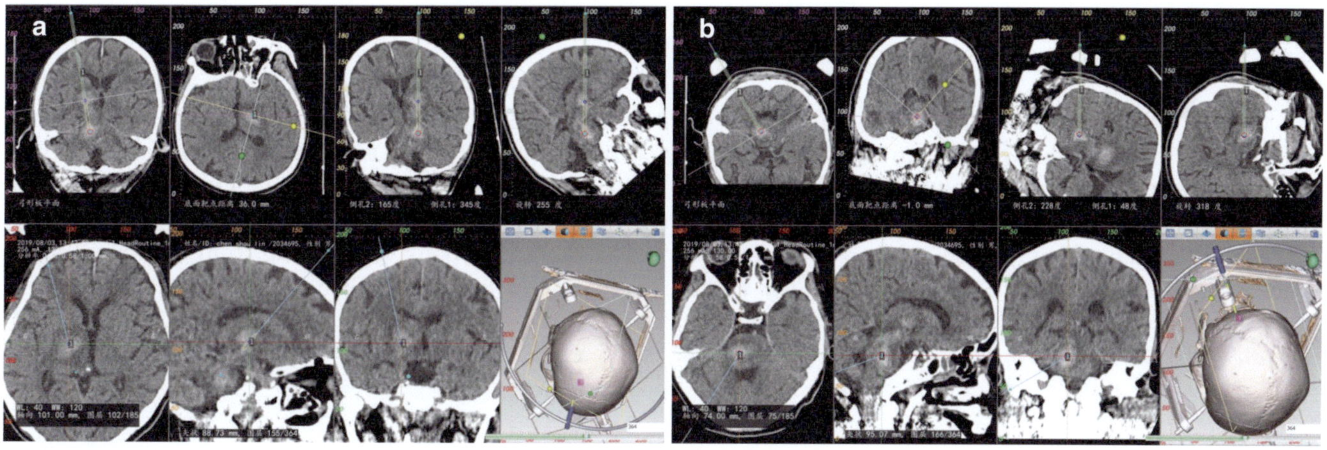

Fig. 14.6 Single target, dual channels: clearing thalamic-pontine hematoma separately through the ring angle and arc angle. (**a**) The pathway avoids puncturing the lateral ventricle for thalamic hematoma. (**b**) The pathway aspirates brainstem hematoma through the middle cerebellar peduncle

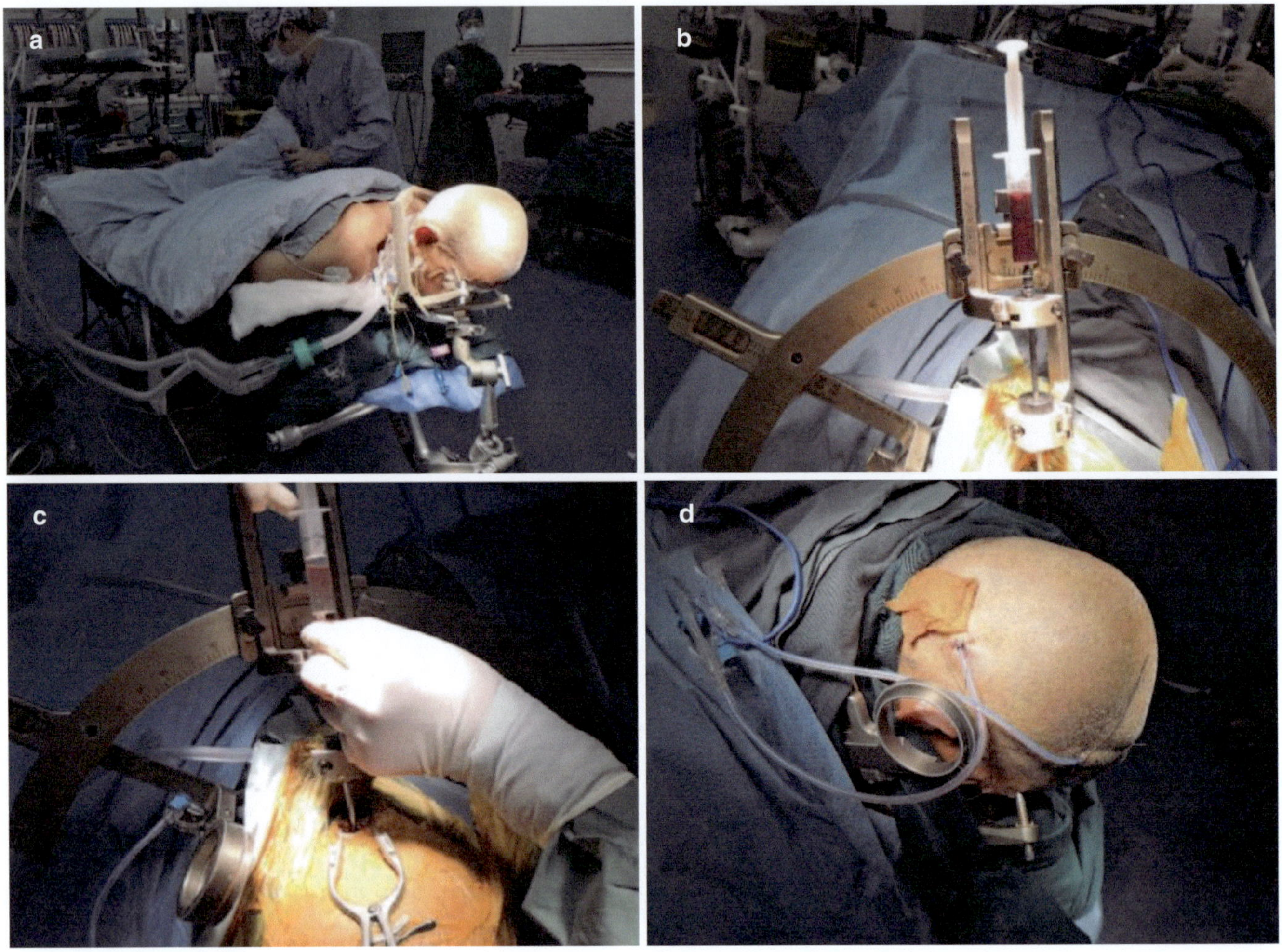

Fig. 14.7 (**a**) Prone position accommodating both puncture paths. (**b**) Puncture of the brainstem hematoma. (**c**) Clear appearance of the irrigation fluid during the surgery. (**d**) Postoperative catheter placement

120–140 mmHg. On the third postoperative day, the patient's consciousness level was assessed at GCS 1 + T + 3, and a tracheostomy was performed.

One month postoperatively: GCS 2 + T + 3, oxygen mask in place, pupils dilated at 3 mm, sluggish light reflex. Right-sided limb muscle strength at level 3, left-sided limb muscle strength at levels 1–2.

Approximately 2 months postoperatively, the patient was discharged from the intensive care unit to a rehabilitation hospital, with a GCS of 2 + T + 4 at the time of discharge, responsive to strong stimuli, oxygen mask in place, right-sided limb muscle strength at level 3, left-sided limb muscle strength at level 2, and a GOS score of 2.

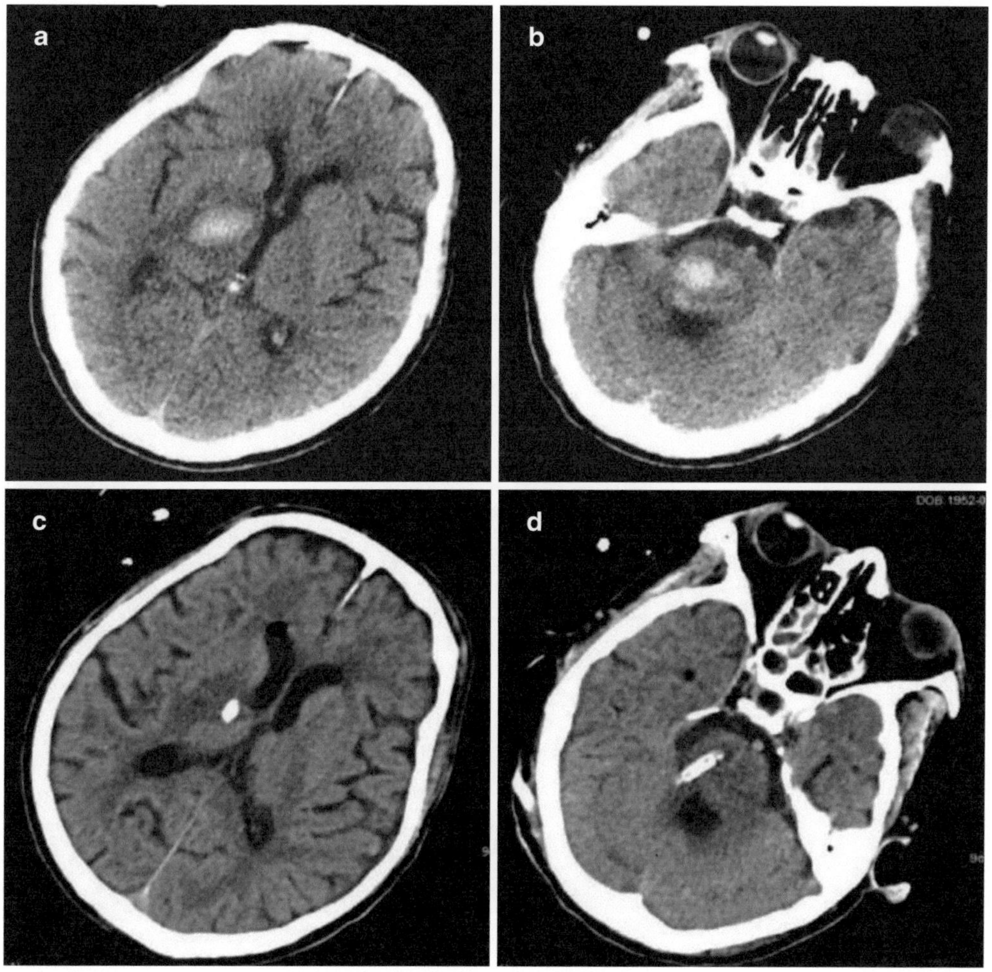

Fig. 14.8 (**a**, **b**) Preoperative CT showing the maximum extent of the hematomas. (**c**, **d**) Corresponding postoperative CT images showing approximately 90% clearance of the hematomas

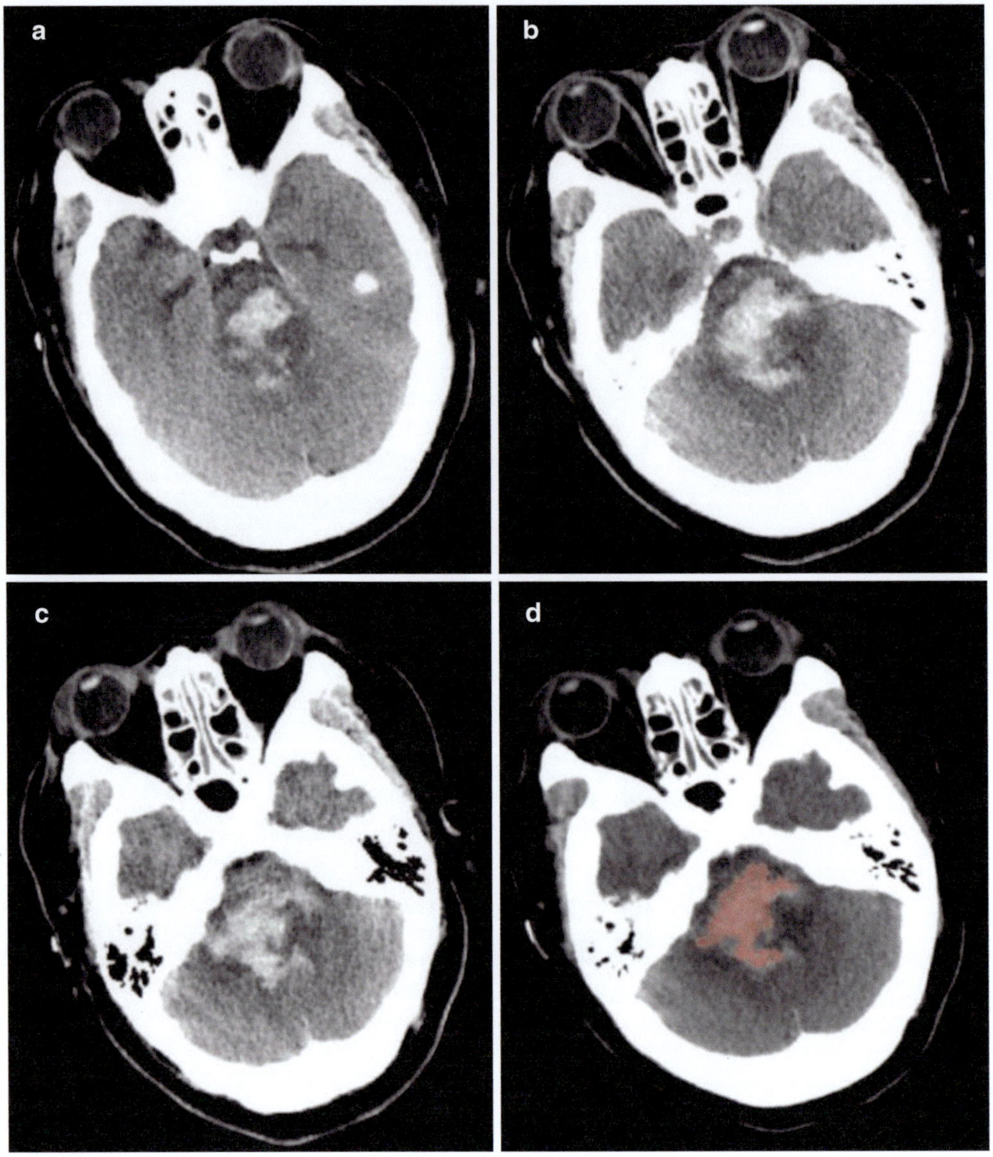

Fig. 14.9 (**a**–**c**) Preoperative CT showing the largest extent of the hematoma, indicating central hemorrhage in the brainstem, predominantly on the right. (**d**) Computer-modeled hematoma volume of approximately 14.8 mL

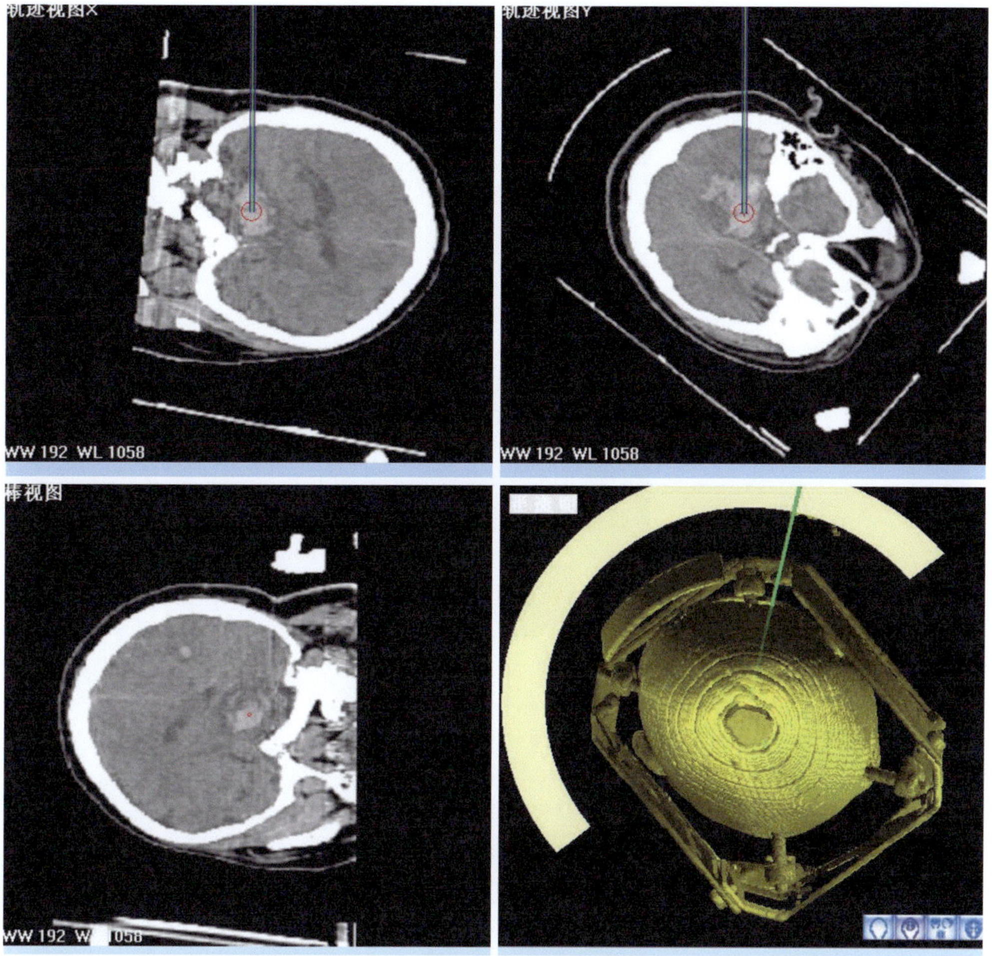

Fig. 14.10 Path planning on the stereotactic navigation software, illustrating the puncture path through the long axis of the hematoma

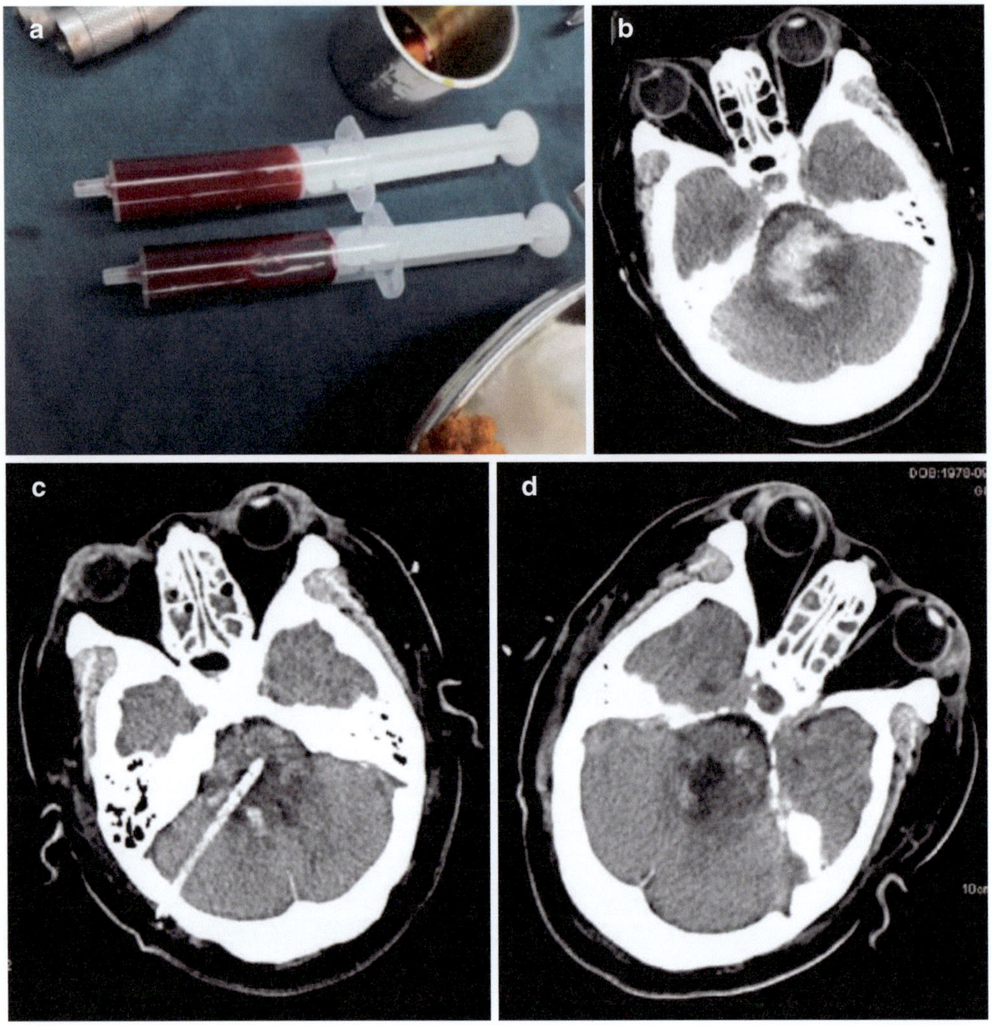

Fig. 14.11 (**a**) A total of 20 mL of hematoma and cerebrospinal fluid mixture was aspirated during the surgery. (**b–d**) Sequential CT images showing the preoperative status, postoperative day 1, and postoperative day 3, indicating a 90% clearance rate of the hematoma

References

1. Neurocritical Care Collaboration Group of the Neurology Branch of the Chinese Medical Association, Neurocritical Care Committee of the Chinese Physicians Association Neurology Branch. Chinese expert consensus on monitoring and treatment of spontaneous large intracerebral hemorrhage. Chin Med J. 2017;97(9):653–60.
2. Fadrus P, Smrcka VT, Svoboda K, et al. Stereotactic evacuation of spontaneous infratentorial hemorrhage with monitoring of intracerebral pressure. Bratislavske Lekadrske Listy. 2004;105(5–6):235.
3. Thiex R, Rohde V, et al. Frame-based and frameless stereotactic hematoma puncture and subsequent fibrinolytic therapy for the treatment of spontaneous intracerebral hemorrhage. J Neurol. 2004;251(12):1443–50.
4. Dun ZP, Zhu SG, et al. Benefits of a frame-based stereotactic surgical planning system for the treatment of spontaneous intracerebral haematomas. J Int Med Res. 2013;41(5):1550–9.
5. Kim MH, Kim EY, et al. Surgical options of hypertensive intracerebral hematoma: stereotactic endoscopic removal versus stereotactic catheter drainage. J Korean Med Sci. 1998;13(5):533–40.

Puncture and Aspiration Evacuation of Brainstem Hemorrhage Via Frameless Stereotactic Brainstem Hematoma

15

Zefeng Wang and Fengqiang Liu

15.1 Overview

Primary brainstem hemorrhage mainly occurs in the pons, accounting for approximately 5%–10% of intracranial hemorrhages [1, 2]. It has a high mortality and morbidity rate compared to other types of stroke, posing a considerable social burden [3, 4]. The onset is rapid, progresses quickly, and often leads to critical conditions, where effective treatment options are limited, and complications in the later stages pose challenges in the treatment of brainstem hemorrhage. The anatomy and function of the brainstem are complex and crucial, and there is still no widespread consensus on the choice between surgical and conservative treatment strategies. Overall, the prognosis is pessimistic, and passive conservative management is often favored [4, 5].

In recent years, minimally invasive techniques such as puncture drainage, aspiration, and endoscopic clearance have been increasingly applied in spontaneous brainstem hemorrhage. Particularly, stereotactic techniques based on precision concepts (including frame-based and frameless techniques) have gained widespread acceptance and have become a hot topic in current research. By accurately designing surgical plans and guiding the puncture, these techniques can safely and effectively evacuate the hematoma, demonstrating significant advantages and gaining increasingly broad applications [6]. Frameless stereotactic (also known as neuro-navigation) technology develops the classical frame-based stereotactic technique. Its advantage lies in the fact that preoperative localization scans do not require the installation of a frame, reducing the inconvenience of patient transportation and avoiding the discomfort of local anesthesia.

Supplementary Information The online version contains supplementary material available at https://doi.org/10.1007/978-981-95-8942-5_15.

Z. Wang · F. Liu (✉)
Department of Neurosurgery, The Second Affiliated Hospital of Zhejiang University School of Medicine, Hangzhou, China

As 90% of brainstem hemorrhages occur in the pons, most can be effectively cleared through a puncture via the middle cerebellar peduncle [1, 3]. The surgery generally uses the Mayfield three-point head fixation system, providing a spacious surgical operating field. Although the positioning accuracy is not as high as frame-based stereotactic techniques, it can meet the hematoma's precise aspiration and clearance requirements. Changing target points and pathways are more convenient than frame-based stereotactic techniques when performing multi-target, multi-channel punctures. This chapter mainly introduces using frameless stereotactic (neuronavigation) surgery to treat brainstem hemorrhage [7, 8].

15.2 Indications and Contraindications

15.2.1 Indications

1. Hematoma located in the midbrain, pons, or extending into the fourth ventricle.
2. Hematoma volume > 5 mL, Type 1 or Type 2 of the "Zhe-Er classification" of Primary Brainstem Hemorrhage, B or C of Type 3 (especially when it is unilaterally and posteriorly located in the brainstem), and clinical GCS score < 12.
3. Patients without a history of hypertension and younger patients should exclude brainstem vascular malformations, cavernous malformations, or aneurysmal bleeding.

15.2.2 Contraindications

1. Brainstem hematoma volume < 3 mL.
2. Clinical GCS score > 12.
3. Secondary brainstem hemorrhage.
4. Patients with signs of brainstem dysfunction, such as bilateral dilated pupils and hypotension.

G. Chen, C. You (eds.), *Surgical Treatment of Primary Brainstem Hemorrhage*, https://doi.org/10.1007/978-981-95-8942-5_15

15.3 Preoperative Preparation and Surgical Instruments

15.3.1 Preoperative Preparation

A routine thin-slice (<2 mm) head CT scan is performed before surgery. The data is transferred to the Brainlab frameless navigation system, and the software (cranial navigation) is activated. The target points and entry points are planned and based on the "Zhe-Er classification" of brainstem hematoma, the surgical pathway, the range of hematoma aspiration, and the depth of drainage tube placement are evaluated. Type 1 and Type 2 hematomas (subtypes A and C) are often approached through the lateral middle cerebellar peduncle approach. For Type 2 (subtype B) and Type 3 hematomas, the lateral middle cerebellar peduncle or the site of rupture at the floor of the fourth ventricle is chosen to access the hematoma cavity.

15.3.2 Surgical Instruments

The surgical instruments include a conventional three-point head fixation system, frameless neuro-navigation system, VarioGuide universal fixation frame, clampable trackball, and navigation probe (Fig. 15.1).

15.4 Surgical Methods, Precautions, and Techniques

15.4.1 Surgical Technique

1. After anesthesia, the patient is placed in the prone position, and the three-point head fixation is applied. The reference frame is fixed, and the navigation camera is adjusted. Surface matching registration is achieved using a laser pen through Z-touch, a non-contact method.
2. Routine disinfection and draping are performed. The VarioGuide universal fixation frame is installed, and the puncture needle tail matches the clampable trackball. Needle tip registration is completed using the navigation system.
3. The scalp incision is made according to preoperative planning. Under direct visualization, the skin is incised, the skull is drilled, and the dura mater and pia mater are opened. Hemostasis is carefully performed at the surgical site.
4. The puncture needle is placed on the VarioGuide frame, and the puncture is performed along the preoperative planned pathway, with real-time monitoring of the navigation image. "Targeted" and "Quantitative" hematoma aspiration is achieved, and a drainage tube is left in place according to preoperative planning (Fig. 15.2, Video 15.1).

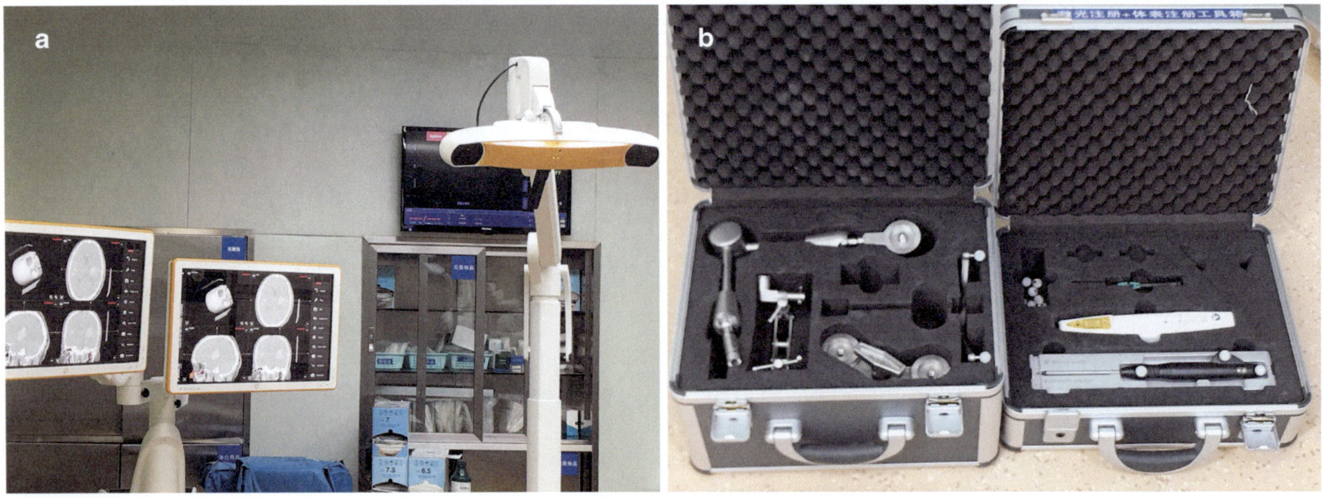

Fig. 15.1 (**a**) Camera and image display monitor; (**b**) instrument accessories, including the VarioGuide universal fixation frame, navigation probe, etc.

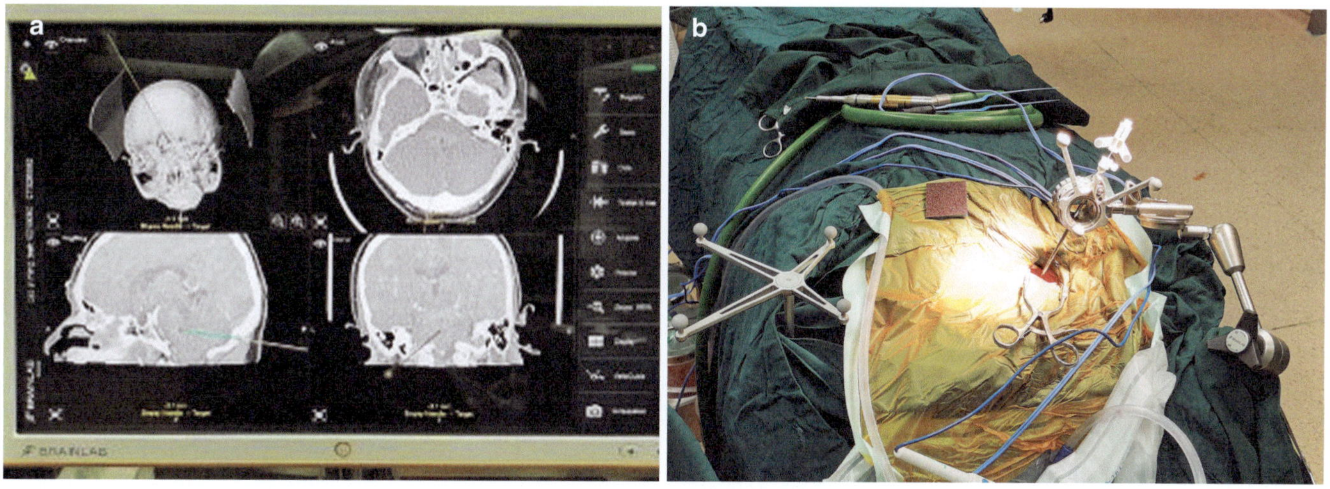

Fig. 15.2 (**a**) Intraoperative operation guided by imaging; (**b**) navigation probe guiding the puncture needle to the target point

15.4.2 Precautions and Techniques

1. Avoiding the transverse sinus and sigmoid sinus as entry points and avoiding important blood vessels, fiber tracts, and nuclei along the puncture pathway.
2. The drainage tube should be placed along the long axis of the hematoma, maximizing the contact area with the hematoma for optimal aspiration and drainage efficiency.

15.5 Postoperative Management and Prevention of Complications

1. Similar to the management of other minimally invasive puncture procedures, blood pressure should be maintained stable during the perioperative period, not exceeding 140/90 mmHg. During anesthesia recovery, avoid severe coughing, continuous sedation, and analgesia. When the drainage tube communicates with the ventricle, it is managed according to the principles related to ventricular drainage.
2. A CT scan should be performed 1 day after surgery or on the same day to determine whether urokinase-assisted drainage should be applied based on the residual hematoma. If the residual volume is less than 3 mL, the drainage tube can be removed within 24 h after surgery.
3. Common surgery-related complications include:
   (a) Rebleeding along the puncture tract or within the hematoma cavity.
   (b) Intracranial infection.
   (c) Obstructive hydrocephalus.
4. Postoperatively, routine admission to the ICU for monitoring and treatment is necessary. During the perioperative period, attention should be paid to analgesia and sedation treatment. After the patient's condition stabilizes, early rehabilitation treatments such as awakening-promoting therapy should be initiated.

15.6 Advantages, Disadvantages, and Lessons Learned

15.6.1 Advantages

1. The frameless navigation system does not require the installation of a stereotactic frame before surgery.
2. Real-time image guidance during the puncture process is more convenient compared to frame-based stereotactic procedures.
3. There are fewer restrictions on patient positioning during the surgery, providing a wider surgical field.
4. Implementing multi-target and multi-channel planning offers more flexibility in changing targets and pathways.

15.6.2 Disadvantages

1. The stability of the guiding frame is not as good as that of frame-based stereotactic systems, requiring smooth and gentle operation during the puncture process.
2. Some navigation products have a cumbersome registration process, and the positioning accuracy and reliability are not as good as frame-based stereotactic systems.
3. The repeatability of preoperative planning and intraoperative referencing is not as good as that of frame-based stereotactic systems.
4. Lack of specialized instruments.

15.6.3 Lessons Learned

Factors affecting prognosis other than hematoma volume include:

1. Age: Older age is associated with higher mortality rates, with a mortality rate over 70% in patients over 70 years old.
2. Medical history: Smoking, alcohol abuse, hypertension, and a history of aspirin use often indicate a poor prognosis.
3. Complications: Preexisting conditions such as coronary artery atherosclerotic heart disease, diabetes, liver or kidney dysfunction, and bronchial asthma suggest a poorer prognosis.
4. Vital signs: Central fever (>39 °C), pulse rate > 120 beats/min, and respiratory rate > 30 breaths/min indicate a poorer prognosis and higher mortality rates.

15.7 Procedure Evaluation and Prospects

Stereotactic puncture and aspiration for the treatment of brainstem hemorrhage allow for early hematoma clearance, shortening the disease course, and achieving decent clinical outcomes. It represents the most promising direction for development. The frameless navigation system has advantages in terms of convenience compared to frame-based systems. However, improvements are still needed in terms of the repeatability and stability of planning/implementation, as well as the development of dedicated instruments.

15.8 Typical Case

15.8.1 Summary of Medical History and Imaging Data

The patient, a male 31 years old, presented with a sudden loss of consciousness for 6 h while playing mahjong. He had a history of untreated hypertension and suffered a left eye globe destructive injury several years ago. On admission, the patient was comatose with a GCS score of 1 + T + 4. The right pupil measured 4 mm with no light reflex, while the left cornea was opaque, and the pupil could not be observed. Tracheal intubation and mechanical ventilation were performed. No pathological signs were elicited. The initial CTA on admission showed no apparent abnormalities (Fig. 15.3).

15.8.2 Procedure and Key Points

1. After obtaining fully informed consent, it was decided to perform a frameless stereotactic puncture and aspiration for the hematoma.
2. The thin-slice sequences from the contrast-enhanced CT scan were imported into the Brainlab navigation workstation for computer simulation and optimization of the puncture pathway. Ultimately, a route through the left paramedian cerebellum was chosen, considering the intraventricular hemorrhage within the fourth ventricle.

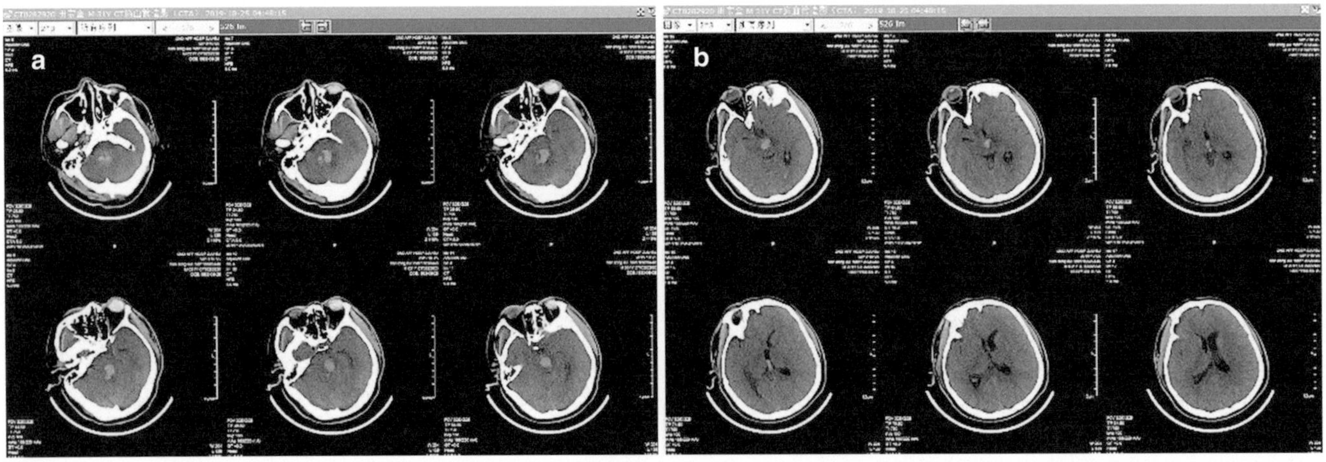

Fig. 15.3 Preoperative CT scan indicating extent of the hematoma

15.8.3 Surgical Procedure

1. The patient was placed in a prone position on the operating table, and the Mayfield three-point fixation head frame was used to secure the patient's head. The localization sphere was then fixed to the head frame. The position of the navigation camera was adjusted to ensure that both the localization sphere and the surgical area were within its field of view.
2. Navigation registration: A non-contact laser scanning probe was used to scan the scalp for surface registration.
3. Preoperative planning was imported, and the entry point on the scalp was identified to guide the scalp incision and drilling.
4. Using the registered trajectory, the hematoma aspiration needle was inserted into the needle probe with a clampable trackball. With the support of the universal bracket and image guidance, the hematoma aspiration needle (4 mm) was placed into the hematoma cavity along the planned pathway, and a "targeted and quantitative" aspiration was performed. Intraoperatively, a total of 12 mL of old blood and bloody cerebrospinal fluid were aspirated (Fig. 15.4).

15.8.4 Preoperative and Postoperative Imaging Comparison

Immediate postoperative CT scan showed satisfactory hematoma clearance (Figs. 15.5 and 15.6).

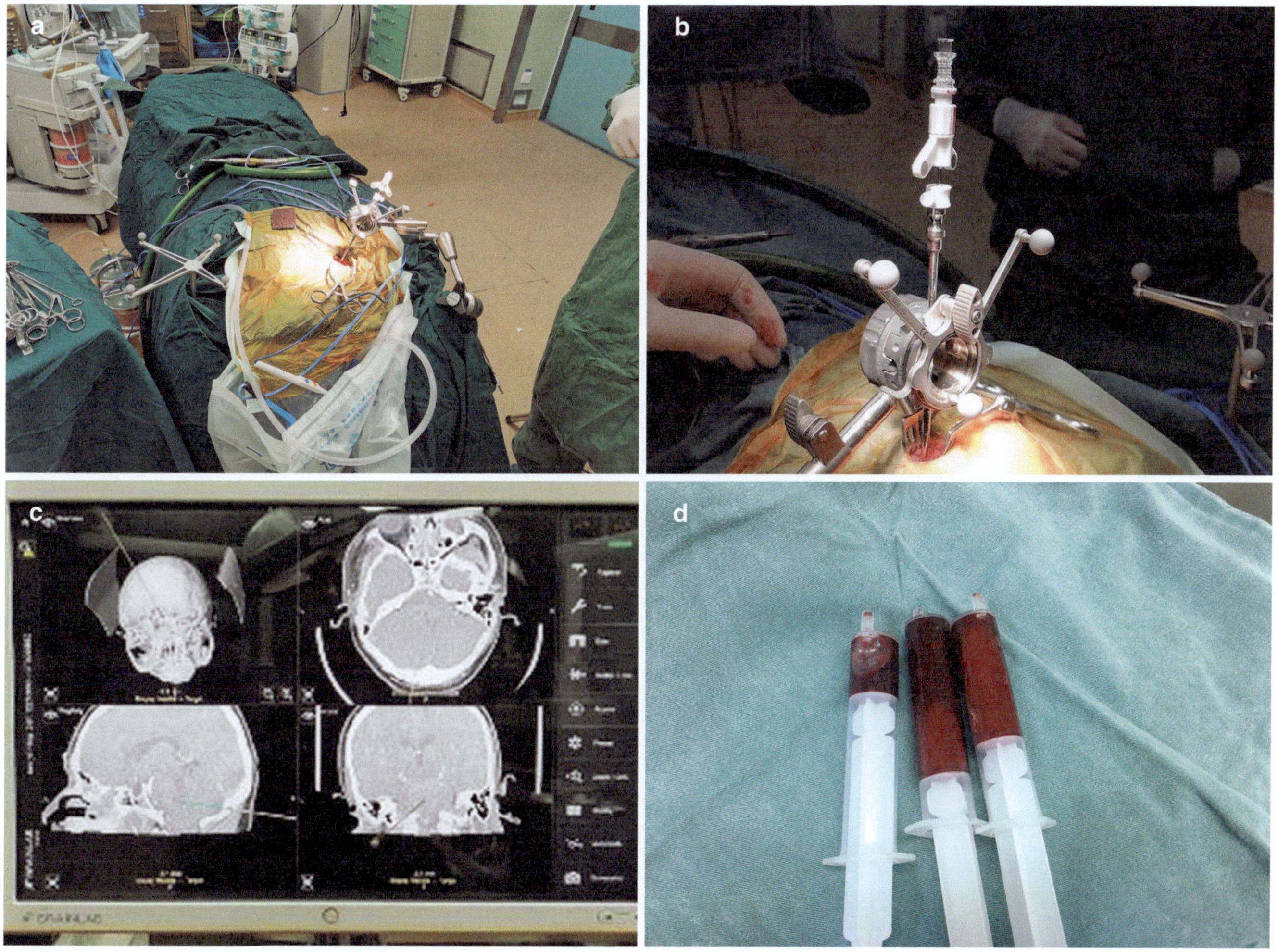

Fig. 15.4 (**a**) Puncture needle reaching the target point; (**b**) navigation probe inserted into the hematoma puncture needle, indicating the position of the needle tip; (**c**) targeted and quantitative aspiration under image guidance; (**d**) hematoma clearance and measurement

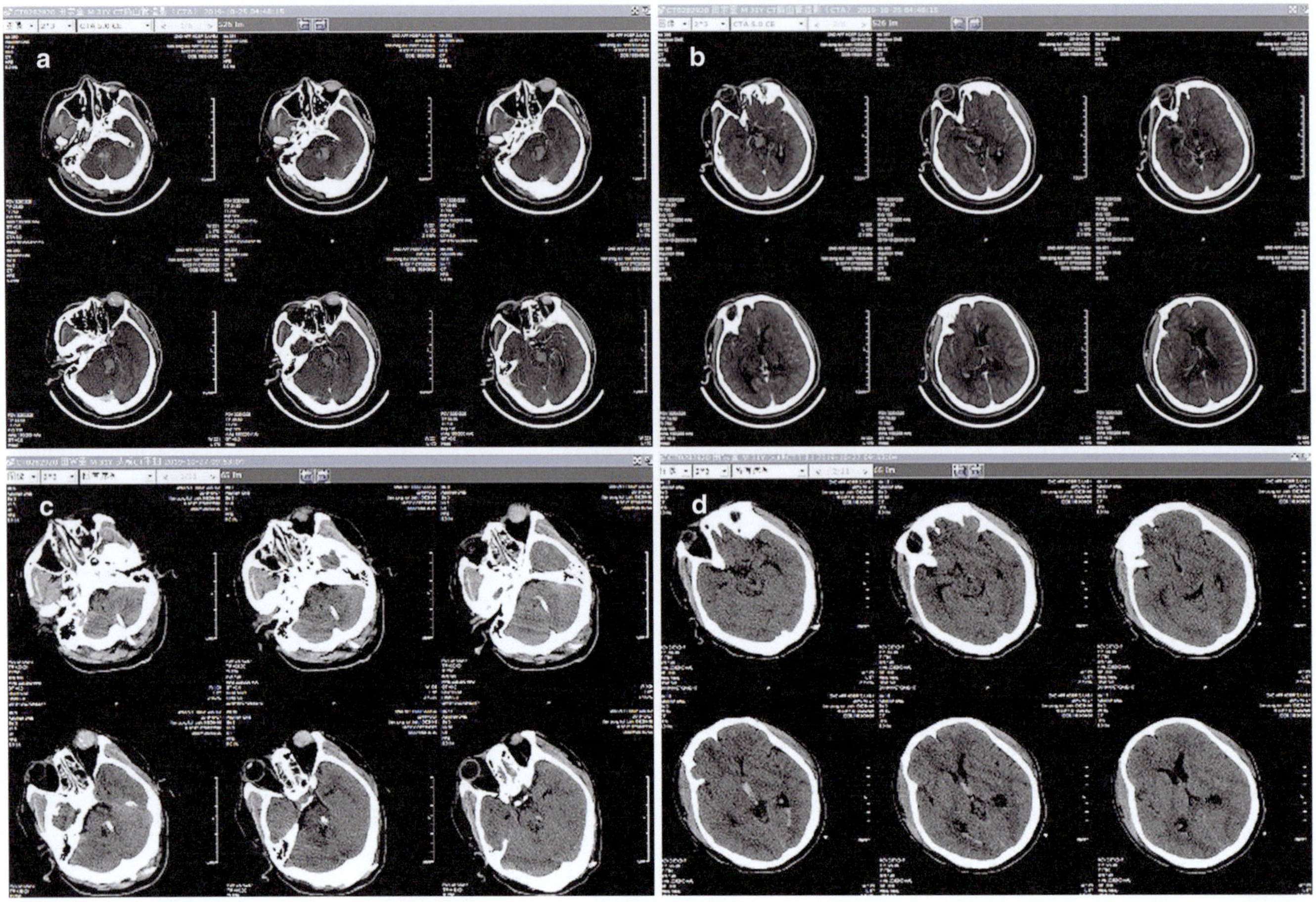

Fig. 15.5 (**a**, **b**) Preoperative volume of the hematoma; (**c**, **d**) postoperative degree of hematoma clearance and position of the drainage tube

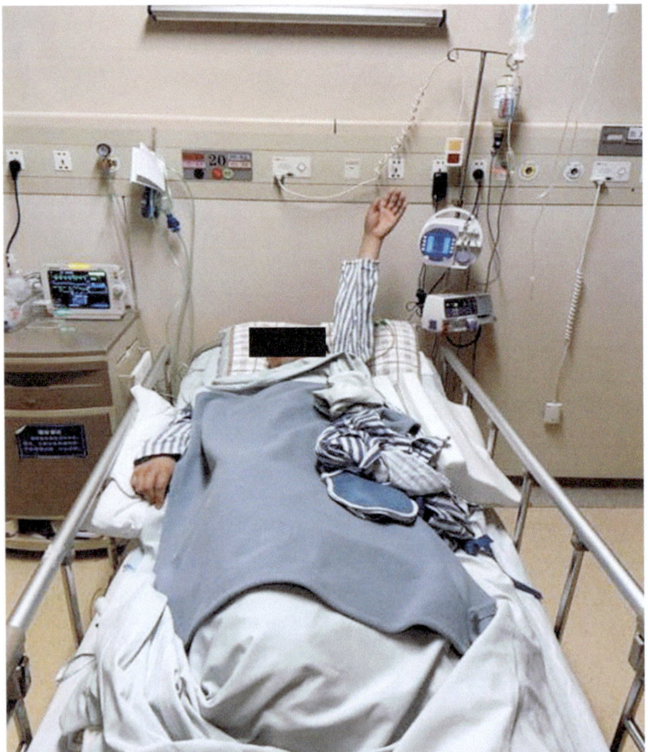

Fig. 15.6 Follow-up video of motor function 2 weeks postoperatively

References

1. Dinsdale HB. Spontaneous hemorrhage in the posterior fossa. A study of primary cerebellar and pontine hemorrhages with observations on their pathogenesis. Arch Neurol. 1964;10:200–17.
2. Freytag E. Fatal hypertensive intracerebralhaematomas: a survey of the pathological anatomy of 393 cases. J Neurol Neurosurg Psychiatry. 1968;31:616–20.
3. Nakajima K. Clinicopathological study of pontine hemorrhage. Stroke. 1983;14:485–93.
4. Balci K, Asil T, Kerimoglu M, et al. Clinical and neuroradiological predictors of mortality in patients with primary pontine hemorrhage. Clin Neurol Neurosurg. 2005;108:36–9.
5. Garnetter S, Roland AN. Primary intracerebral hemorrhage. J Clin Neurosci. 2006;13:511–7.
6. Backlund EO, Holst H. Controlled subtotal evacuation of intracerebral haematomas by stereotactic technique. Surg Neurol. 1978;9(2):99–101.
7. Menon G, Gopalakrishnan CV, Rao BR, et al. A single institution series of cavernomas of the brainstem. J Clin Neurosci. 2011;18:1210–4.
8. Li H, Ju Y, Cai BW, et al. Experience of microsurgical treatment of brainstem cavemomas: report of 37 cases. Neurol India. 2009;57(3):269–73.

16 CT-Guided Bone Marker-Directed Puncture and Aspiration of Brainstem Hematoma

Jinhua Yang, Yuxiong Wang, Shiji Wu, Shiquan Li, and Jieming Li

16.1 Overview

For patients with severe brainstem hemorrhage, it is essential to remove the hematoma as promptly as possible to reduce intracranial pressure and minimize secondary damage to the brainstem tissue. Microscopic hematoma evacuation via craniotomy is a traditional surgical procedure for treating severe brainstem hemorrhage. This technique involves a microscopic craniotomy with neuroendoscopic assistance for hematoma removal [1, 2]. However, these procedures demand a high level of surgical expertise, entail lengthy operation times, involve significant trauma, carry substantial surgical risks, and are costly. As a result, families of patients are often hesitant to pursue this treatment. Consequently, due to technical and resource limitations, most hospitals, both domestically and internationally, have been unable to perform craniotomy with microscopic or endoscopic brainstem hematoma evacuation. As a result, most patients can only receive conservative treatment, which leads to poor prognoses and high mortality rates, presenting a significant challenge in clinical practice [3].

Our relentless pursuit is to develop a technique that not only removes brainstem hemorrhages but also minimizes iatrogenic damage to brain tissue. Therefore, the surgical approach for brainstem hematomas should focus on increasing minimally invasive procedures to improve the quality of life for patients who can be saved. The minimally invasive puncture and aspiration of brainstem hematomas offer several advantages, including a reduction in iatrogenic injuries, lower surgical risks and medical costs, ease of performance and mastery, minimal tissue trauma, rapid hematoma removal, and expedited recovery of neurological function post-surgery. This approach truly embodies the essence of minimally invasive surgery and represents a novel method and concept for treating brainstem hemorrhages with minimal invasion [4, 5]. There are several methods for localizing minimally invasive puncture and aspiration of brainstem hematomas. Currently, various localization techniques are available, including frame-based stereotactic localization and puncture, CT localization combined with bone marker-directed puncture, tetrahedral localization, modified stereotactic localization, 3D printing localization, and navigation localization. Each method has its own advantages and disadvantages; some require expensive medical equipment, while others are complex in their localization processes or have slower localization speeds.

Building on over 10 years of experience in developing the "two-point-three-line-eight-character cross localization" method for the minimally invasive puncture and aspiration of cerebellar hematomas, the Department of Neurosurgery at Gaozhou Chinese Medicine Hospital, affiliated with Guangzhou University of Chinese Medicine, has recently introduced a CT localization technique combined with bone marker-directed puncture using a "three-point-three-line localization" method for the puncturing and aspiration of brainstem hematomas. This innovative technique has been successfully applied in collaboration with several domestic hospitals, treating numerous cases of minimally invasive puncture and aspiration of brainstem hematomas. This chapter focuses on the technical methodology of CT localization combined with bone marker-directed puncture [6].

16.2 Indications and Contraindications

16.2.1 Indications

Currently, there is no unified standard for the indications and surgical criteria for minimally invasive puncture surgery for brainstem hemorrhage, both domestically and internationally.

Supplementary Information The online version contains supplementary material available at https://doi.org/10.1007/978-981-95-8942-5_16.

J. Yang (✉) · Y. Wang · S. Wu · S. Li · J. Li
Department of Neurosurgery, Gaozhou Hospital of Traditional Chinese Medicine Affiliated to Guangzhou University of Chinese Medicine, Gaozhou, China

G. Chen, C. You (eds.), *Surgical Treatment of Primary Brainstem Hemorrhage*, https://doi.org/10.1007/978-981-95-8942-5_16

However, the following conditions are generally deemed appropriate for considering brainstem hematoma puncture surgery:

1. Brainstem hematoma volume > 5 mL.
2. Maximum cross-sectional area of brainstem hemorrhage comprising more than 50% of the same-level brainstem cross-sectional area.
3. The primary location of brainstem hematoma is typically in the pons or midbrain, often exhibiting a lateral bias, relative concentration, and either proximity to the surface or penetration into the ventricle.
4. Patients in a light to deep coma, with a Glasgow Coma Scale (GCS) score of 8 or lower, may present with severe disturbances in vital signs or may not exhibit such disturbances.
5. Patients' families often express a strong desire for surgical intervention, particularly when their financial situation can allow for long-term post-operative rehabilitation.

16.2.2 Contraindications

1. Patients with a brainstem hemorrhage volume ≤ 3 mL, no significant obstruction of the ventricular system, and no impairment of consciousness (i.e., no coma) are not recommended for puncture surgery [7].
2. Patients with large brainstem hemorrhages, significant damage to the vital centers of the brainstem, and bilateral pupils, who have not exhibited no spontaneous breathing for more than 30 min.
3. Patients in extremely poor overall condition who are unable to tolerate puncture hematoma surgery.
4. Patients with severe coagulation abnormalities.
5. Secondary brainstem hemorrhage may occur as a result of anticoagulant treatment, trauma, tumors, bleeding disorders, or other related conditions.
6. Hemorrhage in the medulla oblongata.

16.3 Preoperative Preparation and Surgical Instruments

16.3.1 Preoperative Preparation

Generally, no special preparation is required. For patients with severe brainstem hematomas who are in a deep coma and often exhibit poor respiratory function, immediate tracheal intubation is essential prior to surgery to ensure an open airway. Patients experiencing respiratory failure necessitate mechanical ventilation support. Routine preparation of the scalp area is also important. Rapid preoperative preparations include a thorough assessment of the complete blood count, coagulation time, liver and kidney function, blood glucose levels, electrolytes, bedside electrocardiogram, and any other necessary tests.

16.3.2 Surgical Instruments

Surgical instruments include manual skull drills (Fig. 16.1a, b), electric skull drills (Fig. 16.1c), scalp cones (Fig. 16.1d), rapid skull cones (Fig. 16.1e), and disposable cranial drainage kits (Fig. 16.1f).

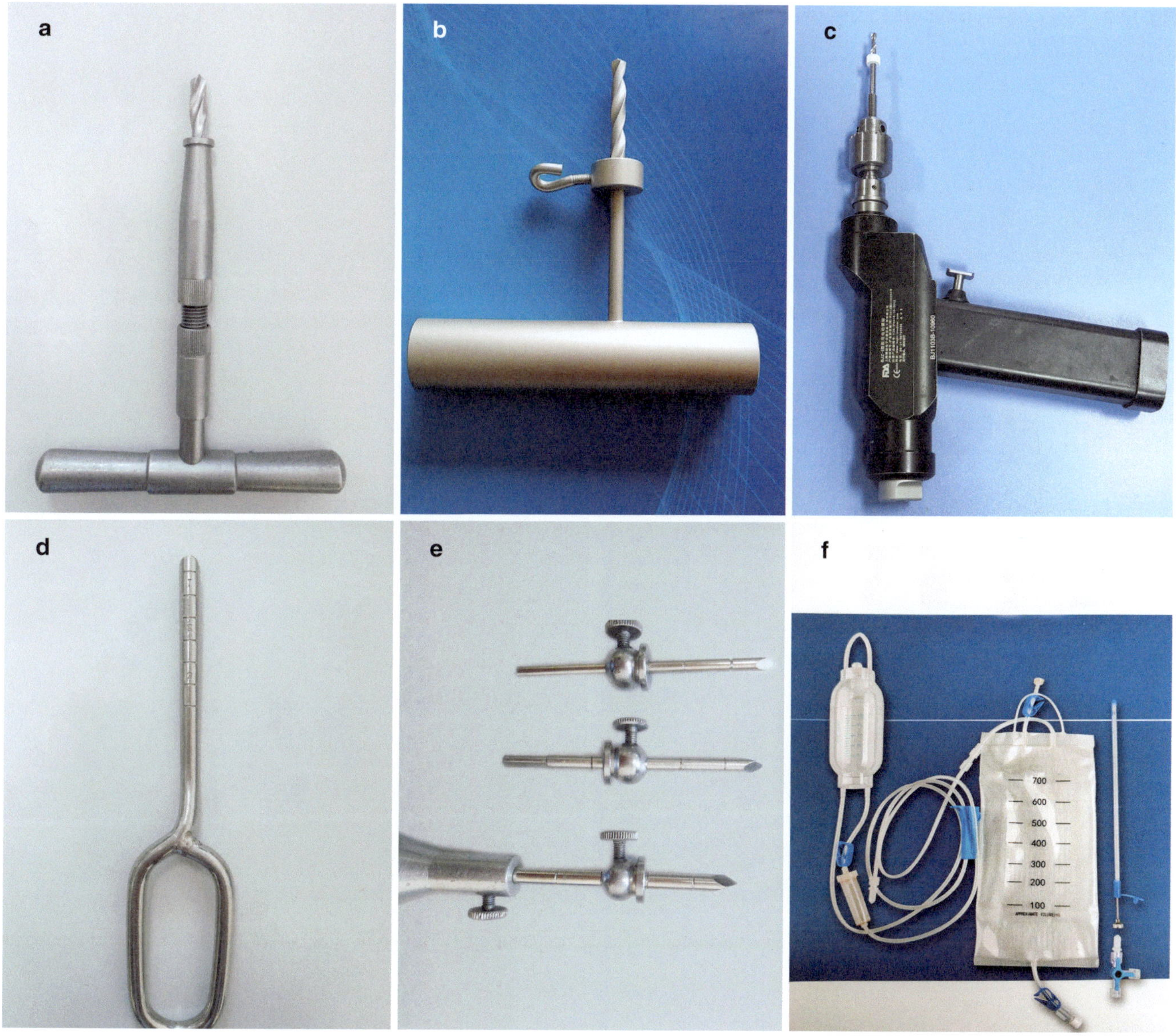

Fig. 16.1 Surgical instruments. (**a**) Manual skull drill; (**b**) manual skull drill; (**c**) electric skull drill; (**d**) scalp cone; (**e**) rapid skull cone; (**f**) disposable cranial drainage kit

16.4 Surgical Methods, Precautions, and Techniques

16.4.1 Surgical Methods

16.4.1.1 Preoperative Positioning

1. Three Points and Three Lines.

   Three points: puncture point at the occiput, center point of the hematoma cavity, and the intersection point of the contralateral zygomatic process of the frontal bone.

   Three lines are drawn: a horizontal line at the occiput (for the directional transverse section), the midline of the brain, and a line extending from the puncture point at the occiput to the intersection point of the contralateral zygomatic process of the frontal bone (the highest point outside and above the orbit) (for the directional longitudinal section).
2. Localization Procedure: Preoperative placement of metal guide wire markers at the right or left occipital puncture point using a CT-guided localization method.

   Place a 5 cm metal guide wire vertically at the middle of the patient's right cerebellum and the left frontal horn, securing them with adhesive tape. Use a colored pen to mark the transverse sinus line on the surface of the scalp at the left or right occipital area (Fig. 16.2).

   After performing a CT scan, identify and select the maximum level of the brainstem hematoma or the designated puncture level for the hematoma. Retrieve the CT

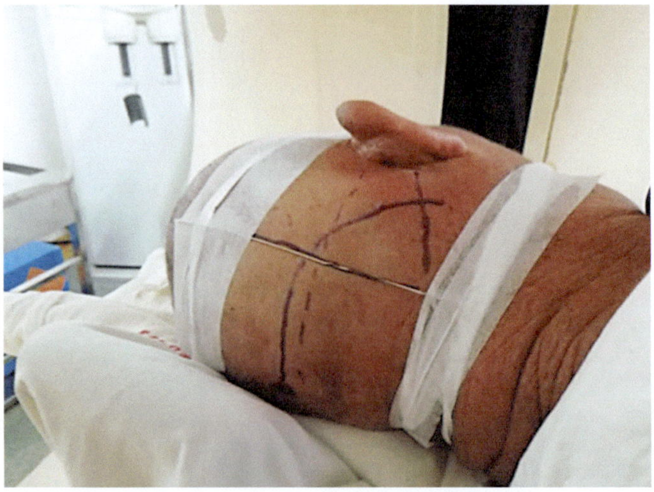

Fig. 16.2 Preoperative placement of metal guide wires in the middle of the cerebellum and the contralateral frontal horn

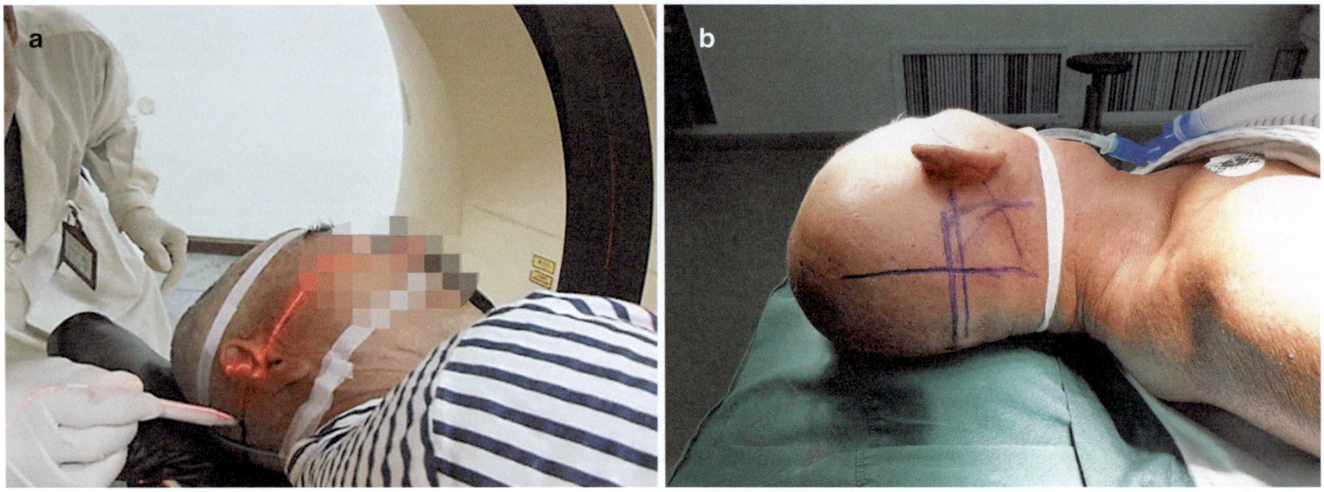

Fig. 16.3 Preoperative localization. (**a**) Drawing the horizontal line at the occiput using CT for positioning; (**b**) marking the transverse sinus and sigmoid sinus

slice thickness data corresponding to that level from the CT machine. With the CT cursor positioned over the patient's head, use a colored pen to draw a horizontal line on the scalp at the puncture site in the occipital area, aligning it with the cursor line (Fig. 16.3a) and mark the locations of the transverse sinus and sigmoid sinus (Fig. 16.3b).

Draw the horizontal line at the occiput (from the external occipital protuberance to the highest point of the ipsilateral zygomatic process of frontal bone—ipsilateral transverse sinus line), draw the midline of the brain (from the midpoint of the nose to the external occipital protuberance), draw the line from the puncture point at the occiput to the intersection point of the contralateral zygomatic process of frontal bone (the highest point outside and above the eye socket), and mark the contralateral frontal area (Fig. 16.4a). Mark the hematoma puncture point (Fig. 16.4b).

On the computer, draw the midline of the brain, draw the directional transverse section and directional longitudinal section (from the puncture point to the intersection point of the contralateral zygomatic process of frontal bone—highest point outside and above the orbit) (Fig. 16.5). Measure the distance from the puncture point to the center point of the hematoma cavity and from the center point of the hematoma cavity to the intersection point of the contralateral zygomatic process of the frontal bone (highest point outside and above the orbit) (Fig. 16.6, Video 16.1).

16.4.1.2 Positioning and Anesthesia

The patient is positioned supine, with a sandbag supporting the shoulder on the side of the puncture, elevated by 15–20°. The head is tilted toward the side of the puncture site. Local infiltrative anesthesia is administered, and the puncture point at the occiput is marked.

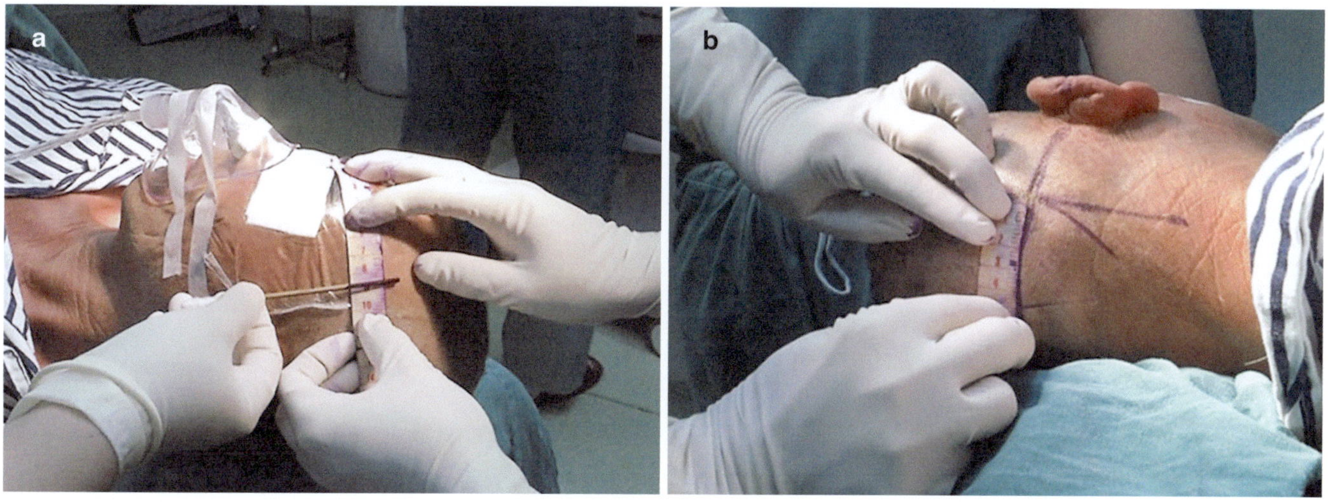

Fig. 16.4 Preoperative localization. (**a**) Drawing the line from the puncture point at the occiput to the intersection point of the contralateral zygomatic process of frontal bone (highest point outside and above the orbit) and marking the contralateral frontal area; (**b**) marking the puncture point at the occiput

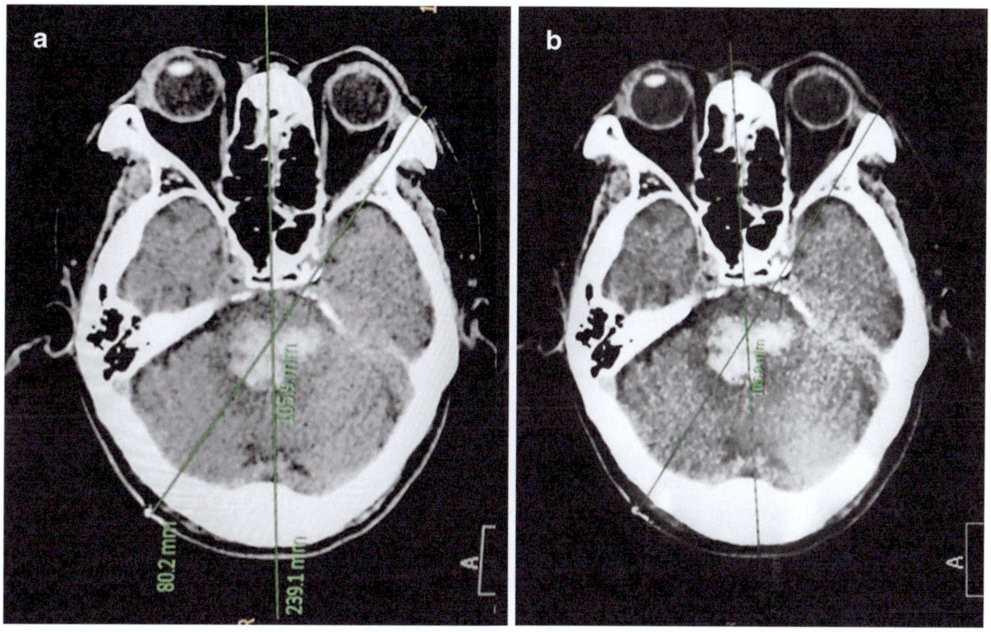

Fig. 16.5 Preoperative localization. (**a**) Drawing the midline of the brain and the directional transverse section from the puncture point to the intersection point of the contralateral zygomatic process of frontal bone (highest point outside and above the orbit) on the computer; (**b**) measuring the distance from the puncture point to the center point of the hematoma cavity and from the center point of the hematoma cavity to the intersection point of the contralateral zygomatic process of frontal bone (highest point outside and above the orbit) on the computer

16.4.1.3 Key Points and Steps of the Surgical Puncture Procedure

1. Routine disinfection and draping should be performed. Administer local infiltrative anesthesia at the preoperative localization point on the occiput using 5 mL of 1% lidocaine.
2. Depending on the degree of ventricular dilation in the patient, perform external drainage on one side of the lateral ventricle using a size F12 external drainage catheter. Position the catheter 4.0–5.0 cm lateral to the midline of the posterior cranial fossa, 1.5 cm below the lower edge of the transverse sinus, and at the preoperative CT localization point on the left or right occiput. Puncture at an angle of 30°. Utilize a high-speed electric cranial drill to penetrate the scalp and occipital bone, or alternatively, employ a scalp cone to pierce the scalp. Subsequently, use a cranial drill cone to penetrate the occipital bone, and rotate the scalp cone to remove bone powder and debris from the orifice in the occipital bone. Finally, employ a rapid cranial cone to puncture the dura mater, which will be indicated by a distinct loss of resistance.
3. During the puncture procedure, the surgeon, guided by an assistant, visually adjusts the puncture point in alignment with the occipital horizontal line (directional transverse section) and the direction of the puncture in relation to the intersection point of the contralateral zygomatic process

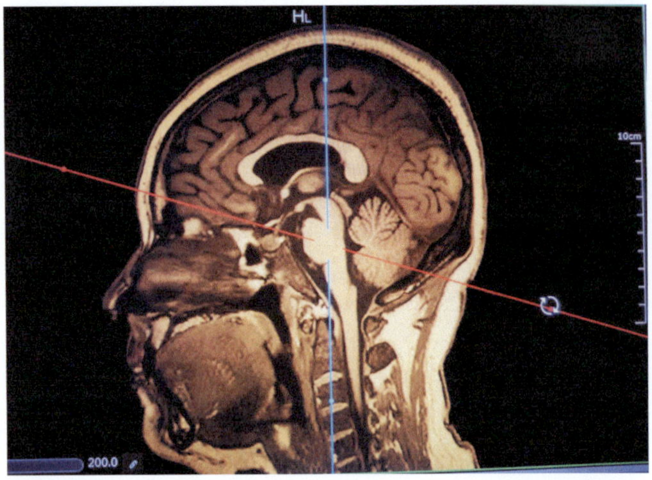

Fig. 16.6 Preoperative localization. Drawing the directional longitudinal section from the puncture point to the intersection point of the contralateral zygomatic process of frontal bone (highest point outside and above the orbit) on the computer

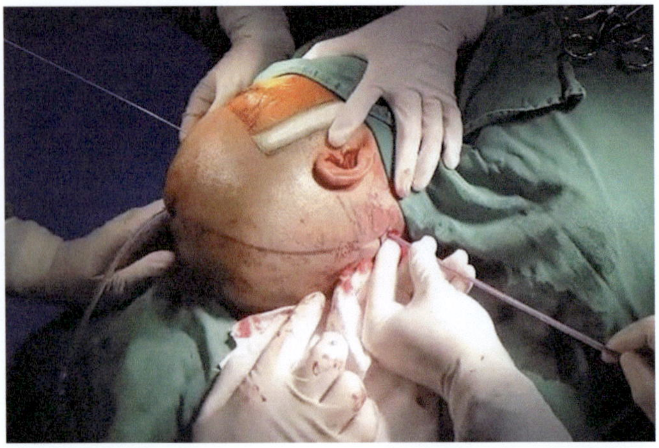

Fig. 16.7 Key points and steps of the surgical puncture procedure. Align the puncture point with the brainstem hematoma and the posterior 1 cm of the contralateral zygomatic process of frontal bone

of the frontal bone (the highest point outside and above the orbit) (directional longitudinal section). To assist the surgeon's visual guidance, a pair of long forceps is employed as a marker at the designated point on the contralateral zygomatic process of the frontal bone clearly indicating the direction of the contralateral puncture. Using a disposable external drainage catheter set (sizes F10–12), align the puncture point on the occiput with the brainstem hematoma and the intersection of the contralateral zygomatic process of the frontal bone (the highest point outside and above the orbit). This alignment should form a "three-point-three-line" configuration along the occipital horizontal line (directional transverse section) and the directional longitudinal section. Next, puncture through the middle part of the infratentorial cerebellum and enter the hematoma cavity in the cisterna ambiens, maintaining a puncture angle of approximately 30° and a depth of 8.5–9.0 cm (Fig. 16.7).

4. After removing the needle core from the drainage catheter, observe the outflow of red-colored cerebrospinal fluid mixed with a small amount of clot. If the pressure is elevated, gradually release the intracranial hematoma through the drainage catheter until the fluid ceases to flow. Utilize a 5 mL syringe to gently aspirate and assess the presence of dark blood clots (Fig. 16.8a). Aspirate approximately 50%–60% of the hematoma volume, depending on the total amount (Fig. 16.8b). Secure the drainage catheter with a 2–0 suture, gently rinse the hematoma cavity with 1–2 mL of 0.9% saline solution through the catheter, and check for any signs of fresh bleeding. Connect a disposable three-way stopcock to a drainage bag externally, and conclude the surgical procedure.

16.4.2 Precautions and Techniques

16.4.2.1 Puncture Precautions

1. Accurate preoperative localization of a brainstem hematoma is crucial, and this localization should be determined by marking the lines during CT scanning.
2. During the puncture, avoid the transverse sinus and the occipital sinus.
3. The direction of the puncture is the foundation of success. The puncture point is located 4.0–5.0 cm lateral to the midline of the brain, 1.5 cm below the lower edge of the transverse sinus. (At this point, there is an approximately 1.0 cm occipital bone horizontal plane. Puncturing beyond this point will encounter the occipital bone slope, which can easily cause serious surgical complications such as respiratory arrest by sliding downward into the medulla.) Direct the puncture towards the hematoma cavity and the contralateral zygomatic process of frontal bone (highest point outside and above the orbit) through the cerebellum, at an angle of approximately 30°, with a depth of 8.5–9.0 cm [8].
4. The location of the puncture into the hematoma plays a crucial role in the prognosis and should not extend into the medulla.
5. The optimal timing for surgery is within 24 h of onset. For patients already experiencing respiratory impairment, puncture is best performed 4–6 h after the onset of symptoms.
6. During the aspiration of the hematoma, closely monitor changes in the patient's vital signs, particularly respiration and heart rate.

16.4.2.2 Puncture Techniques

1. Puncture Site: Select the central region of the infratentorial cerebellum as the entry point for the puncture.

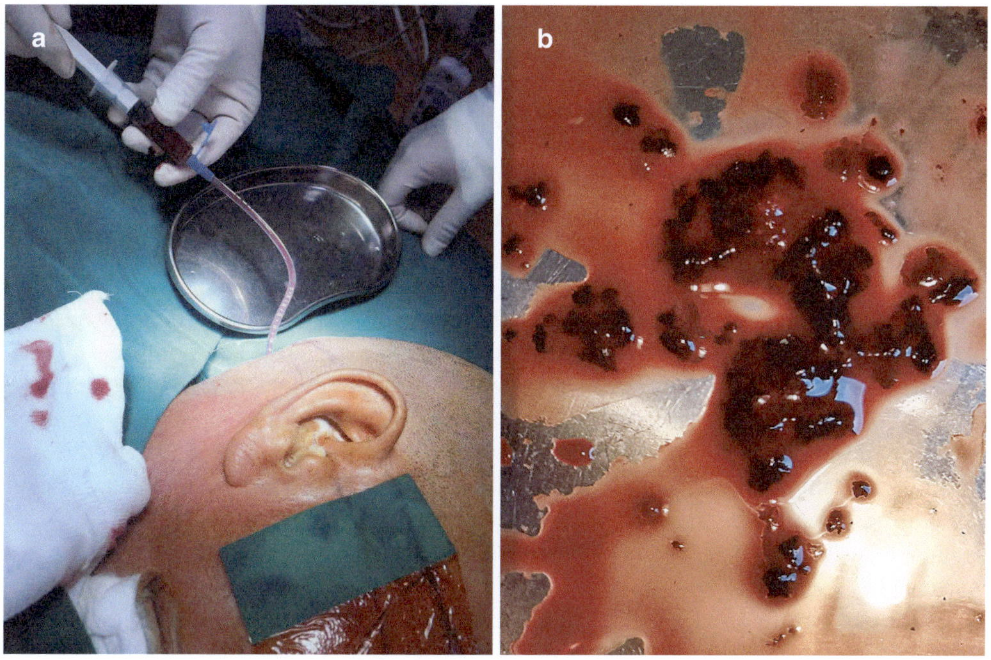

Fig. 16.8 Key points and steps of the surgical puncture procedure. (**a**) Gently aspirate using a 5 mL syringe and observe the presence of dark black blood; (**b**) aspiration volume is 50%–60% of hematoma volume

2. Puncture Direction: Choose the direction through the cerebellum towards the hematoma cavity and the contralateral zygomatic process of the frontal bone (highest point outside and above the orbit).
3. The puncture depth should be 8.5–9.0 cm.
4. The aspiration of the hematoma should be performed slowly, gently, and with minimal force. Utilize a 2 or 5 mL syringe to prevent excessive negative pressure, which may lead to bleeding [9, 10].
5. The amount of hematoma aspirated during the procedure: Aspirating approximately 50% of the brainstem hemorrhage during the initial attempt is sufficient. It is not necessary to remove the majority or all of the hematoma in a single attempt to prevent re-bleeding.

16.5 Postoperative Care and Prevention of Complications

16.5.1 Postoperative Care

1. Transfer the patient to the intensive care unit for monitoring and treatment.
2. For patients with external ventricular drainage, the drainage bag should be elevated by 15–20 cm (measured from the level of the lateral ventricle catheter).
3. Use broad-spectrum antibiotics to prevent infection.

16.5.2 Causes, Prevention, and Treatment of Postoperative Complications

16.5.2.1 Pulmonary Infection

The most common complication postoperatively in brainstem hemorrhage.

16.5.2.1.1 Causes

Brainstem hemorrhage impacts the respiratory center, rendering patients susceptible to respiratory arrest or a diminished cough reflex. Interventions such as tracheal intubation, tracheostomy, and assisted ventilation may also increase the risk of pulmonary infection.

Comatose patients exhibit diminished coughing and sputum clearance capabilities, rendering them more vulnerable to pulmonary infections.

16.5.2.1.2 Prevention and Treatment

Postoperatively, patients should receive enhanced basic care, including turning and back patting, to facilitate sputum clearance.

Patients who are not on a ventilator are advised to be positioned with elevated headrests or in a semi-upright position early on to enhance respiratory mobility.

Patients exhibiting symptoms of infection should undergo early sputum culture and drug sensitivity testing (multiple sputum samples), and sensitive antibiotics should be selected based on the results of drug sensitivity testing. (Patients who undergo tracheotomy in the intensive care unit are at risk of infection with *Pseudomonas aeruginosa, Klebsiella pneumoniae, Escherichia coli, Acinetobacter baumannii,* and others.)

16.5.2.2 Intractable Hiccup and Reflux

16.5.2.2.1 Causes

Brainstem hemorrhage causes damage to the reticular formation and nuclei within the brainstem, impacting the medullary respiratory center, the hiccup center, and the function of the medial longitudinal fasciculus. This damage stimulates the vagus nerve and the phrenic nerve, resulting in intractable hiccups and gastroesophageal reflux. These symptoms may be triggered by factors such as upper gastrointestinal bleeding, gastric distension, or spasms [11].

Excessive use of diuretics can lead to electrolyte imbalances and increased excitability of the vagus and phrenic nerves, resulting in intractable hiccups and reflux.

16.5.2.2.2 Prevention and Treatment

Acupuncture, physiotherapy, and medication injections, such as chlorpromazine, can be used to treat hiccups.

Semi-upright positions during meals and abdominal massage for 20 min in 30 min before meals and 1 h after meals can promote gastrointestinal motility to aid digestion.

Correct electrolyte imbalances, and insert a gastric tube for continuous gastrointestinal decompression in patients with gastric dilation.

16.5.2.3 Stress Ulcer Bleeding in the Digestive Tract

16.5.2.3.1 Causes

Brainstem hemorrhage and cerebral edema can lead to excessive gastric acid secretion due to neuroendocrine disorders, resulting in stress-related gastrointestinal bleeding, manifested as widespread bleeding of the gastrointestinal mucosa.

16.5.2.3.2 Prevention and Treatment

In the event of stress ulcer bleeding in the digestive tract, a gastric tube should be performed to relieve gastrointestinal pressure.

In severe cases, fasting is recommended.

Adrenaline (4–8 mg) and Yunnan Baiyao (1 bottle) in 100 mL of ice-cold saline, administered in two doses via a gastric tube and retained for 30 min, along with intravenous infusion of omeprazole sodium 40 mg once a day for 3–7 days.

16.5.2.4 Hemorrhage at the Puncture Site and Rebleeding

16.5.2.4.1 Causes

Hemorrhage occurs due to vascular injury during the puncture or at the edge of the hematoma.

Rebleeding is often caused by high postoperative blood pressure. Factors such as excessive aspiration volume, excessive suction force, and rapid aspiration during surgery can lead to rebleeding. After a large amount of hematoma is aspirated, negative pressure may be generated within the hematoma cavity, disrupting the intracranial pressure balance formed in the early stages of bleeding, relieving the pressure compressed blood vessels, the subsequent destruction of microthrombus can cause rebleeding [12].

16.5.2.4.2 Prevention and Treatment

During the initial aspiration of the hematoma, it is advisable to avoid excessive speed and volume, and there is no need to completely clear the hematoma in one go.

Slow catheter insertion and minimizing rapid aspiration of the hematoma should be practiced during the puncture procedure.

Emergency hemostasis, even changing surgery mode, is necessary when the aspirated volume exceeds the preoperative calculated amount, and there are changes in the pupil on the operative side, accompanied by altered consciousness and worsening symptoms.

After urokinase thrombolysis, the release of vascular compression may lead to rebleeding.

16.5.2.5 Multi-organ Embolism, Joint Stiffness, and Muscle Atrophy

16.5.2.5.1 Causes

Coma and bed rest after brainstem hemorrhage make patients prone to lower limb venous thrombosis, which can lead to limb swelling and potentially progress to pulmonary embolism, resulting in sudden, short-term death. Prolonged coma can lead to joint stiffness and disuse muscle atrophy, causing joint pain and even dislocation after activity.

16.5.2.5.2 Prevention and Treatment

Comatose patients may undergo hyperbaric oxygen therapy and pharmacological treatments to promote awakening, nourish nerves, and improve brain metabolism.

During the recovery period, active functional exercise, traditional Chinese medicine, and rehabilitation therapy, especially exercises to strengthen the muscles of the neck, back, and limbs with extension and flexion activities of joints, should be emphasized.

16.5.2.6 Electrolyte Imbalance, Anemia, and Malnutrition

16.5.2.6.1 Causes

Dehydration during the acute phase can lead to hyponatremia and hypokalemia. Severe coma can lead to hypernatremia. Anemia and malnutrition may occur in the recovery phase due to reduced food intake and weakened digestive absorption.

16.5.2.6.2 Prevention and Treatment

Monitor electrolyte changes, correct electrolyte imbalances in a timely manner, improve feeding, and pay attention to nutritional supplementation.

16.5.2.7 High Fever and Diabetes Insipidus

16.5.2.7.1 Causes

Early-stage damage to the temperature regulation center and hypothalamic damage. In the middle and later stages, attention should be paid to infectious fever.

16.5.2.7.2 Prevention and Treatment

Treatments such as ice blankets and sub-hypothermia can be used.

Desmopressin may be used in the treatment of diabetes insipidus when necessary, with careful attention to preventing electrolyte imbalances.

16.5.2.8 Intracranial Infection

16.5.2.8.1 Causes

Improper operation and prolonged drainage.

16.5.2.8.2 Prevention and Treatment

Strictly adhere to aseptic procedures, strengthen liquefaction drainage, and timely removal of the drainage tube for brainstem hematoma.

16.6 Advantages, Disadvantages, and Lessons Learned

16.6.1 Advantages

1. This method does not require expensive medical positioning equipment, enabling more primary hospitals to treat severe brainstem hematoma patients according to local conditions.
2. CT localization combined with bone landmark-guided puncture and aspiration of brainstem hematoma offers a simple procedure with high accuracy.
3. The surgical operation is simple, convenient, easy to master, with minimal tissue trauma, and quick removal of the hematoma.
4. It is cost-effective and has low expenses.
5. The surgical trauma is minimal, and postoperative neurological function recovers quickly.

16.6.2 Disadvantages

1. Patients need to be transported to the CT room for scanning to assist with localization, which can be inconvenient for comatose patients during the examination process.
2. The puncture procedure requires the involvement of 2–3 physicians working together.
3. To achieve a more accurate puncture, the physician's visual estimation is needed to guide the puncture plane.

16.6.3 Lessons Learned

1. Preoperative localization should be marked under the guidance of the CT machine's laser positioning line, and the surgical operation should be performed in the operating room.
2. The puncture direction should be well understood, including the horizontal plane formed by the line connecting the external occipital protuberance to the highest point of the ipsilateral zygomatic process of the frontal bone and the coronal section formed by the intersection of the puncture point on the occiput and the contralateral zygomatic process of the frontal bone (the highest point above the orbit). Master the three points: from the puncture point on the occiput to the midpoint of the brainstem hematoma cavity, from the midpoint of the hematoma cavity to the puncture point on the contralateral zygomatic process of the frontal bone, forming a line in a three-point plane [13].
3. It is essential to avoid the transverse sinus (puncture should be performed 1.5 cm below the transverse sinus).
4. The medulla must not be punctured.

16.7 Procedure Evaluation and Prospects

16.7.1 Procedure Evaluation

The advantages of CT localization combined with bone landmark-guided puncture and aspiration of brainstem hematoma through the transcerebellar "three-point-three-line" techniques are as follows: This method utilizes CT guidance and bone landmarks for puncture, providing a scientific, accurate, and practical approach. It offers simplicity, ease of learning and mastery, low medical costs, and high repeatability. Except for a CT machine, there is no need for expensive medical positioning equipment, significantly reducing healthcare expenses. This method is particularly suitable for treating critically ill patients with brainstem hematomas in primary hospitals, facilitating improved rescue success rates in clinical emergencies [14].

16.7.2 Prospects

With the continuous innovation and advancement of minimally invasive neurosurgical techniques, the number of hospitals performing puncture treatment for severe brainstem hematoma and the number of patients receiving such treatment are increasing. The scope of indications and surgical criteria is expanding, leading to better treatment outcomes. More patients with severe brainstem hematomas will benefit from this technique. The future prospects for development are vast, as minimally invasive puncture treatment for severe brainstem hematomas aligns with the trend of scientific development. However, there is still a long way to go despite the heavy responsibility.

16.8 Typical Case

16.8.1 Brief Medical History and Radiological Data

Patient, a 49-year-old male, presented to a local hospital's emergency department on December 19, 2017, with a sudden onset of altered consciousness accompanied by projectile vomiting for 12 h. The diagnosis was brainstem hemorrhage, and urgent tracheal intubation and mechanical ventilation were performed. Due to the large volume of brainstem hemorrhage and critical condition, the patient was later transferred to our hospital. Upon admission, the patient had a body temperature of 38.4 °C, a pulse rate of 89 beats per minute, a respiratory rate of 4–5 breaths per minute (assisted by a ventilator), and a blood pressure of 201/115 mmHg. The patient was deeply comatose with GCS 4, bilateral pupils were constricted with a diameter of approximately 1 mm, and there was no light reflex. Auscultation revealed minimal moist rales in both lungs. The muscle strength of the left limbs was grade 0, while the right limbs exhibited painful extension with muscle strength at grade 1. The bilateral tendon reflexes were diminished, and the bilateral Babinski sign was positive. A head CT scan showed a brainstem hemorrhage measuring 34.38 mm × 25.38 mm with a volume of 9 mL (Fig. 16.9). The patient's blood glucose level was 7.4 mmol/L, and blood routine test showed leukocytosis. The admission diagnoses were the following: (1) Severe brainstem hemorrhage; (2) Grade III hypertension (extremely high-risk group).

The patient had a history of hypertension for 10 years but did not regularly monitor their blood pressure or take medication to control it.

16.8.2 Surgical Procedure and Key Points

After admission, rapid preoperative preparation was conducted, and informed consent was obtained from the patient's family for the surgery. Under assisted ventilation, a head CT scan was performed for localization. The level with the largest extent of brainstem hematoma was selected as the punc-

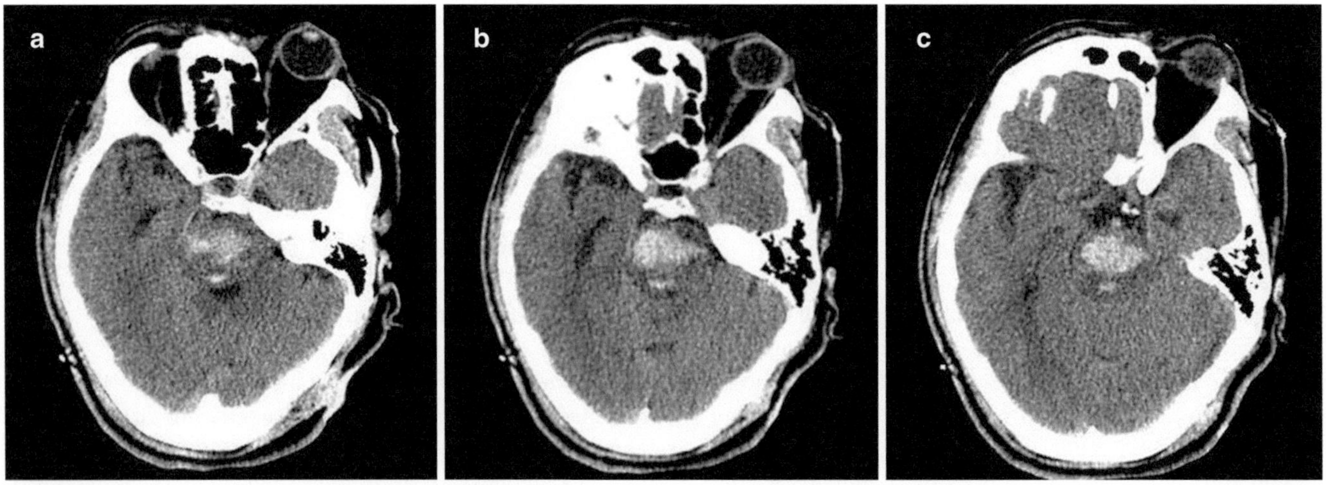

Fig. 16.9 Preoperative head CT scan. The preoperative head CT scan revealed a brainstem hematoma measuring 34.97 mm × 26.38 mm with a volume of 9 mL

ture level. A colored pen was used to mark a horizontal line at the occipital region, the midline of the brain, and the puncture point. The puncture direction and depth were marked on the computer. A disposable external drainage catheter (F12) was inserted using the cranial external drainage kit. The puncture was performed at the right occipital level, aligning with the brainstem hematoma and the intersection of the contralateral zygomatic process of the frontal bone (the highest point above the orbit). The catheter passed through the cerebellum into the cisterna ambiens and reached the hematoma cavity in the brainstem. Approximately 5 mL of the dark blood clot was aspirated (Fig. 16.10), and the drainage catheter was left in place within the hematoma cavity. A three-way stopcock and a disposable drainage bag were connected to ensure continuous drainage of residual blood. The surgery lasted for 30 min, and the patient's vital signs remained stable throughout the procedure [15].

16.8.3 Postoperative Treatment and Imaging Changes Comparison

A follow-up cranial CT scan was performed 12 h after the puncture procedure, revealing that the puncture catheter was located at the center of the brainstem hematoma cavity (Fig. 16.11a). Most of the brainstem hematoma had been cleared (Fig. 16.11b). On postoperative day 3, a subsequent CT scan showed that the brainstem hematoma had been mostly cleared (Fig. 16.12a, b). The brainstem drainage tube was removed the following day, and on postoperative day 3, a tracheostomy was performed. By postoperative day 7, there was a significant improvement in voluntary respiratory strength and cough reflex. The patient was able to open eyes upon stimulation, with both pupils showing sensitivity to light. Eye movement was observed, and the patient was weaned off the ventilator.

At postoperative day 15, there was localized pain response, and limb muscle strength was graded as II–

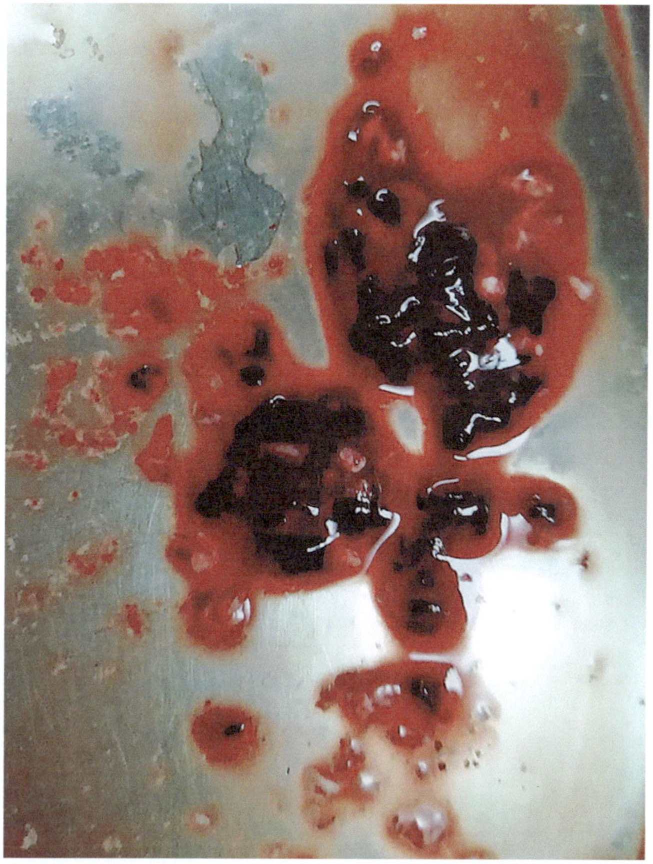

Fig. 16.10 Intraoperative blood clot. Intraoperatively extracted dark blood clot, measuring 5 mL

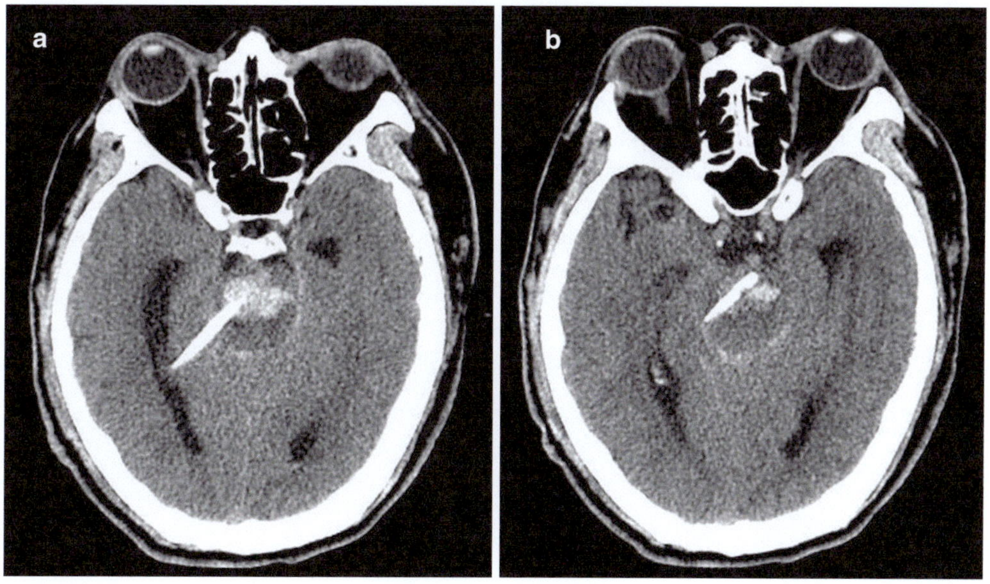

Fig. 16.11 Postoperative 12-h cranial CT scan. (**a**) Postoperative 12-h follow-up cranial CT scan showing the puncture drainage tube located at the center of the brainstem hematoma cavity. (**b**) The brainstem hematoma has been mostly cleared

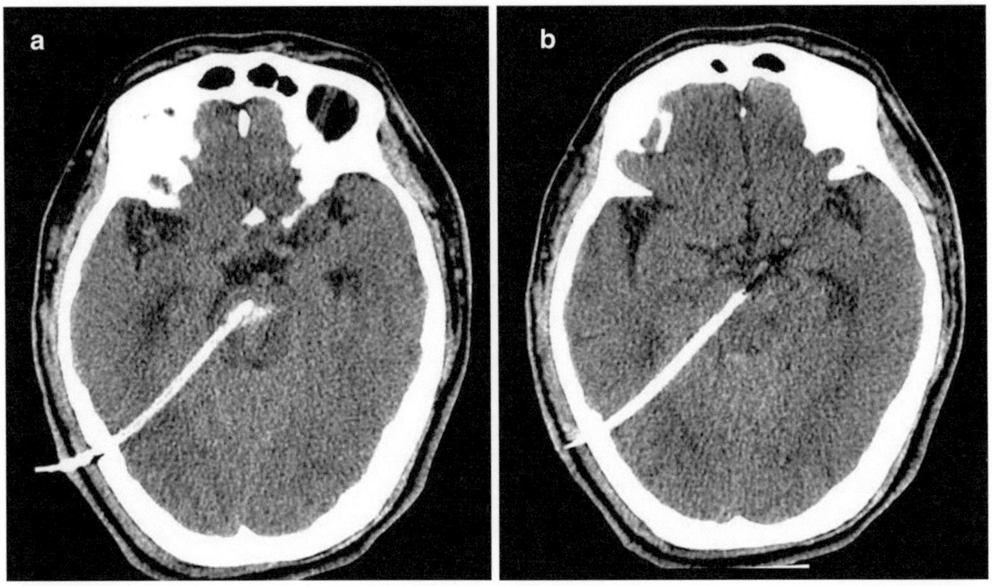

Fig. 16.12 Postoperative 3-day cranial CT scan. Postoperative 3-day follow-up cranial CT scan showing the brainstem hematoma has been essentially cleared. (**a**) Postoperative 3-day cranial CT scan. (**b**) Postoperative 3-day follow-up cranial CT scan showing the brainstem hematoma has been essentially cleared

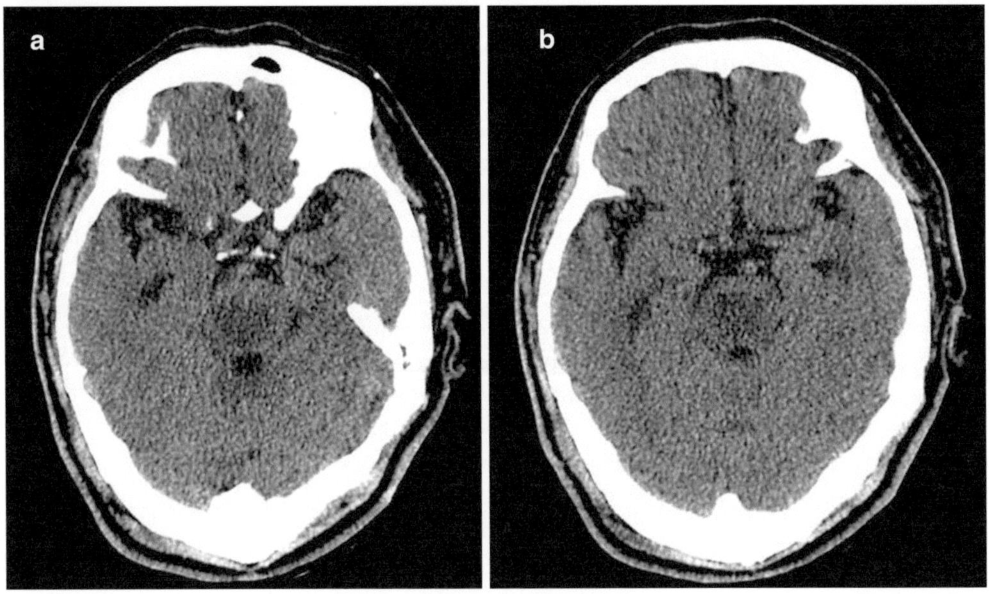

Fig. 16.13 Postoperative 1-month cranial CT scan. Postoperative 1-month follow-up cranial CT scan revealing slight residual edema in the brainstem. (**a**) Postoperative 1-month cranial CT scan. (**b**) Postoperative 1-month follow-up cranial CT scan revealing slight residual edema in the brainstem

III. The patient received treatment including hyperbaric oxygen therapy, traditional Chinese medicine, and rehabilitation therapy. One month postoperatively, a follow-up cranial CT scan revealed a slight residual edema in the brainstem (Fig. 16.13a, b). At 3 months postoperative, a CT scan showed a small liquefaction area in the brainstem (Fig. 16.14a, b). At 6 months postoperative, a follow-up cranial CT scan indicated the absorption and disappearance of both brainstem edema and liquefaction (Fig. 16.15a, b). Nine months postoperatively, a cranial MRI was performed, which showed no abnormalities in the brainstem or other brain tissues. The brainstem had recovered well (Figs. 16.16a, b, 16.17, 16.18, 16.19, 16.20 and 16.21).

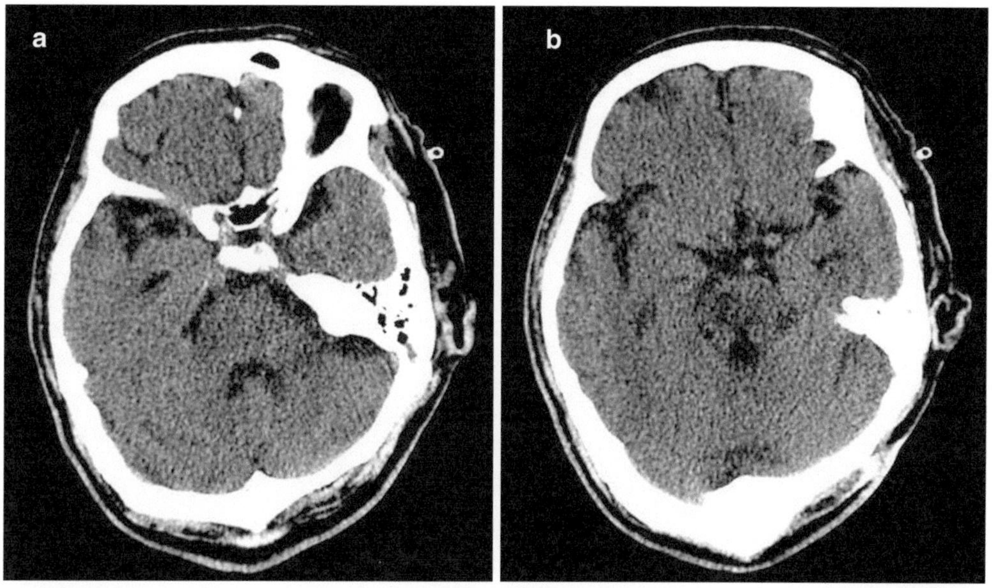

Fig. 16.14 Postoperative 3-month cranial CT scan. Postoperative 3-month cranial CT scan demonstrating a small liquefaction area in the brainstem. (**a**) Postoperative 3-month cranial CT scan. (**b**) Postoperative 3-month cranial CT scan demonstrating a small liquefaction area in the brainstem

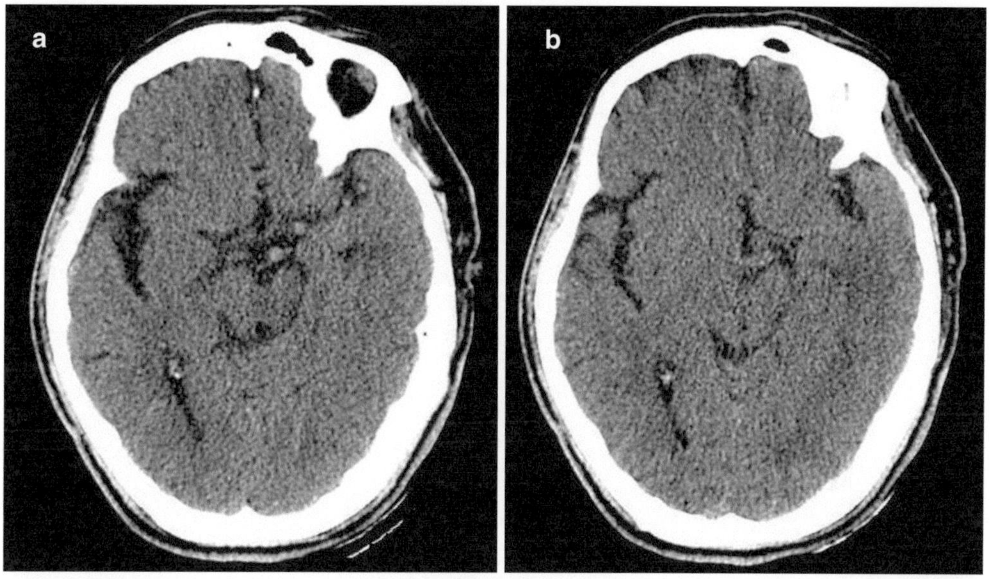

Fig. 16.15 Postoperative 6-month cranial CT scan. Postoperative 6-month follow-up cranial CT scan indicating the absorption and disappearance of both brainstem edema and liquefaction. (**a**) Postoperative 6-month cranial CT scan. (**b**) Postoperative 6-month follow-up cranial CT scan indicating the absorption and disappearance of both brainstem edema and liquefaction

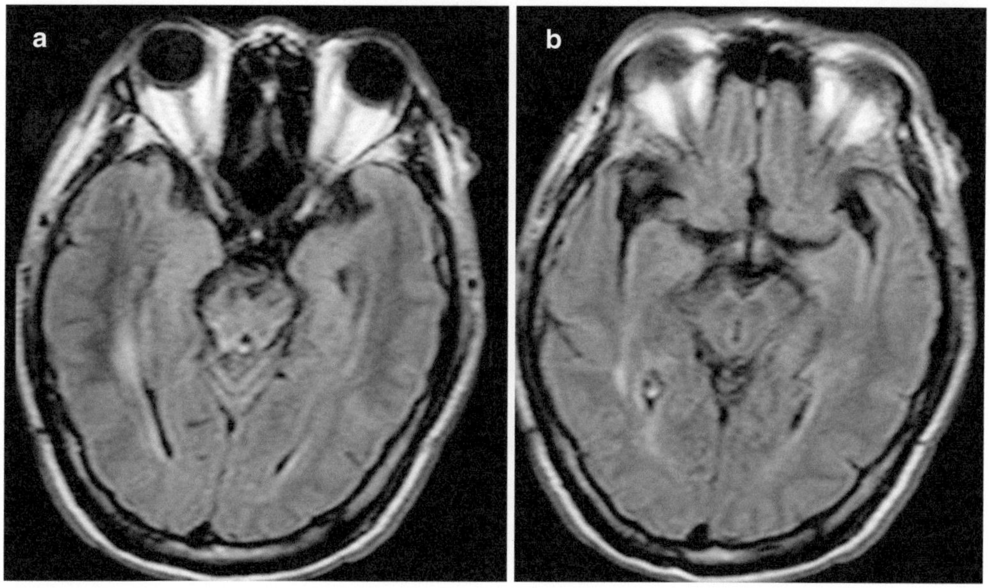

Fig. 16.16 Postoperative 9-month cranial MRI scan. Postoperative 9-month cranial MRI scan showing no abnormalities in the brainstem or other brain tissues. The brainstem has recovered well. (**a**) Postoperative 9-month cranial MRI scan. (**b**) Postoperative 9-month cranial MRI scan showing no abnormalities in the brainstem or other brain tissues. The brainstem has recovered well

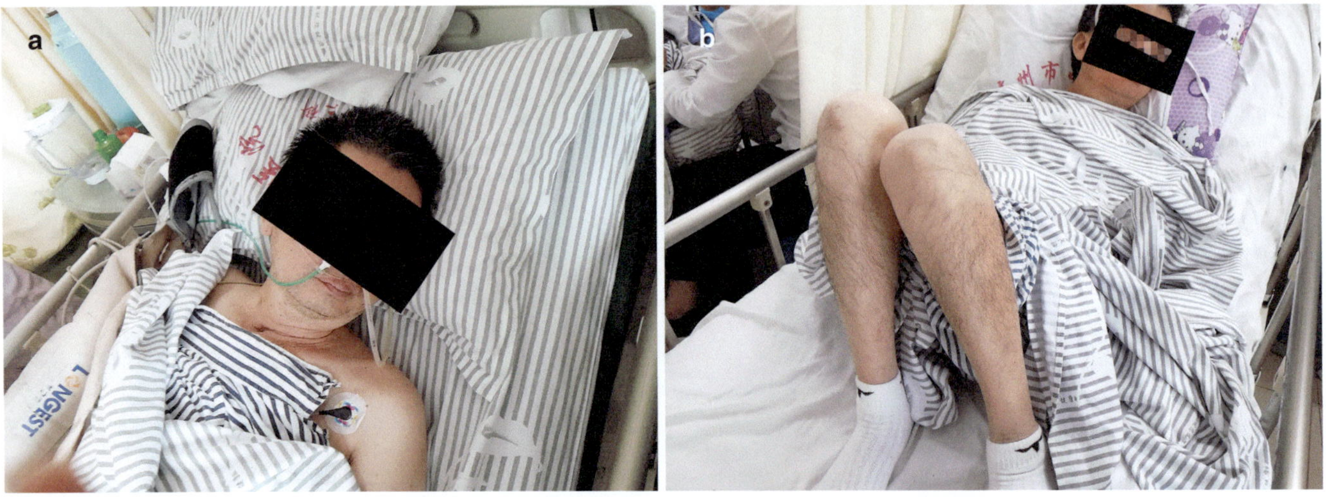

Fig. 16.17 Patient's condition at 1 month postoperatively. (**a**) The patient was conscious and alert 1 month after surgery, able to respond appropriately. (**b**) The patient's limbs were able to move and flex at 1 month postoperatively

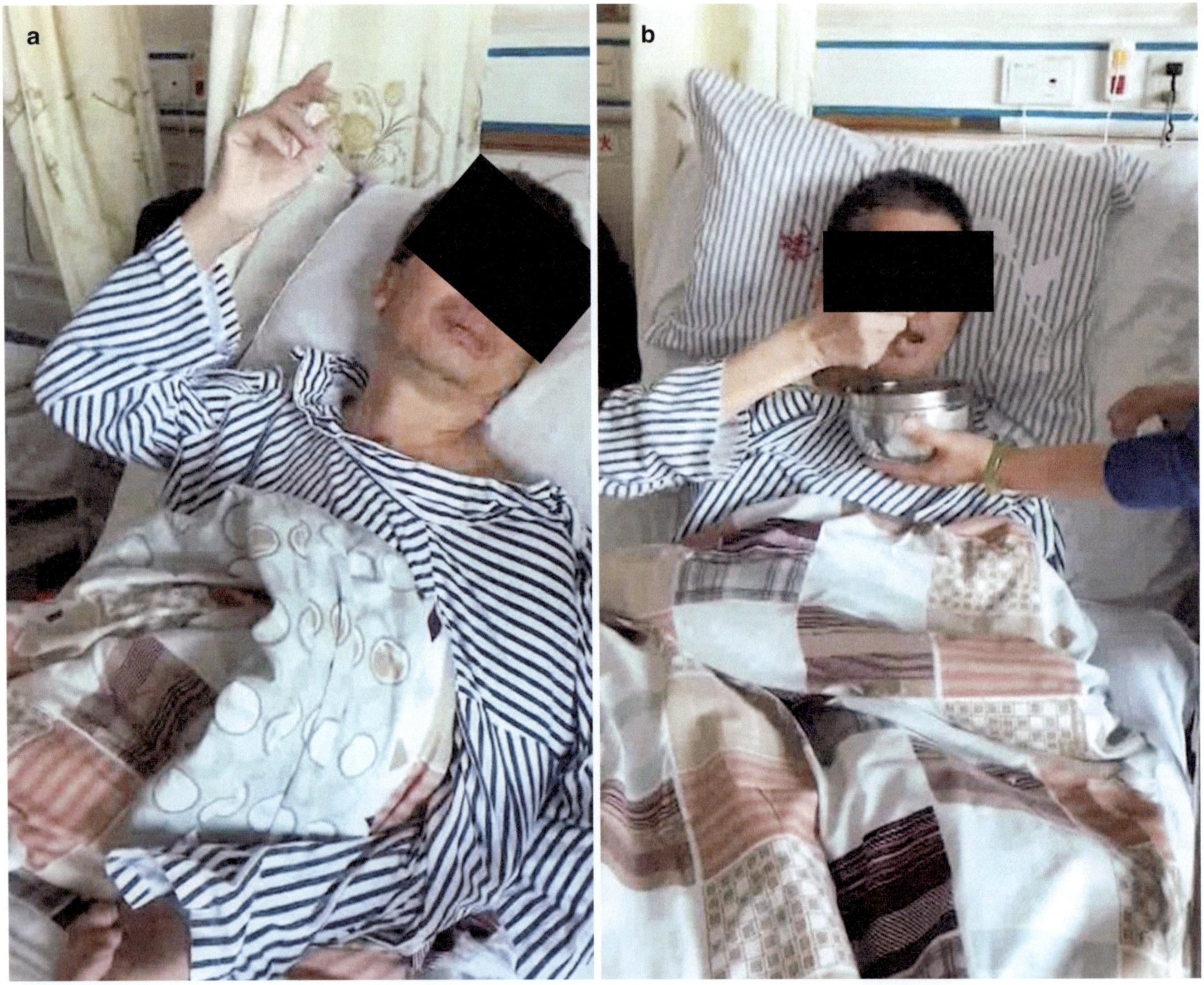

Fig. 16.18 Patient's recovery at 3 months postoperatively. (**a**) The patient's language communication abilities further improved at 3 months postoperatively, with correct responses and enhanced memory. (**b**) The patient was able to eat independently at 3 months postoperatively

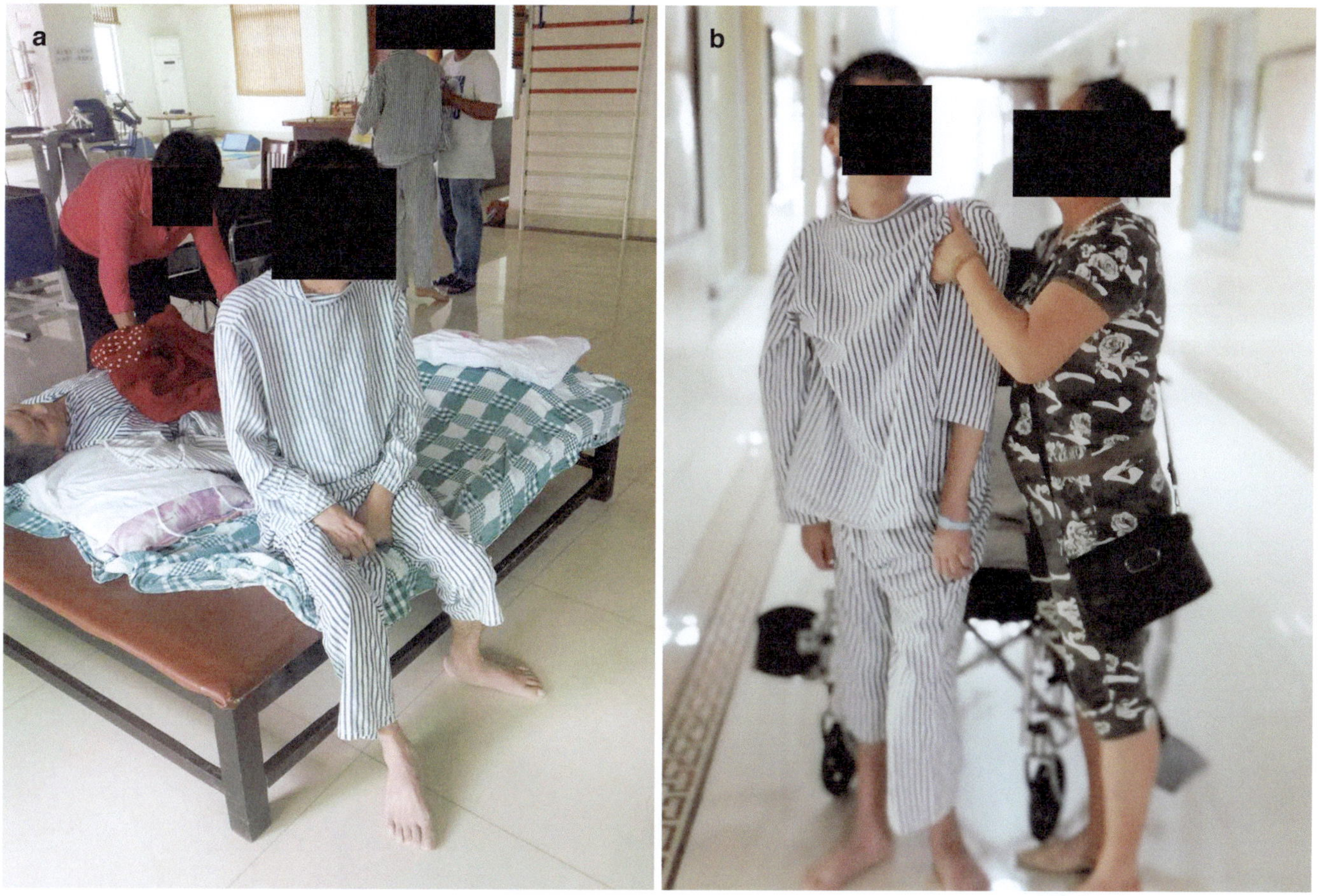

Fig. 16.19 Patient's recovery at 6 months postoperatively. (**a**) The patient's memory and cognitive abilities further recovered at 6 months postoperatively, and was able to sit up independently. (**b**) With the support of family members, the patient could stand and perform simple walking at home at 6 months postoperatively

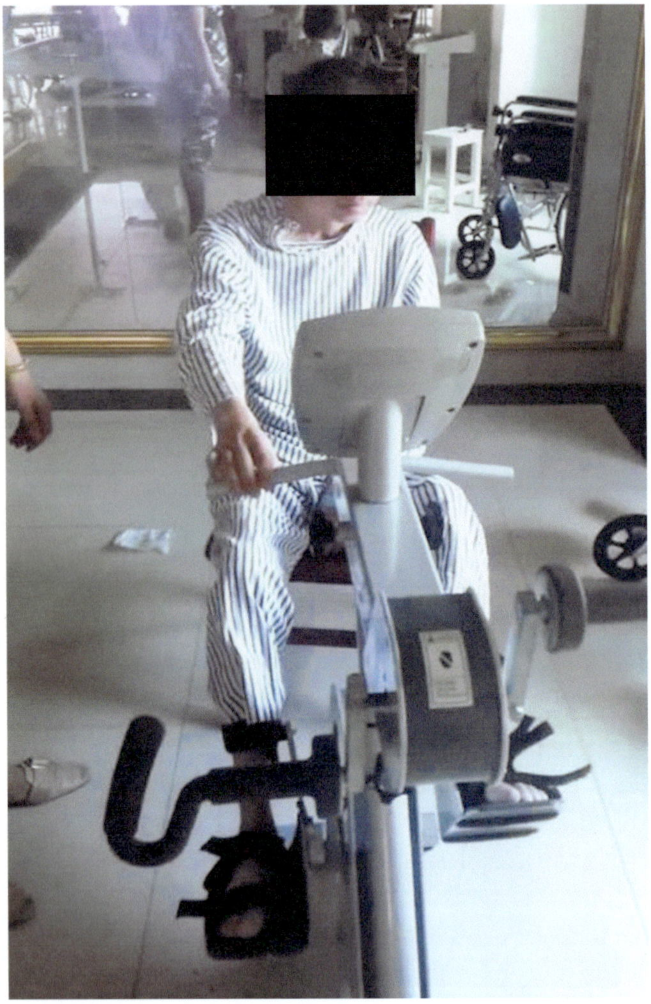

Fig. 16.20 Patient's recovery at 8 months postoperatively. The patient's motor abilities, including walking, further improved at 8 months postoperatively, further engaged in simple cycling exercises

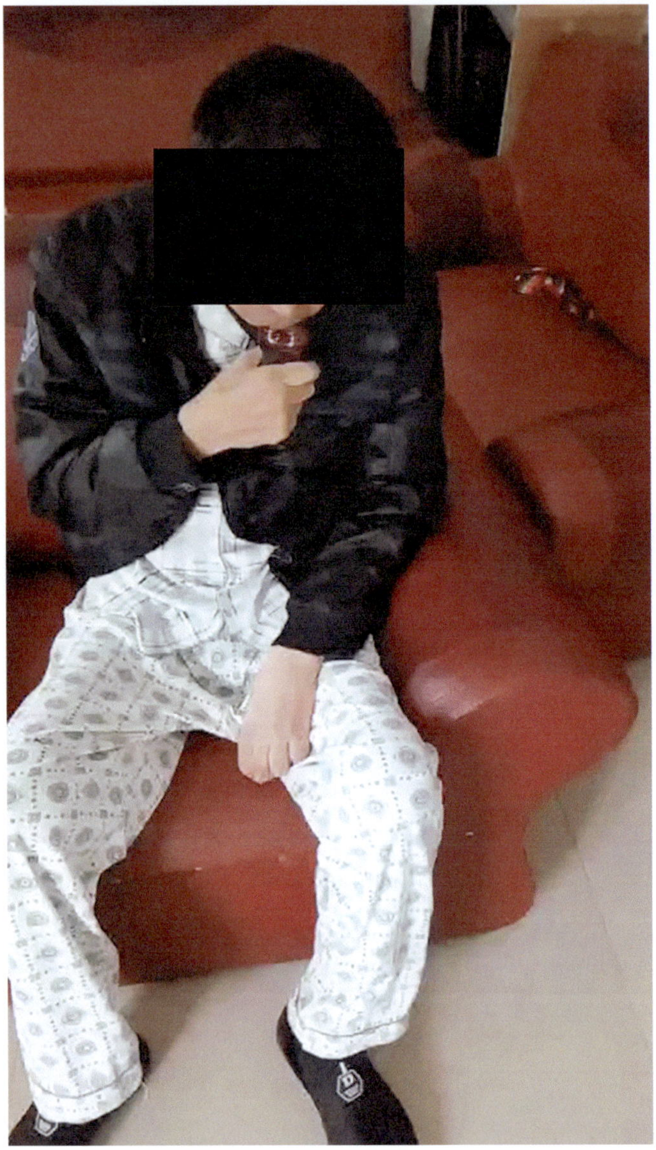

Fig. 16.21 Patient's recovery at 9 months postoperatively. At 9 months postoperatively, the patient's daily living abilities were mostly independent, and cognitive and memory functions had returned to normal

References

1. Almefty KK, Spetzler RF. Management of brainstem cavernous malformations. World Neurosurg. 2015;83(3):317–9.
2. Clinical G, Considerations S. Brainstem cavernous malformations: anatomical, clinical, and surgical considerations. Neurosurg Focus. 2010;29(3):1–22.
3. Gui S, Meng G, Xiao X, et al. Surgical management of brainstem cavernous malformation: report of 67 patients. World Neurosurg. 2019;122:e1162–71.
4. Huang AP, Chen J, Yang C, et al. Brain stem cavernous malformations. J Clin Neurosci. 2010;17(1):74–9.
5. Raison JS, Bourbotte G, Baum TP, et al. Primary brain stem hemorrhage: respective study of 25 cases. Rev Neurol. 2008;164(3):225–32.
6. Ding XQ, Li ZF. Current status and progress in surgical treatment of brainstem hemorrhage. Med Rev. 2017;23(2):4252–5, 4261
7. Li JG, Wang P, Chen BY, et al. Stereotactic surgery for primary brainstem hemorrhage. Chin J Neurosurg. 2009;25(10):919–21.
8. Yang JH, Li ZY, Wang YX, et al. Application and evaluation of the two-point three-line eight-character cross positioning method in minimally invasive puncture and clearance surgery for hypertensive cerebellar hematoma. Chin J Minimally Invasive Neurosurg. 2018;23(3):115–8.
9. Zhou Y, Ao XS, Huang X, et al. Microsurgical treatment of severe brainstem hemorrhage. Chin J Clin Neurosurg. 2010;15(12):721–5.
10. Gao JB, Li WD, Yu B, et al. Observation of the effects of two surgical approaches, transinfratemporal and suboccipital, for the treatment of brainstem hemorrhage under stereotactic navigation. China Med Herald. 2018;15(18):175–7.
11. Li X, Chen J, Zhong L, et al. Stereotactic surgery for severe primary brainstem hemorrhage. Chin J Mod Neurol Dis. 2011;11(3):360–1.
12. Zhang SW, Niu GM, Yuan JH, et al. Comparison of the therapeutic efficacy between stereotactic surgery and conventional conservative treatment for severe brainstem hemorrhage. Chin J Pract Neurol Dis. 2019;22(8):853–8.
13. Zhang YQ, Ye JL, Wu WB, et al. Minimally invasive conical craniotomy for the treatment of 32 cases of severe primary brainstem hemorrhage. Chin J Minimally Invasive Neurosurg. 2017;22(12):562–3.
14. Chen LH, Wei Q, Xu RX, et al. Minimally invasive surgical treatment of primary hypertensive brainstem hemorrhage. J Clin Neurosurg. 2015;12(5):349–54.
15. Zu XW. Stereotactic treatment of severe brainstem hemorrhage using 64-slice CT guidance via the transinfratemporal approach (clinical analysis of 8 cases). J Stereotact Funct Neurosurg. 2011;24(6):371–2.

17 Cubical Stereotactic-Guided Puncture and Aspiration of Brainstem Hematoma

Shujie Sun, Jinbiao Luo, Chao Liu, and Xuan Chen

17.1 Overview

This method utilizes the principles of cubical stereotactic guidance and percutaneous puncture to place a catheter for the aspiration and removal of primary brainstem hematoma.

Based on solid geometry, the system uses a three-dimensional coordinate framework to determine the precise position of a point in space. Combining this principle with cranial anatomy, the "circular-like" skull is enclosed within a cubical space. Using the principle of three intersecting perpendicular planes within the cube, horizontal, coronal, and sagittal planes can be formed, creating a three-dimensional coordinate system centered on that point.

Cubical stereotactic-guided catheter aspiration for primary brainstem hemorrhage involves determining the stereotactic parameters of the hematoma from CT scans and projecting them vertically onto the prefrontal, temporal, parietal, and occipital regions of the head. The intersection points of the three perpendicular planes serve as the central target point for brainstem hematoma. Any straight line formed by the intersection of three perpendicular planes or any two perpendicular planes can be used as the path for puncture and catheter insertion into the skull. The position of the other plane serves as a marker for the depth of reaching the target point within the hematoma. This allows for accurate access to the desired target point within the hematoma.

17.2 Indications and Contraindications

17.2.1 Indications

1. History of hypertension, onset for more than 6 h, with a systolic blood pressure of ≥120 mmHg on admission.
2. GCS score ≤ 8.
3. Hematoma volume ≥ 5 mL.
4. Disturbances in vital signs, such as irregular body temperature, abnormal pupil size, or altered respiration.
5. Informed consent from the patient's family for the surgery.

17.2.2 Contraindications

1. Brainstem hematoma volume < 5 mL.
2. Deep coma, fixed and dilated bilateral pupils, occurrence of autonomous respiratory arrest after onset, blood pressure below 60 mmHg for more than 30 min.
3. Confirmed tumor stroke, arterial aneurysm, arteriovenous malformation, or cavernous angioma by CTA/DSA.
4. Coagulation disorders and hematological diseases.
5. Signs of brainstem functional failure.
6. Severe heart, liver, or kidney dysfunction.
7. Patient's family refusal of surgical treatment.

Supplementary Information The online version contains supplementary material available at https://doi.org/10.1007/978-981-95-8942-5_17.

S. Sun (✉)
Department of Neurosurgery, Shanghai Huangpu Mixed Reality Technology Innovation and Application Transformation Research Institute, Shanghai, China

J. Luo
Department of Neurosurgery, Guangzhou First People's Hospital, School of Medicine, South University of Technology, Guangzhou, China

C. Liu
Department of Neurosurgery, Henan Provincial Chest Hospital, Zhengzhou, China

X. Chen
Department of Neurosurgery, First People's Hospital of Shangqiu City, Shangqiu, China

G. Chen, C. You (eds.), *Surgical Treatment of Primary Brainstem Hemorrhage*, https://doi.org/10.1007/978-981-95-8942-5_17

17.3 Preoperative Preparation and Surgical Instruments

17.3.1 Preoperative Preparation

1. Determination of the surgical site: Coordinate with the CT room or operating room. If possible, perform the procedure under intraoperative CT monitoring. In emergency situations, bedside procedures may be performed.
2. Acquisition of preoperative localization data related to the hematoma: Accurately measure the three-dimensional localization data from CT scans, calculate the size of the hematoma, and measure reference data such as cranial radius, frontal distance, temporal distance, and height distance.
3. Preparation of surgical instruments and supplies: Sterile surgical instruments, disposable cranial drainage bags, disposable medical drainage tubes or ventricular drainage tubes, sterile dressing packs, suture packs, disinfection trays, cranial stereotactic rulers, positioning pens, electrocardiogram monitors, etc.

17.3.2 Surgical Instruments

1. Stereotactic frame: This instrument is used for preoperative localization of brainstem hematomas in stereotactic minimally invasive surgery. It consists of a long board, a short board, and an intermediate board. Its principle is based on the patient's cranial CT images, and it accurately determines the target point of the hematoma and the path of entry into the skull through stereotactic marking lines in a very short time (Fig. 17.1).
2. Directional cranial drill: This minimally invasive surgical instrument is used for drilling through the occipital bone under stereotactic guidance. It can be pre-limited based on the drilling depth (Fig. 17.2).
3. Cranial burr: Used for minimally invasive directional drilling of the skull, it creates a smooth hole in the skull, removes bone debris, and prevents it from entering the intracranial space, ensuring smooth insertion of the cranial lock hole instrument (Fig. 17.3).
4. Cranial lock hole instrument: After directional drilling of the skull, this instrument is used for accurate guidance to establish a channel leading to the intracranial space, facilitating the implementation of minimally invasive directional catheterization surgery (Fig. 17.4).
5. Cranial probe ruler: The cranial probe ruler is used to measure the depth of the drainage tube entering the intracranial space, establishing a pre-channel leading to the hematoma cavity, facilitating intracranial directional catheterization (Fig. 17.5).

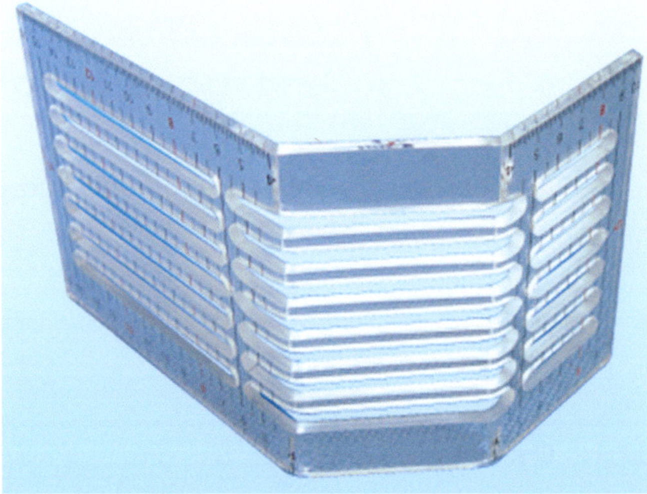

Fig. 17.1 Stereotactic frame

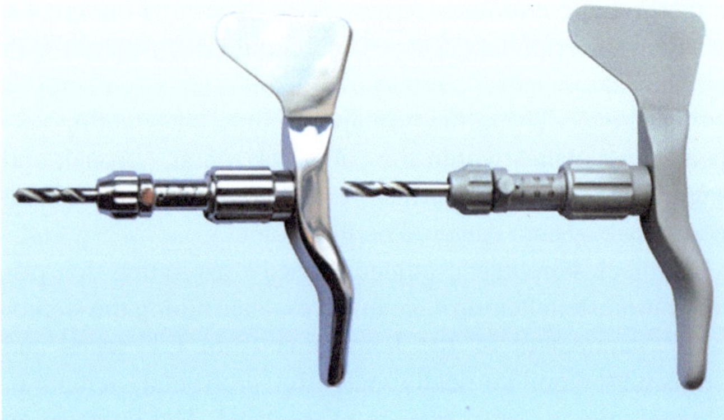

Fig. 17.2 Directional cranial drill

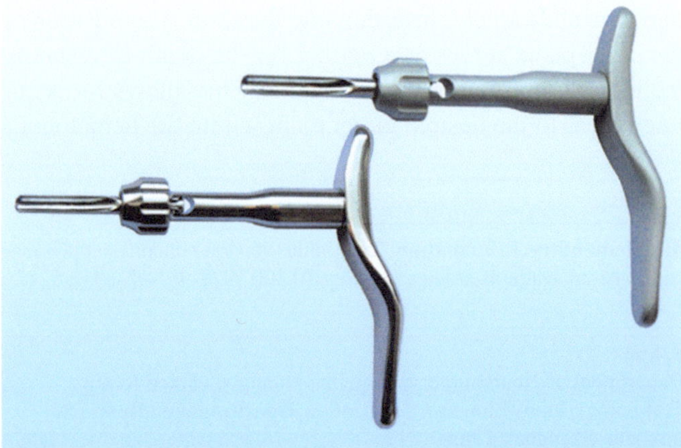

Fig. 17.3 Cranial burr

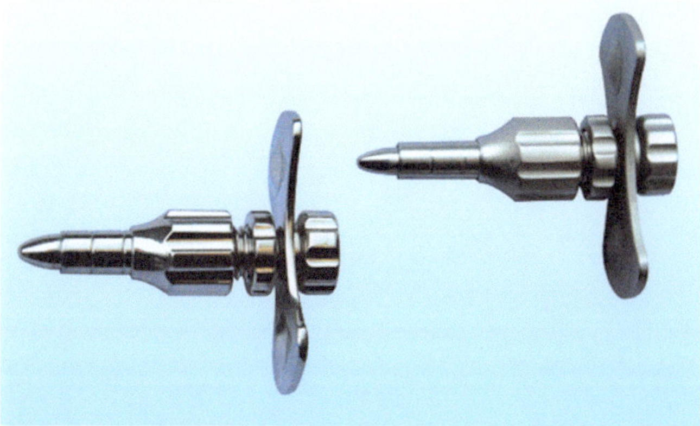

Fig. 17.4 Cranial lock hole instrument

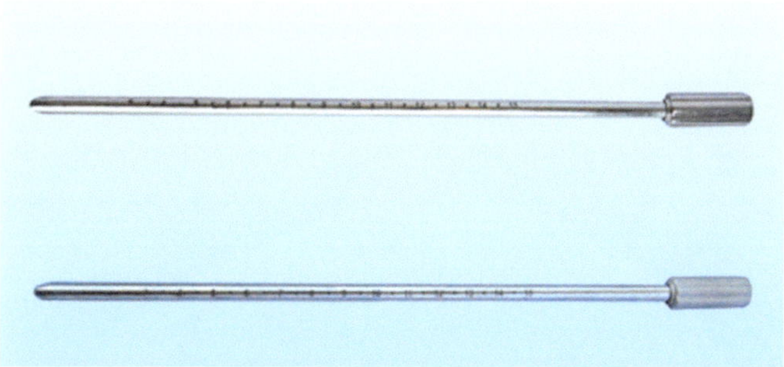

Fig. 17.5 Cranial probe ruler

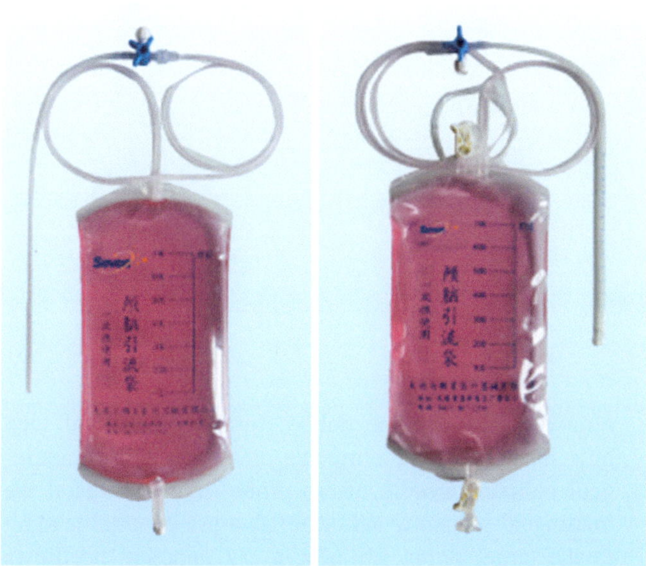

Fig. 17.6 Disposable cranial drainage bag

6. Disposable cranial drainage bag: The disposable cranial drainage bag is designed with a fully sealed and anti-reflux design. It is used in conjunction with the suction tube for brainstem hematoma. It collects residual blood or bloody cerebrospinal fluid after surgery (Fig. 17.6).

17.4 Surgical Methods, Precautions, and Techniques

17.4.1 Surgical Techniques

Based on the skin puncture site, the surgical procedure for cubical stereotactic-guided catheter aspiration can be classified into frontal-occipital, supraoccipital and suboccipital approaches. The suboccipital approach is the most used and is described as follows:

17.4.1.1 Localization Method

1. Draw the basic located line: After skin preparation, with the patient in a supine position and in a calm state, use the midpoint of the glabella as the starting point. Place the short board, intermediate board, and long board of the cranial stereotactic frame against the frontal and parietal regions, respectively. Pass the central strip hole through the starting point and use a cotton swab or pen to draw the mid-sagittal line extending backward through the external occipital protuberance to the posterior neck. Align one edge of the long board of the stereotactic frame with a line connecting the lateral canthus and the external auditory meatus on the surgical side to draw the OM line, which extends to the opposite side at the posterior neck.
2. Mark the projection of the hematoma target and its pathway: In the lateral position, based on the distance between the hematoma target and the OM line observed on CT images, project it onto the temporal side of the head (around 2 cm above the external auditory meatus for pontine hemorrhage). Determine the suboccipital puncture point (approximately 5–6 cm lateral to the midline and 2–3 cm below the projected line of the transverse sinus). Place the short board of the cranial stereotactic frame vertically to the mid-sagittal line and use a pen to draw a line connecting the temporal side point and the suboccipital puncture point to establish the horizontal plane of the hematoma. Depending on the location of the hematoma projection on the frontal or parietal region, draw the appropriate sagittal line using the stereotactic frame to establish the sagittal plane of the hematoma. The intersection of the aforementioned sagittal and horizontal planes represents the path for puncturing the brainstem hematoma, with a depth of 9–10 cm (Fig. 17.7).

17.4.2 Surgical Steps

1. Transfer the patient to the minimally invasive operating room or hybrid operating room (resuscitation can also be performed at the bedside in the intensive care unit), position the patient appropriately, connect the oxygen tube, perform cardiac monitoring, establish intravenous access,

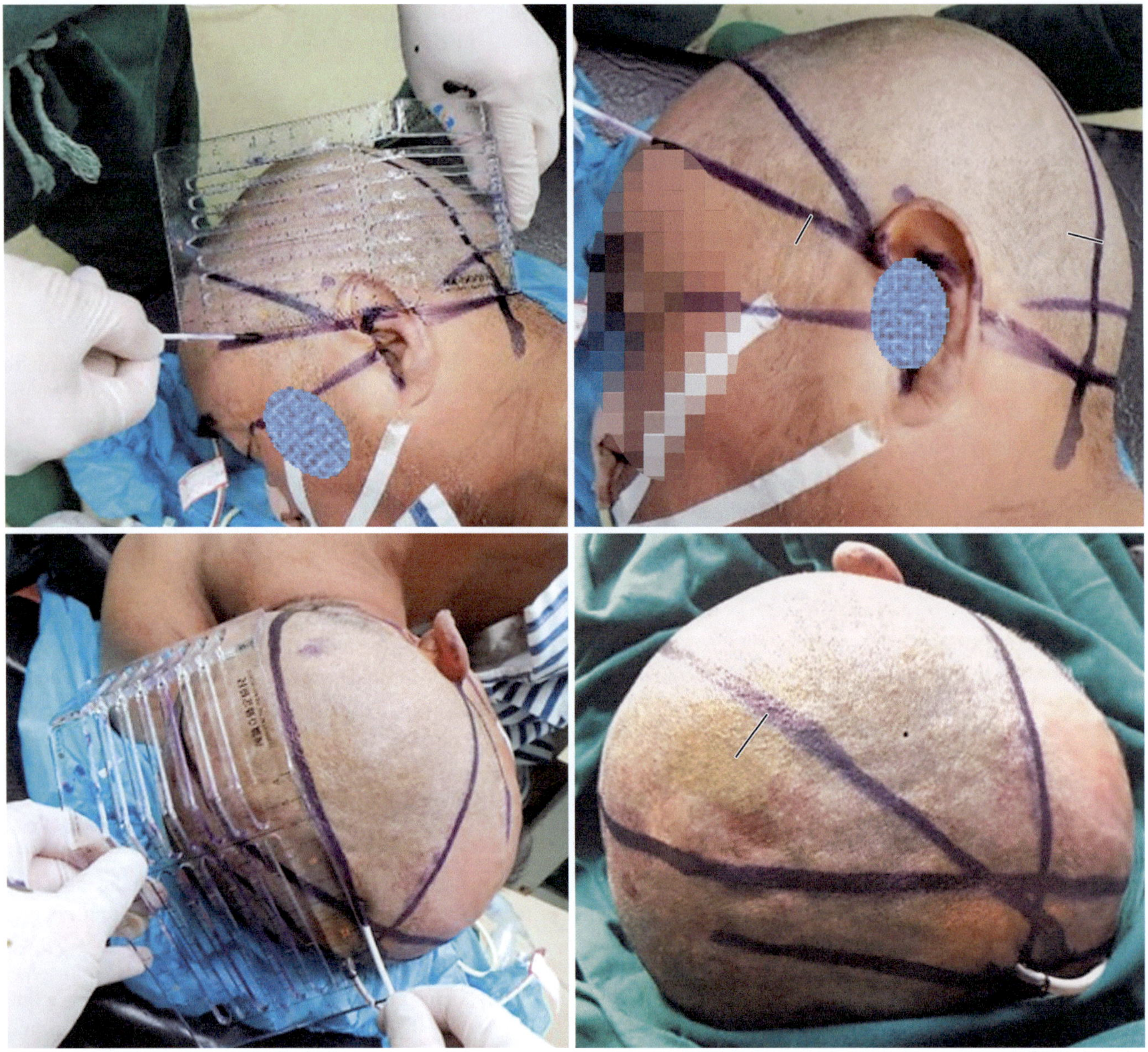

Fig. 17.7 Stereotactic frame drawing horizontal and sagittal lines

observe and record pupil size and vital signs, and continuously monitor their changes during the procedure.

2. After marking the head located lines, perform routine disinfection and drape the surgical area.
3. Perform ipsilateral ventricular puncture and catheterization or place an intracranial pressure probe to measure intracranial pressure. Set up a ventricular drainage system or connect an intracranial pressure monitoring device.
4. Administer local or general anesthesia. Use a surgical blade to make an approximately 0.5 cm incision at the suboccipital puncture point. Create a subcutaneous channel to occipital bone using a cranial burr and use a directional cranial drill to penetrate the occipital bone. Use the cranial burr to expand the drilling hole and remove residual bone debris. Install the cranial lock hole instrument, puncture the meninges with a meningeal puncture needle, use a probe ruler to expand the meningeal incision, and establish a pre-channel leading to the target point. Initially, use a puncture needle to aspirate a small amount of old blood from the center of the hematoma, then insert the brainstem hematoma suction catheter. After aspirating 2–5 mL of old blood, leave the catheter in the residual hematoma cavity and connect the external end of the catheter to the hematoma drainage bag. After dressing the wound, return the patient to the ward or perform a follow-up CT scan to assess the postoperative drainage of the intracranial hematoma (Fig. 17.8, Video 17.1).

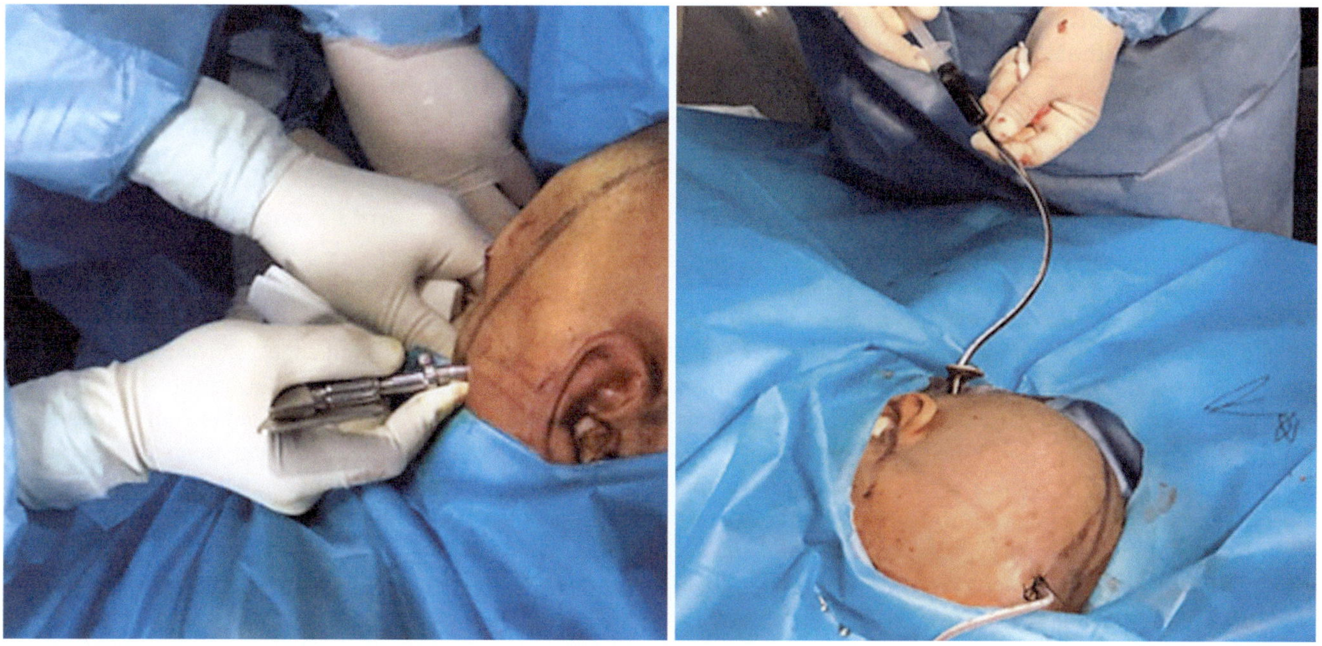

Fig. 17.8 Directional cranial drill, directional catheter placement, and hematoma aspiration

17.4.3 Precautions and Techniques for Surgery

1. When marking the location of brainstem hematoma, it is essential to adhere to the principle of cubical stereotactic localization. CT scanning should strictly follow the OM baseline for positioning.
2. When using the cranial stereotactic frame short board, pay attention to the following: when projecting the lines on the temporal side, the distance line of the cranial radius should overlap with the sagittal line; when projecting the lines on the frontal and parietal sides, the radius line of the short board should be parallel to the OM line.
3. When starting to drill the skull, make a vertical groove on the surface of the skull bone, and then adjust the direction of the directional skull drill according to the plane direction of the puncture.
4. Adjust the length of the drill according to the thickness of the skull to prevent the drill from penetrating too deeply and damaging the dura mater.
5. During the procedure, the aim is not to completely remove the hematoma in one go. Emphasize a slow, intermittent, non-obstructive aspiration process that focuses on blood drainage without damaging brain tissue.
6. When puncturing the skull bone, avoid damaging the venous sinuses, such as the sagittal sinus, transverse sinus, and sigmoid sinus.
7. When puncturing the brainstem, avoid damaging important neural nuclei such as the brainstem reticular ascending excitatory system, cerebellar dentate nucleus, brainstem facial nucleus, main trigeminal nucleus, and oculomotor nucleus. Also, be cautious of placing the catheter too deep, as it carries the risk of damaging the brainstem.
8. If there is a significant drop in blood pressure or notable changes in vital signs during the surgery, the operation should be stopped until the vital signs stabilize before proceeding.
9. First puncture the lateral ventricle, then puncture the brainstem hematoma. If ventricular drainage is performed, follow the principle of removing the brainstem drainage tube before removing the lateral ventricle drainage tube.
10. If there is poor drainage of residual blood, on the day after surgery, an injection of 20,000–30,000 units of urokinase diluted in 2–3 mL of saline can be administered once a day. The drainage tube can be removed when CT shows residual blood volume $\leq$ 2 mL. Avoid leaving the tube in place for an extended period, and the duration of tube retention should be $\leq$1 week.
11. Emphasize the standardization and sterility of the puncture and catheterization procedure for brainstem hemorrhage, to prevent accidental puncture of intracranial blood vessels and avoid the occurrence of bleeding and infection.

17.5 Postoperative Care and Prevention of Complications

Surgical complications are rare, but occasionally there may be postoperative rebleeding, incision or intracranial infections, and pneumocephalus. Some patients may experience transient hypotension and respiratory arrest during the procedure. Other non-surgical complications may include pulmonary infections, acute renal failure, stress ulcers, pressure sores, cardiac damage, urinary tract infections, and deep vein thrombosis. For patients undergoing surgical treatment, hospitals with the necessary resources recommend intracranial pressure monitoring. If there are changes in the patient's vital signs during the surgery, the operation should be temporarily paused to identify the cause. Once the vital signs stabilize, the decision to continue the surgery can be made. Postoperative management includes reducing intracranial pressure, managing blood pressure, sedation, pain management, prevention and treatment of intracranial and pulmonary infections, maintaining a stable internal environment, nutritional support, and prevention and treatment of epilepsy. Routine cranial CT scans should be performed within 24 h after surgery to assess the surgical outcome and rule out postoperative rebleeding. For patients with recurrent bleeding, the decision to perform a second surgery should be based on the patient's specific condition. In patients with coagulation disorders or significant intraoperative oozing, hemostatic drugs or symptomatic treatment can be applied in the short term (within 24–48 h) after surgery.

17.6 Advantages, Disadvantages, and Lessons Learned

17.6.1 Advantages

This method utilizes three-dimensional data from the patient's head imaging, employing the cubical stereotactic line drawing technique and corresponding surgical instruments for brainstem hemorrhage. The method is simple, with a short operation time, minimal trauma, good therapeutic effects, no blood transfusion required, low medical staff and cost, and is suitable for puncture and catheterization treatment of lateral ventricle and brainstem hematomas. The surgery can be performed in the operating room, and critically ill patients can also be treated at the bedside under local anesthesia, which is conducive to implementation in hospitals at all levels.

17.6.2 Disadvantages

Medical staff need to undergo short-term training to master this technique.

17.6.3 Experience and Lessons Learned

1. The procedure is performed under the cubical stereotactic guidance or guidance of imaging, and the puncture channel should be strictly operated in a sterile manner to avoid skin and intracranial infections.
2. Prior to the surgery, vascular-related examinations (CTA/MRA/DSA) should be performed to exclude vascular lesions in patients with unclear etiology of brainstem hemorrhage, in order to avoid and reduce the risk of intraoperative bleeding.
3. Attention should be paid to avoid damage to important neural nuclei, functional fibers, and venous sinus vessels of the cerebellum and brainstem in the puncture path.

17.7 Procedure Evaluation and Prospects

Brainstem hemorrhage is a critical condition in the nervous system and the most dangerous and prognostically poor disease in the field of neurology. The cubical stereotactic-guided soft channel technique, commonly known as the "oriented soft channel" technique, has the advantages of accurate localization, simple operation, minimal trauma, rapid reduction of hematoma, and fast recovery of neurological function. It is believed that an increasing number of patients with brainstem hemorrhage will receive timely and effective treatment.

17.8 Typical Cases

17.8.1 Case 1

17.8.1.1 Brief Medical History and Imaging Data

A 50-year-old male patient suddenly experienced headache and vomiting, followed by altered consciousness, seizures, and difficulty breathing, quickly leading to coma. He was immediately rushed to the hospital. The patient had a history of hypertension for 10 years. Physical examination: blood pressure 180/95 mmHg, heart rate 60 beats/min, weak breathing, moderate comatose state, pinpoint pupils, fixed eyes, neck stiffness, limb paralysis, and positive Babinski sign in both lower limbs. GCS 4. After neurosurgical resuscitating, the patient received assisted ventilation. CT and CTA examinations revealed primary brainstem hemorrhage with a volume of 5 mL. Admission diagnosis: Brainstem hemorrhage; Grade 3 hypertension (extremely high-risk group).

17.8.1.2 Surgical Procedure and Key Points

The procedure of cubical stereotactic-guided catheter placement and aspiration was performed on this patient 27 h after the onset, with the consent of the family. Prior to the surgery, the patient's entire head was shaved and prepared. Based on the three-dimensional data from the CT imaging, a cubical stereotactic guidance template was placed on the patient's head surface, and different reference lines were drawn using a cotton swab dipped in methyl violet or methylene blue solution (as described in the Localization Method section of this chapter). The entry point on the skin and the target site of the puncture into the right lateral ventricle frontal horn and the suboccipital brainstem were determined, along with the pathway. This allowed for rapid and precise location of the patient's head target (Fig. 17.9).

The patient was transferred to the operating room and placed in a right lateral decubitus position under general anesthesia. Standard neurosurgical draping was performed, ensuring that the drape aperture exposed the entire head with the drawn lines. Initially, a cubical stereotactic-guided puncture was made in the right lateral ventricle frontal horn to insert a ventricular drainage catheter. The catheter was inserted to a depth of 6 cm, and after draining a small amount of cerebrospinal fluid, the fluid column within the catheter fluctuated within a range of 15 cm, indicating stable intracranial pressure. This catheter was left in place for postoperative external ventricular drainage. Subsequently, a drainage catheter was accurately placed into the target center of the brainstem hematoma at the left occipital region. When the catheter reached a depth of 9.5 cm, old blood was observed flowing out from the catheter. Using a 5 mL syringe, 2 mL of the old hematoma was aspirated. The scalp was sutured to secure the drainage catheter within the hematoma cavity, and the external end was connected to a hematoma drainage bag for continuous blood drainage.

Immediately after the surgery, the patient was taken to the CT room for postoperative head examination.

17.8.1.3 Preoperative and Postoperative Imaging Comparison

A postoperative cranial CT scan was performed immediately, revealing 90% clearance of the hematoma. On the first postoperative day, CT showed complete clearance of the brainstem hematoma (Fig. 17.10).

17.8.1.4 Postoperative Neurological Examination Imaging Data

On postoperative day 2, the patient responded to verbal stimuli by opening the eyes, and there was a noticeable pupillary light reflex. Eye movements were observed, and the patient exhibited localized response to painful stimuli. Muscle strength in the limbs was graded as II–III. The brainstem drainage catheter was removed. On postoperative day 4, the ventricular drainage catheter was removed. On postoperative day 7, the patient demonstrated significantly improved voluntary breathing strength and response to cough stimulation, and was successfully weaned off the ventilator.

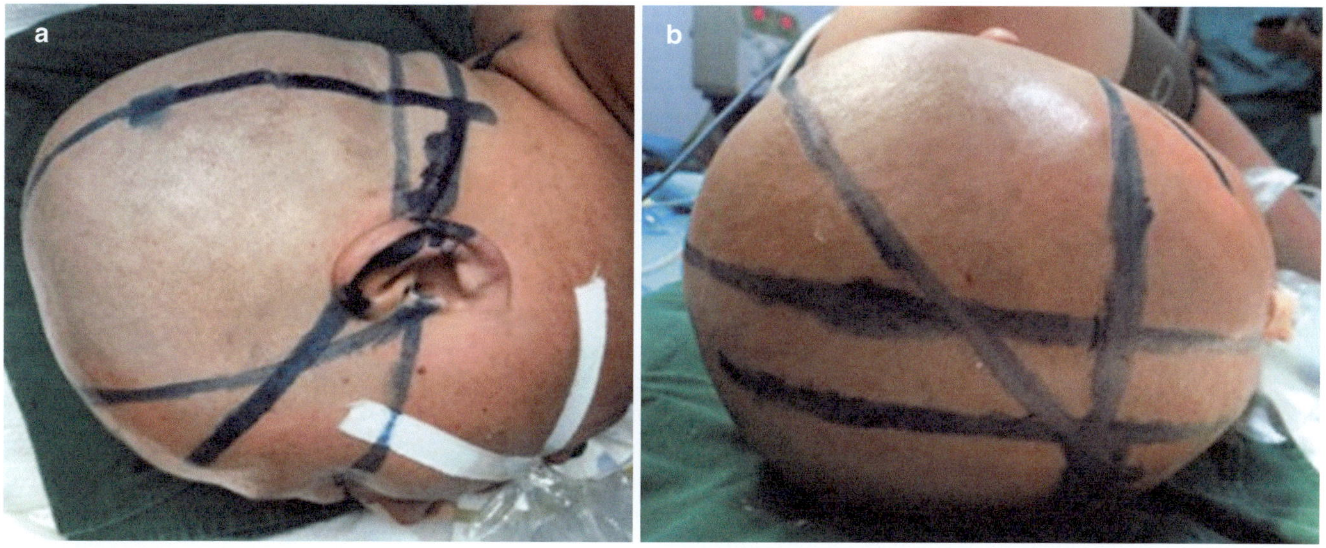

Fig. 17.9 Intraoperative line drawing localization. (**a**) The scalp puncture point of brainstem. (**b**) The scalp puncture point of the right lateral ventricle

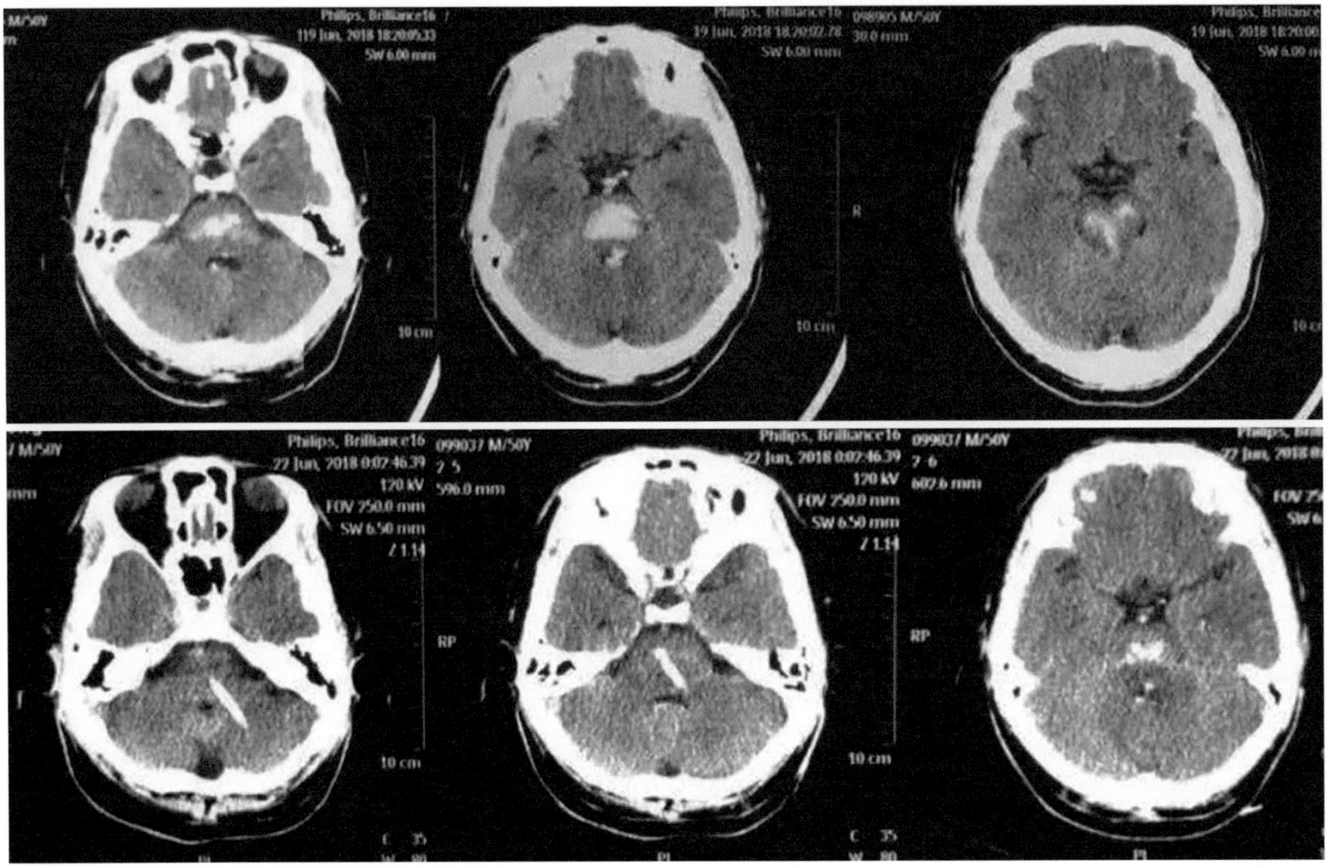

Fig. 17.10 Preoperative and postoperative brain CT

Two months after the surgery, although experiencing hoarseness of voice, the patient regained full consciousness with rehabilitation treatment. The patient was able to walk with assistance. After 3 months of comprehensive rehabilitation treatment, including hyperbaric oxygen therapy, the patient could walk independently with crutches. After 5 months of integrated rehabilitation treatment, the patient could perform basic self-care tasks (Fig. 17.11).

17.8.2 Case 2

17.8.2.1 Brief Medical History and Imaging Data

The patient, a 50-year-old male, presented to the local hospital's emergency department with a chief complaint of "sudden vomiting accompanied by altered mental status and urinary incontinence for 1 h." He had a long-standing history of hypertension. On examination, his body temperature was 36 °C, blood pressure was 210/132 mmHg, pulse rate was 85 beats/min, and respiratory rate was 17 breaths/min. He had altered mental status, bilateral pupils were equally dilated and round with a diameter of approximately 3.0 mm, with sluggish pupillary light reflex. His limbs exhibited increased muscle tone, and bilateral Babinski reflex were positive. A head CT scan revealed a 3 mL pontine hemorrhage extending into the fourth ventricle. The admission diagnosis was brainstem hemorrhage and grade 3 hypertension (extremely high risk).

After 25 h of hospitalization, the patient's level of consciousness deteriorated further. His pupils became constricted and fixed, with the right pupil slightly larger than the left. He developed rapid and shallow breathing, significant decrease in blood oxygen saturation. Immediate interventions were performed, including endotracheal intubation for assisted ventilation, dehydration therapy with mannitol, etc. A second head CT scan showed an increase in the brainstem hemorrhage volume to 10 mL.

17.8.2.2 Surgical Procedure and Key Points

Emergency preparations were made, and the patient was transferred to the operating room. Based on the three-dimensional localization data of the intracranial hematoma provided by the second preoperative CT imaging, a cubical stereotactic guidance line was drawn at the bedside to locate the brainstem hematoma. The patient was positioned in the left lateral decubitus position, and a 2 cm incision was made below the right occipital transverse sinus, entering through

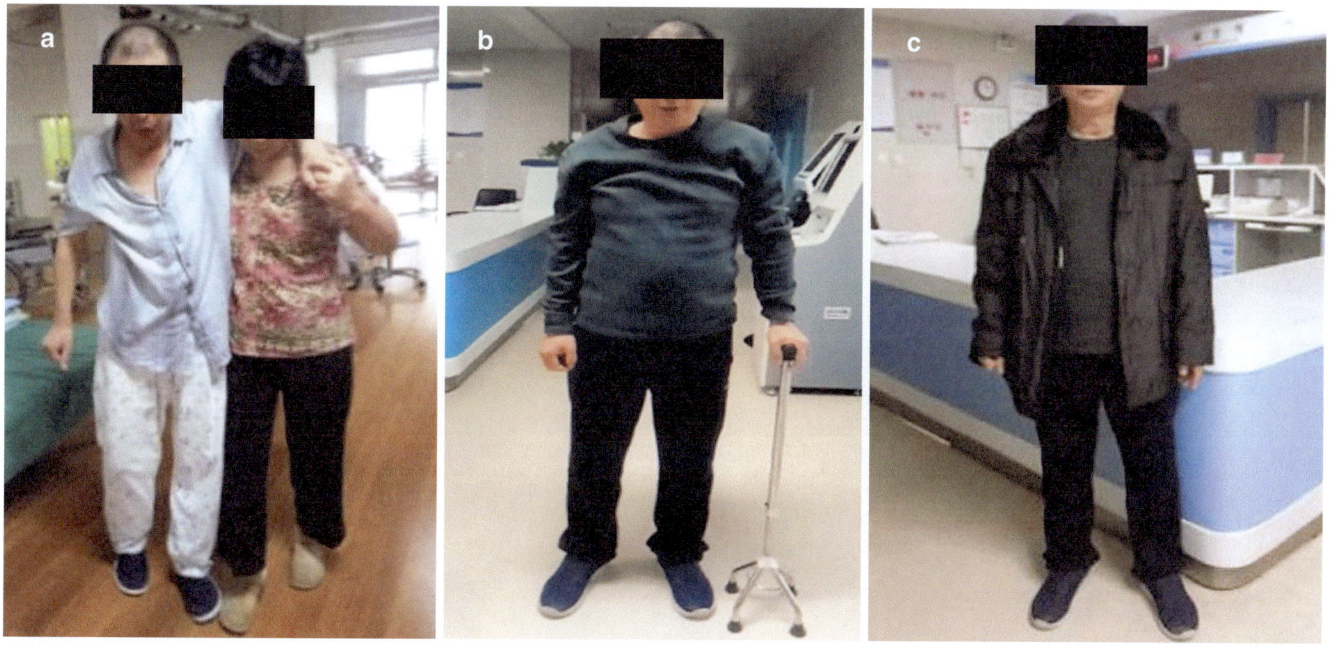

Fig. 17.11 Patient's condition post-surgery. (**a**) 2 months; (**b**) 3 months; (**c**) 5 months

the midbrain brachium conjunctivum. Under 1% lidocaine local anesthesia (5 mL), a cubical stereotactic percutaneous puncture was performed to place a catheter into the cavity of the brainstem hematoma. During the procedure, when 4 mL of old hematoma was aspirated, there was a significant drop in blood pressure, fluctuating between 135–150/80–95 mmHg. The patient exhibited noticeable spontaneous breathing. The catheter was left in place for postoperative drainage to continue removing residual blood within the brainstem for treatment.

17.8.2.3 Preoperative and Postoperative Imaging Comparison

Immediate postoperative head CT scan showed that nearly half of the brainstem hematoma had been cleared (Fig. 17.12). The following day, 2 mL of urokinase (10,000 units per milliliter) was injected into the residual cavity of the hematoma, and continuous drainage was maintained. After 5 h, a repeat CT scan showed that most of the brainstem hematoma had been cleared, and the drainage catheter was removed.

17.8.2.4 Imaging Data and Video of Postoperative Neurological Examination

On postoperative day 5, the patient had confusion but responded to stimuli. On postoperative day 10, the patient could respond when called and was transferred from the EICU to a general ward. On day 20, the patient regained clear consciousness and was transferred to the rehabilitation department for further treatment.

At 2 months postoperatively, the patient was able to walk with assistance. At 5 months postoperatively, the muscle strength of the left limbs was nearly at Grade V, except for difficulty extending the fingers of the left hand. The patient could stand, walk, and ride a motorcycle, and was able to perform basic self-care tasks (Fig. 17.13).

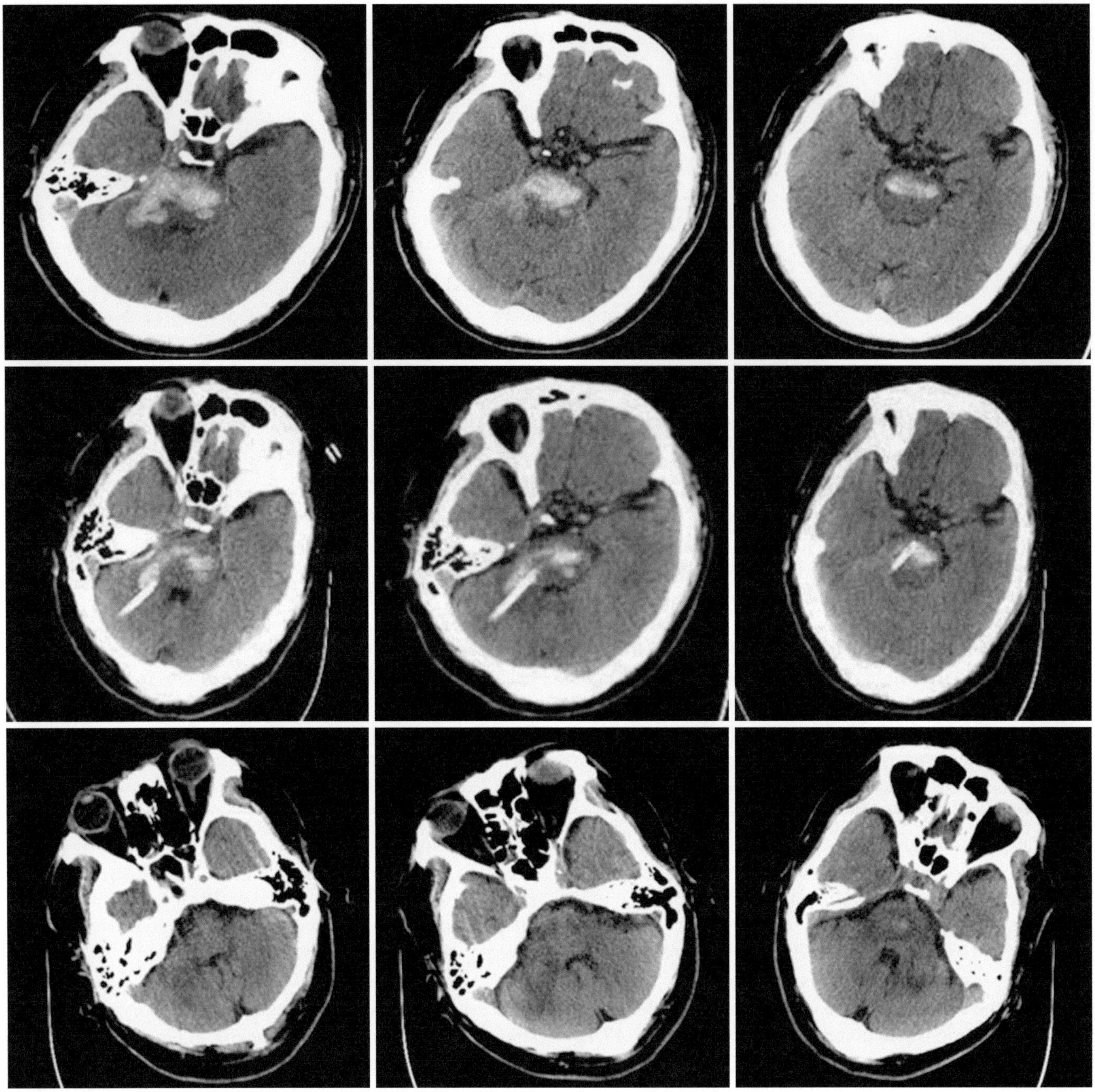

Fig. 17.12 Preoperative and postoperative imaging comparison

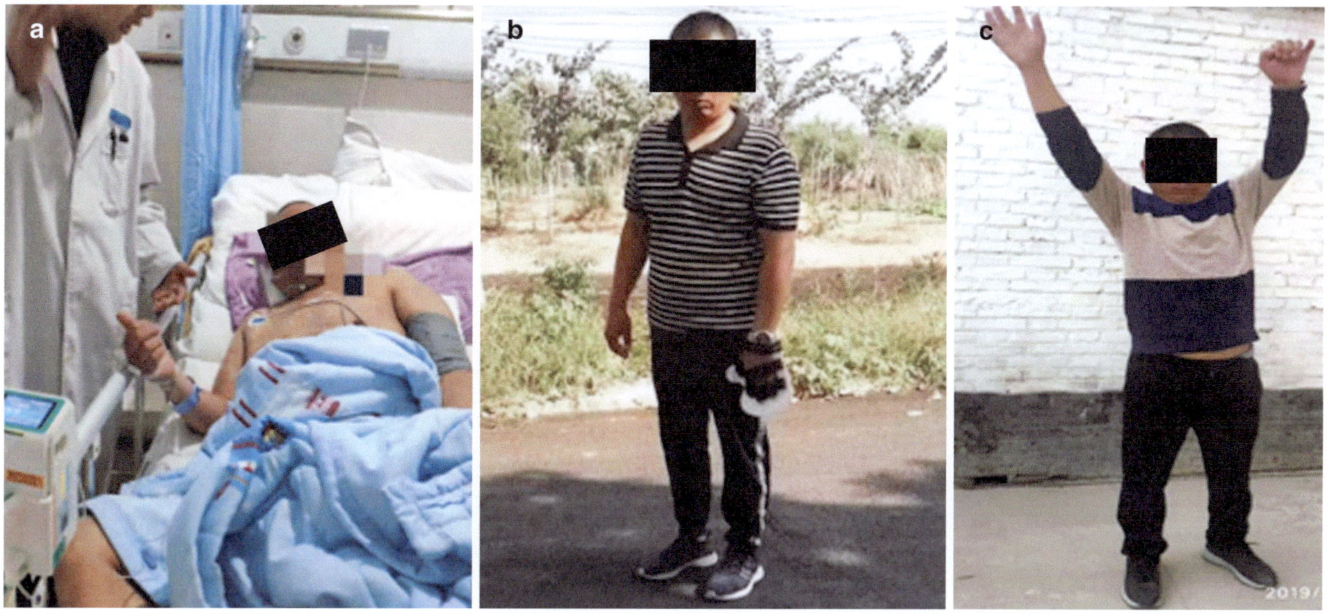

Fig. 17.13 Patient's condition post-surgery. (**a**) Day 10; (**b**) 2 months; (**c**) 5 months

18 Modified Directional Brainstem Hematoma Puncture and Aspiration

Zhenchuan Liu

18.1 Overview

Currently, surgical treatment for spontaneous brainstem hemorrhage remains unconventional. The decision to perform surgery for severe brainstem hemorrhage was balanced and made by experienced surgeons, depending on the patient's condition, the morphology of the brainstem hematoma, potential prognosis, as well as the attitudes, wishes, and economic capacity of the patient's family. Patients with severe brainstem hemorrhage, especially those in a comatose state, have high mortality and morbidity rates. Many surviving patients are bedridden for a long time, or may even in a vegetative state, which poses a heavy burden on both their families and society. The decision to undergo surgical treatment requires in-depth communication between the surgeon and the patient's family, weighing the pros and cons before making a cautious choice. Selective application of the "modified directional intracranial hematoma aspiration" technique can be employed for the clearance of brainstem hematomas in some severe cases. Since October 1996, the author has been performing puncture treatments for primary supratentorial hematomas. In June 2000, the author started performing puncture, aspiration, liquefaction, and external drainage for infratentorial cerebellar hematomas. In 2003, the author began performing puncture, aspiration, liquefaction, and external drainage for fourth ventricle hematomas and brainstem (pons) hematomas via the infratentorial approach, achieving certain clinical efficacy. Since March 2007, training courses on "minimally invasive standardized treatment of cerebral hemorrhage" have been held in China, continuously promoting the clinical application of this technique, which has generated significant response within the industry.

18.2 Indications and Contraindications

Primary brainstem hemorrhage most commonly occurs in the pons, and the hematoma can involve the midbrain and medulla oblongata. Extensive pontine hemorrhage can rupture into the fourth ventricle, subsequently entering the subarachnoid space, the aqueduct of midbrain, and the supratentorial ventricular system, obstructing the circulation of cerebrospinal fluid and leading to acute obstructive hydrocephalus that endangers life. Based on the location of the hematoma, brainstem (pons) hemorrhage can be classified into central, ventral, lateral (left or right), and dorsal types. The clinical condition (consciousness) of brainstem hemorrhage is classified into five levels (Table 18.1).

The need for surgical treatment in patients with brainstem hemorrhage depends on the severity of their clinical condi-

Table 18.1 Clinical classification of brainstem hemorrhage

Grade	Consciousness status	Chief physical manifestation
I	Alert or drowsy	Accompanied (or not) by mild hemiparesis or aphasia
II	Drowsy or confused	Accompanied by varying degrees of hemiparesis (quadriparesis) or aphasia
III	Light coma	Paralysis (quadriparesis), equal pupils, preserved light reflex
IVa	Coma	Paralysis (quadriparesis), equal pupils, pinpoint-like constriction
IVb	Coma	Quadriparesis, unequal pupils, presence of spontaneous respiration
V	Deep coma	Decerebrate or flaccid paralysis, dilated pupils on one or both sides, requiring mechanical ventilation or respiratory control

Supplementary Information The online version contains supplementary material available at https://doi.org/10.1007/978-981-95-8942-5_18.

Z. Liu (✉)
Department of Neurological Intensive Care Unit, Linyi People's Hospital, Linyi, China

G. Chen, C. You (eds.), *Surgical Treatment of Primary Brainstem Hemorrhage*, https://doi.org/10.1007/978-981-95-8942-5_18

tion (grading) and radiological findings. Brainstem hemorrhage without impaired consciousness is generally not suitable for surgery.

18.2.1 Indications

1. Patients with clinical grading of III, IVa, or IVb for brainstem hemorrhage.
2. GCS 4–8 points.
3. Brainstem hemorrhage volume ≥ 5 mL, preferentially considering surgery for dorsal type and/or those rupturing into the fourth ventricle, with discretionary consideration for other types.
4. For lateral and central hematomas, the decision for surgery should be made after comprehensive consideration of the above factors.

18.2.2 Contraindications

1. GCS score ≥ 9 points, hematoma volume < 3 mL.
2. Clinical grade V, GCS 3, and pupil dilation for over 1 h.
3. Structural vascular abnormalities in the brainstem, such as aneurysms, arteriovenous malformations, or cavernous hemangiomas.
4. Patients with unstable hemodynamics, such as malignant hypertension.
5. Severe coagulation disorders.
6. Patients in extremely poor overall condition who are unable to tolerate anesthesia and surgery.

18.3 Preoperative Preparation and Surgical Instruments

18.3.1 Preoperative Preparation

Routine preparation before soft channel surgery for brainstem hemorrhage. Prior to the surgery, it is essential to complete relevant auxiliary examinations, sign the surgical consent form, and conduct skin preparation and preoperative cranial CT localization scans.

18.3.2 Surgical Instruments

1. Items for localization: Standard preoperative cranial CT scans, a 20 cm transparent ruler for students, drafting regulation, an infrared level instrument, a smartphone measurement tool, or protractor software, cotton swabs, and methyl violet.

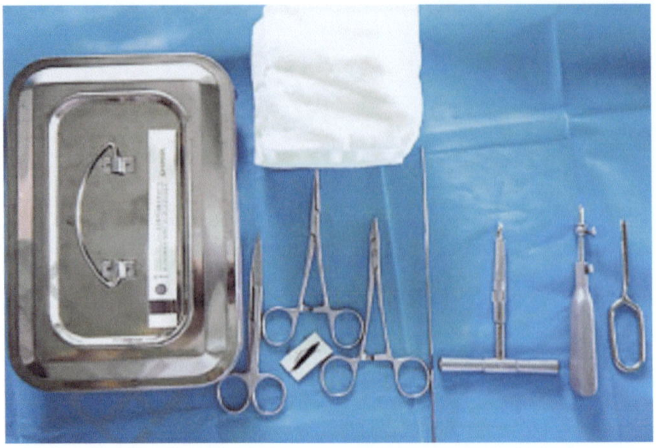

Fig. 18.1 Instruments in the surgical instrument box

2. Instruments in the surgical instrument box: Skull Mitsubishi hand drill (outer diameter 4–4.5 mm), groove hand drill, T-shaped hand drill (outer diameter 4.5–5 mm), outer diameter 2 mm Kirschner needle (guide steel needle), wire cutter, needle holder, hemostatic forceps each one piece (Fig. 18.1).
3. Disposable consumables: 12F disposable cranial external drainage tube (produced by Shandong Dazheng Medical Equipment Co., Ltd.), heparin cap, three-way valve, 5 mL sterile empty needle, 2% lidocaine, disposable wound care kit (drape), sterile gloves, povidone-iodine solution, head cover, gauze, silk thread sutures, adhesive tape, or film.

For the modified directional brainstem hematoma puncture and aspiration, a 12F (outer diameter 4 mm) high-quality silicone drainage catheter is used, with a ball-shaped tip and 2–4 drainage side holes located 0.5 cm from the tip.

18.4 Surgical Methods, Precautions, and Techniques

18.4.1 Surgical Methods

18.4.1.1 Preoperative Localization Method

Surface localization markers are determined using anatomical knowledge and CT images to identify the scalp surface projection range of the posterior cranial fossa. The preoperative localization is performed using cranial surface anatomical landmarks (mainly bony landmarks), requiring higher technical skills due to the narrow space within the posterior cranial fossa.

1. Determining the External Occipital Protuberance Point A: After preparing the patient's head is prepped, in the

supine position, a cotton swab dipped in methyl violet solution is used to mark the midsagittal line. Then, in the lateral decubitus position on the healthy side, with the head slightly flexed toward the sternum, the affected side is exposed to make the midsagittal line parallel to the bed surface. The external occipital protuberance is then accurately marked on the midsagittal line at the posterior midline, identified as point A.

2. Determining the Upper Boundary (Marker) AB Line of the Transverse Sinus Scalp Projection: A line segment is drawn from point A towards the upper half of the mastoid process on the affected side (perpendicular to the midsagittal line originating from point A), with point B being the intersection with the hairline (B corresponds to the boundary between the upper 1/3 and middle 1/3 of the ipsilateral earlobe); the AB line often represents the external scalp projection of the affected side transverse sinus groove.
3. Determining the Outer Boundary (Marker) BC of the Mastoid's Inner Edge: The intersection of the extension of a line connecting the ipsilateral lateral canthus with the inferior wall of the external auditory meatus and the hairline is point C; the BC line represents the inner edge of the mastoid and the outer boundary of the posterior cranial fossa surface projection.
4. Determining the Inner Boundary (Marker) AD of the Posterior Midline: The depression located on the midline of the posterior occipital region, at the junction of the cranial and cervical regions, is point D; the AD line is the posterior midline boundary of the posterior cranial fossa and the inner boundary of the affected side's posterior cranial fossa surface projection.
5. Determining the Lower Boundary (Marker) Skull Base Line: The shortest arc connecting points CD is the skull base line.

The quadrilateral formed by segments AB, BC, CD, and AD represents the external scalp projection of the posterior cranial fossa boundary on the affected side (Fig. 18.2).

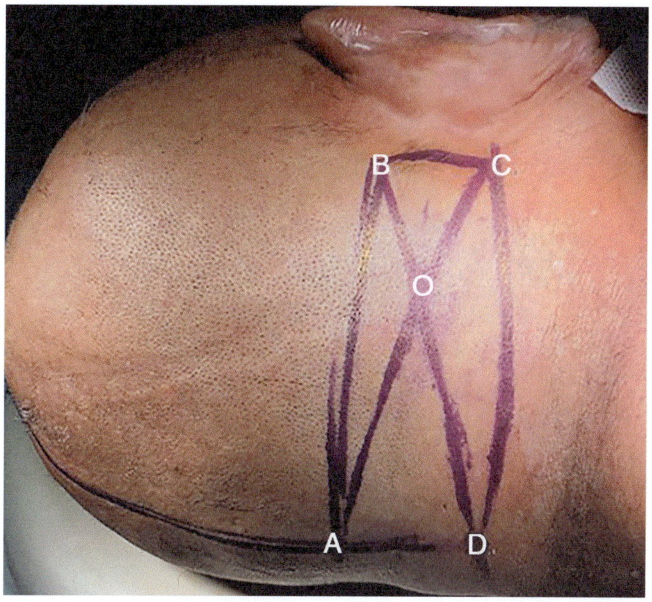

Fig. 18.2 Determining the lower boundary (marker) skull base line AB, BC, CD, and AD represents the external scalp projection of the posterior cranial fossa boundary on the affected side

18.4.1.2 Puncture Surgical Approach (Pathway)

1. Head CT Interpretation: Preoperative standard OM-line cranial CT scans (with bilateral lenses and the external auditory meatus symmetrically appearing on the skull base level) are crucial for the success of puncture surgery. Carefully interpreting the preoperative head CT to determine the basal layer (Fig. 18.3a), puncture layer (Fig. 18.3d), puncture point X, and measuring the distance from point X (scalp) to the distal end of the brainstem hemorrhage (hematoma) to establish the theoretical catheter depth, which typically range between 7.5 and 8.5 cm (Fig. 18.3).
2. Determining Puncture Point X.

   The intersection of the diagonals of quadrilateral ABCD at point O and its vicinity is considered a relatively safe puncture point for brainstem hematoma, avoiding vital anatomical structures.

   Mark the standard and common puncture points for infratentorial hematoma puncture: Point X, the intersection of the line extending from the apex nasi to the central point of the affected side's external auditory pore and line OB, serves as the empirical puncture point for infratentorial hematoma puncture, also applicable to brainstem (pons) hematomas (Fig. 18.4).
3. Determining the Puncture Direction: After determining puncture point X, based on standard head CT observations of the morphology and positional classification of pontine hematomas, establish the end position (destination) for inserting the drainage catheter. From the puncture point (starting point), draw a line passing through the destination and intersecting with the scalp, setting that point as Y, the line XY represents the surgical path for inserting the drainage catheter.

   Dorsal or Fourth Ventricle Penetrating Pontine Hematoma: When puncturing for catheter placement, aim towards the midpoint of the lateral edge of the contralateral (healthy side) supraorbital ridge (processus zygonaticls) and the apex of the ear. This point is Y, and the surgical path is XY.

   Central Pontine Hematoma: When puncturing for catheter placement, aim towards the lateral edge of the

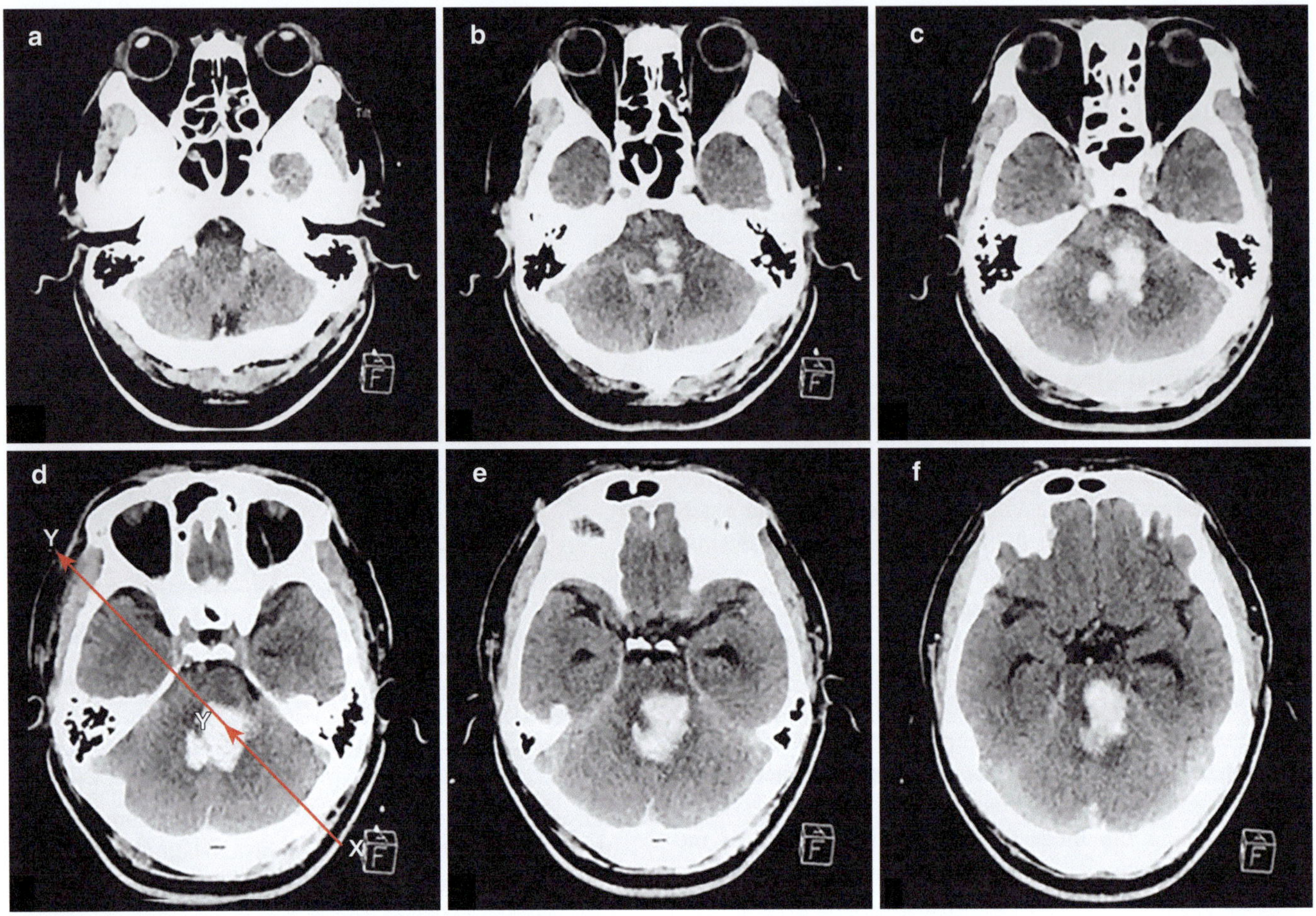

Fig. 18.3 (**a**) Head CT interpretation. (**b**, **c**) Preoperative head CT to determine the basal layer. (**d**) Puncture layer, measuring the distance from point X. (**e**, **f**) Establish the theoretical catheter

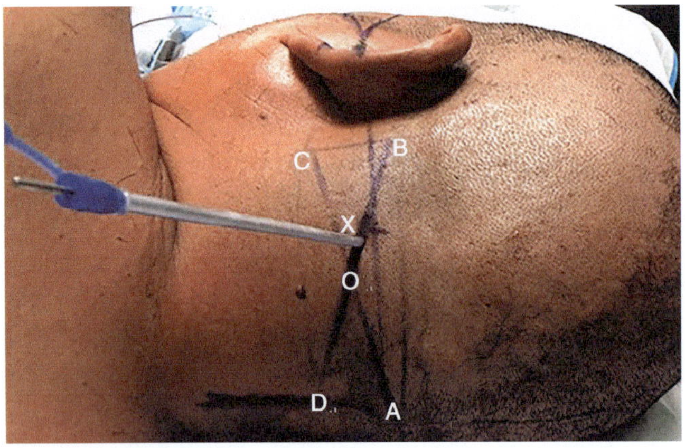

Fig. 18.4 Determining puncture point X

contralateral (healthy side) supraorbital ridge (processus zygonaticls). This point is Y, and the surgical path is XY.

Ventral Pontine Hematoma: When puncturing for catheter placement, aim towards the midpoint of the contralateral (healthy side) supraorbital ridge. This point is Y, and the surgical path is XY.

4. Determining the Orthotopic Scalp Projection Line of the Surgical Path: In the supine position, with a line connecting the lateral canthus and the external auditory pore perpendicular to the bed surface (horizontal plane), use an infrared level to mark the shortest arc passing through points X and Y, intersecting the scalp at the intersection with the largest (midline) sagittal plane (scalp projection line of the superior sagittal sinus), denoted as point E; marked with a methyl violet solution, XEY—this arc segment represents the orthotopic scalp projection line for the puncture surgical path (Fig. 18.5).
5. Determining the Lateral Scalp Projection Line of the Surgical Path: In the lateral decubitus position on the healthy side, mark the midpoint of the lateral edge of the affected side's supraorbital ridge and the apex of the ear as point Z, line segment XZ represents the lateral scalp projection line of the puncture surgical path (Fig. 18.5, Video 18.1).

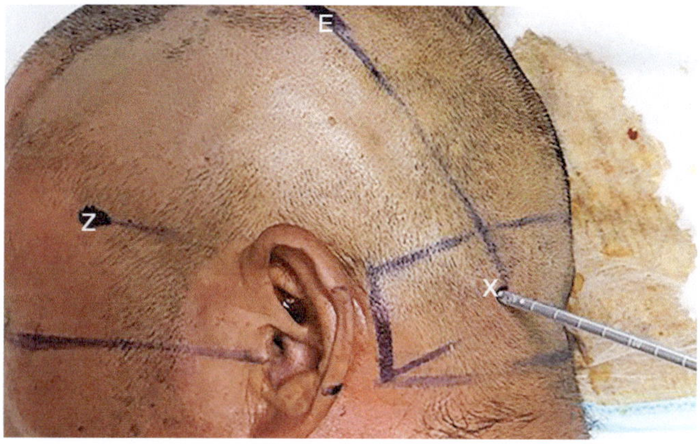

Fig. 18.5 Determining the orthotopic scalp projection line of the surgical path

18.4.2 Surgical Procedure and Steps

Depending on the severity of the patient's condition, the medical environment of the hospital and department, the surgical operation can be performed in the central operating room, the CT hybrid operating room (under CT guidance), the minimally invasive operation room in the neuro ICU, ICU bedside, and other locations.

1. Positioning: Take the healthy side lateral decubitus position, with the head slightly flexed toward the sternum, expose the affected side, and align the midsagittal line with the bed surface.
2. Define the quadrilateral ABCD (same as above) of the body surface projection of the posterior cranial fossa boundary on the affected side.
3. Define the puncture point A (same as above).
4. Define the orthotopic scalp projection line XEY for the puncture surgical path (same as above).
5. Define the lateral scalp projection line XZ of the puncture surgical path (same as above).
6. Anesthesia: After routine preoperative preparation, local infiltration anesthesia + intravenous enhancement anesthesia.
7. Establishment of bone hole: According to the thickness of the scalp at the puncture site, place the limiting device of the bone drill at 3.0–3.5 cm, hold the rapid skull drill with the right hand (the palm of the right hand is on the handle, and the five fingers are clenched to hold the triangular drill body), puncture the scalp through the puncture point (do not slide the scalp in a relaxed state) to Y, that is the longitudinal axis of the drill body, consistent with the lateral and orthotopic projection lines (direction), penetrate the skull and break the dura mater to enter the cranial cavity.

18.4.3 Technical Points

Keep the scalp hole, skull hole, and dural tear on the same path.

1. Catheter preparation: Open the disposable cranial external drainage tube, and moisten the guiding needle with iodine cotton swab and insert the guide needle into the end of the drainage catheter.
2. Catheter placement: The left thumb and index finger continue to press down to fix the local scalp around the puncture point. The right hand slowly rotates and withdraws the skull drill. The right hand pinches and holds the drainage catheter along the scalp hole, skull hole, and dural hole, and places it into the cranial cavity. Release the left hand, remove the drape, pinch and hold the drainage catheter with the right hand, and control the direction with the left hand (the direction of the guide needle is consistent with the lateral and orthotopic projection lines), push forward, deep about 7.5–8.5 cm (individualized, according to preoperative CT measurement).
3. Aspiration: Slowly withdraw the guide needle (do not change the direction of the catheter placement), connect a 5 mL empty syringe for aspiration, and if there is old blood or mixed cerebrospinal fluid, it indicates successful catheter placement. The aspiration volume is determined according to the amount of bleeding, usually 3.0–10.0 mL.
4. Installation of disposable cranial external drainage tube: Disinfect the local area, lay a drape through the drainage catheter (the drape can be cut from sterile gauze), connect the proximal end of the drainage catheter to a three-way valve, then connect a disposable cranial external drainage tube, suture the scalp, fix the drainage catheter, bandage, and suspend the drainage tube with a dropper. The height of the end of the drip tube in the dropper should be between 50 and 150 mm away from the vertical height of the external auditory pore, and positive pressure drainage is used.
5. Implementation of liquefaction drainage: 2–4 h after surgery, the first liquefaction is performed, using a 5 mL empty syringe to prepare urokinase (50,000–100,000 U) or alteplase 1–2 mg, dissolved in 3–5 mL saline, slowly injected into the hematoma cavity through the heparin cap of the three-way valve (routine disinfection), and the three-way valve is closed for 1–2 h before opening, once or twice a day.
6. Re-examination of head CT to dynamically observe the changes of the hematoma, observe the location and shape of the residual hematoma, effectively exert the effect of the hematoma liquefying agents, fully melt the blood

clot, and drain the old blood out of the body through head position changes.

7. Catheter removal: The brainstem hematoma is basically cleared, there is no bleeding in the fourth ventricle, and the aqueduct of midbrain, fourth ventricle, ambient cistern, and quadrigeminal cistern is clear and visible. The cerebrospinal fluid circulation is unobstructed, without hydrocephalus and the drainage catheter can be removed.

18.4.4 About Liquefaction Surgery

In recent years, neurosurgery has been developing towards the direction of minimally invasive, precise and refined surgery. As we all know, drainage is a commonly used method of clinical minimally invasive surgery. The core technology of correct and reasonable application of drainage is liquefaction.

1. First of all, choose standardized, suitable and reasonable drainage products (instruments).
2. Reasonably and efficiently use liquefying agents. The commonly used liquefying agents for extravascular intracranial hematoma in clinical practice are usually urokinase and alteplase.

   At present, the use of liquefying agents is based on factors such as the onset time, size of the hematoma, degree of coagulation of the hematoma, coagulation indicators, and thromboelastography. Generally, urokinase 20,000–100,000 U + 3–5 mL saline, or alteplase 1–3 mg + 3–5 mL saline are used to infuse the hematoma cavity to perform hematoma liquefaction.
3. The position of the patient's head is also one of the factors affecting the liquefaction effect. An appropriate posture is conducive to the liquefaction effect of urokinase.

18.4.5 Precautions and Techniques

1. Minimally invasive surgical treatment of brainstem hemorrhage soft channel clearance is achieved by placing a drainage catheter and implementing suction, liquefaction, and external drainage techniques.

   Regardless of the bleeding (hematoma) in the cerebellum, fourth ventricle, brainstem (pons), and other parts, the infratentorial puncture point is basically fixed for safety and ease of operation. What needs to be changed is the surgical path, that is, the puncture direction, and the key is to determine the Y point.
2. The puncture surgical operation should avoid the transverse sinus and enter along the long axis of the hematoma as much as possible.
3. For the central type of pontine hemorrhage and the pontine hemorrhage near the midline, a left-sided approach is usually selected to place the drainage catheter.
4. Under the condition of comparable therapeutic effect, try to choose the left puncture point, because the left transverse sinus is often thinner than the right and easier to avoid.
5. When a hematoma ruptures into the fourth ventricle, do not excessively drain cerebrospinal fluid to prevent low intracranial pressure and pneumocephalus.
6. Ensure the sealing and integrity of the "disposable cranial external drainage tube" to prevent backflow and use it correctly.

18.5 Postoperative Care and Prevention of Complications

Surgical complications mainly include rebleeding, infection, hypotension, and pneumocephalus, which can occur intraoperatively or postoperatively. Any invasive procedure faces the challenge of complications such as bleeding and infection.

18.5.1 Intraoperative and Postoperative Bleeding

18.5.1.1 Causes of Bleeding

The occurrence and development of brainstem hemorrhage until the formation of relatively stable hematomas is essentially a process of hemodynamic changes. One of the complications during and after modified directional brainstem hematoma evacuation surgery is bleeding, commonly seen along the surgical pathways such as the scalp at the puncture point, diploic veins (venous sinuses), epidural space, subdural space, cerebellar parenchyma, fourth ventricle, subarachnoid space, etc.

Fresh bleeding on dressings, drainage catheters draining fresh arterial blood (coagulated or non-coagulated), significant blood drainage in the collection bag (excluding cerebrospinal fluid, not matching the estimated volume from the head CT), worsening or no improvement in the patient's condition, uncontrollable hypertension, restlessness, altered consciousness, pupil changes, muscle strength and muscle tone changes—all necessitate prompt reevaluation with a head CT.

18.5.1.2 Preventive Measures for Intraoperative and Postoperative Rebleeding

1. Blood Pressure Control: Some scholars suggest maintaining an average arterial pressure not exceeding 130 mmHg

without the need for lowering blood pressure. Within the first 3 days following onset, avoid lowering blood pressure to the normal upper limit of 140/90 mmHg as reduced blood pressure can lead to poor cerebral perfusion, causing cerebral ischemia. Recent studies have shown that excessively high blood pressure can lead to hematoma expansion, even triggering new bleeding. Enlargement of brainstem hemorrhage worsens the patient's condition and jeopardizes their life. Therefore, close monitoring of blood pressure is essential to prevent perioperative rebleeding. The three-word policy of "pressure control, hemostasis, sedation" is an effective preventive measure.

Blood pressure management involves regulating both blood pressure and intracranial pressure to maintain normal cerebral perfusion pressure. The cessation of bleeding results from achieving a balance in the pressure gradient inside and outside the ruptured blood vessel. Controlling blood pressure, especially systolic pressure, and maintaining a relatively high intracranial pressure are advantageous in achieving this equilibrium, playing a certain role in preventing rebleeding and further hematoma enlargement. The use of antihypertensive medications with selective action on cerebral blood vessels to maintain blood pressure within the range of 110–160/70–95 mmHg not only avoids causing organic cerebral ischemia but also aids in hemostasis.

2. Hemostasis: The goal of hemostasis is to stop bleeding, stabilize the hematoma, and prevent further expansion of the hematoma. Hence, the use of hemostatic agents should be immediate to save every second. Once brain (brainstem) bleeding is discovered or confirmed during or after surgery, or if there are risk factors for unstable brain bleeding such as chronic alcoholism, chronic liver disease, hematologic disorders, oral intake of platelet inhibitors, anticoagulants like aspirin, clopidogrel, indobufen, warfarin, or known coagulation disorders, hemostatic agents must be applied promptly.

   Ideal hemostatic agents should:

   Enhance hemostasis in patients with normal coagulation function.

   Act locally at sites of endothelial cell rupture or vessel injury.

   Have antifibrinolytic effects.

   Have a rapid onset, short half-life, and no systemic adverse reactions.

   Snake venom thrombin-like enzymes (batroxobin, ancrod) meet some of these conditions. It is recommended for single-use, with a dosage of 1KU intravenous infusion +1–2KU intramuscular injection.

   Recombinant activated factor VII (rFVIIa) is a vitamin K-dependent glycoprotein and the initiator of hemostasis. It carries a lower risk of causing systemic hypercoagulability and thrombosis, promoting local hemostasis at the site of vascular injury in both coagulation disorders and normal coagulation function individuals. It acts quickly, with a half-life of 2.6 h, aligning with the high-risk period for ongoing brain (brainstem) bleeding, making it an ideal hemostatic agent with potential.

   Depending on the patient's clinical history, other measures that may be considered include intravenous infusion of vitamin K, cryoprecipitate, platelets, plasma, and other blood products.

3. Sedation and Analgesia: For restless patients, sedation and analgesia are beneficial for stabilizing blood pressure. After brainstem hemorrhage, fluctuations in intracranial pressure and blood pressure can cause discomfort and headaches, along with emotional changes such as restlessness, nervousness, and fear, potentially leading to stress-induced hypertension, triggering rebleeding, and further hematoma expansion.

Drugs that may be used include the intravenous administration of diazepam, midazolam, dexmedetomidine, propofol, pentazocine, butorphanol, flupirtine, fentanyl, and measures such as chloral hydrate enemas.

When performing a cone drill puncture for a brainstem hematoma, care should be taken to avoid damaging the vertebral artery and the transverse sinus.

If inadvertent injury to the transverse sinus is noted during surgery, the procedure should be immediately halted. A silicone tube matching the skull hole should be inserted to compress and stop the bleeding, to be removed after 3–5 days; if necessary, hemostasis should be performed under direct visualization through craniotomy.

18.5.2 Postoperative Infection

18.5.2.1 Causes

The main risk factors related to surgical and invasive procedure-associated infections include preoperative hospital stay duration, prepping method and duration, aseptic practices during surgery, the surgical techniques and skills, duration of surgery, use of prophylactic antibiotics, skin disinfection at the surgical site, the operating room environment, and the sterilization of surgical instruments.

Risk factors for secondary intracranial infections following brainstem hemorrhage surgery also include excessive (or prolonged) placement of drainage and monitoring catheters, neglect or improper care of external drainage catheters, overly frequent injection of liquefying agents (urokinase, alteplase) into the intracranial space (hematoma cavity) via drainage catheters, delayed suspicion and diagnosis of intracranial infection, among others.

18.5.2.2 Measures for Preventing Intracranial Infections

Strict adherence to aseptic principles is essential for preventing intracranial infections, including maintaining the sterility of surgical instruments and the surgical environment.

Timely dressing changes postoperatively.

Mastering the techniques and skills of "modified directional minimally invasive evacuation of intracranial hematoma" to promptly remove hematomas and shorten the duration of drainage.

Prompt removal or replacement of drainage catheters and external drainage devices.

The technique of intracavitary infusion of urokinase into brainstem hematomas is an important step, and the dosage must be sufficient while minimizing the frequency of medication administration.

18.5.2.3 Indications of Suspected Intracranial Infections

Fever: The causes of fever need to be differentiated, such as intracranial infections, fever due to absorption of blood, central fever, incisional skin infection, bronchial infection, pulmonary infections, urinary tract infection, central venous catheter infection, intracranial pressure monitoring catheter infection, or infection related to external drainage catheters.

18.5.2.3.1 Exacerbation of Meningeal Irritation Signs

Confirmation is achieved through cerebrospinal fluid routine examination, cytology, biochemistry, culture, and genetic testing, among other measures.

18.5.3 Hypotension and Pneumocephalus

Hypotension occurs when excessive and rapid suctioning of blood and cerebrospinal fluid during surgery, as well as excessive postoperative drainage of blood and/or cerebrospinal fluid, takes place.

Pneumocephalus occurs when gas enters the intracranial space due to improper management during surgical procedures involving transient hypotension, the infusion of urokinase solution into the hematoma cavity during liquefaction procedures, elevating the head of the bed, changes in patient positioning, or even sitting up during a follow-up head CT scan.

Proper use of "disposable cranial external drainage systems" to maintain unobstructed drainage can prevent or reduce the occurrence of complications such as hypotension, pneumocephalus, and intracranial infections.

18.6 Advantages, Disadvantages, and Lessons Learned

The principle of modern neurosurgery is to remove lesions, preserve anatomical structures, and restore function. Under this principle, minimally invasive surgery for treating intracerebral hemorrhage has become a consensus.

Since the early 1990s, puncture therapy for intracerebral hemorrhage has been clinically applied and continuously explored. Over the past two decades, puncture therapy for cerebral hemorrhage has developed and been widely promoted in clinical practice. Particularly in county and city-level hospitals, the soft channel technique for treating cerebral hemorrhage has become one of the important surgical methods for cerebral hemorrhage.

In the surgical treatment of brainstem hemorrhage, precision surgery emphasizing lesion clearance (hematoma) as a means, minimally invasive surgery aiming to maximize the preservation of anatomical structures as the goal, is emphasized to improve efficacy, with the ultimate objective being the maximal restoration of function.

The modified directional soft channel intracranial hematoma evacuation surgery for brainstem hemorrhage is a simple directional surgery guided by cranial CT imaging. It involves using a micro-hole (4–5 mm diameter) tapered cranial drill technique to insert a 12F (4 mm) drainage catheter from the infratentorial scalp to the brainstem (pons) hematoma, establishing a channel for external drainage of the hematoma. Through intraoperative aspiration and postoperative infusion of liquefying agents, the hematoma in the brainstem is liquefied and drained out under the effect of intracranial pressure, emptying the hematoma.

18.6.1 Advantages

1. Easy localization and operation using cranial anatomical landmarks and cranial CT imaging data, enabling operations to be performed at the bedside of critically ill patients with brainstem hemorrhage (e.g., brain herniation, deep coma, or even respiratory arrest) in the intensive care unit, saving crucial time.
2. The specially designed drainage catheter of the "disposable cranial external drainage device" has a smooth ball-shaped end with side holes, causing minimal damage to brain tissue during insertion.
3. The drainage catheter is made of high-quality silicone material with markings, producing no artifacts on CT scans, can be operated under CT guidance. This allows for accurate placement of the catheter within the brainstem hematoma, ensuring thorough hematoma clearance.

4. The direction of the drainage catheter can be adjusted or altered.
5. The injection of liquefaction agents (e.g., urokinase, r-tPA) through the heparin cap on the three-way valve is more convenient. Collection of drainage fluid, cerebrospinal fluid, and other samples through the three-way valve for examination is easier and more reliable.
6. The anti-reflux device helps to prevent intracranial infections.
7. Monitoring intracranial pressure during drainage allows for relative adjustment of intracranial pressure when a brainstem hematoma communicates with the fourth ventricle.

18.6.2 Disadvantages

1. Surgeons need to have a good understanding of cranial anatomy and spatial thinking ability.
2. Novices may lack precision in positioning and puncture direction, requiring precise preoperative mapping of the shortest straight and lateral scalp projection lines, or the completion of the operation under CT guidance.
3. The operation is essentially blind puncturing, even when performed in a mobile CT hybrid operating room. It relies on preoperative localization, intraoperative guidance, and postoperative verification, lacking real-time guidance.

Therefore, to perform puncture surgery for brainstem hematoma through a soft channel effectively, one needs to be familiar with cranial (brainstem) anatomy, grasp the concept of modified directional intracranial hematoma puncture and aspiration, and master the corresponding techniques and skills proficiently.

18.6.3 Experience and Lessons Learned

1. Accurately select commonly used surface puncture points.
2. Collect information from cranial CT scans and conduct a preoperative head CT scan to obtain the most accurate imaging data before surgical procedures.

   Requirements: Strictly base the CT images on the OM line (CT scans can be reconstructed according to standards after a plain scan). Simulate and determine the puncture point (scalp puncture point) on the head CT image, define the location point of the drainage catheter end (destination), and measure the depth, typically between 7.5 and 8.5 cm. The principle is to insert the catheter along the long axis of the hematoma to the far end of the hematoma.
3. Based on the standard morphological and positional characteristics of brainstem hematomas on cranial CT scans, determine the surgical (catheter placement) path and mark (draw) the shortest orthotopic and lateral scalp projection lines of the surgical path.
4. Use a rapid cranial bone drill to pierce the scalp, and penetrate the skull and dura mater in one go, ensuring that the scalp hole, skull hole, and dura mater hole are on the same path.
5. After smoothly inserting the drainage catheter into the cranial cavity under the guidance of a 1.5–2 mm outer diameter guiding steel needle, remove the drape. When inserting the catheter, ensure that the drainage catheter aligns with the orthotopic and lateral scalp projection lines of the surgical path. Verification can be done using an infrared level or a mobile surface positioning software.
6. Regarding catheter depth, a large number of cases and radiological data confirm that the typical depth from the scalp to the edge of the fourth ventricle is 7 cm. The catheter depth for brainstem hematomas depends on the location and size of the hematoma and generally ranges between 7.5 and 8.5 cm (individualized principles should be adhered to for specific patients).
7. When removing the guiding steel needle (Kirschner needle), do not deviate from the planned path (direction).
8. Slowly aspirate using a 5 mm empty syringe to achieve partial decompression and verify the position of the catheter tip within the hematoma cavity.
9. Liquefaction is a core technique. Following the principle of minimal but adequate doses, determine the amount of liquefying agent and liquid based on the size of the hematoma, the duration of the disease, and the patient's condition. Generally, administer 1–2 infusions per day, with each infusion prepared using 2.5–5 mL of saline, 20,000–100,000 U of urokinase, or 1–3 mg of alteplase. If the hematoma in the pons ruptures into the fourth ventricle, more liquefying agent and liquid may be used. If it is a purely central pontine hematoma, the liquid preparation should be less than 3 mL.
10. Re-examine the head CT scan to determine the relationship between the catheter end and the hematoma. During liquefaction, utilize the principles of fluid dynamics to maximize the efficacy of the thrombolytic agent by changing the head position.
11. Re-examine the head CT scan to dynamically observe changes in brainstem hematomas to guide clinical treatment.
12. If necessary, reinsert (replace) the drainage catheter and drainage device based on the latest head CT scan.
13. For brainstem hemorrhage, if there is a blockage in the cerebrospinal fluid circulation, routine external lateral ventricular drainage may be necessary.

Due to the high mortality and morbidity rates associated with severe brainstem hemorrhage, especially in comatose patients, a significant portion of surviving patients may be bedridden long-term or even in a vegetative state. This poses a heavy burden on families and society. Whether to opt for surgical treatment is a serious topic. Surgeons need to engage in comprehensive and in-depth communication with family members, thoroughly weighing the pros and cons of surgical intervention.

After assessment, for some severely affected patients who may benefit from surgical intervention for brainstem (pons) hemorrhage, the application of the "modified directional intracranial hematoma puncture and aspiration" technique for hematoma clearance may be considered.

18.7 Typical Cases

18.7.1 Case 1

18.7.1.1 Brief Medical History and Imaging Data

Patient: Male, 45 years old. Admitted to the emergency room on February 26, 2012, at 17:30 due to a sudden onset of coma lasting for 3 h. Upon examination, blood pressure was 185/105 mmHg, respiratory rate 11 breaths/min, heart rate 95 beats/min, body temperature 36.8 °C. The patient was comatose, with a GCS of 4, exhibiting decerebrate rigidity, irregular breathing, pinpoint pupils with absent light reflex, and a positive Babinski sign bilaterally. Head CT revealed brainstem hemorrhage. Admission diagnosis: Primary brainstem hemorrhage, severe hypertension (grade 3), extremely high-risk group, central respiratory failure. The patient was intubated for mechanical ventilation and received standard neurointensive care and treatment. On the third day of hospitalization, after a discussion with family members, surgical intervention was decided. A follow-up head CT scan showed an estimated hemorrhage volume of approximately 11.0 mL calculated using the Coniglobus formula (Fig. 18.6).

18.7.1.2 Surgical Procedure and Key Points

After local infiltration anesthesia, the patient was positioned in the right lateral decubitus on the operating table with a head cushion, ensuring the head remained in a horizontal position in the maximum sagittal plane. Fine adjustments and verification were made based on the preoperative CT-guided puncture site to allow for entry along the long axis of the hematoma. A grooved hand drill was used to bluntly puncture the scalp at the puncture point, establish a bone hole, and place the catheter. Gentle aspiration was applied, and while slowly rotating the empty needle body, approximately 4 mL of old blood was gently withdrawn (Fig. 18.7). The scalp was sutured, the drainage catheter was secured, a dressing was applied, and a disposable cranial external drainage device was connected before returning to the ward.

18.7.1.3 Postoperative Treatment and Imaging Comparison

Six hours postoperatively, 30,000 U of urokinase with 2.5 mL of saline solution was slowly injected into the hematoma cavity through the heparin cap on the side arm of a three-way valve, followed by supine positioning with the three-way valve closed for 1 h. On the second day post-surgery, another dose of 30,000 U of urokinase with 2.5 mL of saline solution was administered for liquefaction. A follow-up head CT scan (Fig. 18.8) showed partial clearance of the brainstem hematoma and appropriate positioning of the

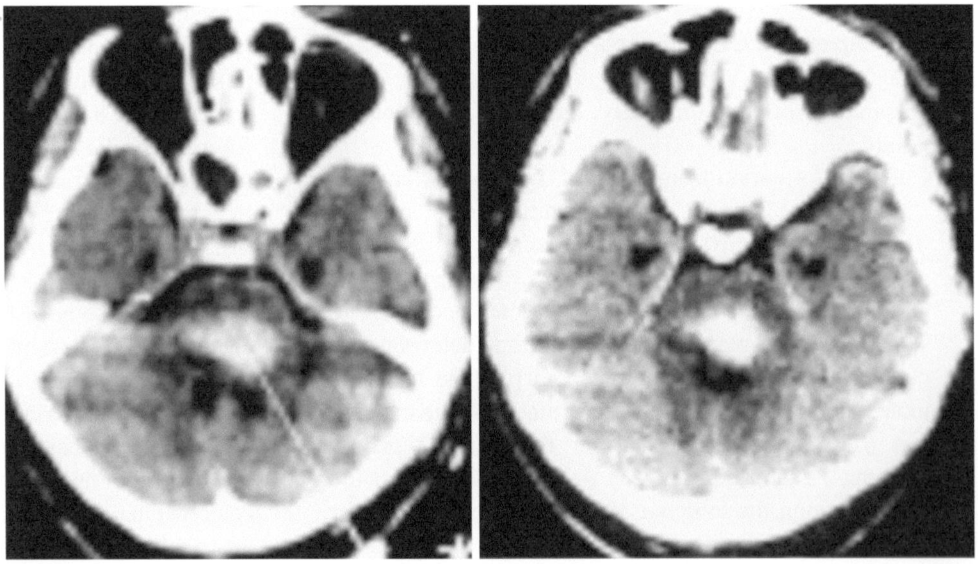

Fig. 18.6 Follow-up head CT scan

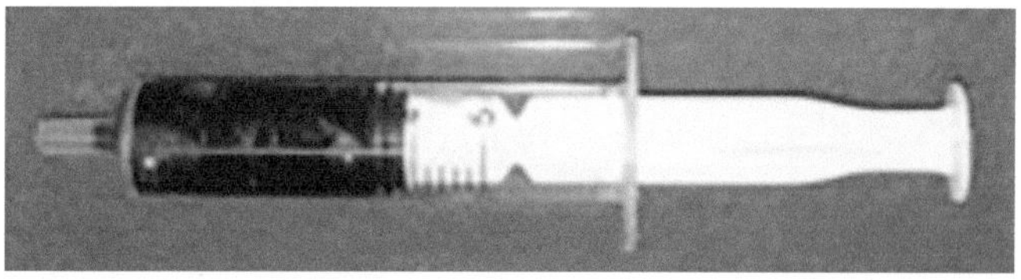

Fig. 18.7 Blood drawn from the puncture point

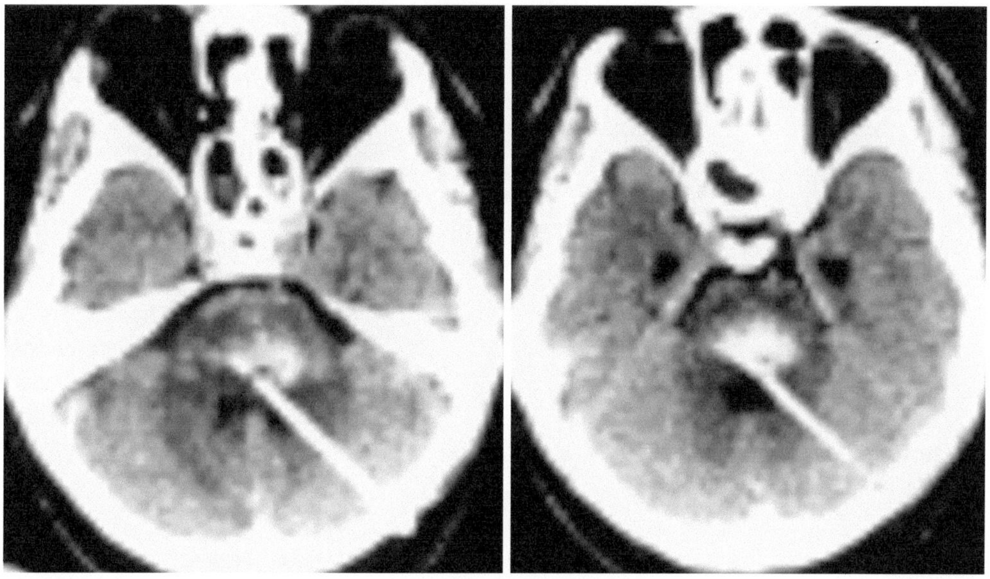

Fig. 18.8 Follow-up head CT scan showing partial clearance of the brainstem

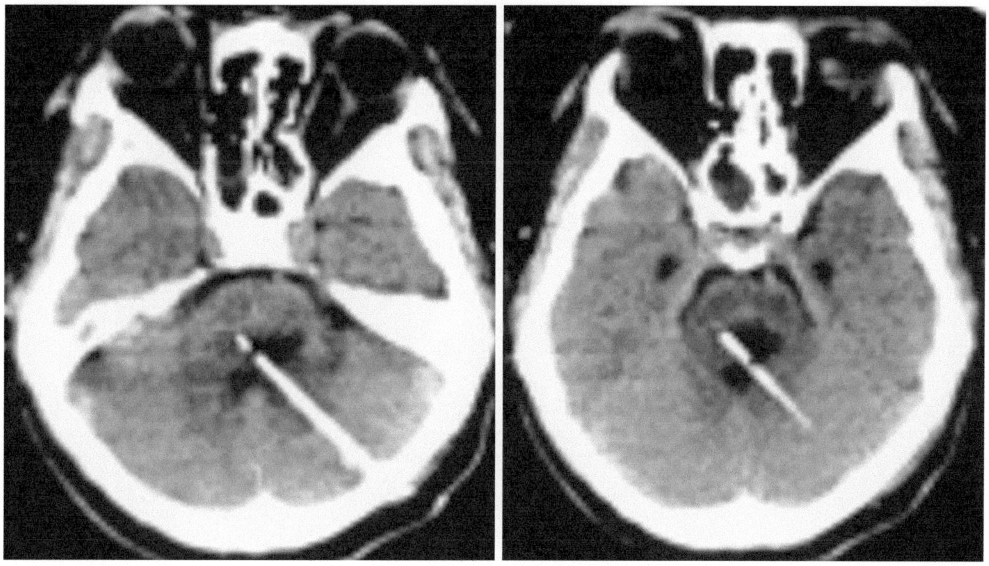

Fig. 18.9 Follow up head CT scan revealing significant clearance of the hematoma

distal end of the drainage catheter. On the third day, a further dose of 30,000 U of urokinase with 2.5 mL of saline solution was used for liquefaction drainage. The drainage tube was opened after closing the three-way valve for 2 h. A follow-up head CT scan (Fig. 18.9) revealed significant clearance of the hematoma, normal cerebrospinal fluid circulation, no hydrocephalus, and minimal brain edema, leading to the removal of the drainage catheter (Fig. 18.10).

Follow-up: Two years later, the patient survived but remained mostly wheelchair-bound and dependent on others for daily activities.

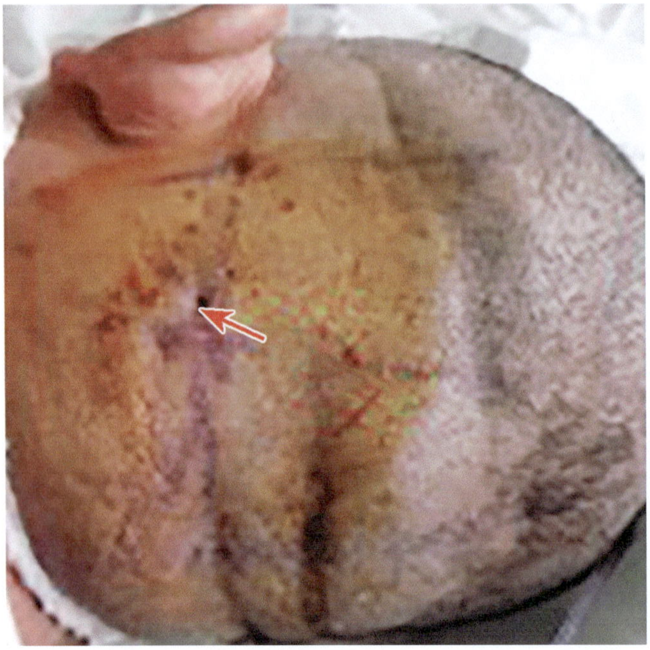

Fig. 18.10 Minimal brain edema, leading to the removal of the drainage catheter

18.7.2 Case 2

18.7.2.1 Brief Medical History and Imaging Data

Female patient, 50 years old. Admitted to the emergency room with sudden coma lasting for 2 h, at a tertiary hospital. History of hypertension for 7 years, irregularly taking antihypertensive medication.

On admission: Temperature: 39.3 °C, Heart rate: 45 beats/min, Respiratory rate: 16 breaths/min (ventilator-assisted), Blood pressure: 185/105 mmHg. Deep coma, bilateral dilated pupils with a diameter of 5 mm, absent light reflex, GCS of 3, cessation of spontaneous breathing, controlled ventilation by the ventilator, flaccid paralysis of all four limbs, muscle strength at 0, no elicited pathological signs.

Admission head CT scan (time: 2017-11-27 11:35, see Fig. 18.11): Massive brainstem hemorrhage extending into the fourth ventricle, involving the midbrain and medulla, leading to secondary expansion of the fourth ventricle with acute obstructive hydrocephalus.

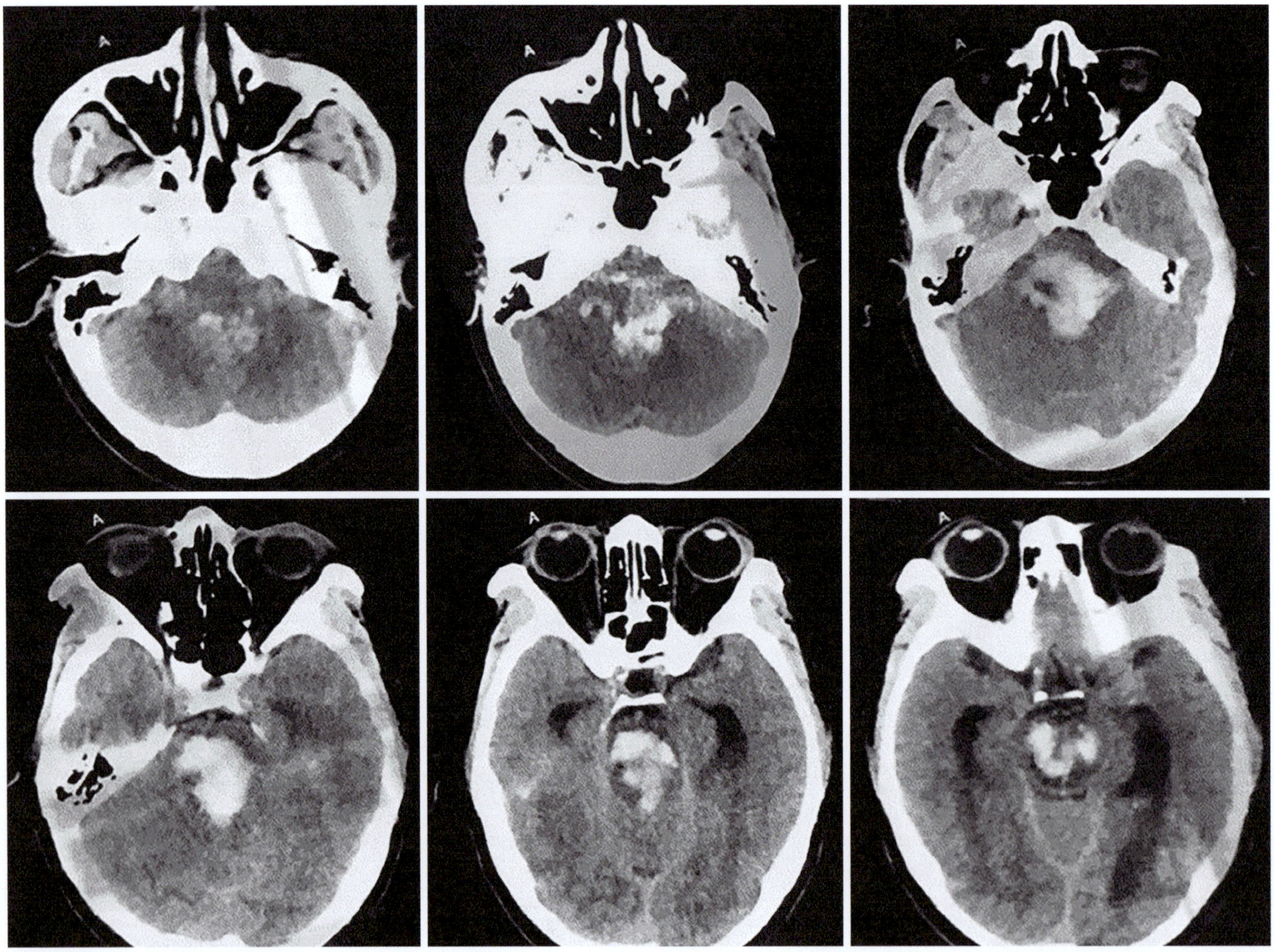

Fig. 18.11 Admission head CT scan

Admission diagnosis: Primary brainstem hemorrhage, hypertension (grade 3, extremely high-risk group), central respiratory failure, stress-related gastrointestinal bleeding, central fever.

18.7.2.2 Surgical Procedure and Key Points

Upon admission, standard neurointensive care and treatment were initiated due to the critical condition of the patient. Despite the severity, the patient's family insisted on surgical intervention. On the same day, a neurosurgeon from the hospital performed a right lateral ventricular puncture and external drainage procedure at the bedside in the ICU to relieve the supratentorial hydrocephalus.

On the second day of hospitalization, the author was consulted, and the patient's family insisted on surgical treatment for the brainstem hematoma. After a thorough discussion with the family, the decision was made to perform a "modified directional intracranial hematoma puncture and aspiration" procedure.

Preoperative skin preparation, reevaluation of head CT scan (standard scan: the lens and external auditory meatus at the same skull base level and symmetric on both sides), and preoperative localization of the brainstem hematoma. The head CT scan showed resolved supratentorial hydrocephalus, with the brainstem hemorrhage (mainly involving the pons) extending into the right thalamus, rupturing into the fourth ventricle, and obstructing cerebrospinal fluid circulation. The estimated hemorrhage volume was approximately 22.7 mL calculated using the Coniglobus formula (Fig. 18.12).

Choosing the left infratentorial approach, the patient was positioned in the right lateral decubitus on the operating table, with a head cushion to maintain the head in a horizontal position within the maximum sagittal plane. Based on the preoperative CT, the puncture point was located (Fig. 18.13a, b), determining the surgical path along the long axis of the hematoma, aimed towards the corresponding point on the contralateral scalp (processus zygonaticls), and drawing the

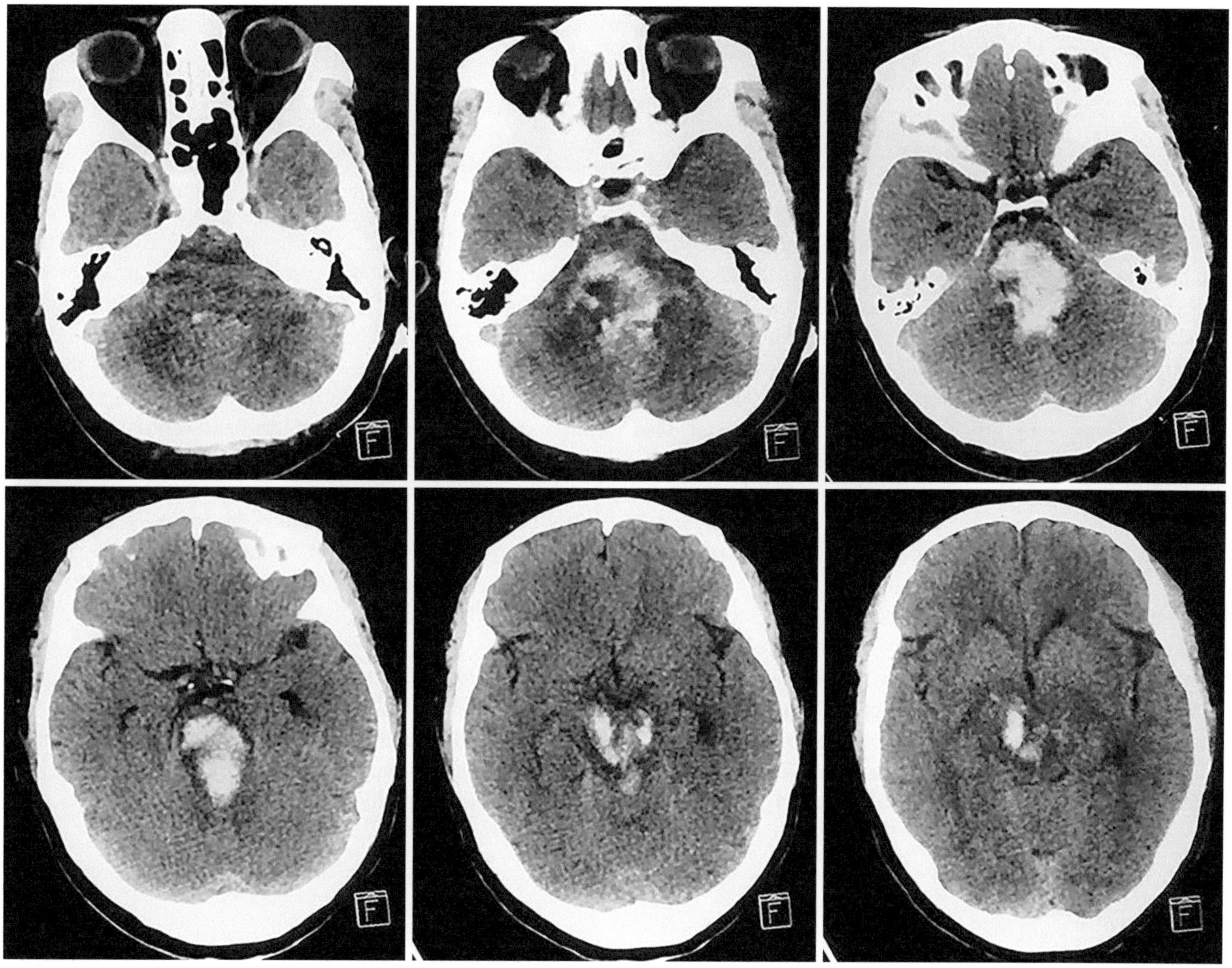

Fig. 18.12 Preoperative skin preparation, reevaluation head CT scan

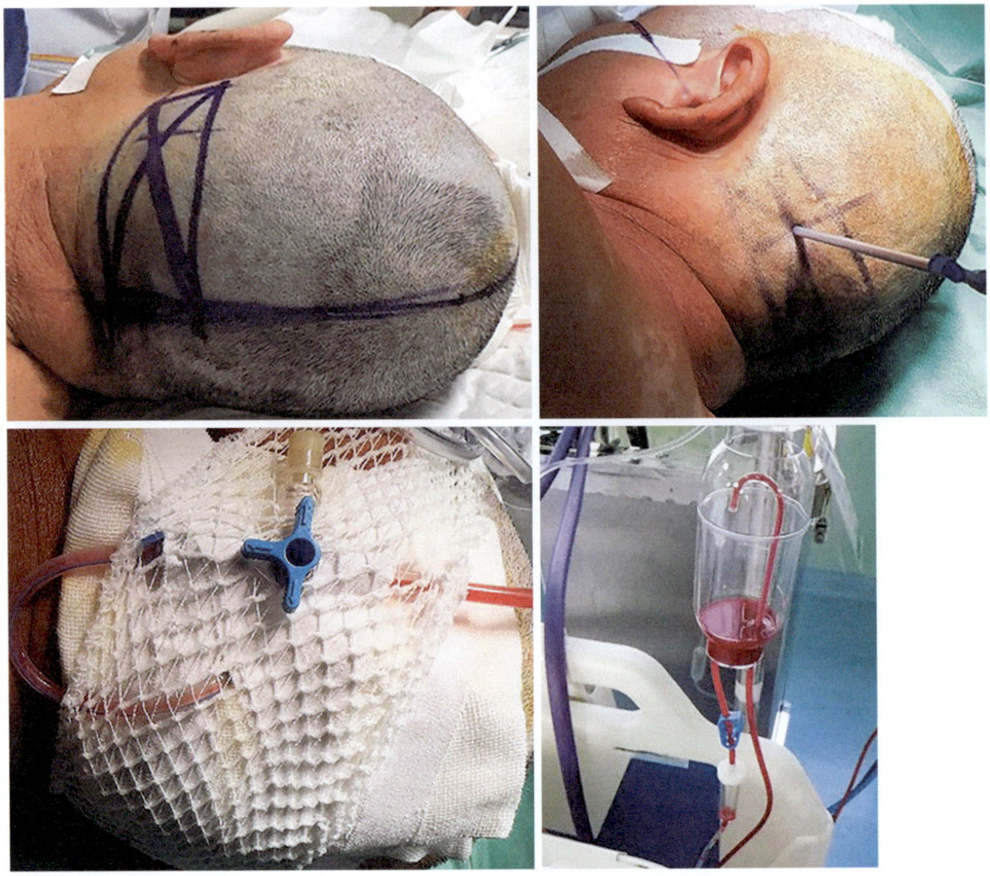

Fig. 18.13 (**a**, **b**) patient positioned in the right lateral decubitus on the operating table, puncture point located by preoperative CT. (**c**, **d**) Old blood slowly aspirated multiple times, catheter secured, dressed, and connected to the drainage device

projection lines of the surgical path on the scalp in orthotopic and lateral views (shortest). A grooved hand drill was used to directly pierce the scalp (deep coma, GCS of 3), penetrate the skull and dura mater, establish the surgical channel, and place the catheter. Gentle suction was applied, while slowly rotating the empty needle, approximately 10 mL of old blood was slowly aspirated multiple times. The catheter was secured, dressed, and connected to the drainage device (Fig. 18.13c, d), and the patient was returned to the ward.

18.7.2.3 Postoperative Treatment and Imaging Comparison

Four hours postoperatively, a hematoma liquefaction external drainage procedure was performed, with urokinase solution infused into the hematoma cavity twice daily (refer to Sect. 18.4); follow-up head CT scans were conducted to monitor hematoma changes.

On the fourth day post-surgery, a head CT scan was performed (Fig. 18.14): The hematoma was mostly cleared, normal cerebrospinal fluid circulation, no hydrocephalus, minimal brain edema, and the drainage catheter was removed.

Postoperatively, with intensive care and comprehensive treatment, the patient's vital signs gradually stabilized and improved.

Three days post-surgery, spontaneous breathing resumed, cough reflex returned, and intermittent ventilator weaning was initiated. Three weeks later, the patient was essentially weaned off the ventilator. Brainstem function was severely damaged as indicated by somatosensory evoked potential testing performed 3 weeks after onset, and hyperbaric oxygen therapy was administered 6 weeks after the onset, along with standard passive rehabilitation treatment.

18.7.2.4 Postoperative Neurological Examination (Fig. 18.15)

Follow-up: Followed up for 26 months, the patient remains alive, in a comatose state, receiving nasogastric feeding, bedridden, and still partially dependent on a ventilator.

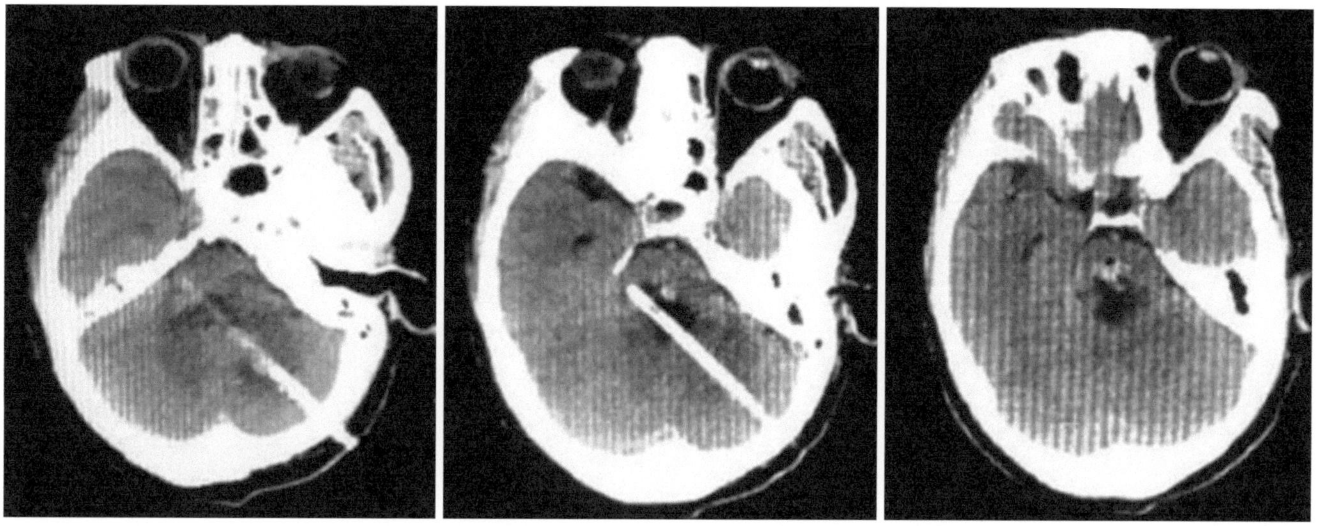

Fig. 18.14 (**a**) Follow-up head CT scans to monitor hematoma changes post operation. (**b**) Head CT scan fourth day post-surgery showing cleared, normal cerebrospinal fluid circulation. (**c**) Drainage catheter removed

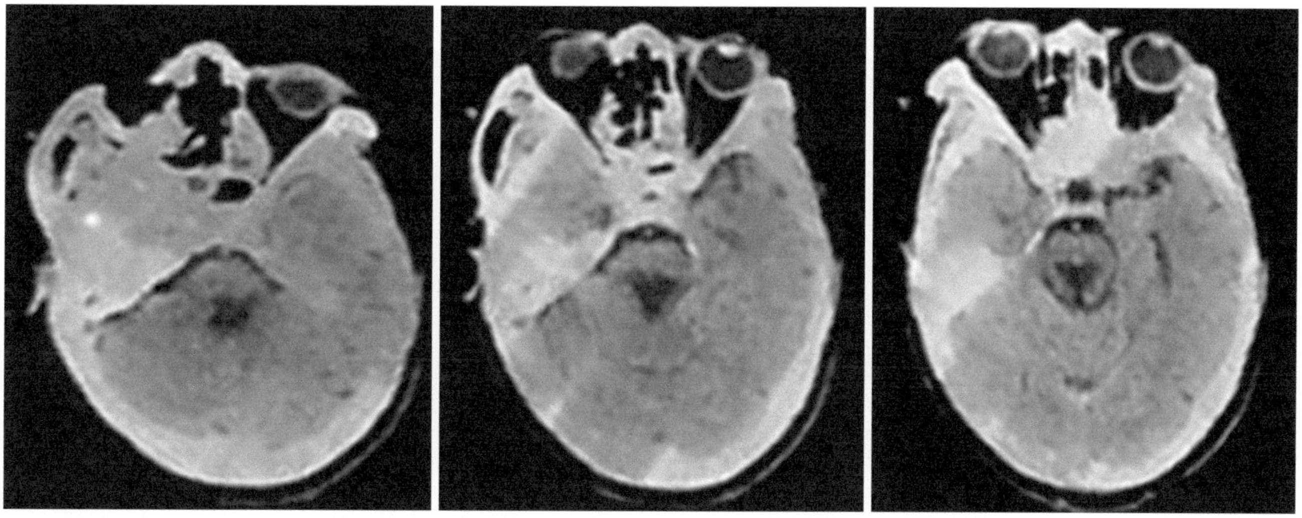

Fig. 18.15 (**a**) Postoperative neurological examination 3 days post-surgery; (**b**) 3 weeks post surgery, (**c**) 26 months post surgery

19 Puncture and Aspiration Evacuation of Brainstem Hematoma Via 3D Printing-Assisted Localization

Zefu Li, Qingbo Wang, and Yu Li

19.1 Overview

With the development of precision medicine, minimally invasive puncture techniques for brainstem hemorrhage, known for their simplicity, safety, swiftness, and minimal tissue damage, have gradually gained recognition. The number of hospitals and specialists applying this technique in clinical practice has also increased [1]. However, accurate and safe puncture of brainstem hemorrhage is crucial to ensure treatment effectiveness and prevent complications. Factors such as CT localization errors, operator deviations, and individual patient differences can lead to deviations in puncture direction and distance, resulting in puncture failure.

3D printing technology utilizes digital design and 3D printing techniques to create personalized templates, introducing a new method for individualized localization of brainstem hematoma puncture [1, 2]. Since the introduction of 3D printing technology in neurosurgical clinical practice, it has provided patients with a personalized and precise treatment approach through reversed design and production of molds for brainstem hemorrhage puncture surgery [1, 3, 4]. This technique minimizes surgical trauma while maximizing the preservation of brain nerve function. Therefore, 3D-printed template-guided puncture is particularly suitable for the intricate and highly neurofunctional region of the brainstem. This chapter focuses on the localization method of 3D-printed minimally invasive puncture technique for brainstem hematoma.

Supplementary Information The online version contains supplementary material available at https://doi.org/10.1007/978-981-95-8942-5_19.

Z. Li (✉) · Q. Wang
Department of Neurosurgery, Shandong Medical and Pharmaceutical University Hospital, Binzhou, China
e-mail: fly8snow@163.com

Y. Li
Department of Neurosurgery, Zhuhai People's Hospital (The Affiliated Hospital of Beijing Institute of Technology, Zhuhai Clinical Medical College of Jinan University), Zhuhai, China

19.2 Indications and Contraindications for Surgery

19.2.1 Indications

Currently, there is no unified standard for surgical indications and criteria for minimally invasive puncture surgery for brainstem hemorrhage, neither domestically nor internationally. However, the following conditions are generally considered as indications for considering brainstem hematoma puncture surgery:

1. Patients aged below 80 years old, especially those between 40 and 70 years old, are more suitable for puncture surgery.
2. Hematoma volume $\geq$ 5 mL.
3. The maximum bleeding area occupies $\geq$50% of the same level of brainstem cross-sectional area.
4. The main part of the hematoma is in the pons or midbrain, biased towards one side and relatively concentrated. Additionally, the hematoma is close to the surface of the brainstem or has penetrated the brainstem surface or ruptured into the ventricle.
5. Patients with shallow to deep coma, GCS <8 but >3, with or without severe signs of vital sign disturbance.
6. Patients' family members have a strong desire for surgery, and the family's financial situation can support prolonged rehabilitation treatment.

19.2.2 Contraindications

1. Patients with small brainstem hemorrhage volume (<3 mL), no obvious obstruction of the ventricular system, and no consciousness impairment are not recommended for puncture surgery.
2. Patients with large hemorrhage volume that severely damages the vital centers of the brainstem and have bilat-

G. Chen, C. You (eds.), *Surgical Treatment of Primary Brainstem Hemorrhage*, https://doi.org/10.1007/978-981-95-8942-5_19

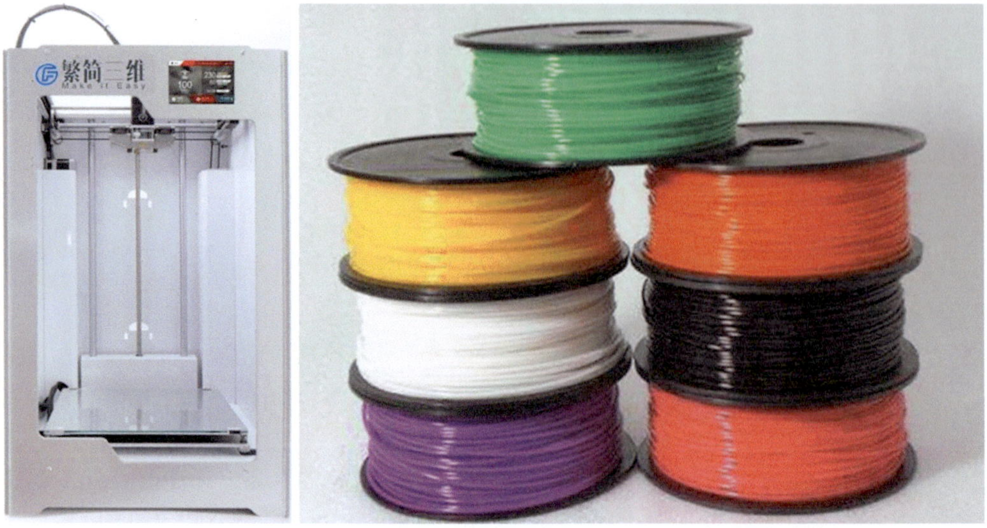

Fig. 19.1 3D printing and PLA printing materials

eral fixed and dilated pupils, accompanied by no breathing for more than 30 min.

3. Patients in extremely poor overall condition who cannot tolerate puncture hematoma surgery.
4. Patients with significant coagulation abnormalities.
5. Medullary hemorrhage.

19.2.3 Surgical Timing

The optimal timing for surgery is within 72 h after the onset of symptoms, although it can sometimes be extended to within 7 days after onset.

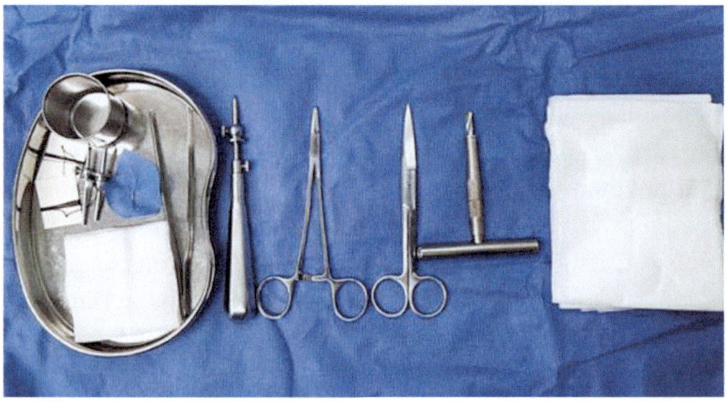

Fig. 19.2 Surgical instrument package

19.3 Preoperative Preparation and Surgical Instruments

19.3.1 Preoperative Preparation

1. 3D Printer: A specialized desktop 3D printer designed for clinical neurosurgery is compact in size, making it suitable for medical offices and teaching purposes. A regular desktop 3D printer can also meet general clinical requirements.
2. 3D Printing Materials: Powder materials, including ceramic and metal powders, filament materials such as PLA and ABS plastics, and liquid materials like photosensitive resin, should be carefully selected based on the clinical needs of the department [5, 6].
3. Data Acquisition: To obtain the cranial CT scan data of the patient with a brainstem hemorrhage in DICOM format, access the CT room and retrieve the data using a CD or DVD, or alternatively, obtain it from the physician's workstation. The scanning mode should have a thickness of ≤1.25 mm; thinner scan layers contribute to enhanced clarity in the details of the 3D reconstruction, resulting in more realistic images.

19.3.2 Surgical Instruments

1. 3D Image Workstation System set, along with a computer.
2. Desktop 3D Printer: One unit, along with PLA (ABS) material or SLA photosensitive resin, and a light-curing laser printer (Fig. 19.1).
3. Sterilized Puncture Surgical Instrument Package: A set of instruments including a needle holder, pointed scissors, a No. 5 "D" shaped hand drill, a triangular hand drill, and forceps (Fig. 19.2).

19.4 Surgical Methods, Precautions, and Techniques

19.4.1 3D Printing Localization Design Method

1. Initiate the E3D software system on the 3D imaging workstation or use software such as 3D-Slicer or Mimics. This article specifically employs the E3D software graphic workstation, which has been developed by the Digital Medicine and Virtual Reality Research Center at Central South University.
2. Import the preoperative DICOM data pertaining to the brainstem hematoma into the 3D image workstation software. Following the successful importation of the data, examine the brainstem hematoma in different 2D sectional views (Fig. 19.3).
3. The threshold segmentation method is utilized within the 3D software for 1:1 reconstruction of the brainstem hematoma model. The threshold for the hemorrhage is set between 50 and 100, whereas the same segmentation approach is employed to reconstruct the soft tissues of the head, with a threshold set between −200 and 3071. After the 3D reconstruction, the brainstem hematoma can be visualized from different angles to show its position within the skull (Figs. 19.4 and 19.5).
4. Based on the 3D reconstructed model of the hematoma, a universal template is used to formulate the optimal puncture path, avoiding critical anatomical structures within the cranial cavity. Generally, the puncture point is selected towards the side where the hemorrhage is located, positioned inferior to the transverse sinus and posterior to the mastoid process. The specific adjustments should be made according to the position of the hemorrhage, and the puncture path should aim towards the center of the hemorrhage. It is advisable for the operating physician to be involved in the planning and design of the 3D surgical strategy to ensure a targeted and precise procedure [1, 4, 7] (Fig. 19.6).
5. When designing the puncture template, it is important to achieve a precise fit to the patient's facial anatomy to avoid puncture errors caused by inadequate adherence. Fixed structures on the face, such as the orbital cavity, frontal arch, external auditory meatus, auricle, and mastoid, are utilized as reference points in the design of the template. The template should be trimmed appropriately while maintaining a tight and secure fit, thereby minimizing its surface area and expediting the production process. The inner diameter of the puncture channel is approximately 5 mm, using a 3/4 cylindrical open design. This allows the template to be completely wrapped in a sterile film, achieving the goal of an aseptic operation. It not only saves the cost of disinfection but also eliminates the waiting time for disinfection [4, 7] (Fig. 19.7).
6. Exporting STL Data: Connect to the network and export the 3D-designed puncture template model data, saving the puncture template data in STL format on the computer desktop for subsequent utilization (Fig. 19.8).

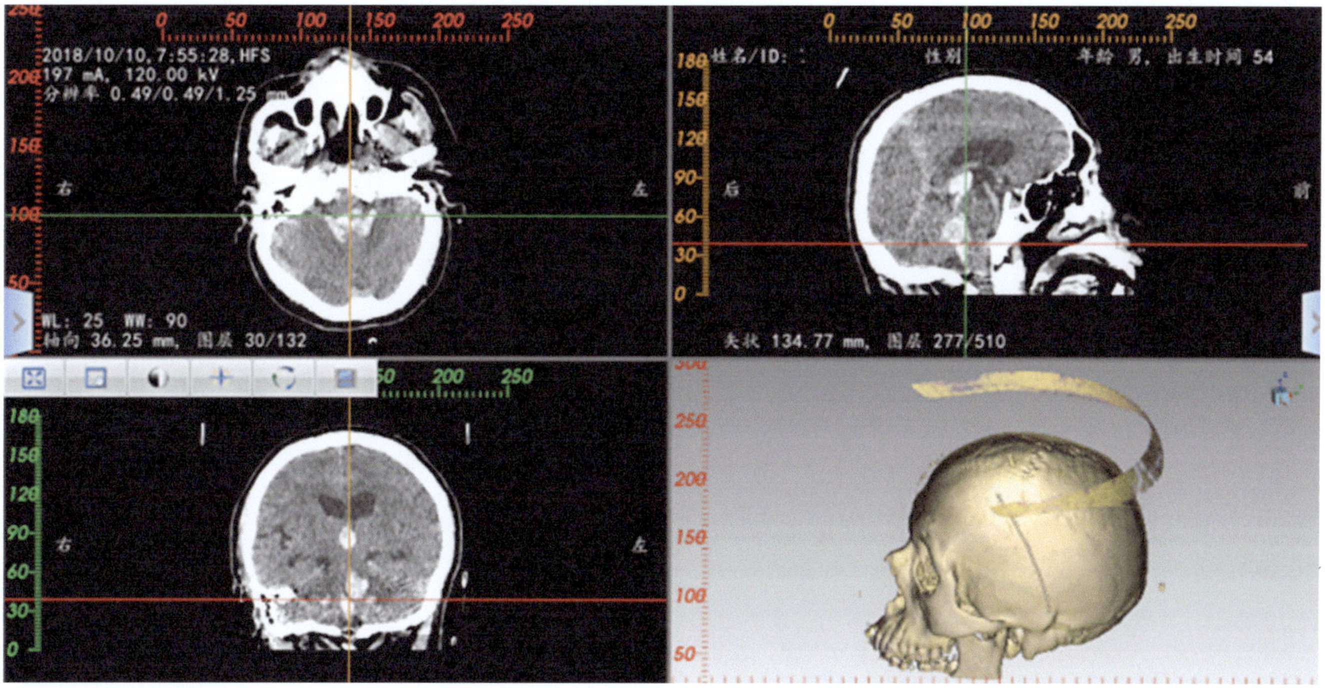

Fig. 19.3 Brainstem hematoma displayed in different sections

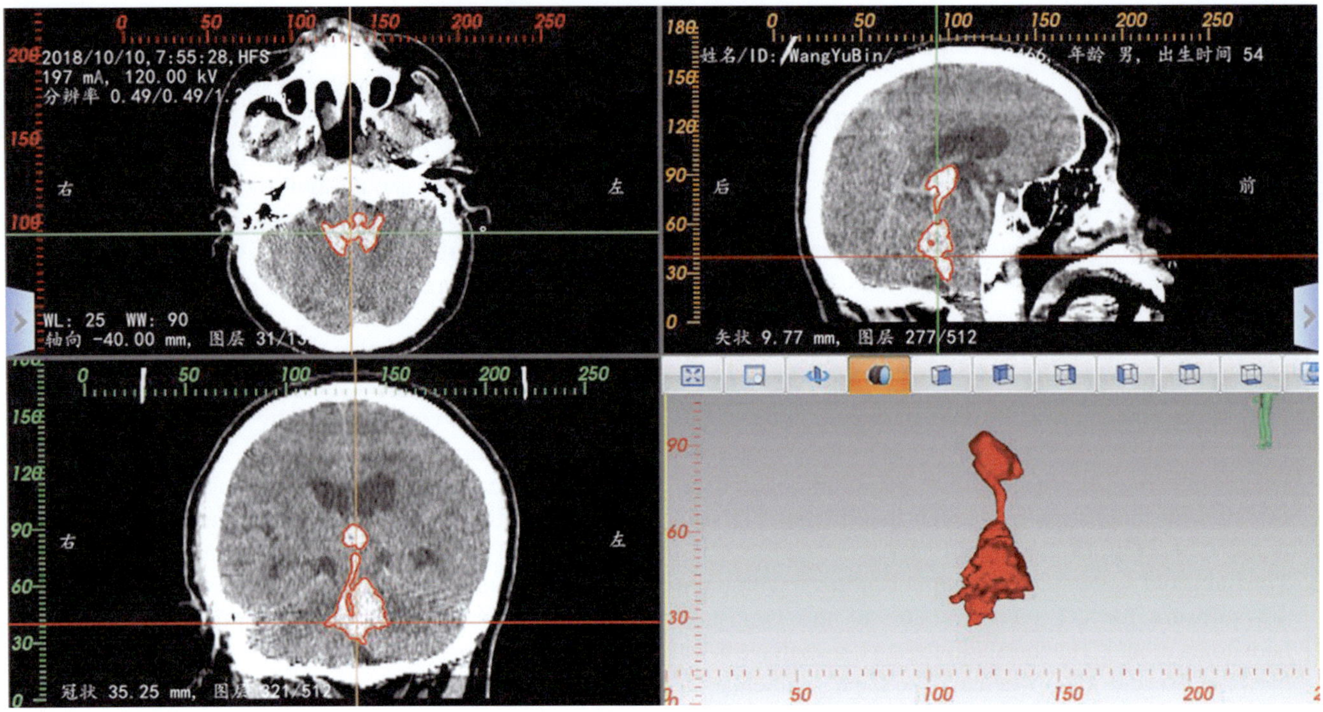

Fig. 19.4 1:1 ratio three-dimensional reconstruction of the brainstem hematoma

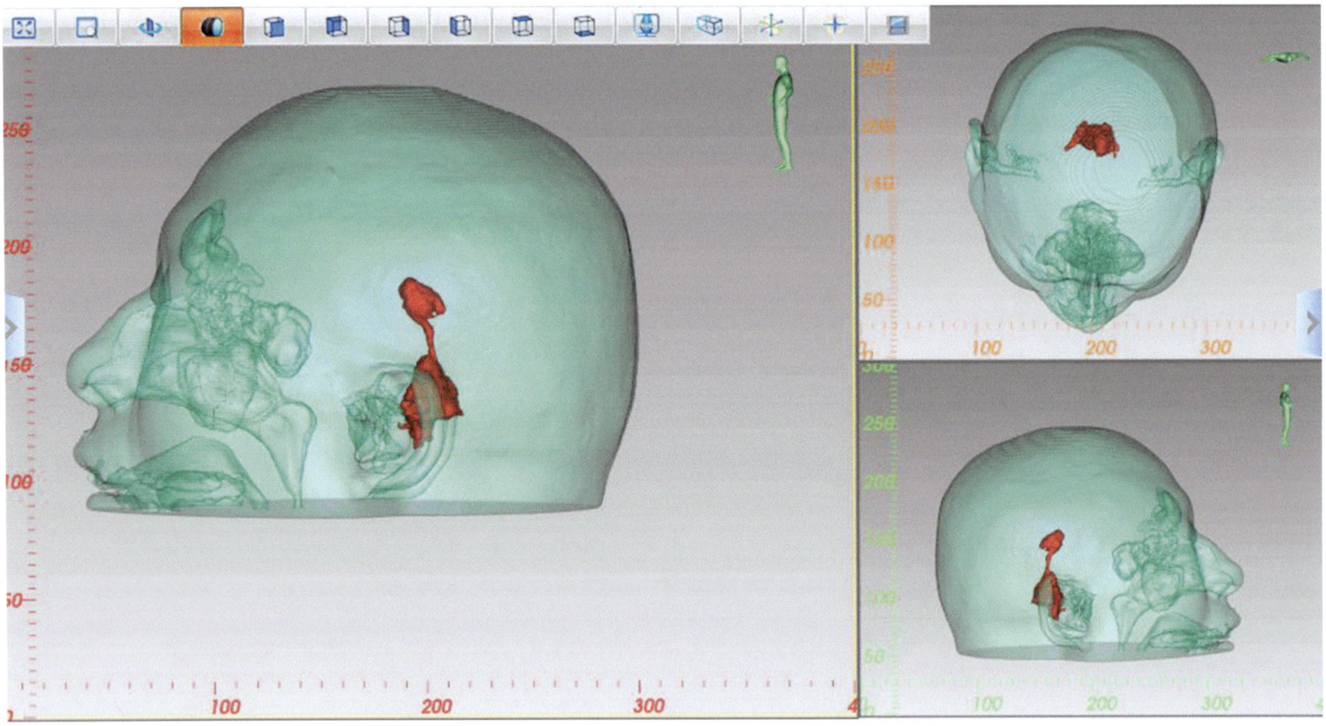

Fig. 19.5 Perspective view of the brainstem hematoma from different angles

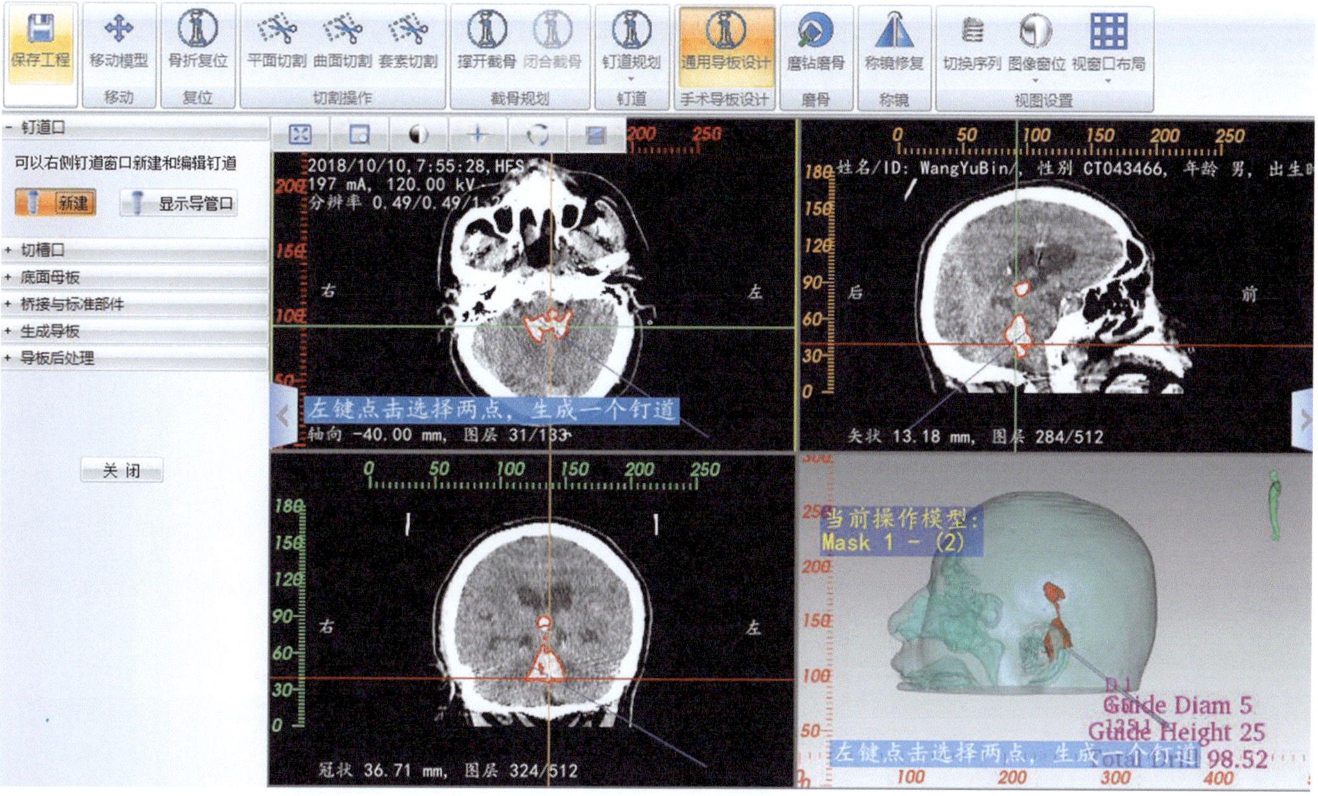

Fig. 19.6 Designing the puncture path

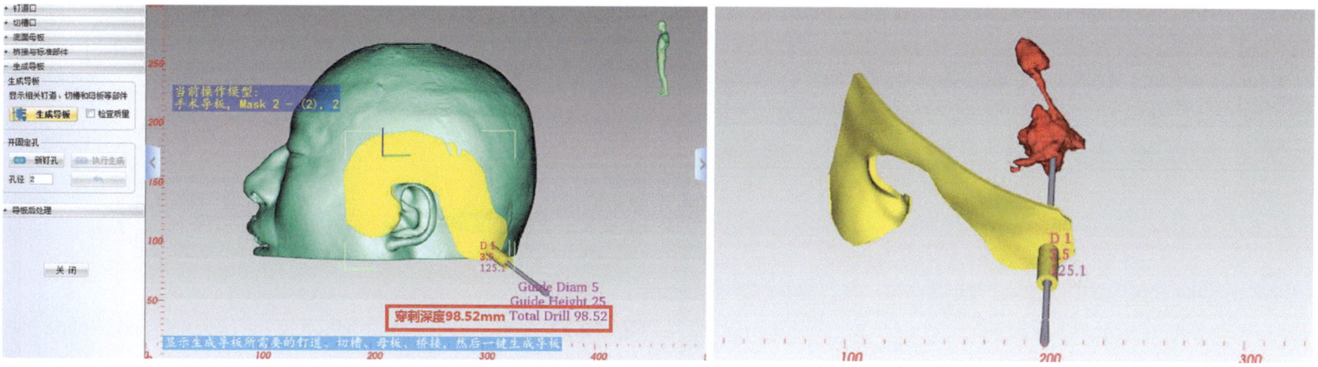

Fig. 19.7 Generating the template and automatically calculating the distance from the outer opening of the catheter to the center of the hemorrhage. The relationship between the trimmed guilde plate and the hematoma

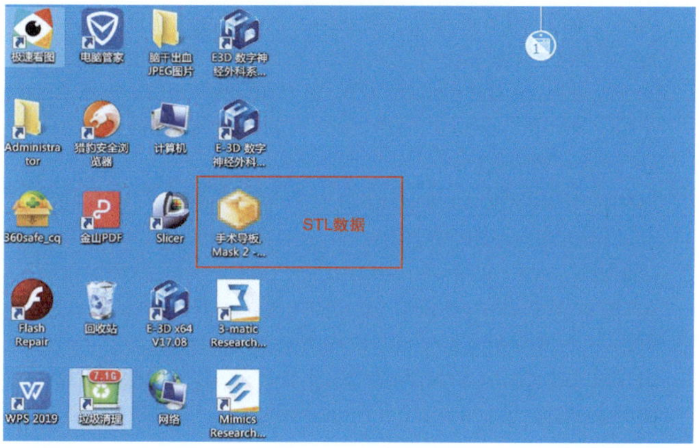

Fig. 19.8 Saving the data on the desktop

7. Open the CURA slicing software that is compatible with the 3D printer and import the puncture template STL data saved on the computer desktop. Set the required parameters for the printer through the slicing software to estimate the working time and consumables needed for printing the puncture template (Fig. 19.9).
8. By adjusting the slicing software parameters, it is possible to produce the GCode file necessary for the printer. Transfer the GCode file to the printer to initiate the printing process and complete the production of the puncture template (Fig. 19.10).
9. Upon completion of the printing process, further process the template to ensure a smooth and secure fit with the patient's face. Verify the compatibility between the tem-

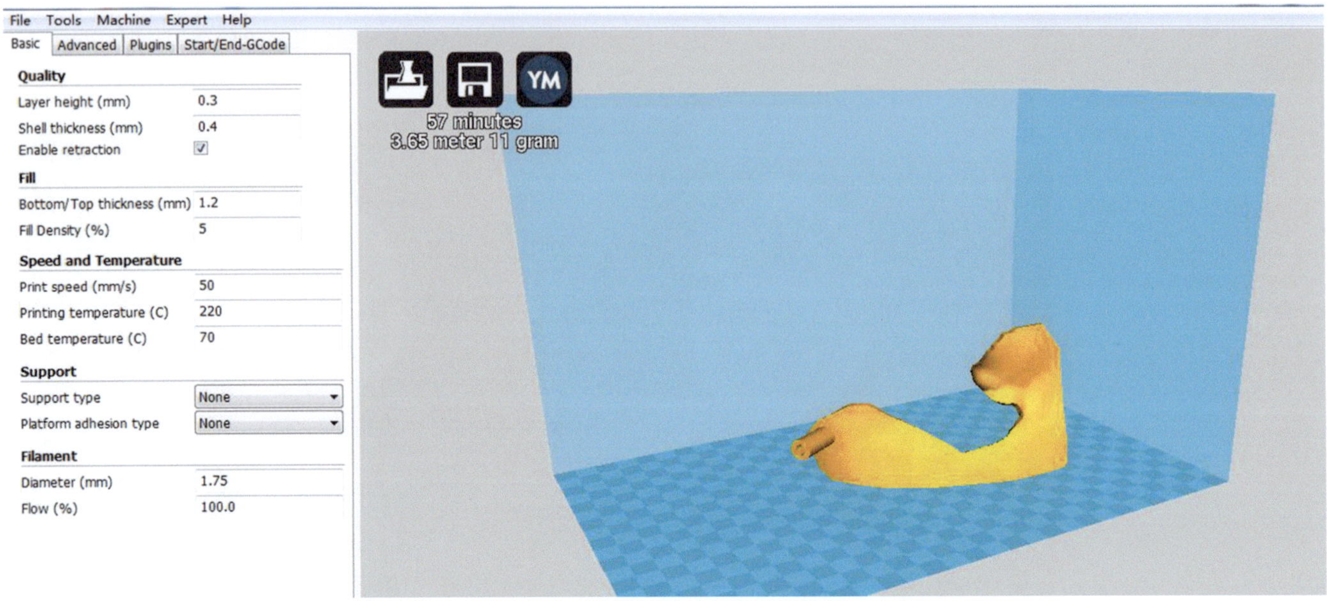
File Tools Machine Expert Help
Basic Advanced Plugins Start/End-GCode
Quality
Layer height (mm) 0.3
Shell thickness (mm) 0.4
Enable retraction
Fill
Bottom/Top thickness (mm) 1.2
Fill Density (%) 5
Speed and Temperature
Print speed (mm/s) 50
Printing temperature (C) 220
Bed temperature (C) 70
Support
Support type None
Platform adhesion type None
Filament
Diameter (mm) 1.75
Flow (%) 100.0
YM
57 minutes
3.65 meter 11 gram

Fig. 19.9 Setting parameters for printing the puncture template

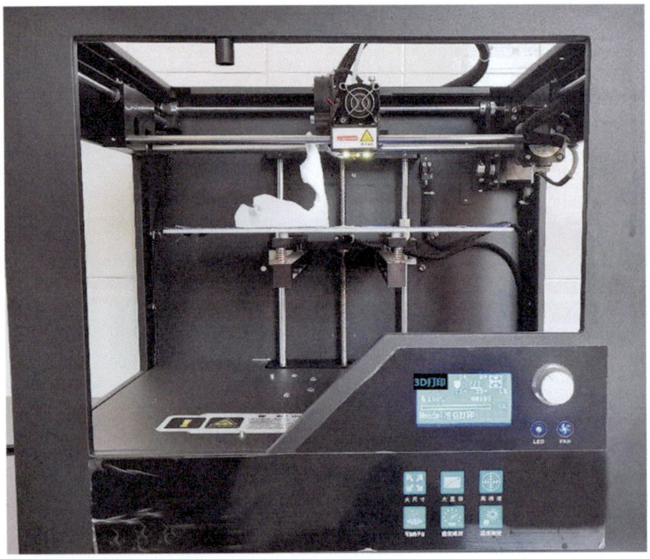

Fig. 19.10 Printing the puncture guilde plate

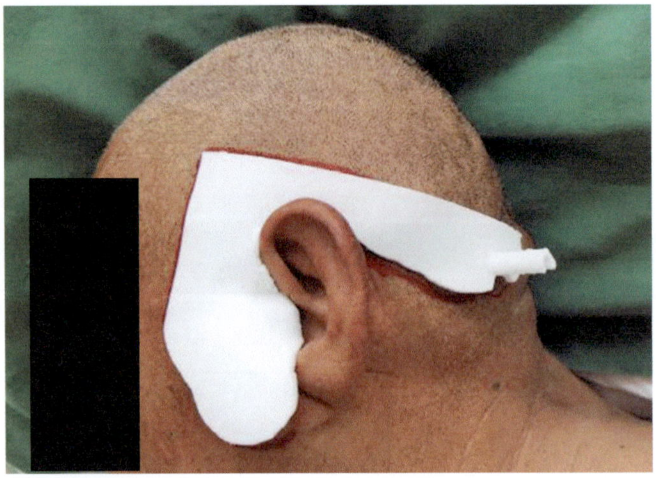

Fig. 19.11 Verifying the information of the puncture guilde plate

plate and the patient's skull, ensuring the accuracy of the template information data prior to its application (Fig. 19.11).

19.4.2 Puncture Surgical Technique

1. The patient is positioned in a lateral decubitus position, with the surgical side oriented upwards, either in a lateral decubitus or lateral prone position. The head is flexed anteriorly to facilitate access to the soft tissues of the occipital-cervical region. After routine disinfection and draping, a puncture template, either a low-temperature plasma-disinfected one or a sterile film-covered one, is used to completely envelop and adhere to the predetermined area of the patient's head, ensuring a precise alignment between the puncture template and the surface landmarks of the patient's head (such as the nasion, brow ridge, eyelid crease, auricle, external auditory meatus, and even wrinkles).
2. Local infiltration anesthesia is performed using 5 mL of 2% lidocaine through the 3D-printed puncture template channel. An incision measuring 0.5 cm is made on the scalp at the designated puncture site, after which a hand drill is employed to penetrate the scalp along the channel of the puncture template until the skull is reached. The drill is rotated to create a bone hole, and then the puncture

template is removed. The "T"-shaped hand drill is used to enlarge the bone hole along the puncture channel by following the path of the drill. The hand drill is rotated clockwise and then withdrawn, while a groove is used to remove bone debris.

3. The dura mater is punctured, and the printed puncture template is subsequently reapplied. A drainage tube is then introduced along the puncture template channel, with the depth determined preoperatively by measuring the distance from the front end of the drainage tube to the external opening of the puncture template channel. Following this, the stylet of the drainage tube is removed, and the drainage tube is slowly aspirated or drained until dark red blood (clots) is observed, indicating that the drainage tube has successfully accessed the hematoma cavity. The initial aspiration volume is approximately half of the hematoma volume. The procedure is then concluded (Fig. 19.12, Video 19.1).

19.4.3 Precautions and Techniques

19.4.3.1 Precautions

1. Make full use of surface landmarks: When applying the 3D-printed puncture template for cranial positioning, it is important to utilize facial surface markers such as the auricle and external auditory meatus. If necessary, additional surface markers like electrode pads can be used to facilitate the accurate alignment of the printed puncture template and facial features, enhancing the precision of the puncture for the hematoma.
2. Avoid puncture path deviation: Due to the relatively thick soft tissues in the occipital region, the skin may stretch and shift when the neck is flexed forward. To prevent deviation of the puncture path during the procedure, after applying the template, the scalp should be directly punctured with a hand drill until reaching the skull, and then a hole should be drilled in the skull for precise positioning.

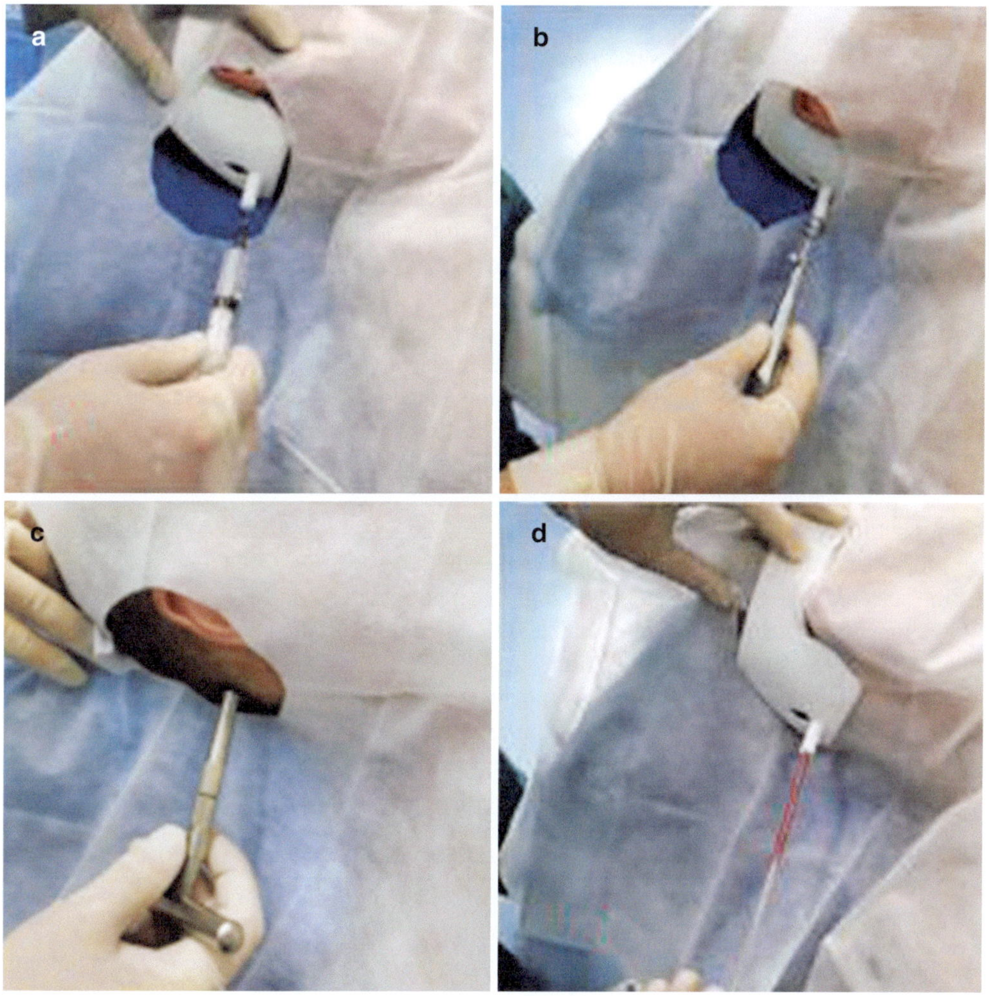

Fig. 19.12 Local anesthesia through the puncture channel, skull penetration along the puncture channel with a hand drill, enlargement of the bone hole with a hand drill, and insertion of the drainage tube along the puncture channel. (**a**) Local anesthesia through the puncture channel, (**b**) skull penetration along the puncture channel with a hand drill, (**c**) enlargement of the bone hole with a hand drill, (**d**) insertion of the drainage tube along the puncture channel

This helps to avoid inconsistencies between the scalp incision and the puncture bone hole, which could lead to path displacement or deviation during the puncture.

3. Prevent extradural hematoma: After successful drilling, it is imperative to puncture the dura mater promptly with the hand drill to avoid excessive bluntness of the drill tip, which could cause dural detachment and lead to an extradural hematoma.

19.4.3.2 Techniques

1. Preoperative verification: The completed 3D-printed puncture template must be verified against the craniofacial region before the procedure. This process involves confirming its fit with the craniofacial anatomy and validating the puncture entry points and directions according to the actual anatomical positioning.
2. Preoperative marking: Preoperative marking is conducted not based on black-and-white 2D CT images but after confirming the accuracy of the puncture template. Lines and markings are made along the periphery of the template and at the puncture channel opening to reduce the time taken to correctly position the template during the procedure and avoid puncture errors caused by template misalignment.
3. Intraoperative puncture: During the puncture procedure, it is important for the assistant or the operator's other hand to stabilize the puncture template to prevent any displacement. The drainage tube should be inserted along the channel of the puncture template, guided by the puncture needle, and gently positioned against the sidewall of the puncture channel to facilitate entry into the hematoma cavity. This technique minimizes the risk of preventing the drainage tube from angling or deviating within the puncture channel, which could compromise the effectiveness of the drainage.
4. Proper selection of drainage tube: The outer diameter of the selected drainage tube should be slightly smaller than the inner diameter of the channel in the 3D-printed puncture template. However, it is essential that the drainage tube is not excessively thin, as this could lead to puncture errors related to displacement during the procedure. A hand drill with a tip size corresponding to a No. 12 drainage tube should be used, along with a No. 5 T-shaped hand drill and a matching No. 12 ventricular drainage tube. These three components should be compatible with each other and provide effective hemostasis for minor oozing occurring within the dura mater and brain tissue along the puncture channel.
5. Appropriate initial hematoma drainage: During the procedure, the negative pressure applied during aspiration should not be excessive to prevent additional bleeding. Generally, a slow aspiration using a 5 mL syringe is recommended. While aspirating, the drainage tube should be rotated to ensure proper contact between the side holes of the drainage tube and the hematoma, thereby facilitating effective drainage. The initial aspiration volume should be approximately half the volume of the hematoma.
6. "Purse-string" suturing of the drainage tube To secure the drainage tube within the hematoma cavity, a "purse-string" suturing technique can be used for scalp closure. Once the desired goal of hematoma drainage is achieved, the drainage tube can be removed, and the "purse-string" suture can be tightened, eliminating the need for additional sutures after the tube is removed.

19.5 Postoperative Care and Prevention of Complications

19.5.1 Pulmonary Infection

Pulmonary infection is one of the main postoperative complications and leading cause of mortality in patients with brainstem hemorrhage. Comatose patients frequently develop pulmonary infections within 3–5 days after brainstem hemorrhage.

19.5.1.1 Causes

Patients with brainstem hemorrhage often experience medullary paralysis, which leads to the loss of swallowing and cough reflexes, making it easier for respiratory secretions and vomitus to be aspirated into the airway.

Prolonged bed rest can lead to the accumulation of respiratory secretions, along with a weakened immune system, increasing the risk of pulmonary infections.

19.5.1.2 Prevention and Treatment Measures

During the acute phase, elevate the head of the bed by 15°, tilt the head to one side, remove dentures if present, position the head slightly downward during vomiting, promptly clear any oral vomitus, and ensure proper oral hygiene.

Regularly suction respiratory secretions while avoiding excessive negative pressure to prevent mucosal damage and decreased oxygen saturation (SpO2). Monitor the patient's response during the suctioning process. If possible, perform suctioning while the monitoring with a pulse oximeter. Use disposable suction catheters, promptly dispose of collected secretions, and thoroughly clean and disinfect the equipment after use.

Maintain tracheal humidification. For patients with a tracheostomy, instill 20 mL of normal saline combined with 80,000 units of gentamicin and 5 mg of trypsin every 15 min at a rate of 2–3 drops, or infuse continuously at a rate of 3 drops per minute. Boil and disinfect the inner tube every 4 h. For patients without a tracheostomy, use 20 mL of normal saline with 5 mg of trypsin and 80,000 units of gentamicin, and perform ultrasonic nebulization 2–3 times. In case of pulmonary infection, select sensitive antibiotics based on sputum bacterial culture and sensitivity. For mouth-breathing patients, cover the oral cavity with moist gauze to maintain airway moisture.

Conduct regular sputum cultures using sterile, disposable suction culture bottles to collect samples. For patients with a tracheostomy, first clean the oral or nasal cavity to prevent external contamination that may affect culture results.

Turn and clean the back every hour. Use appropriate force using the thenar muscles to tap up, down, left, and right, inducing vibrations to break up mucus proteins and facilitate the movement of mucus plugs from the bronchi to the trachea.

Monitor body temperature, respiration, lung sounds, sputum volume, and its characteristics. Take timely and effective measures if any signs of infection are observed.

19.5.2 Upper Gastrointestinal Bleeding

Upper gastrointestinal bleeding caused by stress ulcers is a severe complication of brainstem hemorrhage, often arising within a week of the bleeding and significantly impacting the prognosis.

19.5.2.1 Causes

The excessive stimulation of the sympathetic nervous system during stress leads to the release of catecholamines, resulting in elevated levels of adrenal cortical hormones, increased gastric acid secretion, and heightened gastric protease secretion.

Increased intracranial pressure can elevate blood pancreatic polypeptide levels, leading to increased gastric acid secretion and the development of stress ulcers and bleeding.

19.5.2.2 Prevention and Treatment Measures

Close monitoring of vital signs, especially blood pressure, is essential to prevent hemorrhagic shock.

Temporary fasting or a liquid diet should be implemented while avoiding irritants. Medications such as H2 receptor antagonists and proton pump inhibitors can be used for prevention or treatment.

In cases of severe bleeding, it is crucial to promptly assess the extent of the hemorrhage. If blood volume needs to be replenished, rapidly establish intravenous access and ensure timely and accurate transfusion and fluid therapy. Hospitals with suitable facilities may consider endoscopic hemostasis, surgical intervention, or interventional therapy.

19.5.3 Central Fever

19.5.3.1 Causes

Central fever is caused by damage to the hypothalamic temperature-regulating center. Clinically, it presents as a persistent high fever, with temperatures often exceeding 39 °C, without accompanied by chills.

19.5.3.2 Prevention and Treatment Measures

Pharmacological and physical cooling methods can be used concurrently. Early initiation of selective head cooling with cooling caps is recommended to reduce cerebral oxygen consumption, increase tolerance to hypoxia, alleviate brain edema, lower intracranial pressure, and facilitate the recovery of cerebral function. Close observation of the patient's condition during the cooling process is essential.

Pharmacological cooling methods are available but may not yield satisfactory results.

19.5.4 Urinary Tract Infection

19.5.4.1 Causes

Patients with brainstem hemorrhage often experience urinary dysfunction and may require long-term indwelling catheterization, which increases their susceptibility to urinary tract infections.

Damage to the urethral mucosa during catheterization can disrupt mucosal integrity, providing an environment for bacterial colonization and infection.

Improper catheterization techniques and inadequate disinfection can lead to contamination and subsequent infection.

Underlying conditions, such as prostate diseases and diabetes, can predispose individuals to urinary tract infections.

19.5.4.2 Prevention and Treatment Measures

Strict adherence to aseptic techniques during catheterization procedures, along with proficiency in technical operations, is crucial. Maintain catheter patency, clean the urethral orifice with 0.5% povidone-iodine solution twice daily, ensure perineal hygiene to prevent cross-infection, and closely monitor urine color and output for any abnormalities, taking appropriate action if necessary.

Implement proper care for indwelling catheters. Disinfect the external genitalia twice daily with chlorhexidine, following an inside-out and top-down sequence to maintain perineal cleanliness and reduce the risk of urinary system infections.

To prevent urinary reflux, clamp the catheter before repositioning the drainage bag during patient turning.

19.5.5 Electrolyte Imbalance

19.5.5.1 Causes

Patients with brainstem hemorrhage are prone to electrolyte imbalances due to altered consciousness, inability to eat, vomiting, sweating, and dehydration resulting from medication use, etc. Especially in the early stages of brainstem hemorrhage, reduced food intake and extensive use of diuretics can lead to hyperosmolar dehydration, which often results in hyponatremia and hypokalemia.

19.5.5.2 Prevention and Treatment Measures

Regular monitoring of electrolyte levels during treatment is essential to promptly correct any electrolyte imbalance, which is vital for the successful management of patients with brainstem hemorrhage.

19.5.6 Lower Extremity Deep Vein Thrombosis

Lower extremity deep vein thrombosis (DVT) is a common complication in patients with brain hemorrhage. Once it occurs, DVT becomes an absolute contraindication to limb activity, significantly affecting the rehabilitation process and posing a risk of life-threatening pulmonary embolism.

19.5.6.1 Causes

Factors contributing to lower extremity deep vein thrombosis in patients with brainstem hemorrhage include limb paralysis, prolonged bed rest, surgery, vascular wall damage, coagulation abnormalities, and the hemorrhage itself, all of which complicate the administration of anticoagulant therapy. Assessing and analyzing the high-risk factors for DVT is crucial for the timely implementation of effective preventive measures, improving the recovery outcomes of brain hemorrhage, and reducing the risk of patient mortality.

19.5.6.2 Prevention and Treatment Measures

Assessing and analyzing high-risk factors for lower extremity DVT is essential for the timely implementation of effective preventive measures. Prophylactic measures against venous thrombosis should be taken for paralyzed individuals, including regular passive or active movements of affected limbs, adequate fluid intake to reduce blood viscosity, minimizing venous catheterization to prevent iatrogenic thrombosis, and administering subcutaneous low-dose heparin when necessary, along with monitoring of partial thromboplastin time. Most individuals with DVT do not exhibit obvious symptoms, and their medical history and physical examination lack specificity. Clinical diagnosis primarily relies on non-invasive diagnostic methods, with Doppler ultrasound being the most used technique. A positive result from the ultrasound confirms the diagnosis, and in certain cases, vascular imaging may be performed if necessary. Once a diagnosis of DVT or pulmonary embolism is established, treatment with venous heparin or interventional surgery should be initiated without delay.

19.6 Advantages, Disadvantages, and Lessons Learned

19.6.1 Advantages

1. Personalized Precision Medicine: The use of 3D printing-assisted brainstem hemorrhage puncture and hematoma aspiration allows for tailored customization based on the patient's craniofacial anatomy. This approach effectively avoids critical structures and blood vessels, reducing puncture-related damage and minimizing iatrogenic harm to brain tissue. It maximizes the preservation of neurological function, truly exemplifying the principles of personalized precision medicine [1, 3].
2. Relative Cost-effectiveness: The surgery can be performed under local anesthesia, requiring only an affordable 3D printer which costs a few thousand yuan, a regular computer, and template consumables that cost less than 100 yuan.
3. Shortened Learning Curve for Young Physicians: 3D printing technology facilitates a significant transition from three-dimensional imaging to tangible physical models. Surgeons can simulate operations and establish three-dimensional structures prior to surgery, which assists in surgical planning, teaching, and training. This technology also reduces the learning curve for novice physicians [3, 8].

19.6.2 Disadvantages

1. Software Application Talent Development: Implementing 3D printing technology in clinical settings necessitates specialized training for software technicians. Currently, the learning curve for the freely available 3D-Slicer software is lengthy, and its operation can be cumbersome. While the Mimics software developed by Materialise in Belgium is more user-friendly, the expensive copyright issues have been a persistent challenge for the clinical application of 3D printing in China [9].
2. Cost Issue: As the application of 3D printing technology in clinical settings is still in its early stages, there is no standardized payment mechanism in medical institutions. Additionally, this technology is not covered by medical

insurance, resulting in some hospitals only engaging in research without strong willingness from hospital administrators.

3. Time-consuming Process: The processing time for 3D printing technology can be relatively long. While desktop printers that use PLA materials provide cost-effective printing options, they typically require 2–3 h for completion. Utilizing photosensitive resin for laser stereolithography can reduce printing time, but the expenses associated with the printer and materials are higher [9].
4. Puncture Deviation: When selecting the puncture site in the occipital region, the patient needs to be in a lateral or prone position. Flexion of the occipital neck and the extension of the occipital scalp during the puncture can cause inconsistencies between the preoperative CT scan data and the 3D-printed puncture template, leading to attachment errors. These errors need to be corrected based on the intraoperative head position.

19.6.3 Lessons Learned

1. When cutting the 3D-printed puncture template, it is advisable to retain the reconstructed surface markings of the head. During the surgery, ensure perfect alignment between the 3D template and the surface markings of the head to minimize any deviation in the puncture.
2. The thickness of the 3D-printed puncture template should be no less than 2.8 mm. A template that is too thin may lack adequate support and easily deform, causing positional deviations. The inner diameter of the template channel should be slightly larger than the outer diameter of the drainage tube by approximately 1 mm to prevent movement and deviation within the puncture channel.
3. For areas where surface markings on the head are not prominent, additional markings can be applied, especially in the temporal, parietal, or occipital regions. These additional markings should be arranged in a triangular pattern, avoiding the puncture area to facilitate accurate positioning.
4. If the surgery is not urgent, the 3D-printed puncture template can be disinfected using low-temperature plasma for standby. Avoid placing any objects that may exert pressure on the sterilized template to prevent deformation and render it unusable.
5. By incorporating perforations into the guiding template and adding surface markers on the body prior to CT scanning, or by removing unnecessary parts during the creation of the computer model, printing time can be reduced by approximately 1 h. The area of the reconstructed three-dimensional puncture guide can be appropriately reduced, further decreasing the time required for printing the guide. This enhancement facilitates the placement of the guide during procedures performed in the transoccipital or transtemporal position, making it more convenient for clinical surgeons to perform the surgery.

19.7 Procedure Evaluation and Prospects

19.7.1 Surgical Evaluation

Digital neurosurgery is an emerging interdisciplinary field that combines computer science with neurosurgery. It encompasses various areas such as human anatomy, solid geometry, biomechanics, materials science, informatics, electronics, and mechanical engineering. This field can accurately represent the intricate three-dimensional structures of normal or pathological tissues, allowing for observations and manipulations such as rotations and sectioning. It not only enables the measurement of reconstructed three-dimensional structures to obtain precise anatomical parameters like length, area, volume, and angles but also finds applications in clinical assistance for diagnosis, surgical design, and procedural simulations. It truly represents a significant leap from traditional two-dimensional imaging to tangible physical models [3].

3D printing technology facilitates the three-dimensional reconstruction of brainstem hematomas and simulates the localization and puncture procedures for hematomas, thereby enhancing the safety and precision of surgeries. The puncture approach can vary from transcranial posterior fossa punctures as well as supratentorial occipital or temporal punctures. Due to the relatively minor displacement of soft tissues in the supratentorial and temporal regions compared to the occipital soft tissues, surface markings (or additional surface markings) aid in easier localization.

19.7.2 Prospects

Three-dimensional visualization through 3D printing technology enhances the accuracy of brainstem hematoma punctures and reduces surgical risks. As 3D printing technology advances, coupled with relatively low equipment costs and a shortened learning curve for physicians, it is poised to become an effective tool for enhancing the diagnostic and treatment capabilities of neurosurgeons while reducing surgical risks. The potential applications of this technology in neurosurgery, particularly in cases of primary brain hemorrhage, are exceptionally promising [2, 3, 9].

19.8 Typical Case

19.8.1 Brief Medical History and Imaging Data

1. Patient: Male, 54 years old, admitted to the ICU for "headache, vomiting, decreased consciousness for 2 h." History of hypertension for 7 years, intermittent oral anti-hypertensive medication.
2. Physical examination: BP 260/120 mmHg, light coma, GCS 8, no verbal response, limb flexion in response to pain but unable to localize, muscle strength at level 4, increased muscle tone, positive pathological signs in the left lower limb.
3. Head CT scan shows pontine hemorrhage extending into the ventricular system, approximately 8 mL in volume (Fig. 19.13).
4. Admission diagnosis: (1) Pontine hemorrhage extending into the ventricle; (2) Grade 3 hypertension (extremely high-risk group).

19.8.2 Surgical Procedure and Key Points

After admission, the patient's condition rapidly deteriorated, transitioning from a light coma to a deep coma. Emergency ventricular puncture and external drainage were performed, revealing extremely high intraventricular pressure with bloody cerebrospinal fluid overflow. The patient's consciousness briefly improved to a drowsy state post-drainage tube placement, with peripheral left facial paralysis. A follow-up CT scan was conducted (Fig. 19.14).

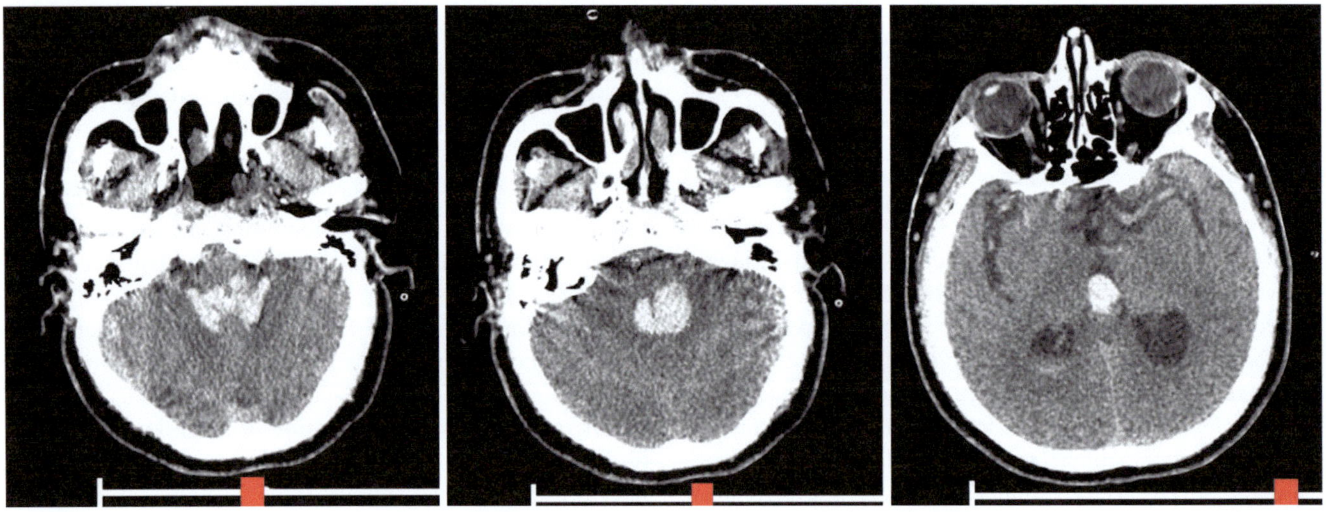

Fig. 19.13 CT scan at admission showing pontine hemorrhage rupturing into the ventricle

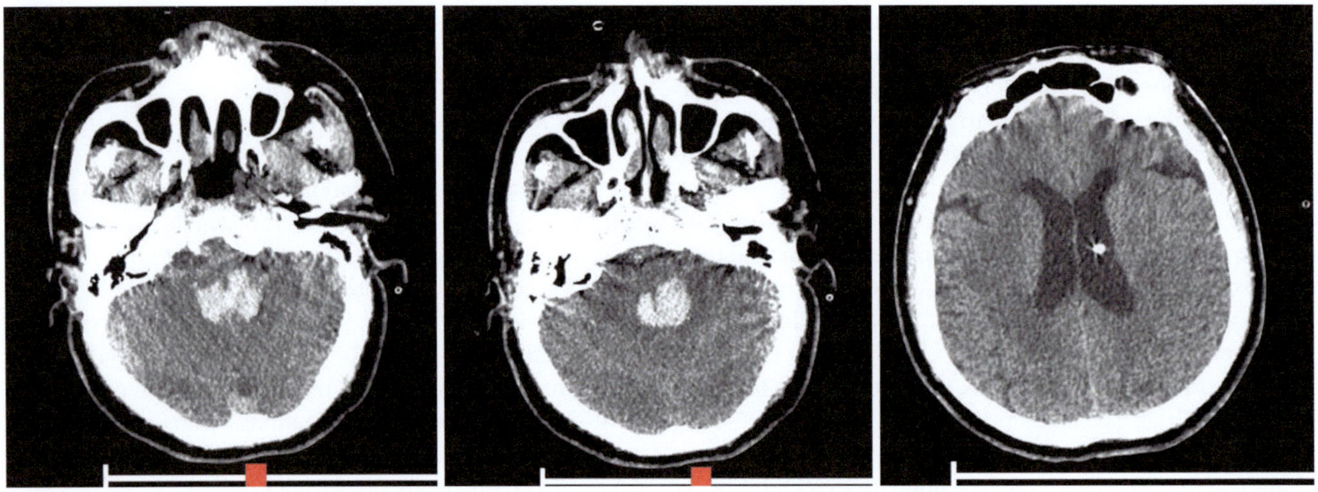

Fig. 19.14 CT scan after ventricular catheterization

The day after the ventricular drainage tube placement, the patient's consciousness deteriorated to a deep coma with pinpoint pupils, SPO2 at 80%. Endotracheal intubation and mechanical ventilation assistance were provided, along with the application of a digitized 3D-designed puncture guide, used for the evacuation of the brainstem and fourth ventricle hematoma during which a 5 mL dark blood clot was aspirated (Figs. 19.15 and 19.16). The patient was then transferred to the ICU for comprehensive rescue treatment.

19.8.3 Postoperative Treatment and Imaging Comparison

A follow-up CT scan and reconstruction of brain tissue, hematoma, drainage tube, and ventricles 16 h postoperatively revealed a residual brainstem hematoma of 1.1 mL (Fig. 19.17). The patient regained spontaneous breathing at 24 h postoperatively. A repeat CT scan at 36 h postoperatively showed significant clearance of the brainstem hema-

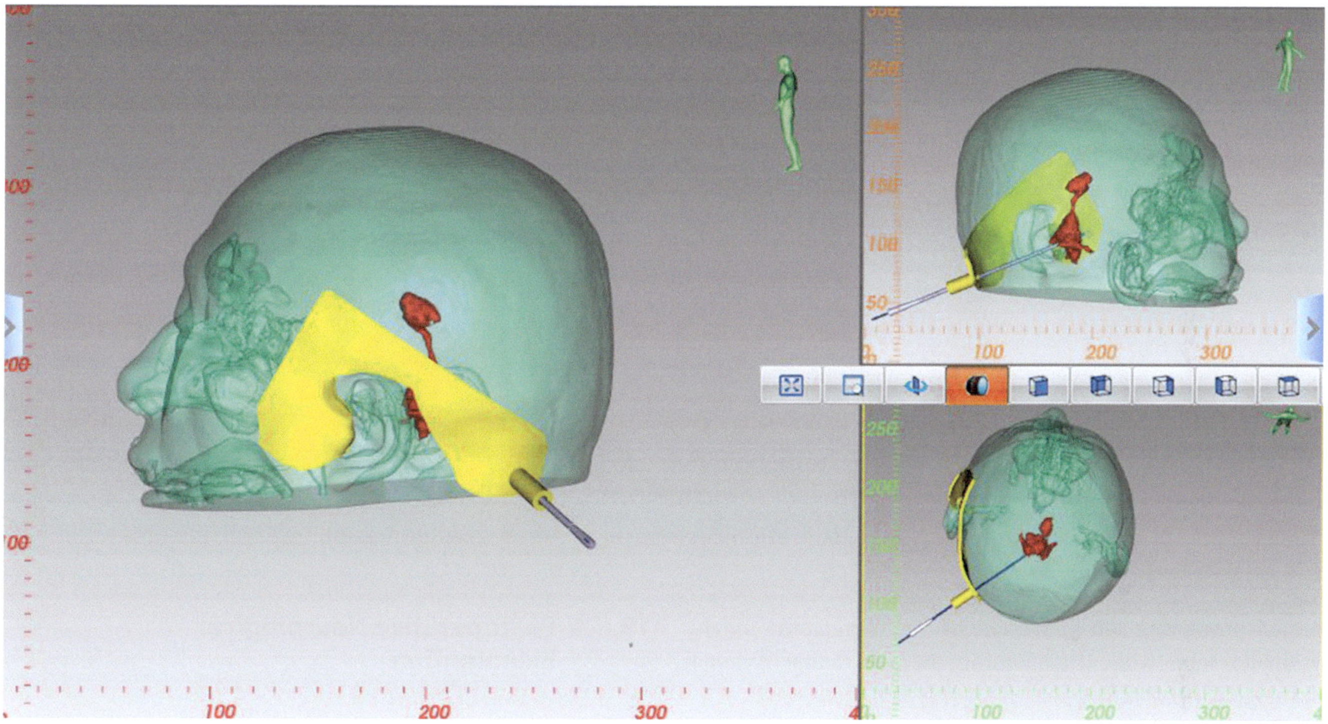

Fig. 19.15 Simulation of puncture surgery design

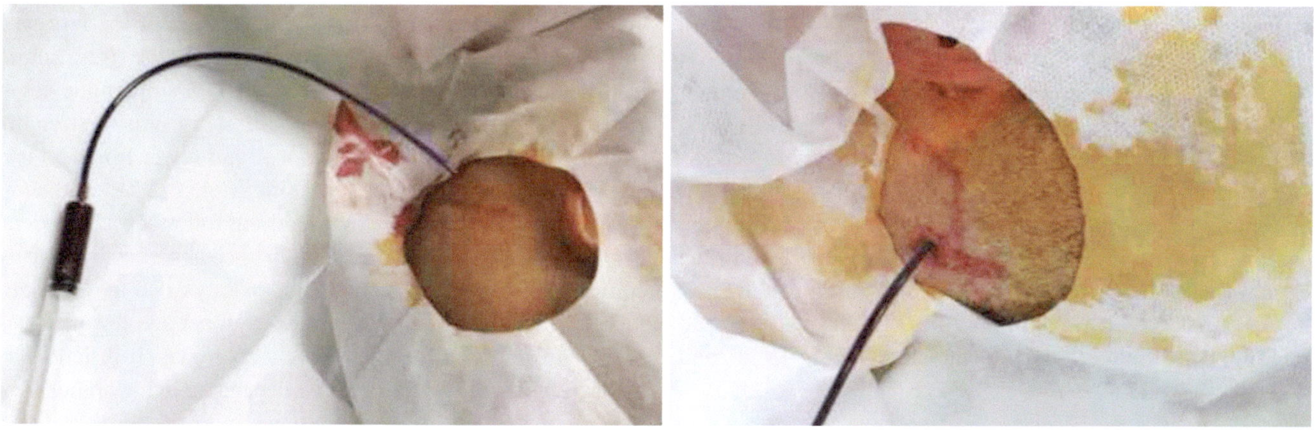

Fig. 19.16 Intraoperative aspiration of a 5 mL dark blood clot

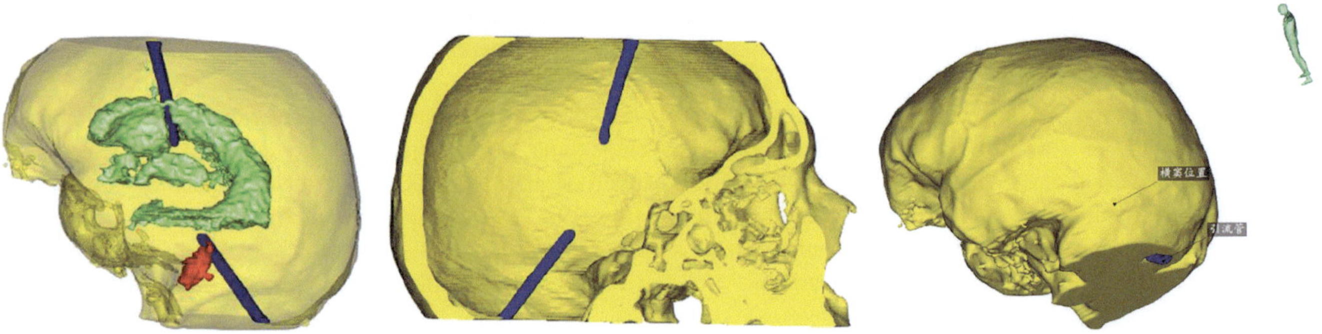

Fig. 19.17 3D reconstruction 16 h postoperatively showing the relationship between the drainage tube and the brainstem, ventricles, and residual hematoma; the drainage tube is positioned 1.5 cm below the transverse sinus

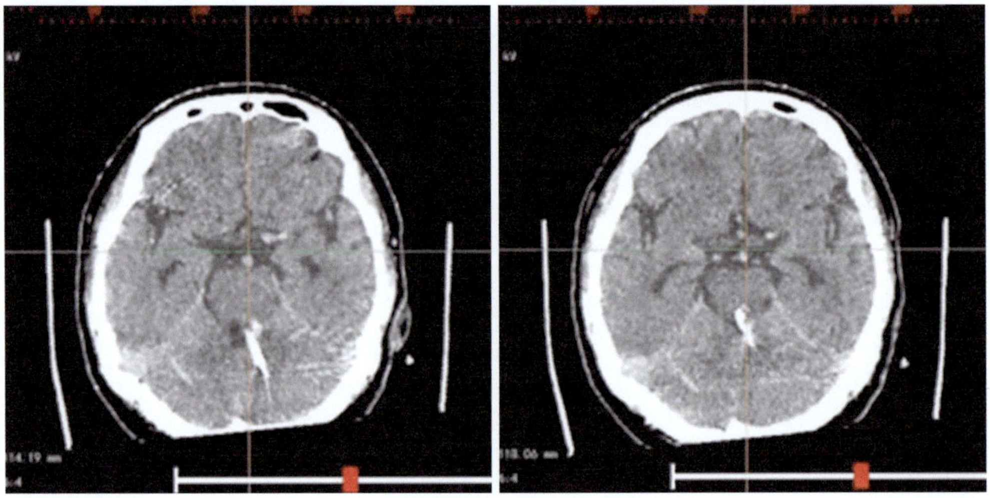

Fig. 19.18 Repeat CT scan on 36 h postoperatively shows substantial clearance of the brainstem hematoma

toma, prompting the removal of the hematoma cavity drainage tube while maintaining the ventricular external drainage (Fig. 19.18).

Tracheotomy was performed and ventilator was weaned 48 h postoperatively. By the third postoperative day, the patient was drowsy with swallowing function, unclear speech, autonomous flexion of the upper and lower limbs on the right side, muscle strength at level IV−, increased muscle tone, and positive pathological signs in the left lower limb. The ventricular drainage tube was removed on the fifth postoperative day for rehabilitation. A follow-up CT scan was conducted 32 days postoperatively upon discharge, revealing residual central facial paralysis on the left side, limited external rotation of the left eye, diplopia, swallowing difficulties, muscle strength at level IV- in the left upper and lower limbs, and incoordination in left limb movements (Fig. 19.19). Follow-up MRI scans at 3 and 6 months postoperatively are shown in Figs. 19.20 and 19.21.

19.8.4 Postoperative Neurological Examination

At 1 month postoperatively, the patient could walk briefly with assistance from family members (Fig. 19.22). At 3 months postoperatively, the patient exhibited incomplete motor aphasia, swallowing difficulties, symmetrical forehead wrinkles, left ptosis, limited abduction of the left eye, shallower left sulci nasolabialis compared to the right, angulus oris deviation to the right upon opening, and tongue deviation to the left upon extension. Additionally, muscle strength was assessed at level IV in the upper and lower limbs on the left side and level V on the right side (Fig. 19.23).

At 15 months postoperatively, during follow-up, the patient displayed good mental status, slightly unclear speech but able to comprehend semantics, central facial paralysis on the left side, muscle strength at level IV+ in the left upper and lower limbs, normal function on the right side, incoordination in left limb movements during walking, and independent living abilities.

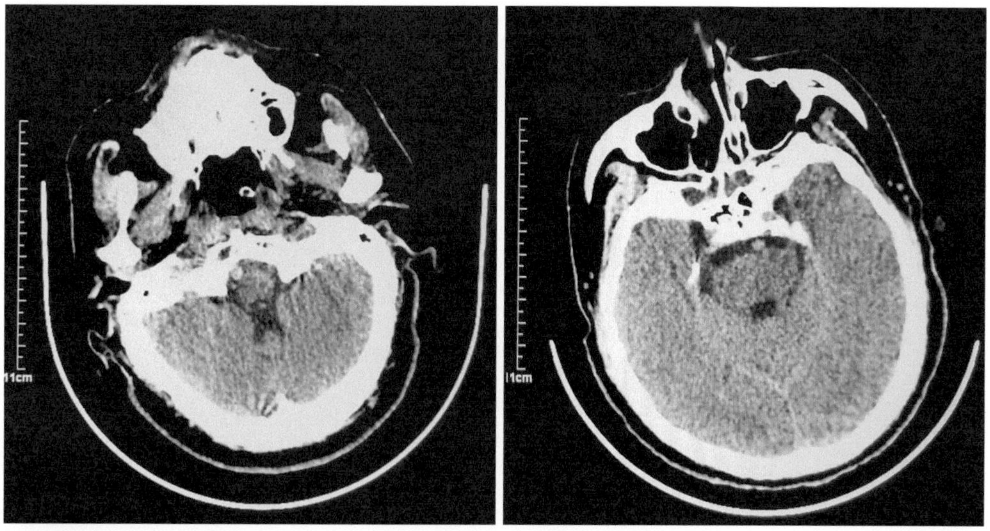

Fig. 19.19 One-month postoperative follow-up CT scan shows a slight liquefaction lesion in the brainstem

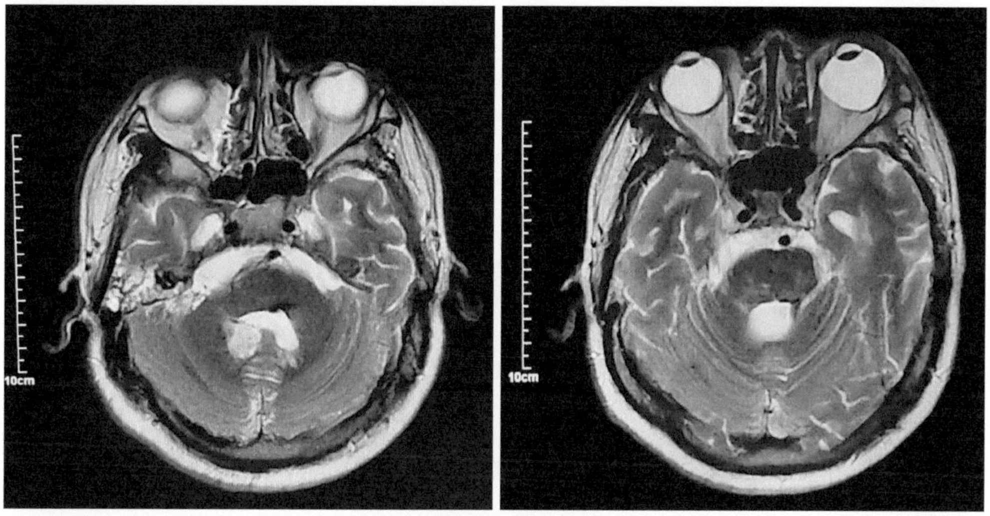

Fig. 19.20 Three-month postoperative follow-up MRI reveals a significant reduction in the liquefaction lesion of the brainstem

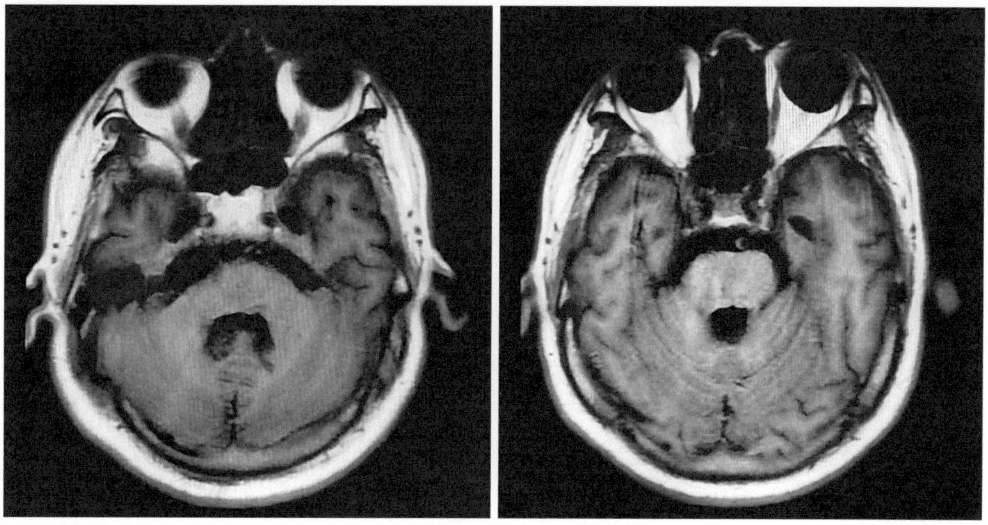

Fig. 19.21 Six-month postoperative follow-up MRI shows the disappearance of the liquefaction lesion in the brainstem

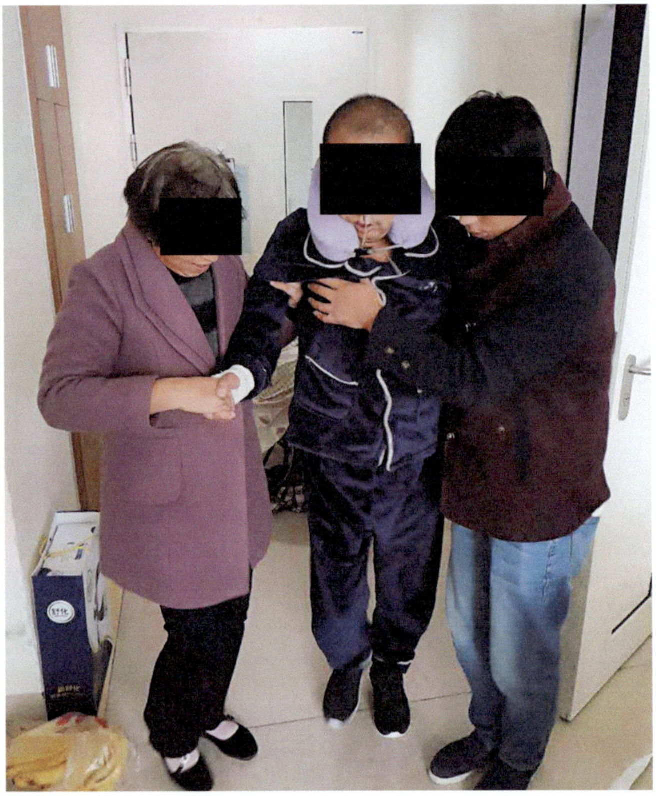

Fig. 19.22 One month after operation, the patient was able to walk with the support of family members

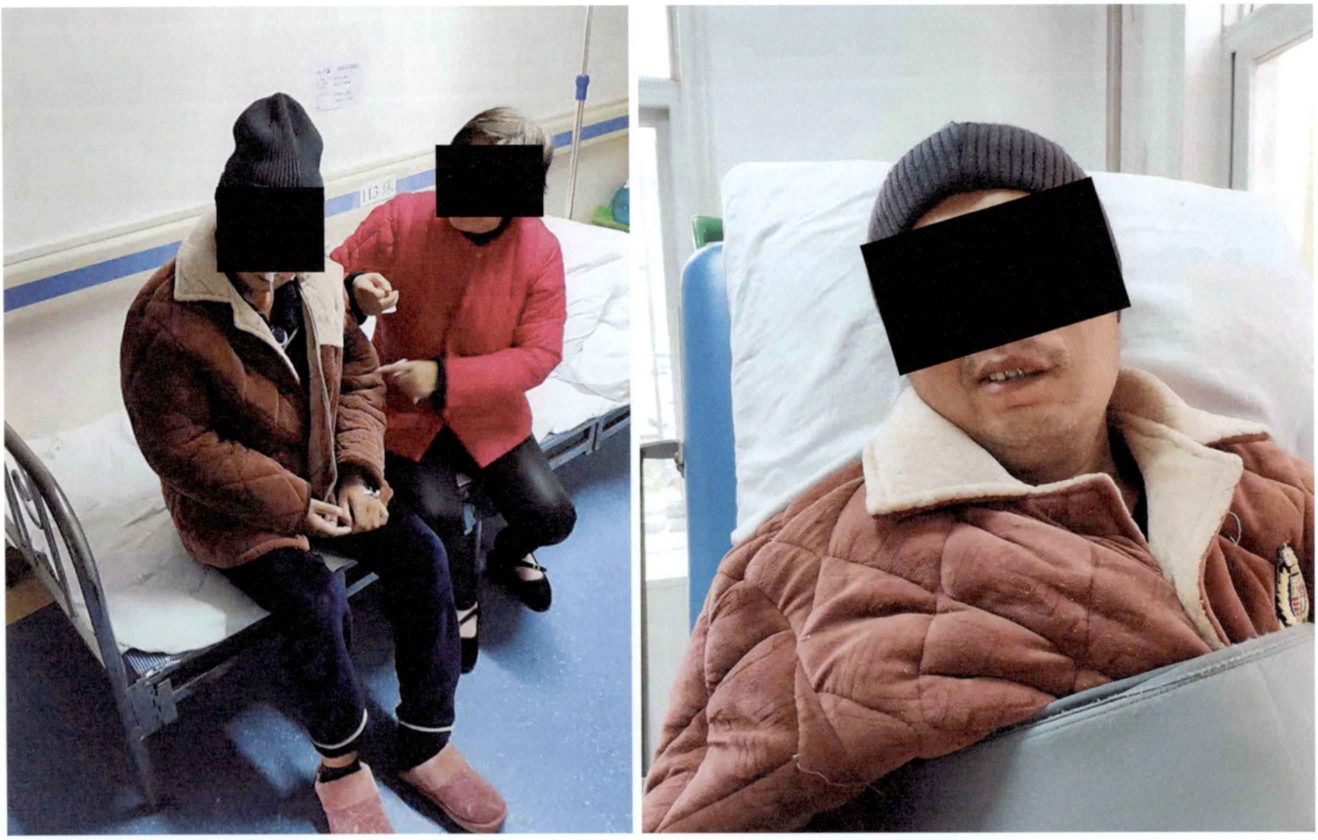

Fig. 19.23 Three months after operation, the patient was able to stand and sit down independently but exhibited incomplete motor aphasia

References

1. Li XL, Ma JX, Li P, et al. 3D printing technology and its application trends. Autom Instrum. 2014;35(1):1–5.
2. Zhou Z, Buchanan F, Mitchell C, et al. Printability of calcium phosphate: calcium sulfate powders for the application of tissue engineered bone scaffolds using the 3D printing technique. Mater Sci Eng C Mater Biol Appl. 2014;38:1–10.
3. Omori S, Murase T, Kataoka T, et al. Three-dimensional corrective osteotomy using a patient-specific osteotomy guide and bone plate based on a computer simulation system: accuracy analysis in a cadaver study. Int J Med Robot. 2014;10(2):196–202.
4. Chung KJ, Hong DY, Kim YT, et al. Preshaping plates for minimally invasive fixation of calcaneal fractures using a real-size 3D-printed model as a preoperative and intraoperative tool. Foot Ankle Int. 2014;35(11):1231–6.
5. Du HP, Li ZZ, Li ZF, et al. Application of 3D printed guide plate technology in minimally invasive puncture and drainage for intracerebral hemorrhage. Chin J Neurol. 2016;15(7):674–7.
6. Zhao J, Wang D, Liu JQ, et al. Current status and issues of 3D printing technology in the medical field. Chin J Mod Med. 2017;27(12):71–4.
7. Kunz M, Ma B, Rudan JF, et al. Image-guided distal radius osteotomy using patient-specific instrument guides. J Hand Surg Am. 2013;38(8):1618–24.
8. Campbell PG, Weiss LE. Tissue engineering with the aid of inkjet printers. Expert Opin Biol Ther. 2007;7(8):1123–7.
9. Hu ZH, Mu S, Wei JB, et al. Current status and prospects of 3D printing in neurosurgery. Mod Med Health. 2019;35(4):553–6.

20 Application of Lateral Ventricle Puncture with External Drainage in Brainstem Hemorrhage

Yinqing Zhang, Jinhua Yang, Chao Sun, and Changhai Peng

20.1 Overview

In some cases of brainstem hemorrhage, hematomas may rupture into the ventricles, obstructing cerebrospinal fluid circulation. The rapid expansion of the ventricular system leads to a sharp increase in intracranial pressure, further worsening the condition of critically ill patients with brainstem hemorrhage and potentially resulting in death. Prompt drainage of the bloody cerebrospinal fluid is essential to prevent secondary brain tissue damage from acute obstructive hydrocephalus. By performing external drainage through lateral ventricle puncture, the accumulation of blood in the ventricles can be effectively cleared. If necessary, after removing the external drainage tube, lumbar drainage can be performed to further drain the bloody cerebrospinal fluid and clear the hematoma [1].

Lateral ventricle puncture with external drainage serves as a palliative emergency surgical procedure for brainstem hemorrhage treatment in primary hospitals lacking conditions for microsurgical craniotomy, neuroendoscopic surgery, direct minimally invasive puncture, or for patients who are unable to undergo these procedures due to their own conditions. It has been used in clinical practice for several decades [2]. Lateral ventricle puncture with external drainage can achieve certain clinical efficacy in treating brainstem hemorrhage ruptured into ventricular system and can serve as an emergency rescue technique in hospitals without the necessary conditions (techniques or equipment) or for patients who cannot be transferred [3].

Y. Zhang (✉)
Department of Neurosurgery, Anxi County Hospital of Traditional Chinese Medicine, Quanzhou, China

J. Yang
Department of Neurosurgery, Gaozhou Hospital of Traditional Chinese Medicine Affiliated to Guangzhou University of Chinese Medicine, Gaozhou, China

C. Sun
Department of Neurosurgery, The Second Affiliated Hospital of Soochow University, Suzhou, China

C. Peng
Department of Neurosurgery, Gaoyao District People's Hospital of ZhaoqingCity, Zhaoqing, China

20.2 Indications and Contraindications for Surgery

20.2.1 Indications

1. Patients with brainstem hemorrhage ruptured to ventricle leading to hydrocephalus [4].
2. GCS ≤ 12, with gradually worsening vital signs and consciousness impairment.
3. During open or minimally invasive surgery for brainstem hemorrhage, ventricular cerebrospinal fluid drainage can be performed to improve surgical exposure and create favorable conditions for the procedure [5].
4. Consent from the patient's family.

20.2.2 Contraindications

1. Deep coma with fixed, dilated bilateral pupils and no spontaneous breathing for ≥ 3 h.
2. Long-term oral anticoagulant therapy, severe coagulation dysfunction, or hematological disorders [6].
3. Severe heart, kidney, or liver failure.
4. The patient's family refusing surgical treatment.

20.3 Preoperative Preparation and Surgical Instruments

20.3.1 Preoperative Preparation

1. Preoperative skin preparation, urgent complete blood count, coagulation function, and biochemistry tests. For patients with unstable respiration, early endotra-

G. Chen, C. You (eds.), *Surgical Treatment of Primary Brainstem Hemorrhage*, https://doi.org/10.1007/978-981-95-8942-5_20

cheal intubation or tracheostomy should be performed, and mechanical ventilation should be provided. The surgical consent form should be signed, and the patient should be transferred to the operating room. In emergency situations, bedside procedures can be performed [7].

2. Based on the patient's preoperative imaging data, mark the puncture site with a marking pen to determine the puncture direction and depth.

20.3.2 Surgical Instruments

Commonly used neurosurgical instruments such as hand drills, pistol drills, and electric drills can be used.

20.4 Surgical Methods, Precautions, and Techniques

20.4.1 Surgical Methods

20.4.1.1 Positioning, Incision, and Puncture Point Localization for Lateral Ventricle Anterior Horn Puncture Via the Frontal Approach

1. The patient is in a supine position with the head elevated by 30–45°. The head should be positioned centrally for anatomical accuracy.
2. Mark the puncture point with a marking pen. There are four possible puncture methods to choose from (Fig. 20.1).

2.5 cm lateral to the midline in the hairline

1 cm in front of the coronal suture, 2.5 cm lateral to the midline.

2 cm inside the hairline, 2 cm in front of the coronal suture, and 3 cm lateral to the midline.

For bald patients, 10–11 cm behind the nasal root, and 2.5–3 cm to the midline.

20.4.2 Operating Steps

1. Perform endotracheal intubation under general anesthesia. Make a vertical incision 3 cm long, located 1–2 cm in front of the coronal suture and 2.5 cm to the midline. After routine disinfection, cover with sterile drapes (Fig. 20.2).
2. Make a straight incision to cut through the scalp layers and periosteum. Use a mastoid spreader to retract it and hand drill or electric drill to create a bone hole. Stop bleeding at the bone edge with bone wax, and after hemostasis of the dura mater with electrocoagulation, make a cross-shaped incision. Insert the puncture needle perpendicularly into the bone hole, aligning the puncture direction with an imaginary line connecting the bilateral external auditory pore. Slowly puncture until reaching the anterior horn of the lateral ventricle, approximately 4–5 cm below the cortex. Remove the stylet, allow cerebrospinal fluid to flow out slowly, release an appropriate amount of cerebrospinal fluid, then suture and secure the drainage tube. To reduce the risk of infection, the drainage tube is usually led out from a separate opening beside the incision, and the surgery concludes with the external drainage bag (see Fig. 20.2) [8].

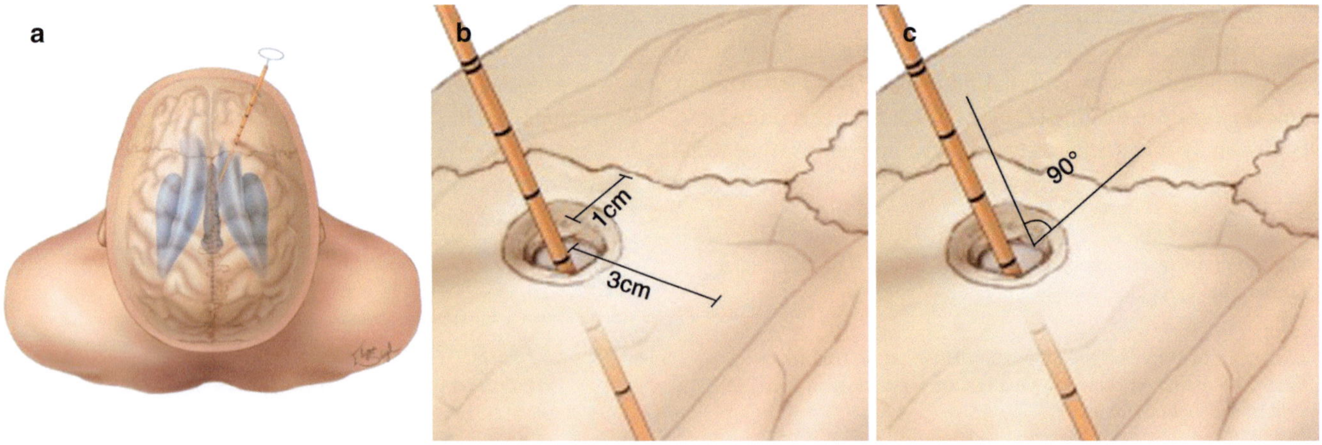

Fig. 20.1 Puncture point diagram for lateral ventricle anterior horn. (**a**) View the relationship between the puncture point and the lateral ventricle from the top of the patient's head, as well as the angle at which the puncture needle enters the ventricle. (**b**) Local enlargement of the bone orifice showing the position of the puncture hole: 1.0 cm in front of the coronal suture, 3.0 cm to the right of the midline. (**c**) Diagram showing the puncture needle making a 90° angle with the skull in the sagittal plane

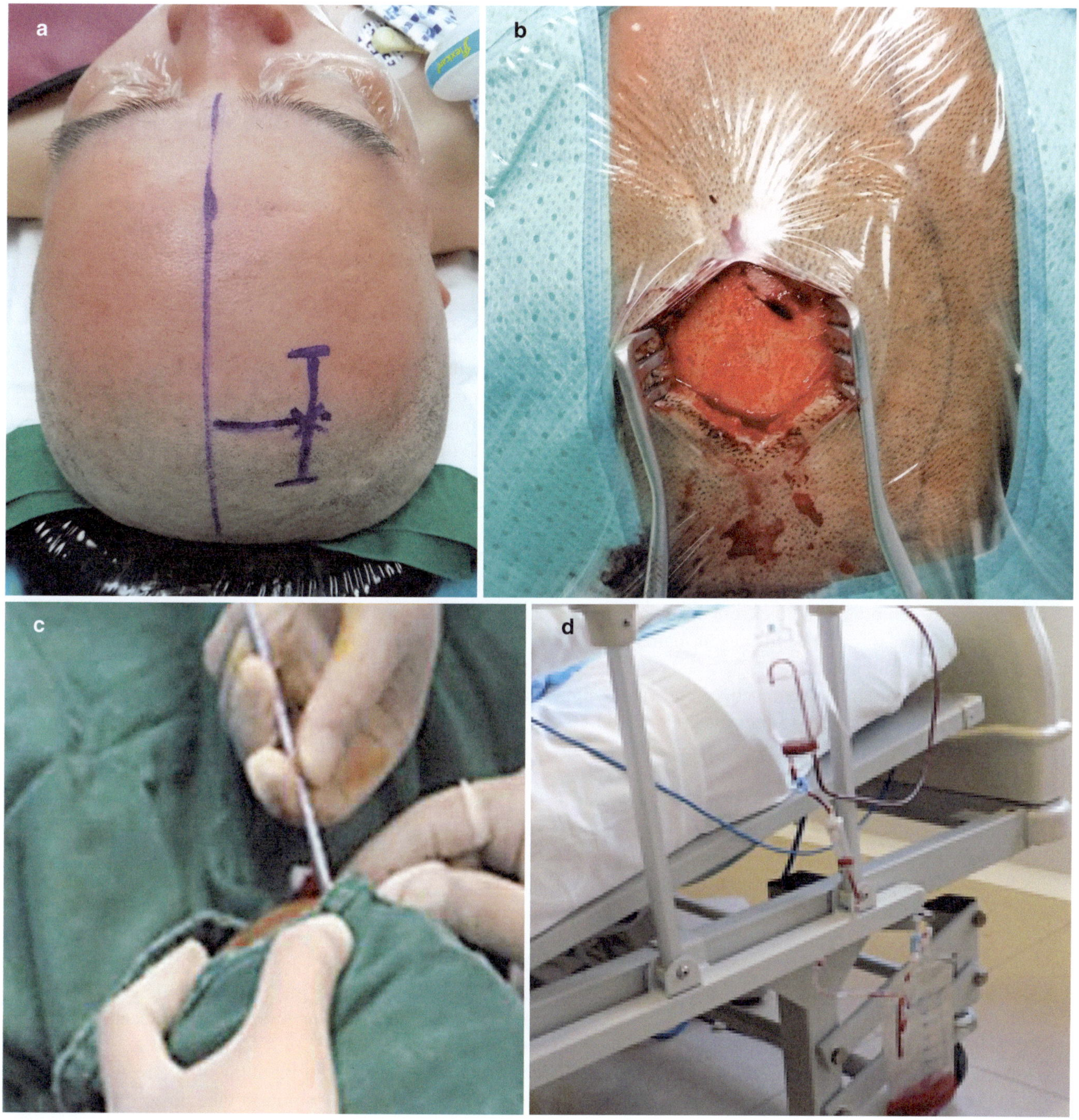

Fig. 20.2 Surgical procedure and post-surgery images for lateral ventricle anterior horn. (**a**) Before the start of the surgery, draw median sagittal line, mark the puncture point 1–2 cm behind the hairline and 2.5 cm to the right of the midline, and outline the incision line along the puncture point. (**b**) Incise the scalp to expose the skull. (**c**) Insert the ventricular puncture tube parallel to the sagittal plane from the drilling hole in the skull, aligning it with an imaginary line connecting the two external auditory hole. Slowly insert the needle vertically. (**d**) Connect the external drainage tube to a drainage bag

20.4.3 Surgical Considerations

1. Strictly adhere to surgical indications and master the puncture technique proficiently. If conditions allow, promptly address brainstem hematomas [9].
2. Placing the external drainage tube in the non-dominant hemisphere (right frontal lobe) is the conventional preferred approach; however, in specific situations, placement on the left side may also be chosen.
3. Maintain strict aseptic techniques to prevent intracranial infections.
4. Select the puncture point correctly, and determine the puncture direction and depth clearly. Incorrect puncture points and directions are often the main reasons for puncture failure; avoid repeated punctures.
5. Do not sway the needle left and right during puncture to prevent brain tissue damage. If changing direction, the needle or catheter must be withdrawn before re-puncturing. Avoid changing directions inside the brain to prevent tissue damage. Slowly and gently insert the drainage tube during the puncture. If there is a feeling of emptiness (about 5 cm), withdraw the needle to observe the flow of bloody cerebrospinal fluid from the drainage tube. Avoid puncturing too deeply to prevent damage to the brainstem or choroid plexus.
6. Do not aspirate or drain too much cerebrospinal fluid upon entering the ventricle to prevent brain tissue collapse, subdural, epidural, intracranial hemorrhage, pneumocephalus, and other complications.
7. Ensure unobstructed drainage. If the drainage tube is blocked, promptly identify and address the cause. If the tube is obstructed by blood clots or brain tissue, gently flush with a small amount of saline. If the blockage persists, replace the drainage tube promptly.

20.4.4 Surgical Techniques

1. The patient should be in a supine position with the head centrally positioned for anatomical accuracy. The head should be elevated by 30–45°. During the procedure, fix the head to minimize movement and avoid misalignment due to even slight head rotation caused by drilling the skull.
2. Understand key anatomical landmarks during the surgery: midline, nasal root, external auditory pore, coronal suture, ipsilateral pupil, and inner canthus. Enlarge the bone hole slightly to prevent the drainage tube's direction from changing due to the edge of the bone hole, leading to a shift in the puncture direction [10].
3. As external ventricular drainage may need to be in place for an extended period, to reduce the risk of cerebrospinal fluid leakage and infection, the distal end of the drainage tube should run under the skin and exit from a separate opening beside the incision.

20.5 Postoperative Care and Prevention of Complications

20.5.1 Complications and Preventions

20.5.1.1 Puncture Site Bleeding

20.5.1.1.1 Causes

Poor control of blood pressure before surgery.

Forcibly inserting a drainage tube without puncturing the dura mater during surgery can lead to local extradural hematoma.

Individual differences may result in damage to blood vessels at the puncture site.

Insertion too deeply.

20.5.1.1.2 Preventive Measures

Strictly control blood pressure before surgery to avoid significant fluctuations.

Precise measurement based on cranial CT scans to prevent shallow insertion that does not puncture the dura mater and deep insertion that may harm brain tissue.

Avoid using diuretics within 6 h of onset, and during surgery, do not excessively or rapidly aspirate or drain cerebrospinal fluid to prevent large fluctuations in intracranial pressure.

Precise preoperative positioning and avoidance of repeated puncture procedures during surgery.

20.5.1.2 Cerebrospinal Fluid Leakage and Local Infection at the Puncture Site

20.5.1.2.1 Causes

Surgical factors: such as inadequate aseptic procedures during surgery, repeated punctures, excessive scalp suture tension, etc.

Factors related to the duration of drainage tube placement: After placing the drainage tube postoperatively, as an insertion of a foreign body, the tube is quickly surrounded by connective tissue. Various proteins in the connective tissue are conducive to bacterial adhesion, particularly Staphylococcus aureus. The "mucous" component of sugar lipids aids in tight bacterial adhesion to the drainage tube wall, evades antibiotic and immune system attacks, and poses a potential risk of infection. The ventricles are in communication with the external environment, making them susceptible to bacterial invasion. Additionally, prolonged placement of drainage tubes can lead to the formation of sinus tracts in the scalp or intracranially, increasing the risk of bacterial retrograde infection and leakage.

Infection-related factors: Since the ventricular system is a weakly defended area of the body, lacking complement and IgM in cerebrospinal fluid, and without phagocytic cells, it is conducive to bacterial growth and reproduction.

Post-surgery operation related factors: such as frequent medication administration and cerebrospinal fluid sampling through the drainage tube, inadequate fixation leading to dislodgement, lack of regular disinfection, dressing changes in the surgical area and drainage tube, and complications like twisting, folding, compression, or blockage of the drainage tube.

Systemic factors: such as severe illness, deep coma, advanced age with comorbidities like diabetes, hypoalbuminemia, lung infections, poor nutritional status, etc.

20.5.1.2.2 Prevention and Treatment Measures

Comprehensive assessment of the basic surgical situation before the operation, strict adherence to aseptic principles during and after surgery, performing surgery in a sterile operating room, and using disposable sterile drainage devices.

Proper fixation of the drainage tube during surgery. After the tube exits the puncture site, it should run subcutaneously for about 5 cm before being securely fixed to reduce cerebrospinal fluid leakage and lower the risk of intracranial infection.

Enhanced postoperative drainage tube care: Ensure the drainage tube remains unobstructed, prevent twisting or folding, perform daily local disinfection and dressing changes, limit the external drainage of cerebrospinal fluid to no more than 10 mL/h, adjust the height of the drainage bottle based on the drainage volume, ensure the sterility of the drainage device, regularly replace it, and record the volume and nature of the drained fluid.

Routine use of antibiotics postoperatively. In cases of intracranial or ventricular infection, the drainage tube should ideally be removed promptly. Daily lumbar punctures for cerebrospinal fluid bacteriological examination should be performed, and sensitive antibiotics should be selected based on culture and sensitivity results. If necessary, continuous drainage through the lumbar cistern tube can be considered, and local medications can be used to control infections.

20.5.1.3 Low Intracranial Pressure, Intracranial Air Accumulation, and Brain Herniation

20.5.1.3.1 Causes

During open drainage, rapid and excessive drainage of cerebrospinal fluid can lead to brain tissue collapse, intracranial negative pressure, low intracranial pressure, intracranial air accumulation, and in severe cases, may result in upward transtentorial herniation.

20.5.1.3.2 Prevention and Treatment Measures

The highest point of the drainage device should be positioned approximately 15–20 cm above the level of the frontal horn of the lateral ventricle to maintain intracranial pressure slightly above normal. The daily drainage fluid should be controlled at around 200–300 mL.

20.5.1.4 Drain Tube Dislodgement and Obstruction

20.5.1.4.1 Causes

Improper fixation of the drainage tube can lead to accidental dislodgement during transportation or bedside care. Tube twisting, folding, compression, or blockage can result in poor drainage.

20.5.1.4.2 Prevention and Treatment Measures

During surgery, to prevent tube dislodgement and reduce infection risk, the tube can be carefully threaded under the galea aponeurotica and then externally fixed. Postoperatively, ensure proper drainage, record the volume and characteristics of drainage fluid, and if the tube is blocked by blood clots or brain tissue, promptly identify and address the cause. Flushing the tube gently with a small amount of saline may help; if the obstruction persists, the tube should be replaced promptly.

20.5.1.5 "Dependence" on Ventricular Drainage

20.5.1.5.1 Causes

In very few patients, where cerebrospinal fluid circulation pathways are established, intracranial pressure is normal, and vital signs are stable, leaving the drain in place for 24 h can worsen symptoms, making it difficult to remove the drainage tube.

20.5.1.5.2 Prevention and Treatment Measures

Gradually increase the drainage tube by 20–25 mmH_2O to allow for adaptation, gradually weaning off the dependence on intracranial pressure, aiming to resolve the issue in about 3–5 days. If the problem persists, a new drainage tube may need to be placed from the other side or a ventriculoperitoneal shunt may be considered.

20.5.2 Postoperative Management

1. Close monitoring of patient consciousness, respiration, pulse, blood pressure, temperature, pupil response, and intracranial pressure.
2. Regular follow-up cranial CT scans to monitor intracranial pressure and adjust the drainage tube height accordingly. Ensure the drainage tube remains unobstructed, maintain the appropriate height (usually 10–15 cm above the level of the frontal horn), maintain sterility of the

drainage device, replace it regularly, and record the volume and characteristics of drained fluid.
3. Postoperative measures include dehydration to reduce intracranial pressure, blood pressure management, sedation, etc.
4. Routine use of antibiotics, regular cerebrospinal fluid bacteriological examinations and sensitivity testing to prevent infection at puncture sites, ventricles, and intracranial areas.
5. Based on the status of intraventricular hemorrhage, daily administration of 20,000–30,000 units of urokinase through the drainage tube to dissolve intraventricular blood clots, promote clearance, and maintain cerebrospinal fluid circulation.
6. Drainage duration typically lasts 3–5 days, not exceeding 7 days. Before removing the drainage tube, conduct a tube clamping trial for 24–48 h, perform a follow-up cranial CT scan, and if the patient's clinical symptoms do not worsen and there is no hydrocephalus present, the tube can be removed.
7. Maintain clear airways, conduct regular sputum bacteriological examinations to prevent lung infections, enhance nutritional support, and address other complications.
8. Initiate early bedside rehabilitation training.

20.6 Advantages, Disadvantages, and Lessons Learned

20.6.1 Advantages

1. The lateral ventricle frontal horn is relatively large, facilitating puncture without choroid plexus.
2. Beneficial for clearing intraventricular hemorrhage, draining cerebrospinal fluid, improving hydrocephalus, reducing intracranial pressure, promoting early restoration of cerebrospinal fluid circulation, enabling circulation flushing of intraventricular hemorrhage, liquefaction, and accelerating drainage of brainstem hematoma.
3. Postoperatively allows dynamic monitoring of intracranial pressure to guide diuretic use.
4. The frontal puncture site is easier to care for and dress than the occipital puncture site.
5. A closed puncture orifice significantly reduces the risk of intracranial and puncture needle site infections.
6. No special equipment required, simple operation, short surgical time, suitable for emergency treatment of brainstem hemorrhage in primary hospitals [11].

20.6.2 Disadvantages

1. Simple external lateral ventricle drainage can only address intraventricular hemorrhage and improve obstructive hydrocephalus in the treatment of brainstem hemorrhage.
2. For severe brainstem hemorrhage cases with large bleeding amounts not rupturing into the ventricular system and without accompanying hydrocephalus, the effectiveness is not significant, requiring craniotomy hematoma evacuation under a microscope or minimally invasive surgery [12].

20.6.3 Lessons Learned

1. Inaccurate puncture site and direction may lead to puncture failure, and repeated punctures causing inadvertent brain tissue hemorrhage.
2. Failure to strictly control blood pressure before surgery and premature use of diuretics can result in significant intraoperative fluctuations in blood pressure and intracranial pressure.
3. Lack of strict aseptic operation during and after surgery and prolonged catheter placement can lead to intracranial infections.
4. External lateral ventricle drainage surgery is performed using a "blind technique" based on external anatomical landmarks, but ventricular anatomy may be altered due to primary diseases, necessitating personalized adjustments based on CT for catheter placement.
5. When drilling bone holes with a hand drill or electric drill, the holes should be slightly larger to prevent deviation of the drainage tube tip due to a too-small hole.
6. Postoperatively, external fixation of the drainage tube under the galea aponeurotica can reduce or minimize the risk of intracranial infection.
7. If three consecutive punctures are unsuccessful, a slight inward and backward tilt or timely head CT re-examination should be performed to correct the drainage tube path.
8. After the successful puncture, excessive or rapid drainage of cerebrospinal fluid should be avoided to prevent complications such as intracerebral hemorrhage, low intracranial pressure syndrome, pneumocephalus, and upward transtentorial herniation.

20.7 Procedure Evaluation and Prospects

20.7.1 Procedure Evaluation

Currently, various techniques such as craniotomy with microscopy, microscopy combined with neuroendoscopy for hematoma evacuation, frame-based stereotactic or frameless neuro-navigation with minimally invasive brainstem hematoma puncture and aspiration, and other positioning techniques like CT-assisted localization have achieved certain clinical efficacy in the treatment of severe brainstem hemorrhage domestically and internationally. However, due to the unique location of brainstem hemorrhage, the surgery is challenging with significant risks, and the iatrogenic trauma caused by surgery cannot be underestimated. While surgery has improved survival rates, the overall quality of life for surviving patients is not ideal. Further exploration and evaluation are needed to determine the clinical efficacy and surgical value. Simple external lateral ventricle drainage surgery may not have a significant effect on brainstem hemorrhage with massive bleeding but not entering the ventricular system and without hydrocephalus. However, for severe cases of brainstem hemorrhage rupturing into the ventricular system, accompanied by intraventricular hemorrhage and obstructive hydrocephalus, external lateral ventricle drainage surgery alone has certain clinical efficacy and value. This procedure mainly involves timely clearance of intraventricular hemorrhage and partial brainstem hematoma (after aspirating intraventricular hemorrhage and allowing brainstem hematoma to flow out of the ventricle again through the hematoma rupture site for external drainage by the lateral ventricle drainage tube), thereby promptly relieving hydrocephalus and restoring cerebrospinal fluid circulation. Additionally, connecting an intracranial pressure monitoring device can monitor intracranial pressure and guide diuretic use.

20.7.2 Prospects

External lateral ventricle drainage for brainstem hemorrhage treatment is simple, easy to master, requires no special equipment, is cost-effective, and minimally traumatic. It is particularly suitable for emergency rescue of brainstem hemorrhage patients in hospitals without the capability to perform brainstem hematoma evacuation surgery, providing valuable time for life-saving treatments (such as transferring to another hospital or consulting higher-level experts). Therefore, this procedure remains an important treatment measure for emergency treatment of brainstem hemorrhage and saving lives in primary hospitals [13].

20.8 Typical Case

20.8.1 Case 1

20.8.1.1 Brief Medical History and Imaging Data

The patient, male, 54 years old, presented to the emergency department with “sudden loss of consciousness.” He had a history of hypertension for over 7 years. On physical examination, his blood pressure was 180/123 mmHg, heart rate was 116 beats per minute, and respiratory rate was 26 breaths per minute. GCS 8, indicating light coma. The pupils were pinpoint with absent light reflex. The patient had neck stiffness, diminished limb reflexes, and positive bilateral Babinski sign. Cranial CT scan revealed a 29.1 mm × 24.7 mm × 40 mm intracerebral hemorrhage in the brainstem (midbrain and pons), estimated 14 mL, extending into the ventricular system. The lateral ventricles were enlarged bilaterally (Fig. 20.3).

20.8.1.2 Surgical Procedure and Key Points

The patient was taken to the operating room after routine preoperative preparations. After successful endotracheal intubation under general anesthesia, the patient was placed in a supine position with the head elevated 30°. The head was positioned in the neutral midline. Standard disinfection and draping were performed. A longitudinal incision of approximately 3 cm in length was made 2.5 cm along the left frontal hairline, 2.5 cm from the midline. The scalp and subcutaneous tissue were sequentially dissected and the periosteum was peeled off. The scalp was retracted, exposing the frontal bone, and a drill was performed. A bone flap was created by drilling a groove at the posterior edge of the bone hole. After thorough hemostasis with bipolar electrocautery, a cruciate incision was made. A disposable external ventricular drain was inserted in the direction of the intersection of the imaginary line connecting the external auditory pore and the sagittal plane. When the needle advanced approximately 5 cm, a distinct breakthrough sensation was felt. The drainage tube was further inserted by 1 cm, the stylet was removed, and a pale red cerebrospinal fluid began to flow slowly. After a suitable amount of cerebrospinal fluid was drained, the distal end of the drainage tube was brought out and sutured in place. After satisfactory hemostasis in the surgical area, the bone hole was filled with gelatin sponge and the scalp was closed layer by layer. The surgery was concluded with the placement of an external drainage bag, and the patient was transferred to ICU for monitoring only (Fig. 20.4).

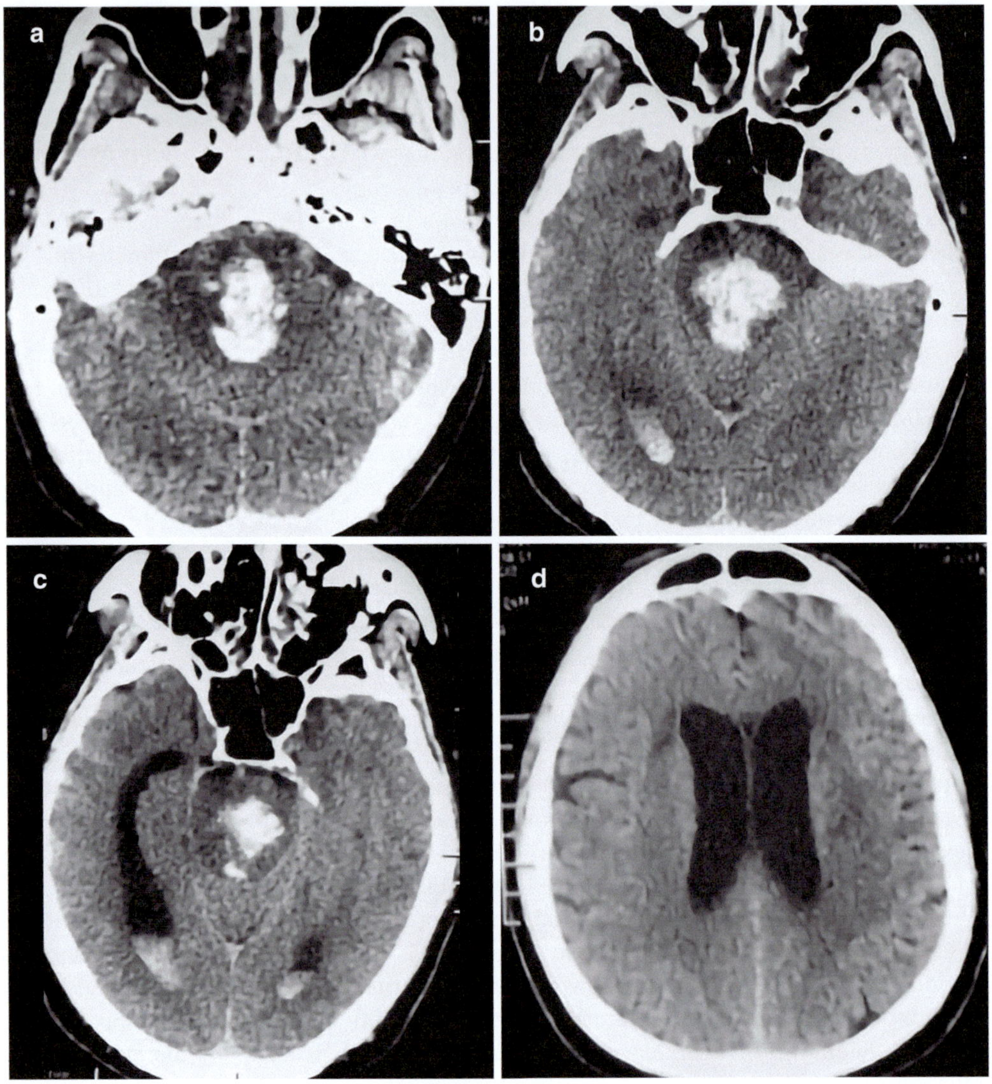

Fig. 20.3 CT scan showing brainstem hemorrhage. (**a**–**c**) Demonstrate the midbrain and pons hemorrhage in this patient, extending into the ventricular system. (**d**) Shows bilateral enlargement of the lateral ventricles

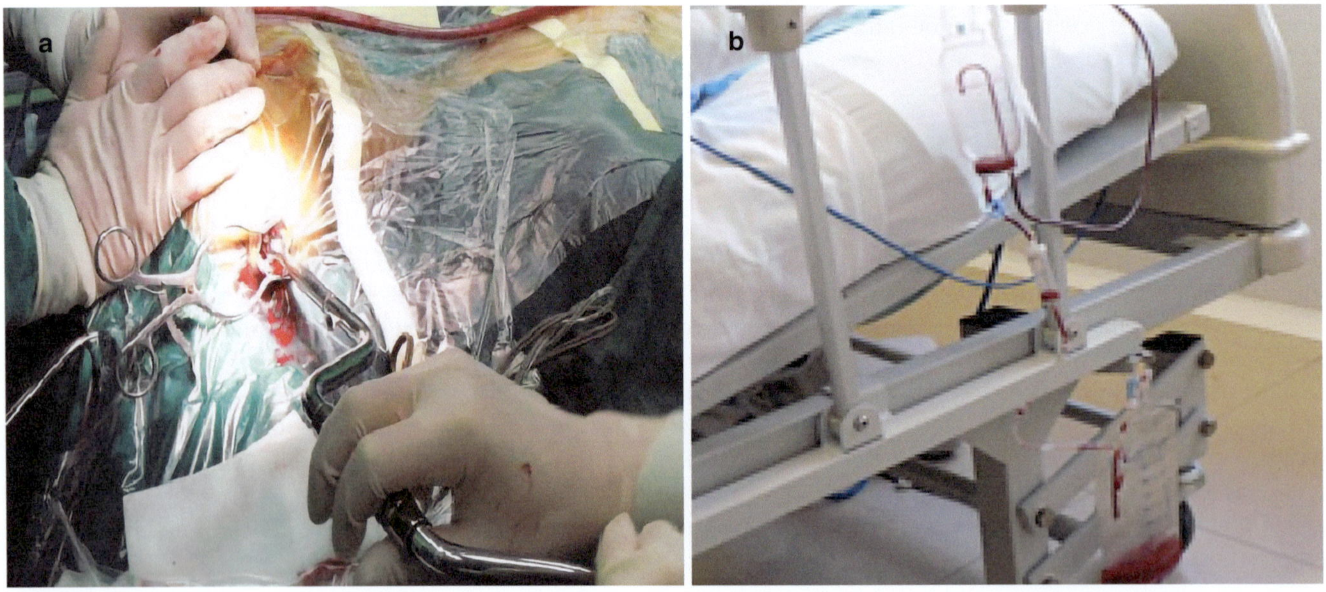

Fig. 20.4 Lateral ventricle puncture procedure. (**a**) Skull drilling and puncture needle advancing toward the intersection of the imaginary line connecting the external auditory hole and the sagittal plane; (**b**) postoperative drainage situation

20.8.1.3 Postoperative Treatment and Imaging Comparison

The patient underwent follow-up cranial CT scans on postoperative day 1, day 10, and 3 months (Figs. 20.5, 20.6, and 20.7), which showed a gradual benign improvement in the amount of intracranial hemorrhage and mass effect. In the past, nonsurgical patients often deteriorated and died within 24 h. However, with aggressive ventricular drainage surgery, GCS of this patient reached 6 at the 3-month follow-up (Fig. 20.8).

20.8.2 Case 2

20.8.2.1 Brief Medical History and Imaging Data

The patient, a 70-year-old male, was admitted to the emergency department with a chief complaint of "sudden onset of altered consciousness for 30 min." He had a history of hypertension for 11 years. On examination, his blood pressure was measured at 220/177 mmHg, heart rate at 116 beats per minute, and respiratory rate at 26 breaths per minute. GCS 8, indicating light coma. The patient had pinpoint pupils with absent light reflex, neck stiffness, decreased limb tendon reflexes, and positive bilateral Babinski sign. Cranial CT scan revealed a 29.1 mm × 24.7 mm × 40 mm intracerebral hemorrhage in the brainstem (midbrain and pons), estimated 14 mL, extending into the ventricular system. The lateral ventricles were enlarged bilaterally (Fig. 20.9)..

20.8.2.2 Surgical Procedure and Key Points

The patient was taken to the operating room after routine preoperative preparation. After successful endotracheal intubation under general anesthesia, the patient was positioned supine with the head elevated 30°. The head was placed in the neutral position. Standard skin disinfection was performed, and a longitudinal incision of approximately 3 cm in

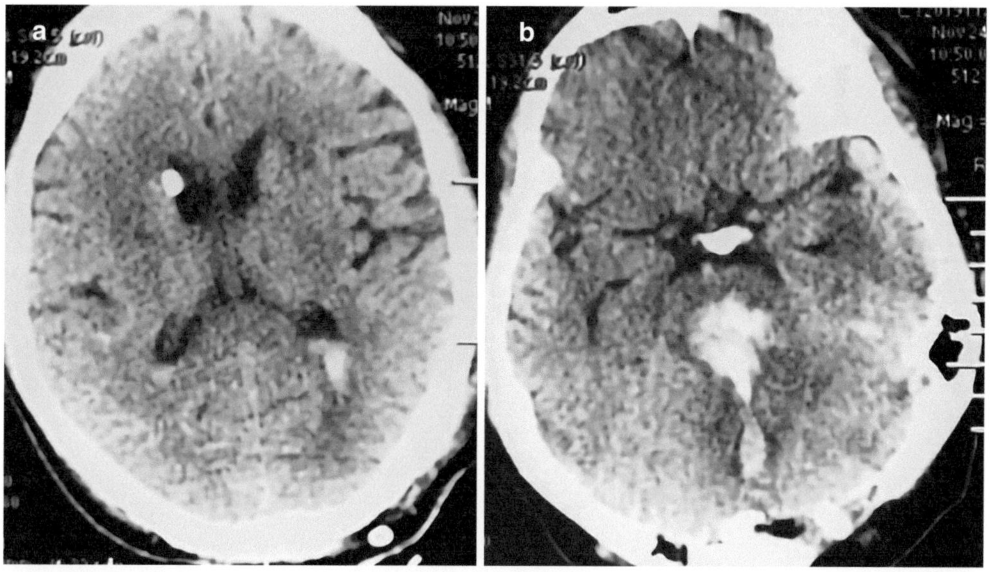

Fig. 20.5 Cranial CT scan on postoperative day 1. (**a**) The drainage tube is located in the left lateral ventricle, and the ventricular dilation has slightly improved; (**b**) decreased brainstem hemorrhage

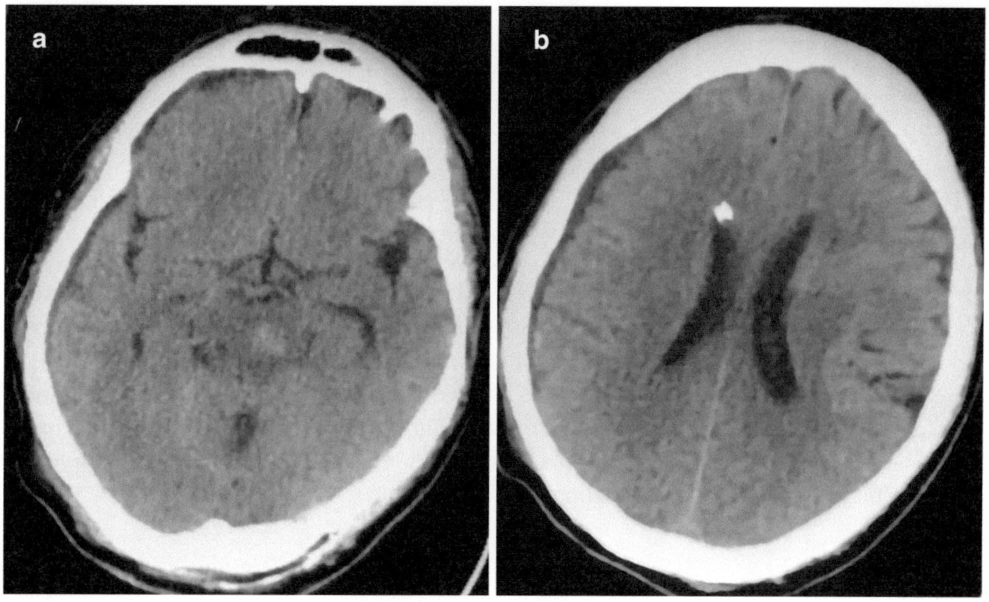

Fig. 20.6 Cranial CT scan on postoperative day 10. (**a**) The drainage tube is located in the left lateral ventricle, and the bilateral ventricular dilation has mostly resolved; (**b**) Marked reduction in brainstem hemorrhage

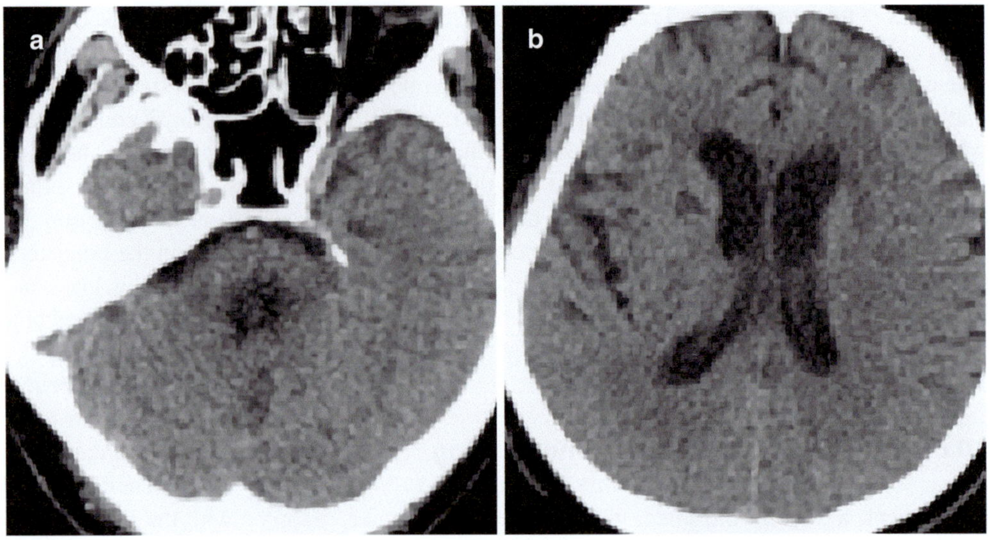

Fig. 20.7 CT scan at 3-month postoperative follow-up. (**a**) Small liquefaction foci in the brainstem are observed; (**b**) no ventricular system dilation

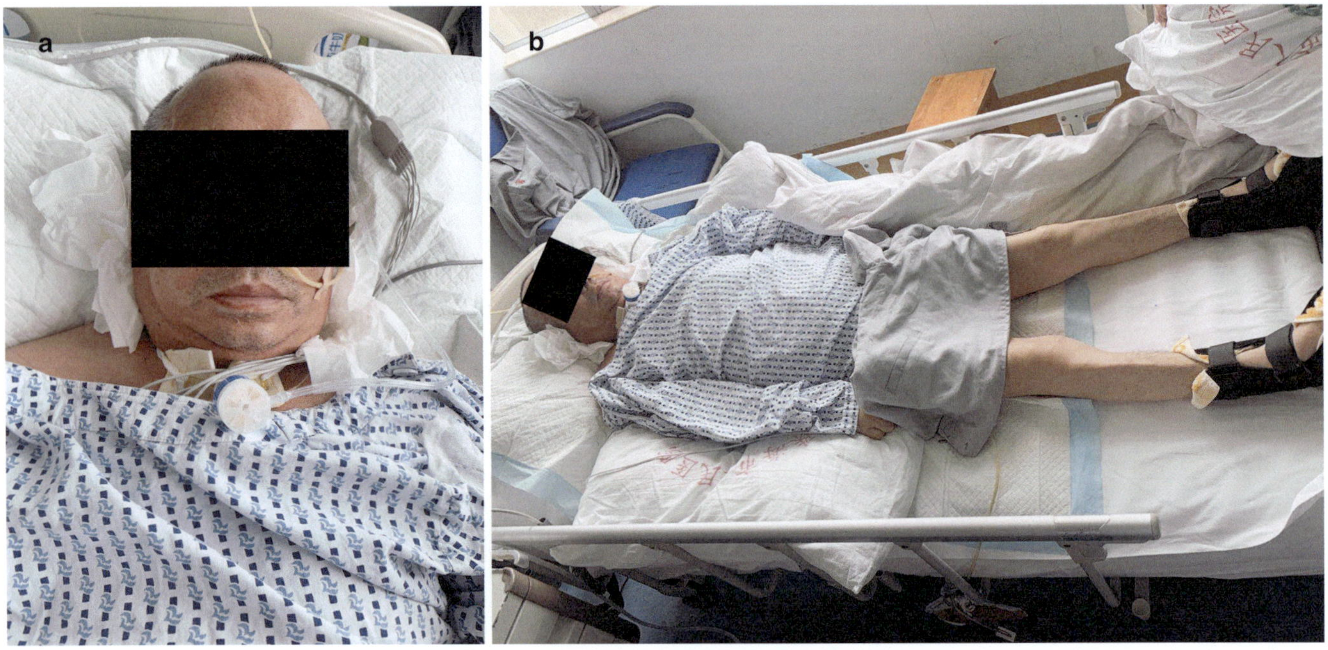

Fig. 20.8 Patient presentation at 3 months postoperatively. (**a**) Patient spontaneously opens eyes; (**b**) GCS 6 (E4V1M1)

length was made 2.5 cm along the left frontal hairline, 2.5 cm from the midline. The scalp and subcutaneous tissue were sequentially dissected, and a bone hole with a diameter of approximately 1.5 cm was drilled using an electric drill. After electrocoagulation for hemostasis of the dura mater, a cruciate incision was made, and the brain surface was coagulated. A puncture needle was inserted parallel to the sagittal plane, aiming at the anterior horn of the left lateral ventricle along the line connecting both external auditory pores. After penetrating approximately 4 cm below the cortical surface with a breakthrough sensation, the stylet was withdrawn, revealing the flow of bloody cerebrospinal fluid. A drainage tube was placed to a depth of approximately 5 cm, and after confirming unobstructed drainage, the drainage tube was fixed, and an additional puncture hole was made near the incision. The incision was sutured, and an external drainage bag was connected for further treatment in NICU.

20.8.2.3 Postoperative Treatment and Postoperative Imaging Comparison

20.8.2.3.1 Postoperative Treatment

1. Maintain unobstructed drainage through the drainage tube. Adjust the height of the drainage bottle according to the patient's condition, with a recommended height of

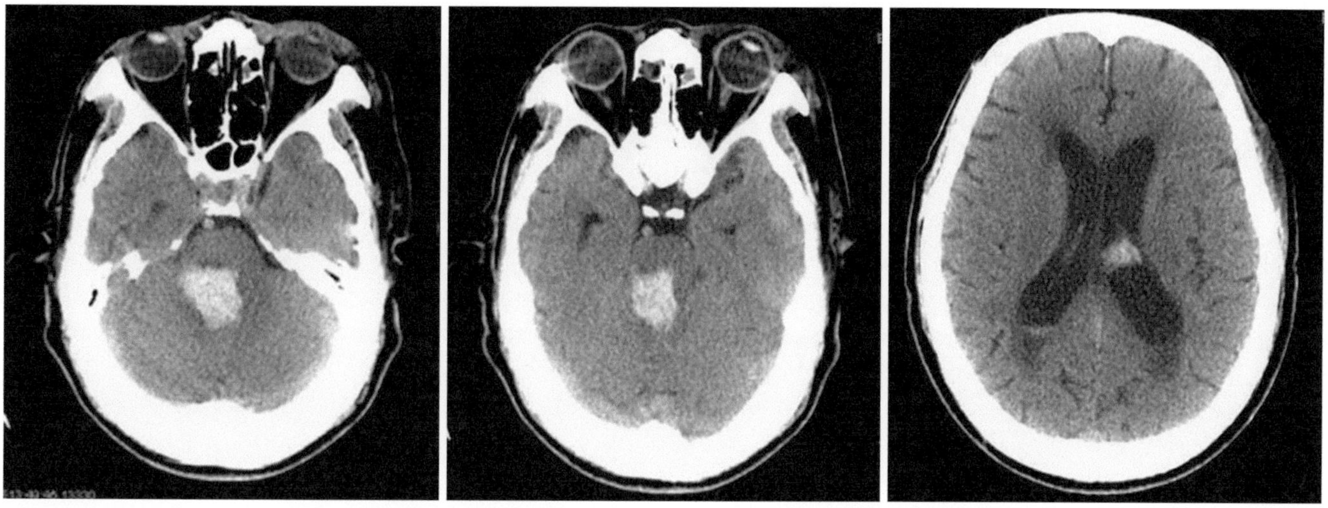

Fig. 20.9 Emergency CT scan showing brainstem hemorrhage (midbrain, pons) with extension into the ventricular system and lateral ventricular enlargement

10–15 cm above the lateral ventricle. Adjust the flow rate using a flow regulator, aiming for a drainage volume of 200–300 mL/24 h.

2. Monitor intracranial pressure closely postoperatively. Monitor routine and biochemical analysis of cerebrospinal fluid, as well as general conditions such as internal environment and electrolyte metabolism, to promptly detect central nervous system infections, if any.
3. Administer medications for infection prevention, neurotrophic support, and diuretics as adjunctive therapy.
4. Perform follow-up CT scans to assess the absorption of the brainstem and intraventricular hematoma. Enhance airway management, considering early tracheostomy for patients expected to have prolonged coma.
5. Administer medications for neurotrophic support and diuretics as adjunctive therapy.
6. After approximately 3 weeks, when the patient's general condition stabilizes, provide hyperbaric oxygen therapy.

20.8.2.3.2 Extubation Criteria

The patient's vital signs are stable, and follow-up CT scans show complete or near-complete clearance of intraventricular hemorrhage, with cerebrospinal fluid biochemical analysis within normal limits and unobstructed cerebrospinal fluid circulation. The drainage tube may be clamped for 24 h before extubation, and extubation can proceed if there is no deterioration in clinical symptoms.

20.8.2.3.3 Postoperative Imaging Comparison

This patient underwent follow-up cranial CT scans at postoperative day 1, day 7, day 10, and 3 months (Figs. 20.10, 20.11, 20.12, and 20.13). The images showed a gradual and favorable improvement in the volume of intracranial hemorrhage and mass effect.

20.8.2.4 Neurological Examination of the Postoperative Patient

At 3 months postoperatively, the patient was able to follow commands, extend the tongue, grip objects and expression to a certain degree. However, he experienced some difficulty with swallowing and required nasogastric tube feeding. Muscle strength in the left limbs was classified as III–IV, while in the right limbs, it was classified as IV–V. The patient was able to walk with assistance.

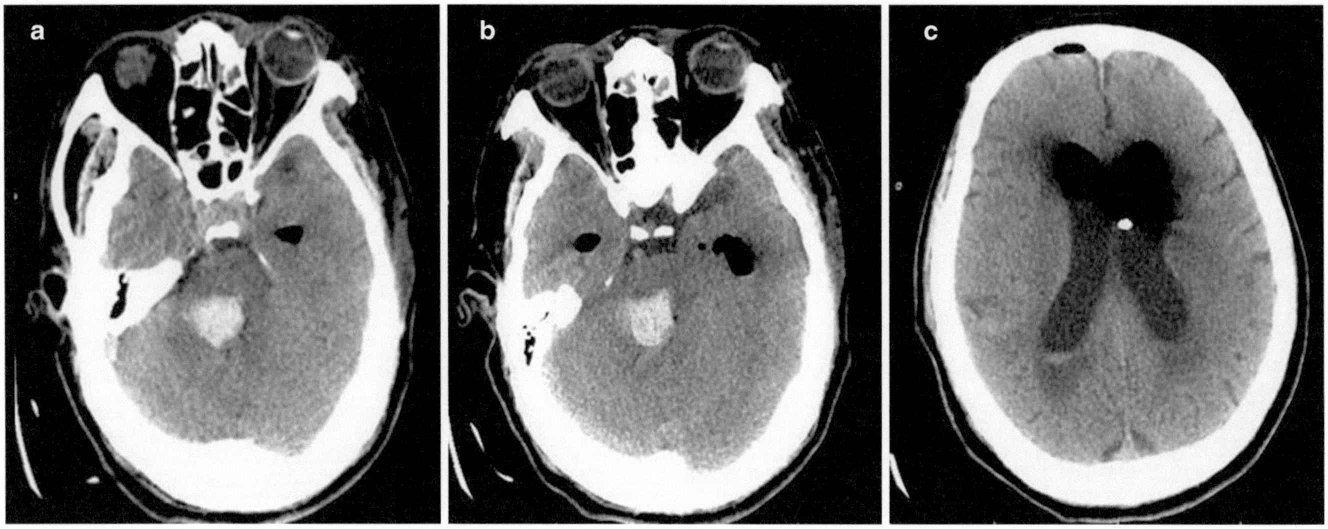

Fig. 20.10 Postoperative CT scan on day 1. (**a**, **b**) Reduced brainstem hemorrhage; (**c**) the drainage tube is located within the left lateral ventricle, with minimal air in the bilateral anterior horns of the ventricles and reduced ventricular dilation

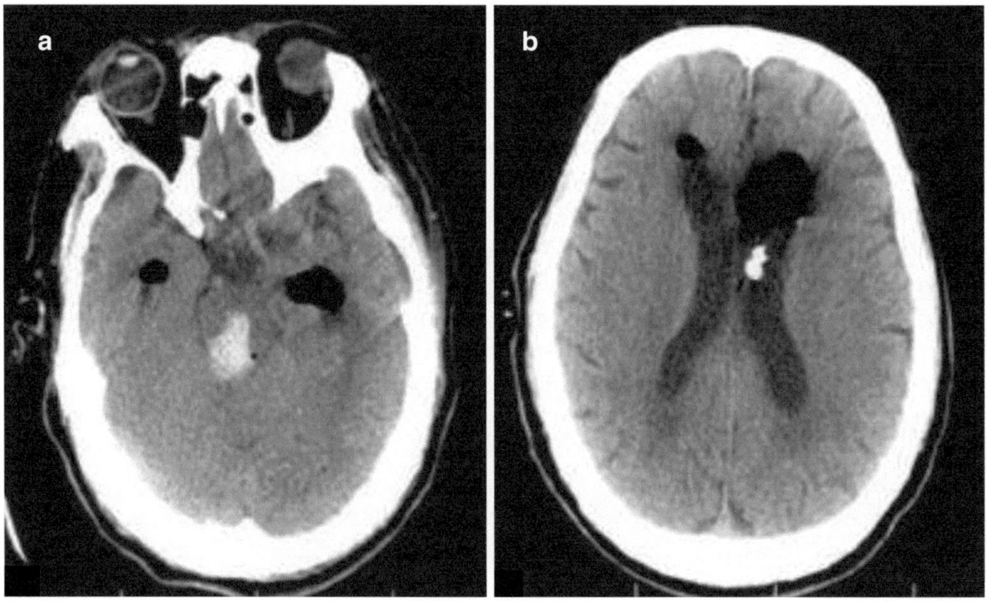

Fig. 20.11 Postoperative CT scan on day 7. (**a**) Marked reduction in brainstem hemorrhage; (**b**) the drainage tube remains in the left lateral ventricle, with a small amount of air in the left anterior horn and near-complete resolution of ventricular dilation

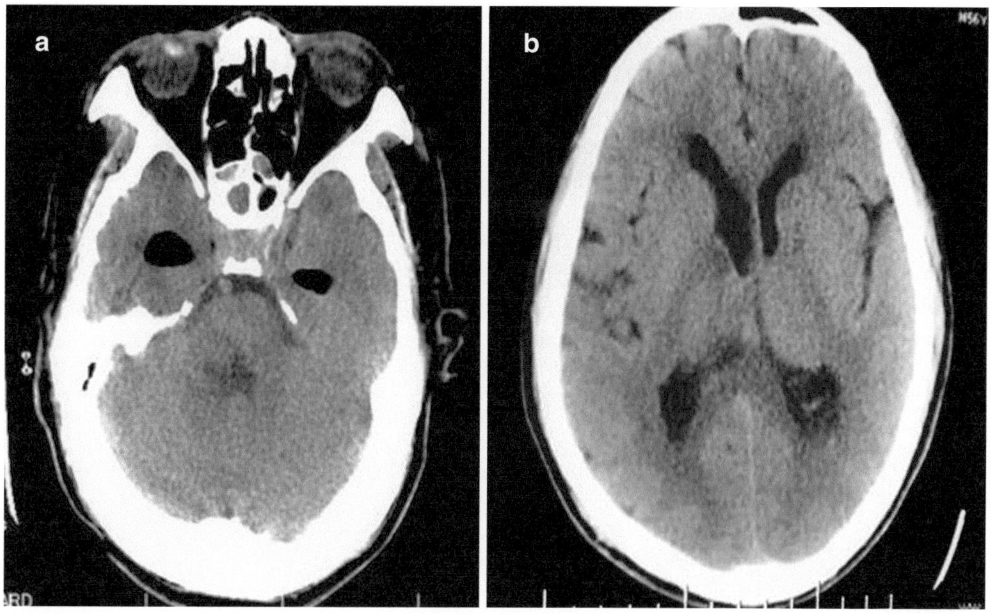

Fig. 20.13 CT scan at 3 months postoperatively. (**a**) Small liquefaction foci in the brainstem; (**b**) no ventricular system dilation observed

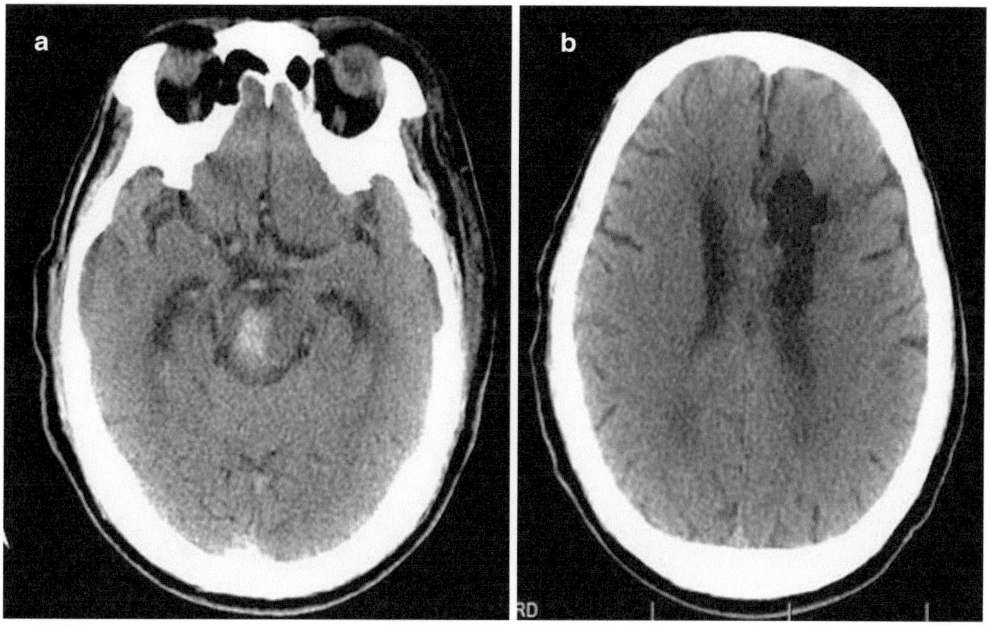

Fig. 20.12 CT scan at 27 days postoperatively. (**a**) Minimal residual blood in the brainstem; (**b**) no ventricular dilation observed bilaterally

References

1. Hemphill JC III, Greenberg SM, Anderson CS, et al. Guidelines for the management of spontaneous intracerebral hemorrhage: a guideline for healthcare professionals from the American Heart Association/American Stroke Association. Stroke. 2015;46(7):2032–60.
2. Peng CH, Chen HM, Xia JB. Observation on the therapeutic effect of lateral ventricular puncture external drainage in the treatment of severe primary brainstem hemorrhage patients. Chin Commun Physician. 2017;33(31):67–9.
3. Zeng GL, Sun JZ, Yuan HG. Clinical analysis of lateral ventricular puncture drainage in the treatment of severe brainstem hemorrhage. Hebei Med. 2015;3:408–9.
4. Peng JH, Huang LQ, Nong SD, et al. Analysis of the predictive value of early changes in hematoma cavity and ventricles on adverse outcomes in patients with primary brainstem hemorrhage. Chin J Neurol. 2019;18(2):127–35.
5. Chen LH, Xu RX. Minimally invasive treatment of primary brainstem hemorrhage. Chin J Neurotrauma Surg Electron Ed. 2016;2(4):252–4.
6. Rowe AS, Rinehart DR, Lezatte S, et al. Intracerebral hemorrhage after external ventricular drain placement: an evaluation of risk factors for post-procedural hemorrhagic complications. BMC Neurol. 2018;18(1):22.
7. Lovasik BP, McCracken DJ, McCracken CE, et al. The effect of external ventricular drain use in intracerebral hemorrhage. World Neurosurg. 2016;94:309–18.

8. Kirmani AR, Sarmast AH, Bhat AR. Role of external ventricular drainage in the management of intraventricular hemorrhage; its complications and management. Surg Neurol Int. 2015;6:188.
9. Ding XQ, Li ZF. Current status and progress in surgical treatment of brainstem hemorrhage. Med Rev. 2017;23(21):4252–5.
10. Li J, Zheng J. Experience in microsurgical treatment of primary brainstem hemorrhage. Chin J Neurosurg. 2017;33(2):184–5.
11. Zhang YQ, Ye JL, Wu WB, et al. Minimally invasive conical skull surgery for the treatment of 32 cases of severe primary brainstem hemorrhage. Chin J Minimally Invasive Neurosurg. 2017;22(12):562–3.
12. Li H, Liu WK, Lin S, et al. Discussion on the treatment of hypertension-related brainstem hemorrhage. Chin J Neurosurg. 2013;29(4):339–41.
13. He ZL, Wang XO. Clinical analysis of lateral ventricular drainage in the treatment of severe primary brainstem hemorrhage. Bethune Med J. 2014;12(2):160–1.

Postoperative Intensive Care Treatment for Primary Brainstem Hemorrhage

21

Yuhai Wang, Wenyan Zhuo, Huasong Wang, Xiaopeng Yang, and Jie Zhu

21.1 Overview

After admission to the neurosurgical intensive care unit (NSICU) following primary brainstem hemorrhage surgery, in addition to routine hemostasis, anti-infection, seizure prevention, and other treatments, a combination of various neurocritical monitoring methods should be used to promptly adjust systemic treatment goals and plans, ensuring that implemented treatment measures effectively maintain the basic life signs of postoperative primary brainstem hemorrhage patients [1–7].

21.2 Definition of Intensive Care Unit

The primary brainstem hemorrhage intensive care unit refers to a specialized multidisciplinary collaborative medical team that possesses fundamental theories, basic knowledge, and basic operational techniques in neurosurgery, as well as expertise in critical care monitoring technology and critical care medicine concepts [1–3]. Utilizing modern critical care medicine principles and monitoring technologies, supported by advanced equipment and instruments, this unit implements effective centralized treatment and care for critically ill brainstem hemorrhage patients [8]. An ideal NSICU can provide rational neurocritical care for patients, including staged treatment for intracranial hypertension, maintenance of cerebral perfusion pressure (CPP), osmotherapy, hypothermia treatment, barbiturate therapy, hyperventilation, decompressive craniectomy, seizure prevention and control, improvement of microcirculation and vasodilation, management of neuroendocrine disorders, hormone replacement, brain protection, and other treatment strategies to comprehensively safeguard brain function [1–3]. Furthermore, comprehensive mastery of critical care monitoring and treatment is essential, including hemodynamic monitoring, organ function assessment, pain management, sedation, fluid resuscitation, mechanical ventilation, nutritional therapy, infection control, deep vein thrombosis prevention, blood glucose regulation, stress ulcer prevention, electrolyte balance, blood purification, and more, to ensure patient safety through the implementation of intensive monitoring and treatment [9–11].

21.3 Emergency Management Process and Monitoring of Critically Ill Patients

Brainstem hemorrhage manifests rapidly, poses a severe prognosis, and has a high mortality rate, making it one of the most fatal and poor prognostic diseases among all types of strokes, requiring prompt intervention and treatment [1, 2]. The emergency management process is outlined in Fig. 21.1 [12].

Y. Wang (✉) · J. Zhu
Department of Neurosurgery, No.904th Hospital of The People's Liberation Army Joint Logistics Support Force, Wuxi, China

W. Zhuo
Department of Neurology, Zhuhai People's Hospital (The Affiliated Hospital of Beijing Institute of Technology, Zhuhai Clinical Medical College of Jinan University), Zhuhai, China

H. Wang
Department of Neurorehabilitation, The Fifth People's Hospital of Zhuhai, Zhuhai, China

X. Yang
Department of Neurosurgery, People's Hospital of Xinjiang Uygur Autonomous Region, Urumqi, China

G. Chen, C. You (eds.), *Surgical Treatment of Primary Brainstem Hemorrhage*, https://doi.org/10.1007/978-981-95-8942-5_21

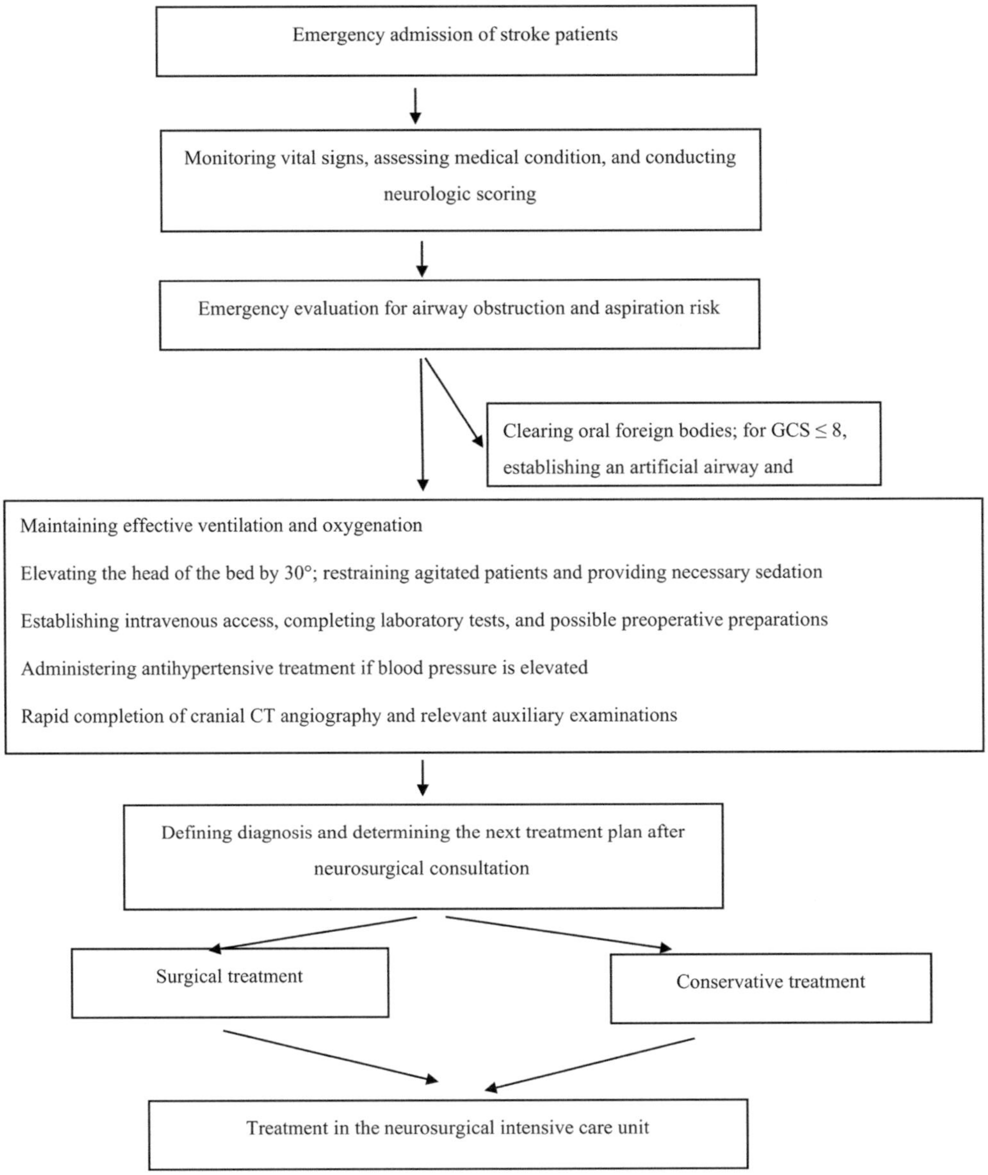

Fig. 21.1 Emergency and intensive care management process for brainstem hemorrhage

21.4 Systemic and Specialized Functional Assessment of the Patient

21.4.1 General Physical Examination and Maintenance of Vital Signs

A systematic general physical examination should be conducted on primary brainstem hemorrhage patients admitted to NSICU [1, 2]. This includes preliminary assessments of the cardiovascular system, respiratory system, hematological system, endocrine system, and overall patient condition [3]. Additionally, monitoring results such as electrocardiography, non-invasive blood pressure, invasive continuous arterial pressure, central venous pressure (CVP), intracranial pressure (ICP), brain temperature, brain oxygenation, liver and kidney function, blood urine osmolarity, coagulation function, body temperature, and peripheral oxygen saturation should be utilized to promptly adjust systemic treatment goals and plans, ensuring that implemented treatment measures effectively maintain the basic life signs of primary brainstem hemorrhage patients [13].

21.4.2 Examination of Primary Brainstem Hemorrhage and Neurological Function Monitoring

21.4.2.1 Neurological Examination and Scoring

After the patient is admitted to the NSICU, a systematic examination of the neurological system should be performed, including assessment of general neurological responses, pupil condition, cranial nerve responses, motor and sensory functions, physiological reflexes, and pathological reflexes [1, 2]. GCS should be evaluated to grasp the patient's basic condition. However, due to factors such as endotracheal intubation and sedation in postoperative primary brainstem hemorrhage patients, GCS may not accurately reflect their basic condition. In such cases, the Full Outline of Unresponsiveness (FOUR) score can be used for comprehensive assessment (Table 21.1) [14].

21.4.2.2 Intracranial Pressure and Cerebral Perfusion Pressure Monitoring

Currently, the commonly used invasive methods for monitoring intracranial pressure include intraventricular and intraparenchymal approaches [1, 2]. Intraventricular catheter placement is considered the gold standard as it allows for the monitoring of intracranial pressure and the potential to lower it by draining cerebrospinal fluid. The surgical placement of intracranial pressure probes must strictly adhere to aseptic procedures, and the monitoring duration typically does not exceed 14 days based on the extent of intracranial edema [15].

21.4.2.3 Cerebral Blood Flow (CBF) Monitoring

Following brain injury, alterations in cerebral blood circulation may occur, such as inadequate perfusion or excessive congestion [1]. Increased intracranial pressure, brain edema, and vascular spasm can contribute to inadequate perfusion. The average cerebral blood flow in normal adults is approximately (50 ± 5) mL/(100 g · min). The average cerebral blood flow in gray matter during rest is (76 ± 10) mL/(100 g · min), while in white matter, it is only (20 ± 4) mL/(100 g · min). Reduced cerebral blood flow can lead to disruptions in protein synthesis and increased anaerobic glycolysis, hindering brain tissue recovery [2]. Therefore, cerebral blood flow monitoring is conducted for patients with post-BSH surgery in the NSICU. Transcranial Doppler ultrasound (TCD) is a common method for CBF monitoring, assessing blood flow velocities in major basal arteries through thin areas of the skull bone using low frequency ultrasound [16]. Changes in arterial mean velocity (MV), pulsatility index (PI), and waveform alterations can indicate conditions such as low cerebral blood flow, high cerebral blood flow, vascular spasm, and cerebral death. The average middle cerebral artery blood flow velocity in normal individuals is (65 ± 17) cm/s, with more severe brain injury correlating with prolonged periods of low blood flow velocity. Elevated blood flow velocity and increased jugular venous oxygen saturation (SjvO2) suggest cerebral congestion, and high blood flow velocity reflects cerebral vascular narrowing and middle

Table 21.1 Full outline of unresponsiveness (FOUR) score

	FOUR score (E)	
	Clinical presentation score	
Eye response	Opens eyes and tracks or blinks in response to command	4
	Opens eyes but does not track	3
	Closes eyes but opens in response to strong auditory stimulus	2
	Closes eyes and opens in response to painful stimulus	1
	No eye opening or response to stimulus	0
	FOUR score (M)	
	Clinical presentation score	
Motor response	Follows commands to move fingers, grip, or make a V-sign	4
	Localizes to painful stimulus	3
	Flexion to painful stimulus	2
	Hyperextension to painful stimulus	1
	No response to painful stimulus or muscle rigidity	0
	FOUR score (B)	
	Clinical presentation score	
Brainstem reflex	Pupillary and corneal reflexes intact	4
	One pupil dilated and fixed	3
	Loss of pupillary or corneal reflex	2
	Loss of both pupillary and corneal reflexes	1
	Loss of pupillary, corneal, and cough reflexes	0
	FOUR score (B)	
	Clinical presentation score	
Respiration	Not intubated, regular respiratory pattern	4
	Not intubated, moist respiration	3
	Not intubated, irregular respiratory pattern	2
	Respiratory rate higher than ventilator setting	1
	Respiratory rate equal to ventilator setting or absent	0

cerebral artery spasm. TCD examinations can assess mass effects and changes in intracranial pressure. Variations in the waveform can be observed in TCD with increased intracranial pressure and decreased cerebral perfusion pressure [17].

21.4.2.4 Neuroelectrophysiological Monitoring

Patients with deep coma following primary brainstem hemorrhage surgery and during NSICU treatment may not be effectively assessed using conventional scoring scales due to sedation and analgesic drug use [1]. EEG monitoring is a valuable method for assessing the consciousness level of critically ill patients [18]. Recent studies have reported a higher incidence of subtle seizures following primary brainstem hemorrhage, thus EEG monitoring can aid clinicians in identifying non-convulsive seizure activity in patients with altered consciousness, or dull and even unconscious, allowing for diagnostic prognostic evaluations during monitoring [19].

21.4.2.5 Neuroimaging Monitoring

Mobile CT technology, intraoperative MRI, and intraoperative ultrasound provide valuable support for perioperative monitoring in neurosurgery. Combining functional MRI, PET, and other metabolic imaging monitoring techniques can effectively guide clinical treatment [20].

21.4.2.6 Other Brain Monitoring Techniques

In addition to the aforementioned brain function monitoring techniques, other clinically applied methods include monitoring brain temperature, brain oxygen levels, and microdialysis [1]. Data obtained through these monitoring methods can help us understand local or global pathophysiological changes in the brain, thereby guiding clinical treatment more effectively [2].

21.4.2.7 Strategies for Controlling Elevated Intracranial Pressure

Various treatment methods targeting elevated intracranial pressure have been developed for brain injury patients; however, these methods may not be suitable for primary brainstem hemorrhage patients [1]. The “Lund concept” attributes high intracranial pressure to disruption of the blood-brain barrier and recommends reducing static pressure and increasing osmotic pressure [2]. Basic treatment measures guided by cerebral perfusion pressure suggest maintaining cerebral perfusion pressure above 70 mmHg to minimize reflexive vasodilation effects and ischemic damage, which has become a standard treatment for high intracranial pressure. Nonetheless, studies indicate that as mean arterial pressure increases, intracranial pressure also rises accordingly [3].

The incidence of elevated intracranial pressure in ICH patients remains unclear. Patients with minimal bleeding may not have high intracranial pressure and may not require treatment, this scenario also applicable to many ischemic stroke patients. However, for patients showing evidence of elevated intracranial pressure, it is essential to utilize ICU monitoring equipment to reduce intracranial pressure gradually, incorporating measures such as head elevation, sedation, and analgesia, followed by the stepwise implementation of invasive clinical interventions [21].

Head Elevation: Elevating the head of the bed by 30° can increase jugular venous return and reduce intracranial pressure. The patient’s head should be maintained in a neutral position to avoid tilting to one side. Head elevation may lower blood pressure and cerebral perfusion pressure in hypovolemic patients, so this measure should be avoided for patients with low blood volume [1].

Cerebrospinal Fluid Drainage: It is recommended to place an external ventricular drainage in primary brainstem hemorrhage patients [2]. Intraventricular catheter placement allows for intracranial pressure monitoring and is an effective method for reducing intracranial pressure. Cerebrospinal fluid can be intermittently and briefly drained based on intracranial pressure levels. The primary risks of ventriculostomy drainage are infection and bleeding, with most studies reporting a bacterial colonization rate rather than systemic infection ranging from 0% to 19%, and the associated incidence of meningitis ranging from 6% to 22% [22].

Osmotic Therapy: For patients with good renal function, difficult-to-control high intracranial pressure, and significant brain edema, the target osmolarity for osmotic therapy is recommended to be 300–320 mmol/L [1]. For elderly patients and those with compromised renal function, the treatment goal may be set at 290–300 mmol/L. Osmotic therapy options include mannitol, glycerol fructose, albumin, synthetic colloids, hypertonic saline, and may be supplemented with diuretics [2].

The choice of osmotic therapy should be based on factors such as intracranial pressure levels, severity of brain edema, cardiac reserve, renal function, and fluid management requirements to determine the optimal strategy. Monitoring plasma osmolarity can help rationalize the treatment approach [3, 23].

21.4.2.8 Analgesia and Sedation

Postoperative patients with primary brainstem hemorrhage may experience pain, restlessness, and agitation, leading to increased blood pressure, elevated heart rate, and anxiety [12, 13]. These factors can increase the risks of rebleeding, elevated intracranial pressure, catheter dislodgement, and inadvertent injuries, necessitating intervention [24]. The objectives of analgesia and sedation in such patients are as follows: (1) to eliminate or alleviate the patient’s pain and physical discomfort, reduce adverse stimuli, and mitigate excessive sympathetic nervous system excitation [25]; (2) to aid in improving patient sleep, minimize or eliminate the patient’s memory of pain during treatment [27, 28]; (3) to alleviate or eliminate patient anxiety, restlessness, and delirium, preventing unconscious behaviors from interfering with treatment and safeguarding the patient's life; (4) to induce and maintain a low metabolic "hibernation" state for an extended period, reducing various stress and inflammatory injuries, lessening organ damage, lowering metabolism, decreasing oxygen consumption, and oxygen demand [29]; (5) short-acting sedation can help patients cooperate with treatment and care [30]; (6) some sedative medications can raise the seizure threshold and inhibit cortical spreading depolarization [31]. It is generally recommended to use short-acting sedative drugs with manageable side effects, such as propofol, midazolam, and dexmedetomidine. However, it is essential to be well-versed in the advantages and disadvantages of various medications and make informed choices regarding sedative and analgesic drugs [32]. The use of the Bispectral Index (BIS) and the Critical-Care Pain Observation Tool (CPOT) can guide the administration of sedative and analgesic medications for patients.

21.4.2.9 Nutritional Therapy

Early initiation of nutritional therapy is recommended [1]. Enteral nutrition should commence within 24–48 h of onset, aiming to achieve energy targets within 48–72 h [2]. A comprehensive assessment should be conducted based on clinical factors such as weight loss, disease severity, previous nutritional intake, comorbidities, and gastrointestinal function [3]. Commonly used nutritional risk screening and assessment tools like the Nutritional Risk Screening 2002 (NRS2002) can help determine the appropriate nutritional support strategy based on the degree of nutritional risk [33]. For patients requiring prolonged enteral nutrition (>4 weeks), percutaneous endoscopic gastrostomy may be considered if conditions permit. In critically ill patients during the stress period, an energy supply target of 20–25 cal/(kg·d) is recommended, with protein providing 16% of energy, fat providing 20%–35%, and the rest carbohydrates, with a caloric nitrogen ratio of around 130:1. For parenteral nutrition, a glucose-lipid ratio of 5:5 and a caloric nitrogen ratio of 100:1 are recommended, with a minimum carbohydrate requirement of 2 g/(kg·day) during parenteral nutrition to maintain blood glucose at appropriate levels, intravenous fat emulsion at 1.5 g/(kg·day), and mixed amino acids at 1.3–1.5 g/(kg·day) [34–36].

21.4.2.10 Blood Glucose Control

For diabetic and non-diabetic patients, hyperglycemia can predict a high mortality rate at 28 days [1]. Central nervous system injury causes stress, hypothalamic damage, and increased catecholamines can trigger stress hyperglycemia, with proportions reaching 30%–70% [2]. Elevated blood glucose can further lead to poor patient outcomes and increased mortality rates. Additionally, hypoglycemia (blood glucose <4.4 mmol/L) should be avoided. Regular monitoring of blood glucose is essential, with perioperative patients maintaining blood glucose levels between 5 and 7.2 mmol/L, and postprandial blood glucose not exceeding 10 mmol/L at 2 h [3]. Controlling blood glucose can involve preparing appropriate concentrations of insulin for intravenous infusion or bolus administration, with glucose and insulin mixed infusion to prevent hypoglycemia. Insulin dosages should be adjusted daily based on blood glucose monitoring results. For patients receiving regular enteral nutrition, long-acting insulin may be considered for blood glucose control when necessary. Vigilance is crucial to prevent diabetic ketoacidosis (DKA) and hyperosmolar non-ketotic state (HONK) resulting from poor blood glucose control. Due to its osmotic diuretic effect, elevated blood glucose levels can lead to hypovolemia in cases of DKA and HONK. In the event of these complications, physiological saline should be supplemented at a rate of 15–20 mL/(kg·day) to address volume depletion, and insulin should be promptly administered to control blood glucose. Close monitoring of blood potassium levels is necessary following insulin infusion, and sodium bicarbonate therapy may be administered when blood pH <7.0 or in the presence of life-threatening hyperkalemia [1, 2].

21.4.2.11 Temperature Control

Brain temperature is a significant factor in ischemic brain injury [1]. Experimental studies have shown that reducing body temperature can improve brain damage by redistributing oxygen and decreasing glucose metabolism, thereby enhancing brain tolerance to oxygen. Fever can lead to poor outcomes, and therapeutic temperature reduction has been extensively studied as a strategy for controlling intracranial pressure and neuroprotection in acute brain injury [2]. Lowering body temperature to 32–34 °C is effective in reducing refractory high intracranial pressure, but prolonged low body temperature (24–48 h) can increase the incidence of complications such as lung infections, blood coagulation disorders, and electrolyte imbalances. There is also a risk of intracranial pressure rebound when body temperature is restored [3].

21.4.2.12 Prevention of Deep Vein Thrombosis and Pulmonary Embolism

Deep vein thrombosis and pulmonary embolism are common preventable causes of disability and death in ICH patients [1]. Preventing and treating venous embolism complications in patients without an increased risk of intracranial rebleeding poses a clinical challenge. Anticoagulants, antiplatelet agents, heparin and heparin analogs, and mechanical methods such as intermittent pneumatic compression and elastic stockings are commonly used methods for preventing venous thrombosis in patients with cerebral ischemia, each supported by varying levels of evidence [2].

Another treatment method involves placing a filter in the inferior vena cava, which can reduce the incidence of pulmonary embolism in deep vein thrombosis patients in the initial weeks but may increase the long-term occurrence of deep vein thrombosis and embolism [3].

References

1. Broderick J, Connolly S, Feldmann E, et al. Guidelines for the management of spontaneous intracerebral hemorrhage in adults: 2007 update: a guideline from the American Heart Association/American Stroke Association Stroke Council, High Blood Pressure Research Council, and the Quality of Care and Outcomes in Research Interdisciplinary Working Group. Circulation. 2007;116(16):e391–413.
2. Hemphill JC III, Greenberg SM, Anderson CS, et al. Guidelines for the management of spontaneous intracerebral hemorrhage: a guideline for healthcare professionals from the American Heart Association/American Stroke Association. Stroke. 2015;46(7):2032–60.
3. Chinese Society of Neurosurgery. Expert consensus on critical care in neurosurgery (2013). Chin J Cerebrovasc Dis. 2013;10(8):436–48.
4. Atkins D, Best D, Briss PA, et al. GRADE Working Group. Grading quality of evidence and strength of recommendations. BMJ. 2004;328(7454):1490.
5. Guyatt GH, Oxman AD, Vist GE, et al. GRADE: an emerging consensus on rating the quality of evidence and strength of recommendations. BMJ. 2008;336(7650):924–6.
6. The GRADE Working Group. GRADEpro:an introduchon to the system [EB/OL]. [2017-09-19].
7. Guyatt GH, Schünemann HJ, Djulbegovic B, et al. Guideline panels should not GRADE good practice statements. J Clin Epidemiol. 2015;68(5):597–600.
8. Chinese Society of Critical Care Medicine. Guidelines for analgesia and sedation in intensive care unit patients (2006). Chin J Surg. 2006;44(17):1158–66.
9. Balas M, Buckingham R, Braley T, et al. Extending the ABCDE bundle to the post-intensive care unit setting. J Gerontol Nurs. 2013;39(8):39–51.
10. Barr J, Fraser GL, Puntillo K, et al. Clinical practice guidelines for the management of pain, agitation, and delirium in adult patients in the intensive care unit. Crit Care Med. 2013;41(1):263–306.
11. Vincent JL, Shehabi Y, Walsh TS, et al. Comfort and patient-centred care without excessive sedation: the eCASH concept. Intensive Care Med. 2016;42(6):962–71.
12. Pain terms: a list with definitions and notes on usage. Recommended by the IASP Subcommittee on Taxonomy. Pain. 1979;6(3):249.
13. Puntillo KA, Max A, Timsit JF, et al. Determinants of procedural pain intensity in the intensive care unit. The Europain® study. Am J Respir Crit Care Med. 2014;189(1):39–47.
14. Chanques G, Jaber S, Barbotte E, et al. Impact of systematic evaluation of pain and agitation in an intensive care unit. Crit Care Med. 2006;34(6):1691–9.
15. Chanques G, Sebbane M, Barbotte E, et al. A prospective study of pain at rest: incidence and characteristics of an unrecognized symptom in surgical and trauma versus medical intensive care unit patients. Anesthesiology. 2007;107(5):858–60.
16. Battle CE, Lovett S, Hutchings H. Chronic pain in survivors of critical illness: a retrospective analysis of incidence and risk factors. Crit Care. 2013;17(3):R101.
17. Perpiñá-Galvañ J, Richart-Martínez M. Scales for evaluating self-perceived anxiety levels in patients admitted to intensive care units: a review. Am J Crit Care. 2009;18(6):571–80.
18. Tate JA, Devito Dabbs A, et al. Anxiety and agitation in mechanically ventilated patients. Qual Health Res. 2012;22(2):157–73.
19. Fraser GL, Prato BS, Riker RR, et al. Frequency, severity, and treatment of agitation in young versus elderly patients in the ICU. Pharmacotherapy. 2000;20(1):75–82.
20. Boyko Y, Jennum P, Toft P. Sleep quality and circadian rhythm disruption in the intensive care unit: a review. Nat Sci Sleep. 2017;9:277–84.
21. Pisani MA, Friese RS, Gehlbach BK, et al. Sleep in the intensive care unit. Am J Respir Crit Care Med. 2015;191(7):731–8.
22. Boyko Y, Jennum P, Nikolic M, et al. Sleep in intensive care unit: the role of environment. J Crit Care. 2017;37:99–105.
23. Cooke M, Chaboyer W, Schluter P, et al. The effect of music on discomfort experienced by intensive care unit patients during turning: a randomized cross-over study. Int J Nurs Pract. 2010;16(2):125–31.
24. Gorji HM, Nesami BM, Ayyasi M, et al. Comparison of ice packs application and relaxation therapy in pain reduction during chest tube removal following cardiac surgery. N Am J Med Sci. 2014;6(1):19–24.
25. Sanders RD, Maze M. Contribution of sedative-hypnotic agents to delirium via modulation of the sleep pathway. Can J Anaesth. 2011;58(2):149–56.
26. Weinhouse GL, Schwab RJ, Watson PL, et al. Bench-to-bedside review: delirium in ICU patients—importance of sleep deprivation. Crit Care. 2009;13(6):234.
27. Figueroa-Ramos MI, Arroyo-Novoa CM, Lee KA, et al. Sleep and delirium in ICU patients: a review of mechanisms and manifestations. Intensive Care Med. 2009;35(5):781–95.
28. Litton E, Carnegie V, Elliott R, et al. The efficacy of earplugs as a sleep hygiene strategy for reducing delirium in the ICU: a systematic review and meta-analysis. Crit Care Med. 2016;44(5):992–9.
29. Akansel N, Kaymakçi S. Effects of intensive care unit noise on patients: a study on coronary artery bypass graft surgery patients. J Clin Nurs. 2008;17(12):1581–90.
30. Voigt LP, Reynolds K, Mehryar M, et al. Monitoring sound and light continuously in an intensive care unit patient room: a pilot study. J Crit Care. 2017;39:36–9.
31. Wu NH, Wu JQ. Current situation of noise pollution in intensive care unit and countermeasures. J QiluNurs. 2013;19(23):54–6.
32. Ryu MJ, Park JS, Park H. Effect of sleep-inducing music on sleep in persons with percutaneous transluminal coronary angiography in the cardiac care unit. J Clin Nurs. 2012;21(5–6):728–35.
33. de Jong A, Molinari N, de Lattre S, et al. Decreasing severe pain and serious adverse events while moving intensive care unit patients: a prospective interventional study (the NURSE-DO project). Crit Care. 2013;17(2):R74.
34. Jaber S, Bahloul H, Guétin S, et al. Effets de la musicothérapie en réanimation hors sédation chez des patients en cours de sevrage ventilatoire versus des patients non ventilés [Effects of music therapy in intensive care unit without sedation in weaning patients versus non-ventilated patients]. Ann Fr Anesth Reanim. 2007;26(1):30–8. French.
35. Friesner SA, Curry DM, Moddeman GR. Comparison of two pain-management strategies during chest tube removal: relaxation exercise with opioids and opioids alone. Heart Lung. 2006;35(4):269–76.
36. Sauls J. The use of ice for pain associated with chest tube removal. Pain Manag Nurs. 2002;3(2):44–52.
37. Bradt J, Dileo C. Music interventions for mechanically ventilated patients. Cochrane Database Syst Rev. 2014;2014(12):CD006902.
38. Rahmani A, Naseri M, Salaree MM, et al. Comparing the effect of foot reflexology massage, foot bath and their combination on quality of sleep in patients with acute coronary syndrome. J Caring Sci. 2016;5(4):299–306.
39. Robleda G, Roche-Campo F, Sendra MÀ, et al. Fentanyl as preemptive treatment of pain associated with turning mechanically ventilated patients: a randomized controlled feasibility study. Intensive Care Med. 2016;42(2):183–91.

22 Surgical Complications and Countermeasures for Primary Brainstem Hemorrhage

Hongtian Zhang, Jinhua Yang, Siying Ren, Guofeng Wu, and Junjun Liang

22.1 Overview

Due to the vital physiological functions and the designation of the brainstem as the "forbidden zone of life" within the central nervous system, complications following surgical treatment for primary brainstem hemorrhage remain numerous and severe. Such complications pose a serious threat to the patient's life. Therefore, it is of great clinical significance to effectively prevent and treat complications arising from severe brainstem hemorrhage surgery. Prognosis is generally poor when the hemorrhage occurs in the upper part of the midbrain, possibly due to the involvement of the hypothalamus. Conversely, pontine hemorrhage has a relatively better prognosis, whereas medullary hemorrhage, due to its direct compression of the respiratory and cardiac centers, often leads to a critically severe condition. Notably, an early, profound, and prolonged coma, along with a high incidence of complications, is commonly observed after the onset of brainstem hemorrhage, resulting in a mortality rate exceeding 80%. The prevalence of severe disability and a vegetative state is also considerably high. Within the reticular formation of the brainstem lie numerous regulatory centers, such as the cardiovascular motor center, blood pressure reflex center, respiratory center, and vomiting center, which play a crucial role in maintaining essential life activities such as normal respiration and circulation. Hence, it is referred to as the "vital center." Following brainstem hemorrhage, damage to the autonomic nervous system and disruption of the neurohumoral regulatory function can lead to various clinical complications, including pulmonary infection, gastrointestinal bleeding, and electrolyte imbalance. Moreover, considering that many patients with brainstem hemorrhage have a history of chronic diseases such as hypertension, diabetes, and coronary heart disease, it is highly likely that these patients will experience concurrent dysfunction in organs such as the heart, lungs, and kidneys.

H. Zhang (✉) · J. Liang
Department of Neurosurgery, Chinese PLA General Hospital, Beijing, China

J. Yang
Department of Neurosurgery, Gaozhou Hospital of Traditional Chinese Medicine Affiliated to Guangzhou University of Chinese Medicine, Gaozhou, China

S. Ren · G. Wu
Department of Emergency, Affiliated Hospital of Guizhou Medical University, Guiyang, China

22.2 Surgical Complications and Countermeasures

22.2.1 Postoperative Hemorrhage

Postoperative hemorrhage is a common complication.

22.2.1.1 Causes

1. Patients with brainstem hemorrhage often have extremely high blood pressure, with an average systolic pressure above 190 mmHg. Prolonged exposure of the blood vessels to high-pressure blood flow leads to pathological and physiological changes, damaging the elastic fibers of the blood vessels and increasing the likelihood of recurrent bleeding.
2. Within 6 h after the initial hemorrhage, the hematoma has not yet stabilized. The probability of hematoma enlargement or rebleeding within 6 h of brainstem hemorrhage is significantly higher than that of supratentorial hemorrhage.
3. After surgery for primary brainstem hemorrhage, patients often experience significant fluctuations in blood pressure. If the airway is not promptly cleared, the gastric tube improperly placed, or mannitol misused, the likelihood of rebleeding increases.
4. Due to the deep location of the brainstem hematoma and the limited operative space, it may be difficult to fully expose the bleeding site in the brainstem, resulting in

G. Chen, C. You (eds.), *Surgical Treatment of Primary Brainstem Hemorrhage*, https://doi.org/10.1007/978-981-95-8942-5_22

incomplete hemostasis. Additionally, if some small bleeding arteries are not completely sealed off, the bleeding within the arterial vessel may temporarily cease. However, rebleeding can occur with the blood pressure fluctuations that are common in primary brainstem hemorrhage patients after surgery.

5. High blood pressure postoperatively can lead to rebleeding. Factors such as excessive suction volume, excessive suction force, or rapid suction during the surgery all can contribute to rebleeding. The initial suction volume during surgery has a significant impact on rebleeding. After a large amount of hematoma is aspirated, negative pressure may develop within the hematoma cavity. This disrupts the intracranial pressure balance established during the early stage of cerebral hemorrhage, relieving the pressure on compressed blood vessels. The disruption of microthrombi can cause rebleeding.
6. Recurrent bleeding can occur after urokinase thrombolysis, as the release of vascular compression can trigger rebleeding.
7. Patients on anticoagulants like aspirin, or those with a history of alcohol abuse or liver dysfunction, are prone to coagulation disorders and rebleeding.

22.2.1.2 Countermeasures

1. The benefit of aggressive blood pressure reduction for brainstem hematoma is still inconclusive. However, controlling blood pressure to around 150–160 mmHg may be appropriate while ensuring adequate cerebral perfusion pressure. Further prospective studies are required to confirm these approaches, but maintaining stable blood pressure without significant fluctuations should be the fundamental requirement to reduce rebleeding.
2. The optimal timing for surgery is around 6 h after the onset of hemorrhage. Performing surgery during the acute phase allows for easier removal of the hematoma, though small bleeding arteries are unstable and perihematoma edema has not fully stabilized, increasing the risk of blood vessels rebleeding after the hematoma is relieved. Additionally, unlike supratentorial hemorrhage, even a small amount of oozing appears significant in brainstem hemorrhage due to the limited volume of the brainstem. Therefore, the timing of surgery should be around 6 h after the onset of bleeding.
3. Gentle surgical manipulation is essential. The suction device's primary function is to adsorb the hematoma rather than completely aspirating it. Use tumor forceps to gently crush the hematoma and remove it. If the hematoma is tightly adhered to the brain tissue, it should not be forcefully separated to avoid damaging the perihematoma edema and causing new bleeding.
4. The initial aspiration of the hematoma should not be too rapid or excessive. Avoid pursuing complete hematoma removal in a single attempt.
5. During the puncture procedure, insert the catheter slowly and avoid rapid aspiration of the hematoma. If the aspiration volume exceeds the preoperative calculation and there are changes in the pupil on the surgical side, accompanied by altered consciousness and worsening symptoms, immediate hemostasis is required, or even a change in the surgical approach.
6. For patients with coagulation disorders and platelet dysfunction, surgical treatment should be considered after correcting the condition.

22.2.2 Residual Hematoma

Excessive residual hematoma is a relatively common complication.

22.2.2.1 Causes

1. Limited visual field during surgery may lead to residual hematoma.
2. Inadequate surgical skills and lack of experience in operating in confined spaces.
3. Incorrect choice of surgical approach.

22.2.2.2 Countermeasures

1. When clearing the hematoma, proceed in a specific direction, place a cotton pad after clearance, and then proceed in a different direction. During hematoma clearance, maximize exposure of the hematoma cavity by utilizing position, microscope angles, and head rotation.
2. Choose appropriate surgical instruments, such as a 1.5 mm suction device and the smallest diameter tumor forceps. Coordinate both hands, with the tumor forceps serving as a tool for dynamic traction. Of course, complete clearance of the hematoma while protecting the brainstem tissue requires accumulated experience.
3. Select an appropriate surgical approach using the two-point localization method. Draw a straight line between the center of the hematoma and the shallowest point of the hematoma from the brainstem. This line serves as the basis for selecting the surgical approach. Common approaches for brainstem hemorrhage include the subtemporal transtentorium approach, posterior midline cerebellomedullary fissure approach, and retrosigmoid approach. Ninety percent of hematomas are located in the pons. For hematomas predominantly located on one side in the lower part of the pons, the retrosigmoid approach

can be chosen. For hematomas involving the upper part of the pons and extending into the midbrain, the subtemporal transtentorium approach can be used. For hematomas extending into the fourth ventricle or involving the lower part of the pons and extending into the medulla, the posterior midline cerebellomedullary fissure approach is selected.

22.2.3 Puncture Site Bleeding

22.2.3.1 Causes

1. Unfamiliarity with local anatomy.
2. Insufficient analysis of preoperative imaging data and inadequate surgical planning.
3. Rough and excessive force during puncture and catheter removal.
4. Elderly patients with vascular degeneration, prone to bleeding.

22.2.3.2 Countermeasures

1. Thoroughly understand and master the relevant local anatomy before surgery.
2. Carefully analyze the preoperative imaging data for precise localization, avoiding vascular areas as much as possible.
3. Perform puncture and catheter removal with gentle and slow movements.
4. Pay heightened attention during the surgical process for elderly patients.

22.2.4 Cerebrospinal Fluid Subcutaneous Fluid Leakage and Intracranial Infection

22.2.4.1 Causes

1. Inadequate sealing of the mastoid air cells during bone handling.
2. Unwantertight closure of the dura after opening.
3. Insufficient aseptic awareness and inadequate cleaning of the surgical field.
4. Prolonged surgical operation time.
5. Poor alignment and inadequate wound healing of the skin and subcutaneous tissues.
6. Inadequate skull base repair during surgical procedures involving bone removal.

22.2.4.2 Countermeasures

1. For approaches involving the mastoid air cells, such as the retrosigmoid approach and subtemporal approach, it is necessary to ensure a tight seal with bone wax, muscle, or fat.
2. The dura should be sutured in a watertight manner. If the dura shrinks or cannot be sutured in place, use a superficial fascia or muscle for meticulous repair.
3. Perform gentle surgical manipulation during the procedure to reduce mechanical injury and minimize the presence of residual bone fragments, hematomas, and other debris in the surgical field. Flush the surgical field repeatedly, and in cases of prolonged operation time or a higher risk of infection, the prophylactic use of antibiotics is recommended.
4. If bone removal (such as petrous bone) is performed during the procedure, a dead space outside the dura should be closed with fat grafting. Then, the skull base should be meticulously sealed with biological glue or cyanoacrylate combined with gelatin sponge.

22.2.5 Brainstem Dysfunction (Most Severe Complication)

Brainstem dysfunction is the most severe complication.

22.2.5.1 Causes

1. The hematoma causing mass effect and compressing the brainstem. Furthermore, secondary injuries can result in brainstem edema and damage to important functional nuclei.
2. Excessive force during surgery leading to additional damage to brainstem tissue.
3. Disruption of the transition zone between the hematoma and normal tissue, exacerbating brainstem dysfunction.
4. Damage to crucial blood supply vessels and venous outflow during the surgical procedure.
5. The medulla oblongata houses the respiratory and cardiovascular centers, making postoperative respiratory and/or circulatory failure common and a significant cause of mortality. Sudden respiratory arrest leading to death on the third day after surgery in patients with brainstem hemorrhage, may be attributed to brainstem edema or swelling.

22.2.5.2 Countermeasures

1. Surgery is the only way to relieve the mechanical compression of the hematoma. Clearing the hematoma during the safe period and reducing secondary damage is also a strategy. During surgery, important functional nuclei such as the facial colliculus, obex, reticular ascending fibers, and corticospinal tract should be avoided as much as possible. This requires a thorough understanding of the anatomy of the brainstem before the operation.
2. Perform surgical manipulations with gentle movements, strictly avoiding the use of large-caliber suction devices and bulky instruments. Use hemostatic sponges to protect

the surrounding normal brainstem tissue around the hematoma.

3. Deep-seated operations may overlook potential secondary injuries around the hematoma. Adjust the field of view and observe carefully during the procedure. Take great care to protect blood vessels and avoid using bipolar coagulation, focusing on hemostatic compression instead.
4. Damage to the transition zone between the hematoma and brain tissue is a significant cause of postoperative brain edema. During microscopic surgery, efforts should be made to minimize damage to the brain tissue edema zones. Avoid excessive suction during hematoma evacuation to prevent damage to the edema zone. If small blood clots are tightly adhered within the hematoma cavity, there is no need to forcefully remove them. For venous bleeding, compression with Surgicel is sufficient, while for arterial bleeding, identify the bleeding artery and use low-intensity bipolar coagulation for gentle hemostasis.
5. Brainstem hemorrhage, especially in the lower part of the pons, requires close monitoring even after respiratory recovery postoperatively. It is recommended to monitor for at least 5–7 days post-medulla oblongata surgery. In patients with respiratory failure, even after recovery and discharge, early precautions should be taken to avoid aspiration or colds, especially pulmonary infections, which can easily lead to central respiratory failure.

22.2.6 Cranial Nerve and Nucleus Damage

22.2.6.1 Causes

1. Damage to nuclei caused by the location of the hemorrhage, particularly in the tegmentum and pericentral gray matter, which are prone to cranial nerve and nucleus damage.
2. Microscopic operations, although minimally invasive, can cause certain damage to nerve fibers that have not reached the surface of the brainstem, as incisions are necessary.
3. Specific surgical approaches may increase the probability of cranial nerve damage within the field of view.
4. Damage to nuclei and nerve tissue contained within the corresponding brainstem tissue during hematoma evacuation.
5. Potential secondary injuries to important brainstem tissue surrounding the hematoma during the surgical procedure.

22.2.6.2 Countermeasures

1. Hemorrhage itself, due to mechanical injury, compression, and the release of toxic substances during hematoma resolution, inevitably causes damage to the brainstem tissue. Therefore, it is imperative to emphasize early surgical intervention in brainstem hemorrhage patients to relieve pressure and reduce the likelihood of secondary damage.
2. When incising along the longitudinal fibers of the brainstem, it is advisable to use a sharp blade or a non-contact laser knife to open the brainstem, while making every effort to avoid cauterization.
3. The subtemporal approach is prone to damaging the trochlear and oculomotor nerves and should be handled with care. The retrosigmoid approach is susceptible to damaging the posterior cranial nerves, facial and acoustic nerves, trigeminal nerves, and nuclei. The posterior midline approach, when incised from the bottom of the rhomboid fossa, is at risk of damaging the facial nerve nucleus, vagus nerve, or hypoglossal trigone. Adequate preoperative preparation and the selection of a safe entry point into the brainstem can reduce the probability of damage.
4. When incising the brainstem, it is important to avoid selecting crucial functional areas and to operate within the hematoma cavity as much as possible, thus reducing the chance of damaging surrounding normal brainstem tissue.

22.2.7 Motor and Sensory Dysfunction

22.2.7.1 Cause

Damage to the basilar part of pons, medullary pyramids, and cerebral peduncles of midbrain can result in severe motor and limb sensory impairments. Postoperative lesions in the midbrain not only cause sensory and motor impairments but also primarily affect eye movement function due to the involvement of the oculomotor nucleus and the medial longitudinal fasciculus. The basilar part of pontine contains a large number of ascending and descending fiber bundles, and damage to this area can lead to consciousness disorders, limb paralysis, and vegetative state. Medullary damage is mainly characterized by crossed paralysis of the limbs. Difficult-to-recover complications mainly include disturbances in deep and superficial sensory functions. Similarly, the cerebral peduncles serve as a pathway for motor fibers, and damage to this area can also result in motor dysfunction.

22.2.7.2 Countermeasures

If the hematoma is located in the region where these fiber bundles converge, the ideal approach is to rely on fiber bundle reconstruction to determine whether the hematoma is causing compressive or destructive damage. If it cannot be determined, a surgical approach that avoids the fiber bundles should be chosen to enter the hematoma cavity. Reducing secondary damage to the fibers in these locations is the most important measure.

22.2.8 Long-Term Complications

22.2.8.1 Cause

1. Hydrocephalus: If the hematoma ruptures into the fourth ventricle or if the hematoma is located higher and ruptures into the aqueduct of Sylvius, it can block the opening of the aqueduct and lead to obstructive hydrocephalus postoperatively.
2. Pulmonary infection: Many brainstem hemorrhages result in damage to the nuclei and nerves associated with the posterior cranial nerves, leading to decreased swallowing and coughing abilities and an increased risk of aspiration, which can cause recurrent pulmonary infections. Additionally, patients with brainstem hemorrhage often remain in a prolonged coma and require tracheostomy and prolonged bed rest, which can also increase the risk of pulmonary infections.
3. Facial paralysis, oculomotor dysfunction, and corneal ulceration. These are clinical manifestations resulting from the impairment of cranial nerves or nuclei associated with eye and facial movements.

22.2.8.2 Countermeasures

1. Promptly perform ventriculoperitoneal shunting for obstructive hydrocephalus to rapidly relieve symptoms.
2. Maintain a stable internal environment: Ensure normal ranges of water and electrolytes, maintain acid-base balance, and provide adequate supply of calories and various nutrients. In cases of swallowing difficulties to prevent aspiration, enteral nutrition via nasogastric tube should be administered.
3. Ensure sufficient oxygen supply: If inadequate ventilation occurs postoperatively, provide timely artificial assistance or control of respiration until effective breathing is restored to avoid hypoxia-related damage.
4. In patients with brainstem hemorrhage, the duration of nasogastric tube feeding can be appropriately extended. Within1 year after brainstem hemorrhage, it is advisable to avoid activities that involve forceful sneezing, coughing, and laughing. Implement measures to keep warm and reduce the probability and risk of catching a cold. Additionally, early intervention with neurorehabilitation training should be initiated to promote neurological recovery.

22.3 Non-surgical Complications and Countermeasures

22.3.1 Postoperative Fever

Postoperative fever can manifest as high fever, primarily due to the imbalance of temperature regulation in the midbrain and the lower part of the hypothalamus, as well as the result of hypermetabolism. On the other hand, it is also related to the presence of infection. Patients who undergo minimally invasive puncture for brainstem hemorrhage may experience postoperative fever under the following four conditions:

22.3.1.1 Postoperative Infectious Fever

22.3.1.1.1 Cause

1. Postoperative pulmonary infection is the main cause of infectious fever.
   (a) Patients with brainstem hemorrhage accompanied by consciousness disorders and swallowing difficulties may develop aspiration pneumonia or atelectasis pneumonia due to vomiting or obstruction of the airway by oral secretions.
   (b) Patients in the EICU may develop pulmonary infections due to healthcare-associated infections resulting from improper mechanical ventilation measures or cross-infections caused by prolonged hospital stays.
2. Postoperative urinary tract infection is a secondary cause of infectious fever. The infecting bacteria are mainly Gram-negative rods residing on the skin and mucous membranes. Patients with indwelling urinary catheters for more than 1 week should be cautious to prevent urinary tract infections, especially female patients.
3. Intracranial infection is relatively rare and is mainly caused by improper aseptic operations during surgery and postoperative inadequate and prolonged drainage.

22.3.1.1.2 Countermeasures

1. Elevate the head of the bed by 30° whenever possible. For patients with consciousness disorders, a lateral position should be adopted with the corners of the mouth lowered to facilitate the expulsion of pharyngeal secretions. After vomiting, any foreign objects remaining in the oral cavity should be suctioned out using a bedside suction device to prevent inhalation into the trachea.
2. To prevent reflux during nasogastric feeding, the feeding speed should not be too fast, and attention should be paid to maintaining an appropriate temperature. Prior to nasogastric feeding, thorough suctioning should be performed. After nasogastric feeding, elevate the head of the bed by 30° for 2 h. Avoid suctioning during this time to minimize the risk of vomiting. In cases of gastric reflux, the daily amount of nasogastric feeding can be appropriately reduced, and in many severe cases, temporary fasting may be necessary. When removing the tube, a small amount of gas should be injected to prevent food from falling into the trachea during withdrawal.
3. Strengthen respiratory care and oral hygiene for patients unable to eat due to consciousness disorders. Turning and back patting should be performed every 2–3 h. Special

attention should be given to suctioning issues. If excessive sputum cannot be completely suctioned out in patients with concurrent pneumonia, even with the use of large quantities of antibiotics, satisfactory control of pneumonia may not be achieved.

4. In cases of severe pulmonary infection resulting in high body temperature and thick, difficult-to-expectorate sputum, as well as a lack of rapid recovery in consciousness within a short period of time, or in cases of ineffective drug treatment or signs of suffocation, consideration should be given to performing a tracheostomy to facilitate sputum clearance, intratracheal administration of medication, and reduce mucosal damage caused by pharyngeal suctioning.
5. Actively treat brainstem hemorrhage, control cerebral edema, and strive for early recovery of consciousness to facilitate early control of pulmonary infection.
6. In the presence of pulmonary infection, broad-spectrum antibiotics must be administered. Respiratory tract infections that occur concurrently with severe brainstem hemorrhage are often caused by nosocomial pathogens, with Gram-negative bacteria being the most common (accounting for approximately 50%–60%), such as *Escherichia coli*, *Klebsiella pneumoniae*, *Pseudomonas aeruginosa*, etc. *Staphylococcus aureus* accounts for approximately 10%, while *Streptococcus pneumoniae* is less common (5%).
7. To reduce urinary tract infections, urinary catheterization should be avoided as much as possible. If catheterization is necessary, strict disinfection should be carried out, and a closed drainage system with disinfection should be utilized. Asymptomatic bacteriuria generally does not require treatment to avoid the development of drug-resistant bacterial colonization. Symptomatic cases can be treated with antibiotics based on susceptibility testing. Most cases of bacteriuria are resolved after catheter removal or the addition of antibiotics.
8. During surgery and postoperatively, adhere to strict aseptic surgical procedures. Drainage tubes should not remain in place for an excessive amount of time, and whenever possible, they should be removed within 3 days after surgery.

22.3.1.2 Postoperative Central Fever

22.3.1.2.1 Cause

High fever and diabetes insipidus. This is mainly due to damage to the temperature regulation center in the acute phase of brainstem hemorrhage and dysfunction of the hypothalamic temperature regulation center. Clinical manifestations include persistent high fever, with body temperature often exceeding 39–40 °C, absence of sweating, high trunk skin temperature but cool extremities, no accompanying chills, and no corresponding changes in heart rate with temperature changes. Antipyretic medications are ineffective.

22.3.1.2.2 Countermeasures

1. The primary approach for reducing fever is physical cooling, which can be achieved through methods such as tepid sponge baths, alcohol sponge baths, cold compresses with ice packs, and cooling blankets.
2. For patients with suitable physical conditions, resembling hibernation subnormothermia therapy can be considered. The earlier the treatment starts, the better the effects will get, preferably within 6 h after the onset of symptoms. The recommended temperature range for hypothermia is 32–34 °C, and the duration is 3–5 days. Within half an hour after administering hypothermic medications, the patient should not be turned or moved. If the blood pressure drops below 60 mmHg, the medication should be discontinued. In elderly patients with weak constitutions, the use of antipyretic drugs should be approached with caution to prevent collapse.
3. When conditions permit and there are appropriate indications, subnormothermia therapy can be considered. There have been reports suggesting a link between central fever and dysfunction of dopamine receptors in the brain. Therefore, the use of dopamine receptor agonists, such as bromocriptine, may be effective.
4. In cases of diabetes insipidus, desmopressin may be administered as necessary, with attention to preventing electrolyte imbalances.

22.3.1.3 Postoperative Dehydration Fever

22.3.1.3.1 Cause

1. Excessive dehydration and inadequate fluid replenishment after brainstem hemorrhage surgery can lead to blood concentration and compromised temperature regulation in the intracranial center, resulting in fever.
2. Excessive dehydration can also cause difficulties in sputum expectoration due to insufficient body fluids, increasing the risk of infectious fever. In cases where patients experience unexplained fever, dry skin, decreased urine output, and increased hematocrit during the treatment process, the possibility of dehydration fever should be considered.

22.3.1.3.2 Countermeasures

1. Adjust the dosage of medications for dehydration.
2. Implement physical cooling measures.

22.3.1.4 Postoperative Absorption Fever

22.3.1.4.1 Cause

This refers to fever caused by the release of various heat-generating factors during the process of blood absorption, commonly occurring within the first 1–2 weeks after onset. It is mostly mild to moderate fever and does not present with signs of septicemia or symptoms of hypothalamic dysfunction.

22.3.1.4.2 Countermeasures

The main approach for management is physical cooling.

22.3.2 Pulmonary Infection

22.3.2.1 Cause

Following brainstem hemorrhage, the respiratory center is most vulnerable to impairment, leading to respiratory arrest. Tracheal intubation, tracheostomy, and mechanical ventilation are often required, and tracheostomy patients lack the nasal hair filtering function, which increases the risk of respiratory tract infection.

22.3.2.2 Countermeasures

1. Emphasize turning and percussion to facilitate sputum drainage.
2. For patients without mechanical ventilation, it is recommended to elevate the head of the bed or even maintain a semi-sitting position early on to enhance respiratory mobility.
3. For patients with symptoms of infection, early sputum culture and drug sensitivity testing should be performed (multiple samples of sputum should be collected). Select appropriate antibiotics based on the results of the drug sensitivity test (common pathogens in patients with tracheostomy in the intensive care unit include *Pseudomonas aeruginosa*, *Klebsiella pneumoniae*, *Escherichia coli*, and *Acinetobacter baumannii*).

22.3.3 Postoperative Neurogenic Pulmonary Edema (NPE)

22.3.3.1 Cause

In addition to respiratory tract infections, brainstem hemorrhage can lead to complications in the respiratory system, including neurogenic pulmonary edema (NPE). NPE is caused by damage to the hypothalamus, resulting in the release of a large amount of sympathetic neurotransmitters, peripheral vasoconstriction, increased blood pressure, and the transfer of blood from high-resistance peripheral circulation to low-resistance pulmonary circulation. This leads to increased capillary hydrostatic pressure in the pulmonary artery, damaging the capillaries and causing fluid to leak into the alveoli. Recent studies have shown that NPE is mainly caused by hypoxia. The incidence of NPE is closely related to the severity of the condition, and patients with brainstem hemorrhage have a higher incidence of NPE. NPE often presents as a sudden onset.

22.3.3.2 Countermeasures

1. Timely treatment is crucial, as most cases result in death within 24 h. Therefore, early administration of high-concentration oxygen is recommended.
2. Nifedipine, at a dosage of 10–20 mg sublingually, is now recommended. It can rapidly reduce peripheral and pulmonary artery pressure and has a good effect on NPE. Dobutamine treatment can improve myocardial contractility and accelerate cardiac blood flow, often being the preferred medication for NPE treatment.

22.3.4 Postoperative Digestive System Complications

22.3.4.1 Cause

1. Upper gastrointestinal bleeding often occurs after brainstem hemorrhage and is one of the severe complications. The more severe the condition, the higher the incidence of gastrointestinal bleeding. Patients with gastrointestinal bleeding have a poor prognosis, with a mortality rate of over 50%.
2. The causes of gastrointestinal bleeding include ulcers, hemorrhagic erosions, hemorrhagic gastritis, acute exacerbation of chronic ulcers, and others. Gastrointestinal bleeding mostly occurs in the first 1–2 weeks after brain hemorrhage.

22.3.4.2 Countermeasures

The key to preventing and treating upper gastrointestinal bleeding is to protect the gastric mucosa, reduce and neutralize gastric acid, and maintain a gastric pH above 4, along with active treatment of brainstem hemorrhage. Specific measures include:

1. For intractable hiccups and reflux, acupuncture, physical therapy, and medications such as chlorpromazine can be used for symptomatic relief. For reflux, a semi-sitting position is recommended during meals, and abdominal massage for 20 min before meals and 1 h after meals can promote gastrointestinal motility and aid digestion.
2. For stress-related gastrointestinal ulcer bleeding, which manifests as extensive gastric bleeding, gastric decompression should be performed using a nasogastric tube to relieve gastrointestinal pressure. In severe cases, fasting is necessary. Administer epinephrine at a dosage of 4–8 mg and Yunnan Baiyao (a traditional Chinese medicine) mixed with 100 mL of frozen saline solution, divided into two doses, injected through the gastric tube and retained for 30 min. Additionally, intravenous infusion of Losec (omeprazole sodium) at a dosage of 40 mg once a day for 3–7 days is recommended.
3. Correcting hypoxia is essential to improve oxygen supply to the body. Ensuring the patency of the respiratory

tract and optimizing lung function are the primary considerations. Oxygen supply should be carefully managed in critically ill patients with brainstem hemorrhage.

4. Maintain water, electrolyte, and acid-base balance. Although upper gastrointestinal bleeding is a local manifestation in the stomach, it is part of a systemic response, and the homeostasis of the body directly or indirectly affects it. Adequate and effective blood volume should be maintained, but excessive fluid can cause damage to the heart and lungs. Arterial pH can also affect gastric mucosal pH, as acidemia can increase gastric mucosal acidity. Therefore, maintaining water, electrolyte, and acid-base balance is one of the preventive measures for upper gastrointestinal bleeding.
5. Provide early nutritional support. The gastric mucosa requires energy for regeneration and mucus secretion to protect the mucosa. Enteral nutrition plays a role in promoting gastrointestinal recovery, stimulating visceral and hepatic circulation, improving mucosal blood flow, preventing mucosal acidosis and osmotic disorders, etc. For patients with brain hemorrhage, early enteral nutrition should be initiated. Formula feeding should be started within 24–48 h, gradually increasing from 25 to 100 mL/h. Antioxidants such as glutathione, vitamin E, and beta-carotene can be added. Dietary fiber can improve colonic mucosal nutrition to prevent enterogenic infections, with a daily requirement of at least 10 g. When oral intake is not feasible, adding glutamine to parenteral nutrition can facilitate gastric mucosal growth and provide essential energy for the gastric mucosa.
6. Hemostatic agents such as carbacol and thrombin can be used. Gastric lavage with ice-cold water (100–200 mL) mixed with 4–8 mg of epinephrine can also be performed.
7. Surgery should be considered if the above hemostatic measures are ineffective. Early endoscopic examination should be performed, and endoscopic hemostasis or surgical treatment can be attempted.

Furthermore, it is necessary to closely observe the patient's condition, including the examination of vomit and stool characteristics, monitoring changes in consciousness and body temperature, and assessing skin coloration. Blood pressure and pulse should be monitored, and regular follow-up tests should be conducted, such as red blood cell count, hemoglobin level, and hematocrit. Proper care of the gastric tube should be ensured, including the aspiration of gastric fluid for visual inspection before medication administration or feeding. If necessary, a fecal occult blood test should be performed.

22.3.5 Postoperative Pulmonary Embolism and Deep Vein Thrombosis of the Lower Extremities

22.3.5.1 Postoperative Pulmonary Embolism

22.3.5.1.1 Causes

1. Patients with brainstem hemorrhage often remain in a comatose state due to impaired reticular formation function. The combination of limb dysfunction and prolonged bed rest leads to reduced blood circulation, resulting in a hypercoagulable state and a high risk of deep vein thrombosis formation, leading to acute pulmonary embolism.
2. Acute pulmonary embolism refers to the clinical, pathological, and physiological syndrome caused by the blockage of pulmonary arteries or their branches by endogenous or exogenous emboli, resulting in impaired pulmonary circulation. It is characterized by a high incidence rate, high misdiagnosis rate, and high mortality rate. The untreated mortality rate of pulmonary embolism is 25%–30%, while timely diagnosis and treatment still result in a mortality rate of 2%–8%. The clinical manifestations of pulmonary embolism are diverse, with nonspecific symptoms and signs ranging from asymptomatic to hemodynamic instability, and even sudden death.

22.3.5.1.2 Countermeasures

1. Thrombolytic therapy is the primary method for treating acute pulmonary embolism. It can rapidly dissolve partial or complete thrombi, restore pulmonary tissue perfusion, and is currently the thrombolytic method used in clinical practice for acute pulmonary embolism. Recombinant tissue plasminogen activator (rt-PA) is commonly used, as it has fibrin-specificity, strong thrombolytic effects, a short half-life, and reduces the risk of bleeding complications.
2. Anticoagulant therapy plays a crucial role in the treatment of acute pulmonary embolism and effectively prevents thrombus reformation and recurrence. It should be combined with thrombolytic therapy. Common heparin, warfarin, or novel anticoagulant drugs are preferred anticoagulants.

22.3.5.2 Deep Vein Thrombosis of the Lower Extremities

Deep vein thrombosis (DVT) of the lower extremities manifests as unilateral limb swelling due to abnormal coagulation of blood within the deep venous system, leading to venous reflux obstruction. Symptoms include lower limb edema, superficial venous dilation, local skin temperature elevation, pain in the affected limb, and obvious thickening compared to the corresponding area of the healthy limb. If left untreated, it may progress to pulmonary embolism, resulting in sudden death within a short period.

Lower extremity DVT is a common complication of brainstem hemorrhage. The process of deep vein thrombosis formation in the lower extremities is not easily detected and can lead to life-threatening pulmonary embolism if the thrombus embolizes. The occurrence of lower extremity DVT after brainstem hemorrhage is not only related to impaired limb mobility, the use of vasoactive drugs, body dehydration, and hypercoagulable states but also closely associated with factors such as advanced age, obesity, diabetes, and vascular sclerosis.

22.3.5.2.1 Causes

1. Impaired limb mobility: Patients with brainstem hemorrhage often experience coma and prolonged bed rest, resulting in reduced blood flow.
2. Use of vasoactive drugs: Drugs such as mannitol, piracetam, and antibiotics with strong vascular irritability, when used repeatedly and for a long time, can cause vascular wall damage and increased vascular permeability. Endothelial injury can lead to the release of various vasoactive substances, promoting platelet aggregation and adhesion, and facilitating thrombus formation.
3. Dehydration: Dehydration drugs like mannitol and furosemide are commonly used to treat brain edema. Patients with brainstem hemorrhage may experience repeated vomiting, resulting in significant loss of gastric fluid and reduced blood volume, leading to blood concentration and a hypercoagulable state. Additionally, stress-induced gastrointestinal bleeding, hyperglycemia, and/or hypothalamic dysfunction, such as fever and diabetes insipidus, can cause fluid loss and increase blood viscosity.
4. Coagulation mechanism: Patients with brainstem hemorrhage may have an activated coagulation system due to lung infections or stress, which can lead to a hypercoagulable state. The use of hemostatic drugs can also promote blood coagulation, increasing the risk of thrombus formation. Hypercoagulability, acidosis, and bleeding can all shorten clotting time and contribute to the development of deep vein thrombosis.

22.3.5.2.2 Countermeasures

22.3.5.2.2.1 Prophylactic Measures for DVT

1. Preventive care: Intermittent use of calf muscle pumps or compression, such as soleus muscle and lower limb massage. Early assistance with limb movement for patients, passive limb massage for comatose or hemiplegic patients to promote blood flow and prevent stasis. Use pneumatic compression therapy to compress superficial veins to facilitate deep venous blood return. Also, elevate the lower limbs by 20°–30°, ensuring the distal end is higher than the proximal end, and avoid using knee pillows and excessive hip flexion, which may affect venous return.
2. Minimize femoral vein punctures and lower limb venous infusions, especially on the paralyzed side, to avoid repeated punctures in the same location and reduce the occurrence of venous inflammation. Strengthen surveillance during infusions to detect medication leakage early and change puncture sites promptly. While closely monitoring the patient's condition, observe the skin temperature, color, edema, and dorsalis pedis artery pulsation of the lower limbs. If local redness and swelling at the puncture site are noticed, elevate the limb promptly and apply 95% ethanol or 50% magnesium sulfate wet packs.
3. During diagnosis and treatment, minimize the prolonged use of hemostatic drugs to prevent blood from remaining in a hypercoagulable state. If necessary, administer subcutaneous injections of low molecular weight heparin calcium for anticoagulation, intravenous infusions of low molecular weight dextran to promote blood circulation and coagulation, and increase venous tone. Additionally, closely monitor high-risk populations (such as the elderly, obese, and those with diabetes and cardiovascular diseases), especially controlling blood sugar levels when they are elevated.

22.3.5.2.3 Management and Measures After DVT Formation

1. Limb care: After confirming lower extremity DVT through vascular color Doppler or angiography, the patient should remain strictly bedridden with the affected limb elevated by 20°–30°, avoiding compression or massage of the affected limb. Prohibit any compressive operations or examinations on the affected limb to prevent embolism from causing thrombosis in other areas, exacerbating the condition, or even endangering life. Meanwhile, monitor the swelling of the affected limb and measure its circumference at the same site every morning to assess the resolution of edema.
2. Treatment principles include non-surgical and surgical methods. During the acute phase, thrombus dissolution is the main focus, while reducing lower limb venous congestion and improving quality of life are emphasized in the mid to late stages.

Non-surgical treatment: Includes general measures, thrombolysis, anticoagulation, and anti-aggregation therapy.

1. General measures: Bed rest, limb elevation, and the use of diuretics to alleviate limb swelling. Once systemic symptoms and local tenderness are relieved, light activities can be initiated.
2. Thrombolytic therapy: Suitable for patients within 72 h of onset. Commonly used drugs include urokinase,

recombinant streptokinase, and recombinant tissue plasminogen activator, administered intravenously over 7–10 days.

3. Anticoagulation therapy: Suitable for small thrombi. Heparin and coumarin anticoagulants are used to prevent thrombus propagation and promote thrombus dissolution. Typically, heparin is administered first, followed by coumarin drugs, usually warfarin, for about 3–6 months.
4. Anti-aggregation therapy: Drugs such as dextran and *Salvia miltiorrhiza* can expand blood volume, dilute blood, and reduce viscosity.

Surgical treatment: Commonly used for lower extremity deep veins, especially if thrombosis in the iliac vein does not exceed 48 h. Even for patients with prolonged disease and signs of femoral cyanosis, thrombectomy should be performed to salvage the limb. Fogarty catheter thrombectomy is commonly used, followed by anticoagulation and anti-aggregation therapy postoperatively to prevent recurrence.

22.3.6 Postoperative Brain-Heart Syndrome

Brain-heart syndrome refers to the occurrence of myocardial ischemia, myocardial infarction-like symptoms, or arrhythmias accompanied by stroke after a cerebral infarction, in the absence of coronary artery disease and corresponding electrocardiographic changes. The condition and electrocardiogram gradually return to normal or remain mildly abnormal as stroke symptoms improve. Cardiac damage is quite common during brainstem hemorrhage, causing myocardial damage, arrhythmias, and acute myocardial infarction. Elevated levels of GOT, LDH, CPK, and CK-MB isoenzyme have significant diagnostic value.

22.3.6.1 Mechanism

The mechanism behind neurogenic cardiac dysfunction and ECG abnormalities is multifaceted and can be formed through various aspects:

1. Hypothalamus-Pituitary-Adrenal Cortex System: The hypothalamus includes the preoptic nucleus, supraoptic nucleus, paraventricular nucleus, tuber cinereum funnel, and mammillary body, with the latter two being the primary sites. Hemorrhage in the brainstem often involves important nuclei of the hypothalamus and brainstem, leading to an imbalance in the sympathetic and parasympathetic nervous systems. Damage to the hypothalamus increases blood cortisol levels via the pituitary-adrenal axis, causing increased heart rate and elevated blood pressure. Excessive cortisol leads to electrolyte imbalances, especially decreased serum potassium, disrupting myocardial repolarization, resulting in ST-T changes and the appearance of U waves on the ECG. Decreased serum potassium can increase myocardial excitability, leading to premature contractions, and in severe cases, ventricular tachycardia or ventricular fibrillation.
2. Sympathetic-Adrenal Medullary System: Affected hypothalamus can stimulate catecholamine synthesis through the sympathetic-adrenal medullary system directly or via cortisol, leading to toxicity and causing endocardial damage. Excitement and hyperactivity of the sympathetic nervous system increase plasma concentrations of adrenaline and noradrenaline, causing systemic hypertension, exacerbating myocardial ischemia and hypoxia, resulting in myocardial fiber degeneration and subendocardial ischemia leading to left ventricular strain, prolonged Q-T interval, arrhythmias, or conduction abnormalities, among various ECG abnormalities.
3. Vagus Nerve Cortical Representation Area and Brainstem-related Vagal Nuclei and Ganglia: The orbital surface of the frontal lobe has a vagus nerve cortical representation area 13, stimulation of which can cause ECG abnormalities; damage to the upper brainstem can lead to sinus tachycardia, transient premature contractions, or myocardial ischemia; damage to the lower brainstem can lead to sinus bradycardia or myocardial ischemia; ECG abnormalities are evident in deep brain, ventricular, or midbrain hemorrhages. In animal experiments, stimulation of the floor of the third ventricle or the cerebral arterial circle (sensory reflex area) can cause ECG and arrhythmias.

In summary, the brain-heart syndrome is formed by the neurohormonal regulation abnormalities at multiple levels of the nervous system, with the neural mechanism being predominant.

22.3.6.2 Countermeasures

1. Etiological Treatment: Actively treat the underlying disease.
2. Protect Cardiac Function: Nourish the myocardium and improve myocardial metabolism.
3. Prevent Iatrogenic Injury: For patients with poor cardiac function, use furosemide for dehydration before using mannitol.
4. Pay Attention to Maintaining Fluid and Electrolyte Balance.
5. Ectopic arrhythmias can be classified into active and passive types. The former is related to the release of catecholamines by the cardiac sympathetic nerves, treated with beta-blockers or left stellate ganglion blockage; the latter is related to increased acetylcholine release by the vagus nerve, treated with postganglionic anticholinergic drugs such as atropine.

6. The main causes of death in brain-heart syndrome are arrhythmias and heart failure. More attention is focused on cerebral hemorrhage treatment, neglecting the treatment of secondary cardiac damage. Combined with symptoms such as aphasia and consciousness disorders, patients may not be able to describe symptoms well, delaying the timing of treatment. Therefore, during the acute phase of brainstem hemorrhage, cardiac function monitoring should be strengthened. While treating brainstem hemorrhage, attention should also be paid to the cardiac condition to avoid blind dehydration, excessive fluid infusion, and prolonged use of hemostatic agents.

22.3.7 Postoperative Fluid and Electrolyte Imbalance and Malnutrition

22.3.7.1 Causes

1. During the acute phase, hyponatremia and hypokalemia may occur, while severe cases of coma can lead to hypernatremia, requiring prompt correction and electrolyte monitoring. Approximately 5%–30% of patients with brainstem hemorrhage develop hyponatremia, primarily due to changes in antidiuretic hormone secretion and free water retention. Involvement of the thalamus can result in cerebral salt-wasting syndrome characterized by decreased extracellular fluid volume, negative sodium balance, and nitrogen retention. This syndrome is associated with hyponatremia without intracellular water accumulation but with a decrease in extracellular fluid due to the excretion of a large amount of sodium in the urine, leading to high urinary sodium and reduced blood volume. Antidiuretic hormone levels in the blood remain normal. Hyponatremia occurring within 2 weeks after brainstem hemorrhage is often caused by cerebral salt-wasting syndrome.
2. During the recovery phase, anemia and malnutrition may occur due to reduced food intake and weakened digestive and absorptive functions.
3. Severely ill patients with brainstem hemorrhage who have consciousness disorders, difficulty swallowing, reduced food and water intake, and undergo dehydration treatment are prone to develop hyperosmolar syndrome.

22.3.7.2 Countermeasures

1. For patients with hyponatremia, it is important to monitor their serum sodium levels, urinary sodium, urine specific gravity, and blood and urine osmolality. If possible, monitor the concentration of antidiuretic hormones in the blood. Intravenous administration of 3%–5% hypertonic saline and oral sodium chloride solution can be used while replenishing blood volume. The rate of sodium supplementation should not be too fast, with a maximum increase of 0.7 mmol/L per hour, and the daily change in blood sodium should not exceed 20 mmol/L. Inappropriate sodium supplementation may lead to central pontine myelinolysis.
2. For patients with hypernatremia, sodium intake should be restricted. Severe cases may require gastric lavage with water and intravenous infusion of 5% glucose solution to correct hypernatremia gradually, avoiding the risk of cerebral edema.
3. Enhance postoperative nutritional supplementation and feeding.

22.3.8 Prolonged Coma After Surgery

22.3.8.1 Causes

1. Coma: Brainstem hemorrhage causes central nervous system damage, leading to deep and prolonged coma in patients.
2. Prolonged coma can result in joint stiffness and disuse atrophy of muscles.

22.3.8.2 Countermeasures

1. Short-term coma patients can undergo hyperbaric oxygen therapy and receive medications to promote awakening, improve neural nutrition, and enhance brain metabolism. Long-term coma patients require measures to prevent complications such as infections in various body parts, deep vein thrombosis, and pulmonary embolism.
2. Prevent and treat joint stiffness and muscle atrophy. During the recovery phase, active functional exercises should be emphasized, especially strengthening the muscles of the neck and lower back and performing range-of-motion exercises for limb joints. Rehabilitation, traditional Chinese medicine, acupuncture, and physical therapy can also be employed for treatment.

23 Postoperative Recovery and Traditional Chinese Medicine Treatment for Primary Brainstem Hemorrhage

Zhiqiang Zhang, Yanling Gan, Jie Zhan, Yong Xu, Zhanneng Ren, Qibiao Weng, and Zeyu Li

23.1 Hyperbaric Oxygen Therapy for Primary Brainstem Hemorrhage After Surgery

Hyperbaric oxygen therapy is a treatment method for hypoxic diseases and related conditions, utilizing pure or high-concentration oxygen inhalation in a high-pressure environment exceeding atmospheric pressure. It has been clinically implicated for over 50 years. Medical hyperbaric oxygen chambers have two types: pure oxygen chambers and air pressurized chambers. In pure oxygen chambers, patients directly inhale the oxygen after it is pressurized and stabilized. These chambers have the advantages of small size, low cost, and easy to transport. However, it is important to note that synthetic fibers are prohibited inside the chamber, and individuals entering the chamber must wear cotton clothing (Fig. 23.1a). Alternatively, air pressurized chambers use compressed air. After stabilization, patients receive oxygen through masks or oxygen tents. In severe cases, artificial respiration may be required. The advantages of air pressurized chambers include enhanced safety, larger size allowing multiple patients to receive treatment simultaneously, a more comfortable therapeutic environment, and the ability to accommodate medical personnel inside the chamber, which is beneficial for the treatment of critically ill patients and those with unstable conditions. However, air pressurized chambers are larger in size, less portable, and more expensive (Figs. 23.1b, 23.2 and 23.3).

The application of hyperbaric oxygen therapy after surgery for brainstem hemorrhage has been shown to promote the recovery of neurological deficits. Following the rupture and bleeding of blood vessels in the brainstem, the blood supply to the brainstem tissue is disrupted, leading to functional impairments. Although surgical treatment can address acute issues such as relieving hematoma-induced compression, it is challenging to improve the functional impairments caused by ischemia in the brainstem. A critical goal in the postoperative recovery of brainstem hemorrhage is to enhance the blood flow and oxygen delivery to the affected brainstem tissue. Experimental evidence has shown that in an environment with 2–2.5 times atmospheric pressure, breathing pure oxygen reduces the lactate/pyruvate ratio in the blood and cerebrospinal fluid of individuals and animals, indicating sufficient oxygen supply to the brain tissue. This effect is particularly pronounced in ischemic brain tissue during hyperbaric oxygen therapy, where the decrease in the lactate/pyruvate ratio in the blood and cerebrospinal fluid is more significant. In 1974, Hayakawa discovered that animals breathing pure oxygen in an environment with 2 times atmospheric pressure experienced a decrease in blood flow in the carotid artery but an increase of 18% in the vertebral artery flow. This finding holds great significance for the treatment of brainstem cerebrovascular diseases, as hyperbaric oxygen therapy can provide ample oxygen to the brainstem tissue.

Furthermore, hyperbaric oxygen therapy has been demonstrated to reduce intracranial pressure, with a 15% decrease in intracranial pressure when breathing pure oxygen at atmospheric pressure, a 36% decrease at 2 times atmospheric pressure, and a 40% decrease at 3 times atmospheric pressure. Brainstem hematoma are often accompanied by cerebral edema and increased intracranial pressure. Hyperbaric oxygen therapy can augment the effect of dehydrating medications, thereby further reducing intracranial pressure and aiding in the recovery of brainstem function.

Z. Zhang (✉) · Y. Gan · J. Zhan · Y. Xu · Z. Ren · Q. Weng
Department of Neurosurgery, The Second Affiliated Hospital of Guangzhou University of Chinese Medicine, Guangzhou, China

Z. Li
Department of Neurosurgery, Shandong Medical and Pharmaceutical University Hospital, Binzhou, China

G. Chen, C. You (eds.), *Surgical Treatment of Primary Brainstem Hemorrhage*, https://doi.org/10.1007/978-981-95-8942-5_23

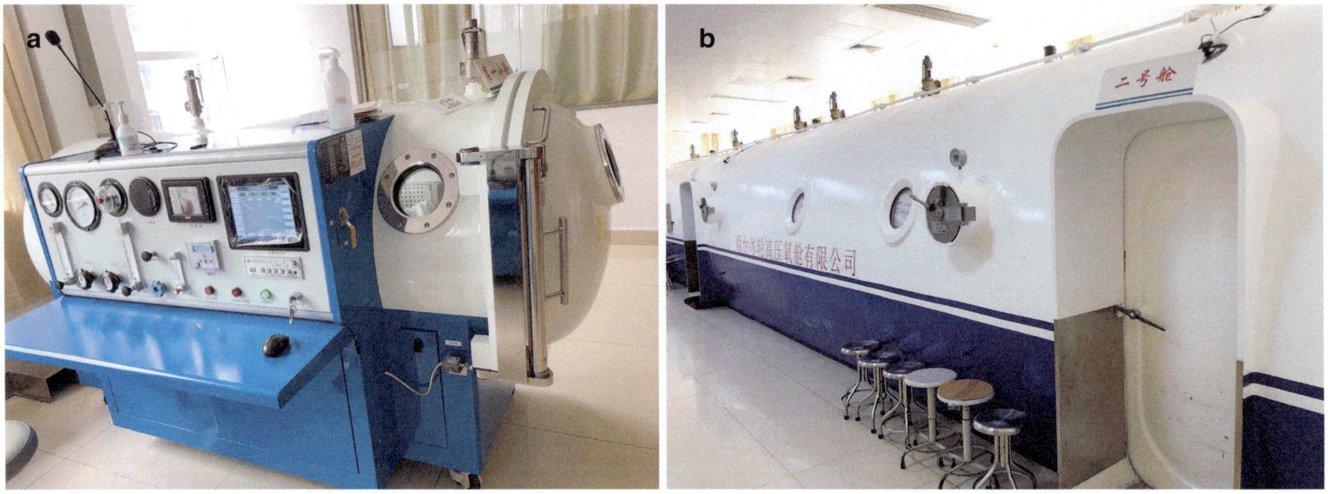

Fig. 23.1 Hyperbaric oxygen chambers. (**a**) Medical hyperbaric oxygen pure oxygen chamber. (**b**) Medical hyperbaric oxygen air pressurized chamber

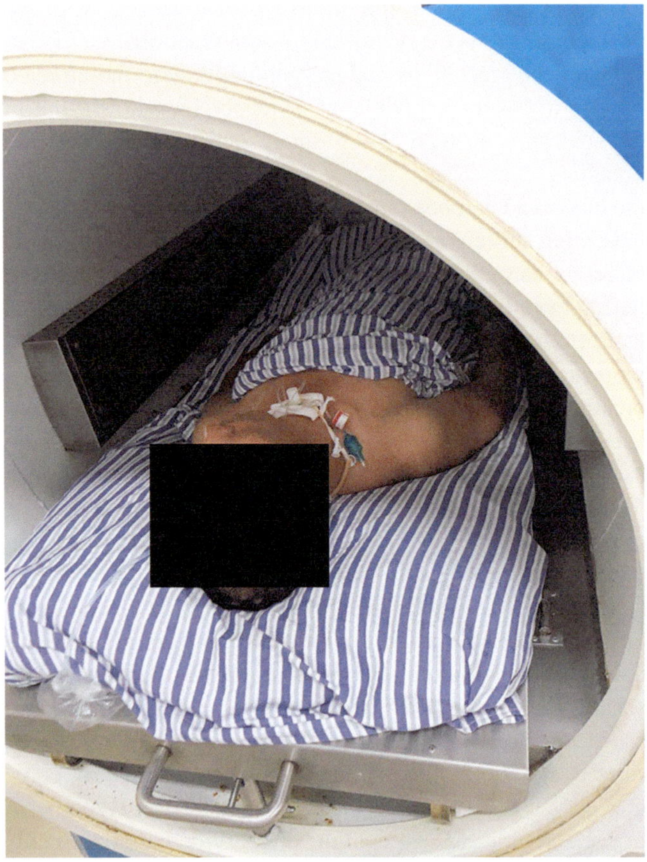

Fig. 23.2 Hyperbaric oxygen therapy administered to patients with stable vital signs after brainstem hemorrhage surgery as early as possible

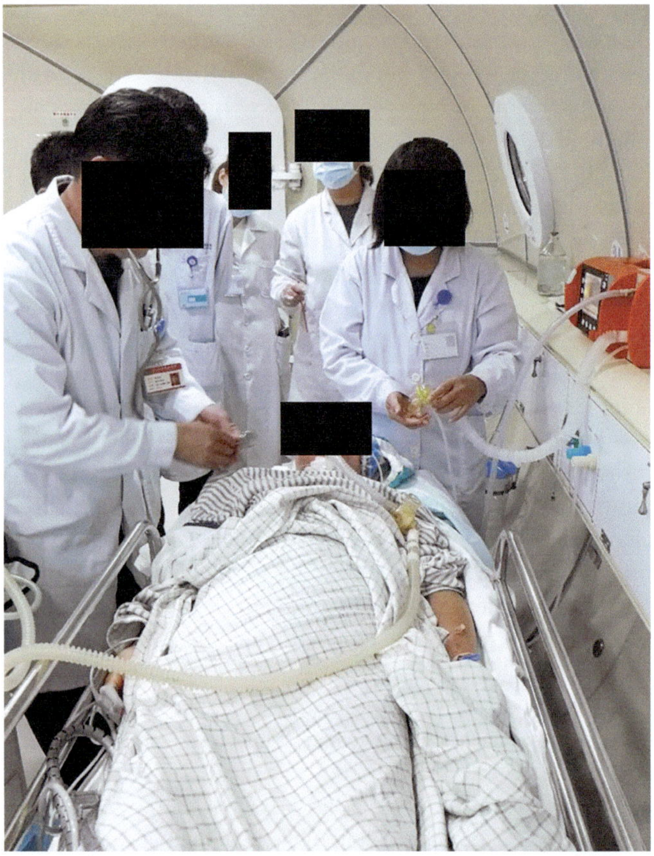

Fig. 23.3 In the acute phase, critically ill patients should preferably be placed in a multi-person chamber with healthcare personnel present. The chamber should be equipped with pneumatic ventilators, suction devices, and necessary rescue equipment and medications

23.1.1 Indications and Contraindications

23.1.1.1 Indications

1. The brainstem hemorrhage is relatively localized, and the patient's vital signs are basically stable.
2. The brainstem hematoma has been surgically removed, and the patient's postoperative condition is stable.
3. No formation of focal brain herniation.
4. The patient shows no signs of worsening local bleeding.
5. There are no signs of systemic bleeding.

23.1.1.2 Contraindications

1. The brainstem hemorrhage is extensive and has ruptured into the subarachnoid space.
2. The brainstem hematoma is large and has not been treated surgically.
3. Vital signs are unstable, and there is severe impairment of consciousness.
4. Brain herniation has occurred.
5. The patient is restless, convulsing, and unable to cooperate with oxygen therapy.
6. Blood pressure is too high, exceeding 200/110 mmHg.

23.1.2 Treatment Mechanism and Timing Selection

Regarding the oxygen supply following brainstem hemorrhage surgery, hyperbaric oxygen therapy is currently recognized as the most economical, reliable, and safe method that cannot be replaced by any other method. The timing of initiating treatment after brainstem hemorrhage surgery is crucial. Treatment administered during the optimal therapeutic window yields significantly better outcomes, while delays in intervention may compromise efficacy.

Combining hyperbaric oxygen with other medications is extremely effective for emergency and early treatment of brainstem hemorrhage edema. Treatment with hyperbaric oxygen after brainstem hemorrhage surgery may last for weeks for mild cases and may take several months for severe cases. For patients in a vegetative state, therapy may extend to over 6 months.

23.1.2.1 Treatment Mechanism

23.1.2.1.1 Increase in Blood Oxygen Content

Under hyperbaric oxygen therapy, blood oxygen content increases, rapidly improving the hypoxic state of hemorrhagic brain tissue.

23.1.2.1.2 Reduction of Cerebral Edema and Intracranial Pressure

During hyperbaric oxygen therapy, cerebral blood vessels constrict, leading to a reduction in cerebral blood flow. At 2 atmospheres absolute pressure, cerebral blood flow decreases by 21%, while at 3 atmospheres absolute pressure, it decreases by 25%. This constriction also reduces fluid leakage from blood vessels. Additionally, hyperbaric oxygen therapy corrects hypoxia, reduces lactate production, restores brain tissue energy metabolism, and reduces swelling of brain nerve cells, thereby lowering intracranial pressure. Hence, hyperbaric oxygen therapy is highly effective in preventing and managing cerebral edema after cerebral hemorrhage.

23.1.2.1.3 Effect on Cerebral Blood Flow

Under hyperbaric oxygen therapy, blood flow in the carotid artery decreases while blood flow in the vertebral artery increases. Breathing pure oxygen at 2 atmospheres absolute pressure has been shown to increase vertebral artery blood flow by 18%. Blood flow to the reticular activating system and brainstem does not decrease, and the elevated oxygen partial pressure is conducive to the awakening of comatose patients and the maintenance of vital functions.

23.1.2.2 Selection of Treatment Timing

For general patients with stable vital signs and no active bleeding on head CT or MRI scans, hyperbaric oxygen therapy can be initiated 6–8 h after cerebral hemorrhage.

Most scholars advocate initiating hyperbaric oxygen therapy 7–10 days following cerebral hemorrhage or surgical intervention, considering this period to be optimal for achieving the best therapeutic outcomes.

23.1.2.3 Treatment Protocol and Precautions

23.1.2.3.1 Treatment Protocol

In the acute phase, critically ill patients are best treated in multi-person chambers. These patients should be accompanied by medical staff to ensure close monitoring of vital signs during treatment. Equip the chamber with pneumatic ventilators, suction devices, and necessary rescue equipment and medications. Initially, lower treatment pressures are recommended, typically 1.8–2.0 ATA. Treatment pressure can be adjusted based on the patient's condition, tolerance, and observed improvements over successive treatment sessions.

23.1.2.3.2 Notes

1. During the course of hyperbaric oxygen therapy, it is emphasized to integrate comprehensive treatment, namely hyperbaric oxygen therapy + X protocol. Hyperbaric oxygen therapy serves as an adjunctive treatment, and should not replace routine postoperative treatment for brainstem hemorrhage.
2. During hyperbaric oxygen therapy, the rate of pressurization and depressurization should be slow, especially for patients with intracranial hypertension. Decompression should be performed as slowly as possible, combined

with the use of diuretics and corticosteroids to prevent rebound increases in intracranial pressure.
3. If the patient's condition worsens during hyperbaric oxygen therapy, the therapy should be immediately stopped CT or MRI scan should be performed to assess for ongoing bleeding for timely intervention.
4. Each treatment session should not exceed a long duration, typically controlled within 60–90 min, and indirect oxygenation should be employed.
5. Patients should not bring matches, lighters, or other flammable or explosive items into the chamber, nor wear synthetic clothing to prevent fires.
6. Patients should avoid consuming gas-producing foods such as soy products and potatoes before entering the chamber. They should empty their bowels and bladder before entering.

23.2 Postoperative Rehabilitation Treatment for Primary Brainstem Hemorrhage

Rehabilitation medicine considers common functional impairments after brainstem hemorrhage surgery, including disorders of consciousness, motor functions, sensory perception, cognition, speech, sleep, and urinary and fecal control. Rehabilitation medicine is an important branch of medicine that promotes the recovery of patients from illness, injury, or disability. It mainly utilizes rehabilitation measures to treat functional impairments caused by brainstem hemorrhage. For patients who temporarily or permanently reducing or losing their ability to live and work, these measures aim to restore their function to the maximum extent possible, creating conditions for them to return to society. Moreover, rehabilitation efforts are designed to minimize neurological damage after brainstem hemorrhage surgery, reduce the disability rate after surgery, and optimize the patient's ability in daily life, ultimately improving their overall quality of life.

While timely rescue and treatment of brainstem hemorrhage are essential, early initiation of effective rehabilitation intervention is equally critical. For postoperative brainstem hemorrhage patients with various functional impairments, it is important to start scientific and effective rehabilitation education, assessment, and treatment early, actively manage modifiable factors that affect the recovery of functional impairments after brainstem hemorrhage surgery, and reduce various postoperative complications. A multidisciplinary, function-oriented collaboration should provide patients with systematic, comprehensive, safe, efficient, and high-quality rehabilitation treatment to facilitate their early return to work and integration into family and society.

23.2.1 Rehabilitation Assessment

23.2.1.1 Comprehensive Assessment of Neurological Deficits

National Institutes of Health Stroke Scale (NIHSS) The NIHSS is the most widely used neurological assessment scale internationally. It includes 11 assessment items, and a higher score indicates a more severe degree of neurological impairment.

Scandinavian Stroke Scale (SSS) The SSS evaluates the severity of neurological deficits in various aspects, such as consciousness, orientation, eye movements, language, facial palsy, upper limb muscle strength, hand muscle strength, lower limb muscle strength, and walking ability. It is a commonly used quantitative assessment tool in neurological specialty for evaluating the severity of neurological deficits.

23.2.1.2 Assessment of Consciousness Disorders

Glasgow Coma Scale (GCS) The GCS is the most frequently used scale for assessing consciousness disorders internationally. It was developed by Jennett and Teasdale at the University of Glasgow's Institute of Neuroscience. It consists of three major components: eye-opening response (E), verbal response (V), and motor response (M). It includes 15 sub-items, and the total score ranges from 3 to 15. The highest score is 15, indicating clear consciousness, while scores between 12 and 14 indicate mild consciousness impairment, scores between 9 and 11 indicate moderate consciousness impairment, and scores below 8 indicate coma. A lower score indicates a more severe consciousness impairment.

Coma Recovery Scale-Revised (CRS-R) The CRS-R is a sensitive assessment scale that categorizes six subscales—visual, auditory, motor, verbal, communication, and arousal levels—to diagnose and differentiate between vegetative state and minimally conscious state. The CRS-R demonstrates good content validity, acceptable standardization, and scoring procedures. It serves as a gold standard for evaluating patients with consciousness disorders. Within the motor function subscale, "functional object use" is a key item for distinguishing between a vegetative state and a minimally conscious state.

Evoked Potentials (EP) EP is used to assess the correlation between certain neural pathway damage and the degree of consciousness impairment and prognosis. Commonly used EPs in clinical practice include somatosensory evoked potentials (SEP) and brainstem auditory evoked potentials (BAEP). In SEP, the N20 component (parietal postcentral gyrus) is more clinically relevant as it is associated with the conscious cortical loop. BAEP reflects the functional status of the auditory pathway from the cochlea to the brainstem, particularly pathways below the midbrain and pons.

23.2.1.3 Comprehensive Assessment of Motor Function

Fugl-Meyer Assessment (FMA) FMA is a commonly used comprehensive physical function assessment scale in clinical settings. It includes evaluations of movement, balance, sensation, joint range of motion, and pain. The total score is 226, with movement accounting for 100 points, balance for 14 points, sensation for 24 points, joint range of motion for 44 points, and pain for 44 points. FMA is known for its detailed and quantitative content, high reliability, validity, and sensitivity. It is suitable for assessing upper and lower limb function in patients with brainstem hemorrhage.

Brunnstrom's Movement Function Assessment Brunnstrom categorizes the recovery of motor function after stroke into six stages, based on changes in muscle tone and movement patterns in the upper limb, hand, and lower limb. This scale has the advantages of being concise, time-saving, highly compliant, and having strong repeatability. It is suitable for predicting clinical rehabilitation outcomes.

Ueda's Toshi Assessment This assessment method is based on Brunnstrom's scale and consists of 12 levels that have been standardized, ensuring high reliability. Its characteristic is the significant correlation between functional impairments in the affected lower limb and mobility. The grading of the lower limb has a 50% impact on walking ability, making it suitable for assessing upper and lower limb function in patients with brainstem hemorrhage.

Rivermead Mobility Index (RMI) RMI is a simple and quantitative method used in rehabilitation to assess the degree of movement impairment and treatment progress in patients. It focuses on evaluating comprehensive mobility in daily life situations.

23.2.1.4 Assessment of Balance and Coordination Function

Berg Balance Scale (BBS) BBS is a commonly used balance assessment scale in stroke rehabilitation. It can assess the subject's balance ability in both static and dynamic conditions and predict the risk of falls in normal situations. The total score is 56, and a score below 40 indicates a risk of falling.

Timed Up and Go Test This test measures the time it takes for the subject to stand up from a chair, walk 3 m forward, turn around, and return. It also observes the subject's dynamic balance during the walking process. This method is simple to administer and can be used to predict the risk of falls in the subject.

Balance Measurement Devices Balance measurement devices can objectively assess the subject's static and dynamic balance function. They have the advantages of objective and quantifiable parameters, as well as high reliability and validity. However, during the assessment process, subjects need to actively cooperate, and their safety should be ensured to prevent accidents. Balance Performance Monitor, Balance Master, Smart Balance, and Equitest are commonly used balance testing instruments abroad.

23.2.1.5 Walking and Gait Analysis

Rancho Los Amigos Gait Analysis (RLA) Eight-Point System The RLA is a gait observation and analysis method designed by the Rancho Los Amigos National Rehabilitation Center in California, USA. It provides detailed and systematic observations, allowing for a comprehensive analysis of the performance of each joint or body part during different phases of the gait cycle. This method assists rehabilitation therapists in identifying any abnormalities and determining when these abnormalities occur during a patient's walking.

Four-Phase Analysis This method involves two double-support phases, one single-support phase, and one swing phase. It is the most commonly used qualitative gait analysis method.

Holden Walking Function Classification This classification system divides the walking function into six levels and is an objective grading method with good reliability and high accuracy. It is particularly suitable for assessing lower limb function in post-stroke patients with motor impairments.

Footprint Analysis This method involves using corridors or therapy halls with surfaces that can leave footprints as the walking path. A 45-m wide and 1100-cm long path is used, with a horizontal line drawn 250 cm from each end, and the middle 600 cm is used for formal gait measurements. Footprint measurements are taken to assess parameters such as step length, stride length, step width, and foot angle, as well as calculate gait speed and cadence. This method is a simple, quantitative, objective, and practical clinical rehabilitation assessment method.

Gait Analysis Systems These systems utilize gait analysis devices to collect kinematic parameters, kinetic parameters, energy parameters, and other data to conduct an in-depth and detailed analysis of a subject's gait. While these instruments are relatively expensive and not yet widely accessible, they offer advantages such as objectivity and precise quantification, making them particularly suitable for clinical rehabilitation research.

23.2.1.6 Cognitive Function Assessment

Mini-Mental State Examination (MMSE) The MMSE, developed by Folstein et al., assesses cognitive function using various aspects such as orientation, memory, attention, calculation, naming ability, repetition, three-step command, reading and writing skills, and visuospatial and constructional abilities. It is a simple tool used to evaluate cognitive function and determine the severity of cognitive impairment. The total score is 30, and the criteria for determining normal cognitive function are as follows: high school education or above, score > 27; middle school education, score > 24; primary school education, score > 20; illiterate, score > 17.

Montreal Cognitive Assessment (MoCA) The MoCA, developed by Nasreddine et al. at the Montreal Neurological Institute, Canada, assesses various aspects including visuospatial and executive abilities, naming, memory, attention, language, abstraction, and orientation. It is primarily used for elderly patients with an education level of 7 years or more. The total score is 30, and a score of ≥26 is considered normal.

23.2.1.7 Swallowing Function Assessment

Water Swallowing Test by Warita This test involves having the patient drink 30 mL of warm water as they normally would, and then observing and recording the time taken to swallow the water, as well as any coughing or difficulties experienced during swallowing. The grading scale for evaluation is as follows: Grade 1: The patient can swallow 30 mL of water smoothly within 5 s. Grade 2: The patient can swallow 30 mL of water in more than 5 s, divided into two swallows without coughing. Grade 3: The patient can swallow 30 mL of water in more than 5 s in one swallow but with coughing. Grade 4: The patient can swallow 30 mL of water in more than 5 s, divided into multiple swallows with coughing. Grade 5: The patient frequently coughs, and it is difficult to swallow the entire amount within 10 s.

Saito Swallowing Function Classification This classification system consists of seven levels. Level 7 represents normal swallowing function without any difficulties, indicating no need for rehabilitation. Level 6 indicates mild problems during swallowing, requiring modifications in food consistency, such as eating soft food due to insufficient chewing. However, there is minimal residue in the oral cavity, and there are no swallowing errors. Level 5 represents oral phase problems, mainly moderate to severe swallowing disorders during the oral phase, requiring improvement in chewing consistency, prolonged meal times, increased oral residue, and the need for reminders or supervision during swallowing without any swallowing errors. Level 4 represents occasional swallowing errors, where swallowing with conventional methods results in occasional errors, but adjustments in posture or portion size can prevent these errors. Level 3 represents water swallowing errors, where even compensatory methods cannot control water swallowing, changing food consistency has some effect, and eating only allows food to be swallowed, but the intake of energy is insufficient. In most cases, parenteral nutrition is required, and long-term management of the whole body may require consideration of gastrostomy. If appropriate swallowing methods are adopted, it is possible to ensure the supply of water and nutrition through direct swallowing training. Level 2 represents food swallowing errors, where changing food consistency has no effect, and water and nutrition are primarily supplied intravenously. Level 1 represents saliva swallowing errors, where saliva causes swallowing errors, preventing food and water intake, and direct swallowing training is not possible.

Video Fluoroscopic Swallowing Study (VFSS) The VFSS, initially proposed by Mosher, utilizes X-ray fluoroscopy to evaluate swallowing disorders. It is considered the "gold standard" for diagnosing swallowing disorders and determining the mechanisms of oropharyngeal dysfunction. This method allows for a detailed assessment and analysis of the entire swallowing process, making it the most comprehensive, reliable, and valuable swallowing function assessment method available.

23.2.1.8 Activities of Daily Living (ADL) Assessment

Barthel Index (BI) and Modified Barthel Index (MBI) BI and MBI are currently the most commonly used ADL assessment scales internationally. The former sensitively reflects changes in patient conditions or functional progression, suitable for clinical efficacy observation and prognosis judgment. The latter, based on BI, weights the levels, maintaining the original 10 items but subdividing each assessment item into 5 levels, enhancing the accuracy and sensitivity of the assessment.

Functional Independence Measure (FIM) FIM is a widely used functional assessment scale internationally. It not only evaluates physical function but also assesses speech, cognition, and social function. It has high retest reliability and validity in terms of surface, content, and construct.

Rapid Disability Rating Scale (RDRS) RDRS, proposed by Linn in 1967 and revised in 1982, includes 18 items, each scored from 0 to 3, with a total score of 54. The higher the score, the more severe the disability. It is suitable for patients living in hospitals and communities, especially for the elderly.

23.2.1.9 Sleep Disorder Assessment

Pittsburgh Sleep Quality Index (PSQI) PSQI is one of the most widely validated and used scales for assessing sleep disorders. It is mainly used to evaluate the sleep quality of patients with organic or non-organic sleep disorders. PSQI assesses the sleep quality of subjects over the past month, consisting of 19 self-evaluation and 5 peer-evaluation items. The 19th self-evaluation item and 5 peer-evaluation items are not included in the scoring. Only 18 self-evaluation items that contribute to scoring are discussed here. These 18 items form 7 components, with each component scored on a scale of 0–3. The cumulative score of each component constitutes the total PSQI score, ranging from 0 to 21. A higher score indicates poorer sleep quality.

Epworth Sleepiness Scale (ESS) ESS, designed by the Epworth Hospital in Melbourne, Australia, is used to assess excessive daytime sleepiness in patients. The scale consists of eight items, each rated as "Never, Rarely, Sometimes,

Often." Participants choose the most appropriate option based on their recent daily life situations, with scores ranging from 0 to 3 for each item. A higher score indicates a more pronounced tendency for sleepiness.

23.2.1.10 Quality of Life Assessment

Medical Outcomes Study Short Form 36 (SF-36) SF-36 comprises 36 items covering eight aspects: physical functioning, role limitations due to physical health problems, bodily pain, general health perceptions, vitality, social functioning, role limitations due to emotional problems, and mental health. The entire assessment takes about 5–10 min, and the Chinese version was compiled by researchers including Fang Jiqian from Zhongshan University. Studies on the quality of life of stroke patients have shown that SF-36 is highly sensitive in evaluating physical and mental health but slightly less sensitive in assessing social functioning.

Stroke Specific Quality of Life Scale (SS-QOL) SS-QOL is a widely used quality of life assessment method in China, developed by American scholar William and others specifically for stroke patients. It includes 49 items covering 12 aspects: family roles, speech, mobility, emotions, personality, self-care, social roles, cognition, upper limb function, vision, energy, and work capacity. The scale has strong targeting, wide coverage, and good reliability and validity.

23.2.2 Rehabilitation Intervention Timing and Intensity Selection

After surgery for brainstem hemorrhage, rehabilitation treatment should adhere to the principles of safety, effectiveness, and gradual progression. When the patient's vital signs are stable, it is advisable to initiate rehabilitation treatment early to promote the recovery of impaired functions in various body systems.

There is no unified understanding of the optimal timing for initiating rehabilitation treatment after brainstem hemorrhage surgery. Generally, clinicians consider the postoperative condition stable 48–72 h after surgery, and rehabilitation treatment can commence simultaneously with clinical diagnosis and treatment. Rehabilitation training intensity should progress gradually. According to the National Stroke Rehabilitation Guidelines issued by the National Brain Injury Prevention Office, stroke patients should undergo at least 45 min of relevant rehabilitation training daily in the initial stage of stroke rehabilitation. Increasing the training intensity within a certain range can enhance the training effectiveness. However, for patients with brainstem hemorrhage, the safety of the patient should be carefully considered, and the tolerance of the patient's postoperative condition should be assessed to flexibly arrange appropriate rehabilitation treatments. It is generally considered feasible for inpatient rehabilitation institutions to conduct rehabilitation training for 3 h per day, 5 days a week, if tolerated by the patient, including physical therapy, occupational therapy, speech therapy, and necessary rehabilitation nursing care.

Actively managing the primary disease and various complications, stabilizing the condition, and alleviating symptoms can eliminate factors that affect the effectiveness of rehabilitation treatment, facilitating the progress of rehabilitation therapy. Additionally, attention should be paid to risk management during the rehabilitation of brainstem hemorrhage to prevent recurrence.

23.2.3 Staged Rehabilitation Treatment

23.2.3.1 Early Rehabilitation Treatment

Currently, most studies suggest that early rehabilitation for stroke patients refers to providing rehabilitation intervention treatment when the condition is relatively stable and no longer progressing. According to the "Chinese Stroke Rehabilitation Treatment Guidelines (2011 Complete Version)," early rehabilitation involves "routine treatment and early rehabilitation treatment in the emergency room or neurology department of the hospital" and "after the acute phase standardized treatment, when vital signs have stabilized, and neurological symptoms no longer progress after 48 h." The key to early rehabilitation intervention is whether the patient's condition is stable.

Rehabilitation Objectives: During this period, patients cannot actively participate in rehabilitation training due to the impact of their condition. Therefore, the purpose of rehabilitation treatment during this period is to use passive activities to promote the recovery of hemiplegic limb strength and muscle tone after brainstem hemorrhage surgery. Proper limb positioning and appropriate position changes are employed to prevent and manage complications such as pressure sores, venous thrombosis in the limbs, osteoporosis, pulmonary infections, and urinary tract infections. These measures also serve to prepare patients for functional rehabilitation training during the recovery period. Additionally, actively managing postoperative risk factors related to brainstem hemorrhage is an important objective of rehabilitation during this period.

Rehabilitation Content: Depending on the actual situation of patients after brainstem hemorrhage surgery, early rehabilitation treatment should include proper limb positioning (also known as limb positioning), regular turning, position changes, and passive activities in bed. Patients should also be encouraged to re-engage with external communication. Proper limb positioning is the most fundamental measure for early rehabilitation intervention after brainstem hemorrhage surgery.

Proper Limb Positioning: Maintaining an anti-spasm position. Proper limb positioning, also known as an anti-spasm position, aims to maintain the good function of limbs, prevent or counteract the appearance of spasm patterns, prevent secondary joint contractures, deformities, or muscle atrophy, and prevent pressure sores, pneumonia, and deep vein thrombosis.

1. Supine Position: Place a pillow under the head to avoid lateral bending, excessive flexion, or extension. Place a pillow behind the shoulder of the affected side to avoid posterior shoulder retraction. Align the affected upper limb on the side of the body, slightly abducted, with the elbow extended, the forearm rotated backward, and the thumb pointing outward. Place a pillow under the affected side hip to avoid posterior hip retraction. Support the lateral side of the affected thigh with a pillow to prevent external rotation of the thigh. Avoid placing a pillow under the affected lower leg or knee to prevent compression of the lower limb veins and excessive flexion or extension of the knee (Fig. 23.4). The supine position should not be maintained for too long.
2. Affected Side Lateral Position: Place a pillow under the head, slightly elevate the trunk, and support it with a pillow behind. The scapula of the affected side should be sufficiently protracted, and the shoulder joint should be flexed forward 90°–130°. The affected side elbow should naturally extend, the forearm should rotate backward, and the hand should be in a dorsal flexion position. The joint of the affected side should naturally extend, and the knee joint can be slightly flexed (Fig. 23.5). The unaffected upper limb should be placed naturally, and the unaffected lower limb should be placed in a step-like position on the pillow.
3. Healthy Side Lateral Position: The head is supported by a pillow, keeping the trunk vertical. Place a pillow under the upper limb, with the scapula of the affected side sufficiently protracted, the shoulder flexed forward 90°–130°, and the elbow and wrist joints naturally extended. The hip and knee joints on the affected side are naturally semi-flexed, placed in a step-like position on the pillow, and the affected foot and lower leg are kept as vertical as possible (Fig. 23.6). The healthy side lateral position is the most comfortable position for patients after brainstem hemorrhage surgery and is beneficial for the recovery of the affected limb.

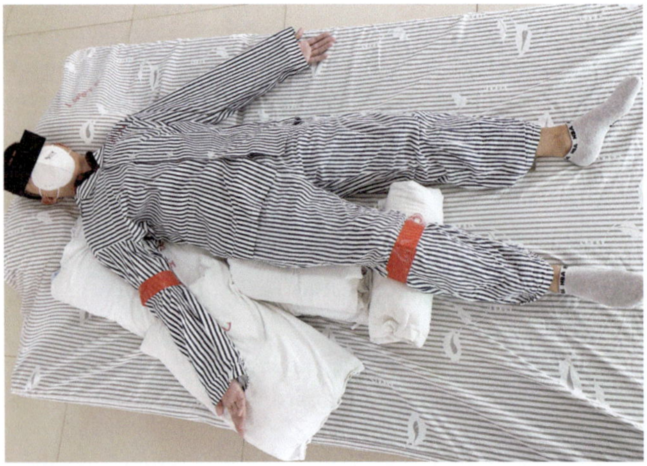

Fig. 23.4 Proper limb positioning in the supine position. Place a pillow under the head, a pillow behind the posterior shoulder of the affected side, place the affected upper limb on the side of the body, slightly abducted, with the elbow extended, the forearm rotated backward, and the thumb pointing outward. Place a pillow under the affected side hip. Avoid placing a pillow under the lower leg or knee of the affected side

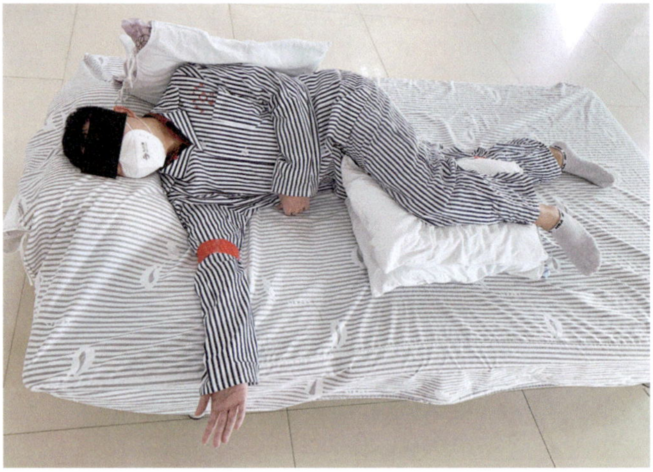

Fig. 23.5 Proper limb positioning in the affected side lateral position. To increase sensory stimulation on the paralyzed side, a lateral position on the paralyzed side is advocated

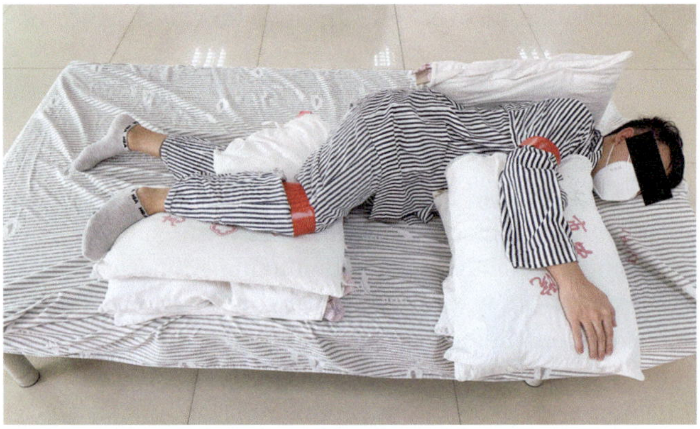

Fig. 23.6 Proper limb positioning in the healthy side lateral position. The head is supported by a pillow, keeping the trunk vertical. Place a pillow under the upper limb, with the scapula of the affected side sufficiently protracted, the shoulder flexed forward 90°–130°, and the elbow and wrist joints naturally extended. The hip and knee joints on the affected side are naturally semi-flexed, placed in a step-like position on the pillow, and the affected foot and lower leg are kept as vertical as possible

Position Changes: The implementation of bed position changes should involve therapists, patients, family members, nurses, and other caregivers. The training principles should proceed in the order of complete passive, assisted, and fully active. Passive position changes: Positions should be adjusted every 1–2 h to prevent lung infections and pressure sores. By continuously alternating between supine, affected side lateral, and healthy side lateral positions, the muscle tone of the patient's limbs can be balanced, preventing and alleviating spasm patterns. Subsequent methods include assisted and active position changes (Fig. 23.7). The training content of position changes includes lateral movement, forward and backward movement, passive healthy side turning, affected side turning and sitting-up training, assisted and active turning and sitting-up training, bed bridging training, and transfer training from bed to wheelchair and wheelchair to bed, among others. The implementation of bed position transfer techniques should pay attention to safety issues during the transfer process and, under the premise of physical conditions permitting, patients should be encouraged to leave the bed as early as possible.

Joint Mobility Training: Joint mobility training can promote limb blood circulation, increase sensory input, prevent restricted joint movement, effectively prevent disuse muscle atrophy, and promote overall functional recovery. Joint mobility training can begin in a completely passive manner, focusing on: shoulder joint abduction, flexion, and external rotation, elbow joint extension, wrist and finger extension, hip joint abduction, flexion, and extension, knee joint flexion and extension, and dorsal flexion and eversion of the foot (Fig. 23.8). Perform 2–3 repetitions for each joint each time. As muscle tone increases, the number of passive joint movements should be appropriately increased. Generally, each joint should be exercised 2–3 times a day. When starting from flaccid paralysis, the range of joint motion should be within 2/3 of the normal range, especially for the shoulder joint, and attention should be paid to joint protection to avoid unnecessary injury and prevent heterotopic ossification. Later, a transition can be made to assisted and fully active methods. Joint mobility training includes not only limb joints but also spinal joint mobility training. Emphasis should be placed on the affected side, while also considering the healthy side for long-term bedridden patients.

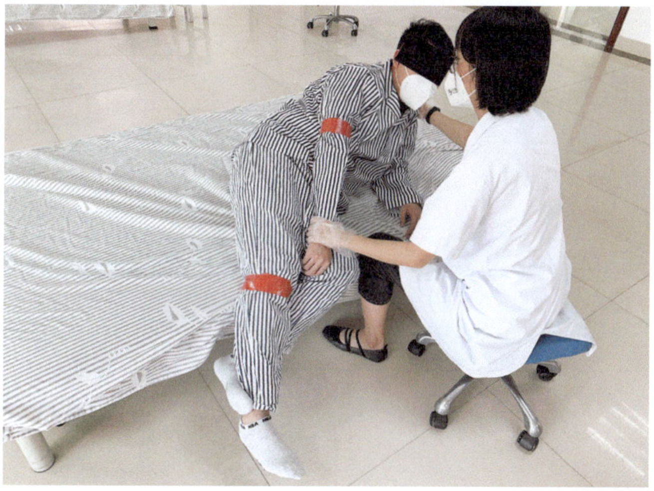

Fig. 23.7 Bed position changes. Therapists assist patients in performing bed position changes and turning to the healthy side

Physical Therapy: Physical therapy involves the application of physical factors such as electricity, heat, sound, and light to the body to prevent and treat diseases. Physical therapy is characterized by a wide range of indications, high safety, and few contraindications, making it widely used in the early rehabilitation of patients after brainstem hemorrhage surgery. At present, in the early rehabilitation stage, commonly used physical therapy includes electrotherapy (direct current, direct current drug iontophoresis therapy, low-frequency pulse therapy, medium-frequency electrotherapy, high-frequency electrotherapy, etc.), magnetotherapy (static magnetic field therapy, magnetic heat therapy, pulsed magnetic field therapy, etc.), light therapy (infrared therapy, visible light therapy, ultraviolet therapy, laser therapy, etc.), ultrasound therapy, heat therapy, cold therapy, hydrotherapy, mud therapy, electromyographic biofeedback therapy, transcranial magnetic stimulation, etc. (Fig. 23.9).

Considering the patient's specific medical condition and functional status, the selection of an appropriate physical modality therapy, the frequency of treatment, the duration of treatment, and the intensity of treatment in the rehabilitation prescription should be determined based on the patient's tolerance and the maximization of functional recovery.

23.2.3.2 Rehabilitation Therapy in the Recovery Period

Patients in the recovery period after brainstem hemorrhage surgery are able to actively move the affected limbs. The affected limbs gradually transition from the flaccid paralysis stage to the spasticity stage, with muscle activity transitioning from co-movement to selective muscle activity. The recovery period after brainstem hemorrhage surgery generally begins around the third to fourth week after onset.

Rehabilitation Goals: During this period, patients are able to positively move the affected limbs and participate to some extent in rehabilitation training. In addition to managing the risk factors associated with brainstem hemorrhage surgery, the goals of rehabilitation therapy should include inhibiting limb spasticity, promoting recovery of isolated movements, improving coordination and selective voluntary movement, forming correct movement patterns, enhancing activities of daily living, and ultimately achieving reintegration into family, society, and work.

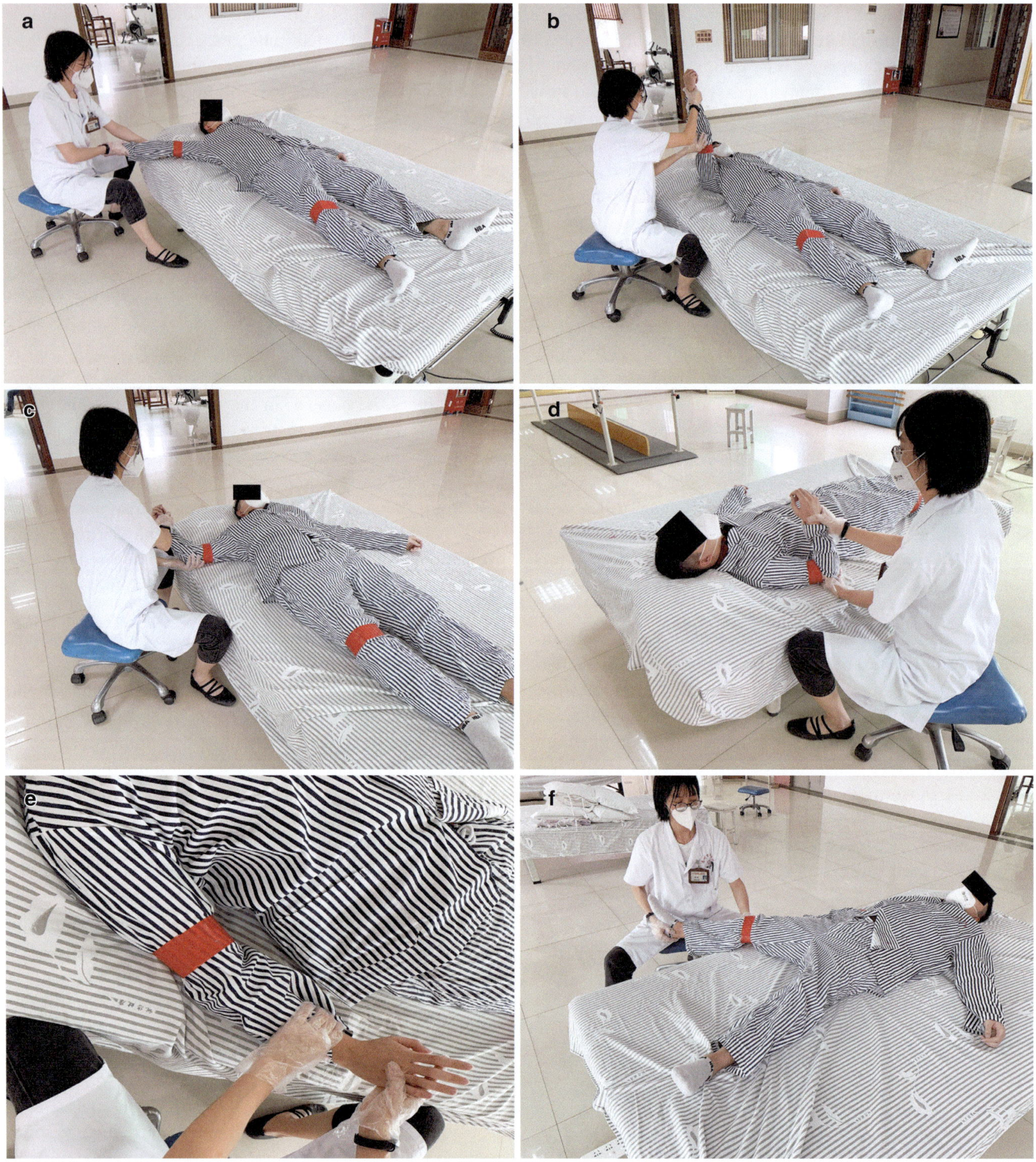

Fig. 23.8 Joint mobility training. (**a**) Shoulder joint abduction; (**b**) shoulder joint flexion; (**c**) shoulder joint external rotation; (**d**) elbow joint extension; (**e**) wrist and finger extension; (**f**) hip joint abduction; (**g**) hip joint flexion and knee joint flexion; (**h**) dorsal flexion of the ankle

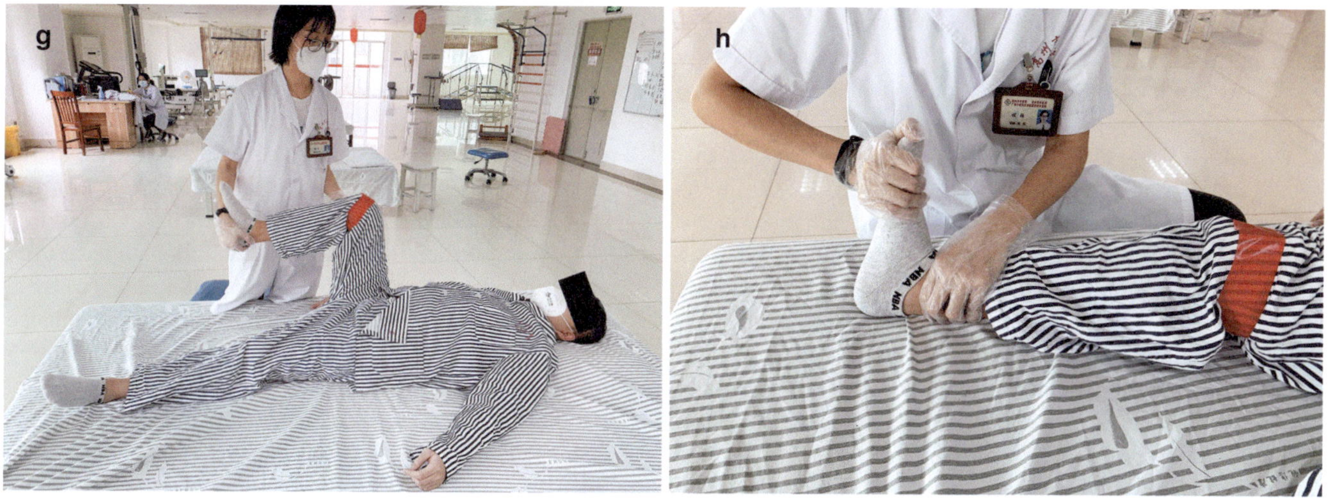

Fig. 23.8 (continued)

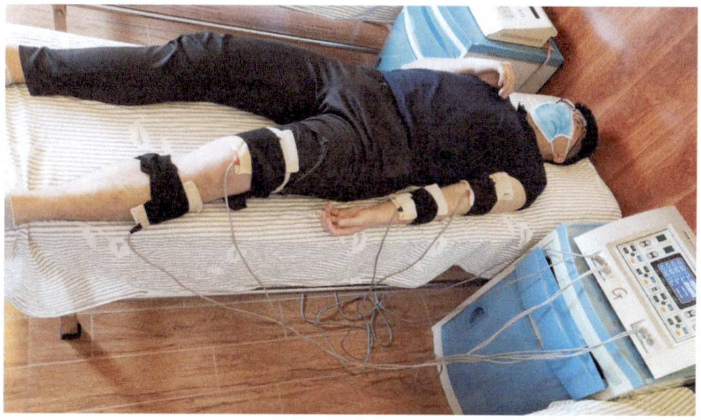

Fig. 23.9 Low-frequency pulse electrotherapy. Stimulate the flexor muscles of the upper limbs and extensor muscles of the lower limbs in patients in the flaccid paralysis stage to increase muscle tone and induce movement

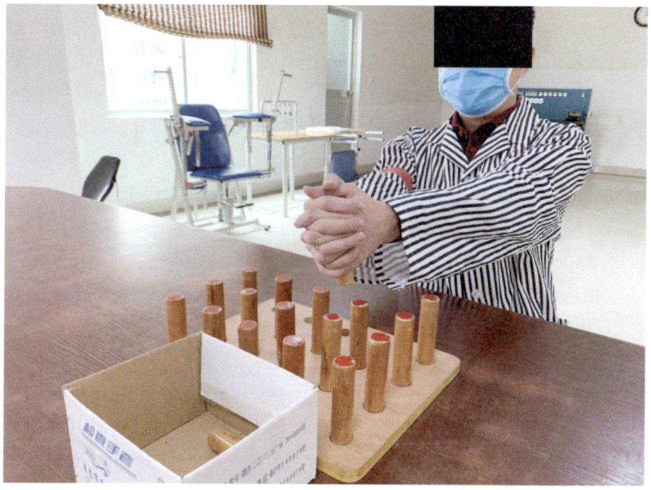

Fig. 23.10 Upper limb functional training. Bobath handshake, gripping a wooden stick with the palm and extending it forward into a box

Rehabilitation Content: Based on the results of rehabilitation functional assessment, individualized rehabilitation training plans are formulated to carry out corresponding rehabilitation therapy for the recovery period after brainstem hemorrhage surgery. Suitable patients are encouraged to actively participate in rehabilitation training. Rehabilitation training mainly includes sitting balance, transfer training, standing, weight shifting, normal movement pattern training, activities of daily living (ADL) training, etc. Rehabilitation training should be progressive, and the rehabilitation plan should align with the patient's goals. Providing appropriate encouragement during training is essential to foster motivation and enhance outcomes.

Exercise Therapy: Various exercises are used for limb activity and correction of abnormal movements in rehabilitation training. Under the guidance and supervision of therapists, patients actively engage in exercise therapy activities. Patients relearn compromised movement functions. Exercises are performed in the order of trunk, scapula, pelvis, and from proximal to distal limbs, including rolling, sitting, standing, and walking basic movements. Basic training also includes muscle strength training, joint mobility training, gait training, balance function training, coordination training, etc.

1. Upper Limb Functional Training: Patients lie supine with their upper limbs extended forward, reaching toward the ceiling; or they touch their forehead, pillow, etc., with their hands. In a seated position, patients practice pointing forward and upward with their hands, gradually increasing the range; in a seated position, the forearm is neutrally positioned on the table, the hand grips a glass, and they attempt to lift it, followed by training to lift an object—extend the wrist—flex the wrist—release the object (Fig. 23.10).

Wrist Extension: In a seated position, with the forearm in a neutral position on the table, extend the wrist to move the back of the hand backward and touch an object, gradually increasing the distance. Forearm Pronation: Grip a cylindrical object and pronate the forearm, causing the end of the object to touch the table; alternatively, train by pressing the back of the hand into clay. Palmar Activity: Grasp and release a cup, ensuring a neutral forearm and wrist extension. Finger Activity: With forearm pronation, practice opposition of the thumb and other fingers. Object Manipulation: Practice picking up small objects from a bowl with the fingers, then pronate the forearm and place the object into another bowl; alternatively, practice gripping the edge of a plastic cup without deforming it and moving it in different directions; or practice picking up small pieces of paper from the opposite shoulder.

2. Bed Mobility Training: The patient crosses their hands with fingers interlocked, extends the upper limbs, and performs exercises of elevation and lateral extension. During the turning motion, the crossed hands extend towards the side of turning, the head lifts and turns towards the same side, the trunk rotates to the side-lying position, then returns to the supine position, and finally turns to the other side (Fig. 23.11). This training should be performed multiple times daily.
3. Seated Training: This includes balance training and endurance training. In an unsupported sitting position at the edge of the bed or on a chair, the hip, knee, and ankle joints are flexed at 90°, with both feet supported on a footstool or the floor, approximately 1 ft width apart. The unaffected upper limb supports the bed or rests on the knee. The therapist assists or guides the patient in adjusting the trunk and head to the midline position, then releases the hands. The patient should be able to maintain this position for a certain period of time before slowly tilting to one side. Subsequently, the therapist guides or assists the patient in returning to the original position and repeats the process. Following this, the patient can interlock their fingers or use the unaffected upper limb to reach forward, backward, left, right, up, and down, in different directions while maintaining good trunk control. This is referred to as automatic seated balance training (Fig. 23.12). When the patient can maintain balance even when subjected to sudden pushing or pulling forces (passive balance), it can be considered that seated balance training has been completed. Subsequent seated training primarily focuses on endurance training.
4. Standing and Walking Training: Research suggests that prolonged bed rest can affect a patient's potential for functional recovery, particularly in terms of neuro-muscular and balance function, and can reduce brain plasticity and

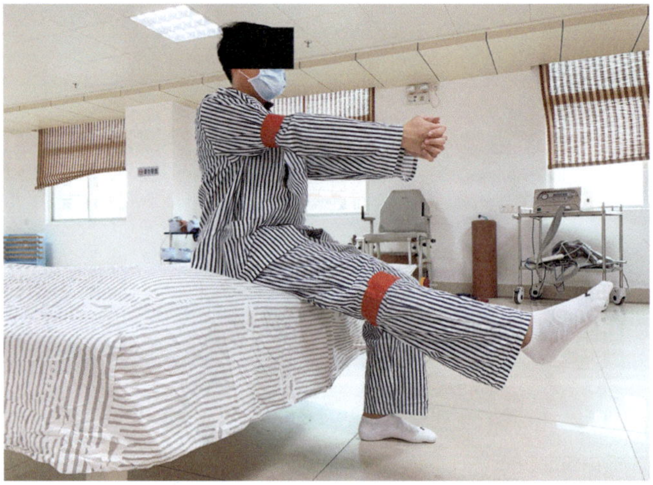

Fig. 23.12 Seated balance training. Reducing support surface to enhance automatic balance ability

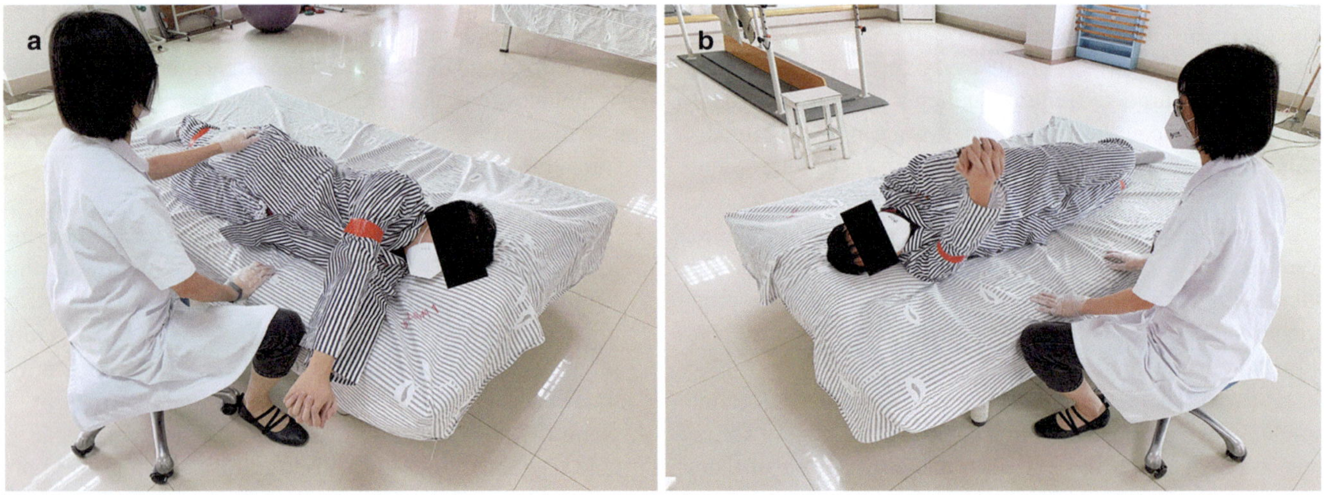

Fig. 23.11 Bed mobility training. (**a**) Turning to the unaffected side; (**b**) turning to the affected side

functional reorganization. Hemiparesis and abnormal gait after brainstem hemorrhage are the major functional impairments in stroke patients and also the primary factors affecting their daily life abilities and quality. For stable patients with brainstem hemorrhage, stable vital signs, and no progression of symptoms within 48–72 h, it is possible to consider early mobilization and utilize equipment for standing and walking rehabilitation training.

The basic elements of walking mainly include the following aspects: (a) The neck, trunk, and paretic lower limbs can resist gravity; (b) The affected lower limb can bear weight and support the body; (c) The center of gravity can move forward, backward, left, and right during standing; (d) The affected lower limb hip joint can flex and take steps. Based on the functional status of patients after getting out of bed following brainstem hemorrhage, targeted early walking training according to the aforementioned basic elements is a clinically simple and effective method for basic walking rehabilitation.

Before walking training, based on the patient's rehabilitation assessment, corresponding muscle strength enhancement training, sit-to-stand training, and parallel bar training should be conducted to prepare for walking exercises. Parallel bars, canes, and crutches can be used for standing, weight shifting, single-leg support, marching in place, or stepping exercises. Once the patient can achieve automatic standing balance and the affected leg can bear more than half of the body weight and take steps forward, walking training can be initiated (Fig. 23.13). In the initial stages of training, it should be done in small amounts and multiple times, then gradually progressed to avoid excessive fatigue or occurrences of foot inversion.

Occupational Therapy: Upper Limb and Hand Function Training: Utilize rollers, sliding boards, inclined sand boards, and Bobath ball exercises for gross upper limb movements (Fig. 23.14). Employ activities such as lacing shoes, cutting paper, and weaving to train bilateral coordination. Use tasks like writing, picking up small objects, and screwing to train the fine motor skills of the affected hand.

Activities of Daily Living (ADL) Training: Train patients to utilize residual functions and assistive devices to independently perform personal hygiene, eating, dressing, and other tasks to achieve self-care.

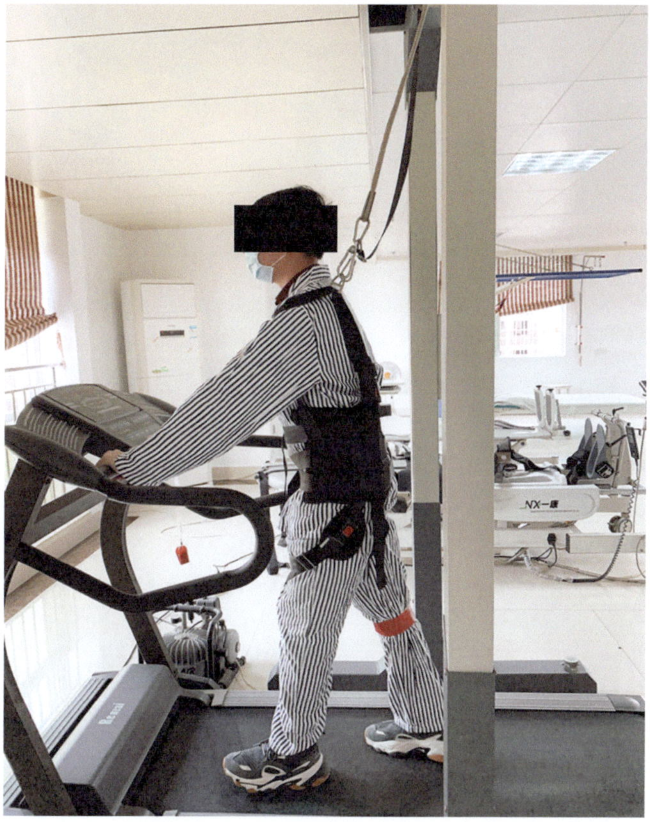

Fig. 23.13 Walking training. Treadmill walking training to consolidate gait

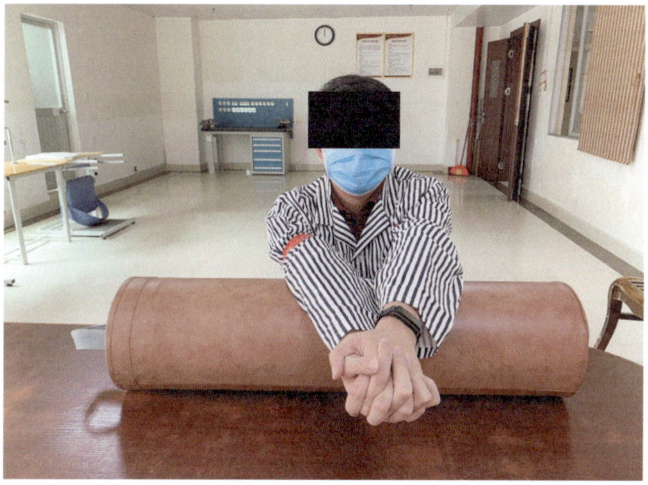

Fig. 23.14 Occupational therapy. Rolling training facilitates elbow extension

Swallowing Training: Swallowing disorders are common symptoms in patients with brainstem hemorrhage, often severely affecting their physical and psychological health. The water swallow test is a commonly used clinical screening method, while Videofluoroscopic Swallow Study (VFSS) is considered the "gold standard" for evaluating swallowing function. The goal of treating and managing swallowing disorders is to enable patients to safely, adequately, and independently ingest sufficient nutrition and fluids. For patients with swallowing disorders, training to enhance the strength and coordination of perioral muscles is conducted (Fig. 23.15). Various stimuli such as ice stimulation are applied to induce and facilitate the disappearance or reduction of swallowing reflexes. Swallowing electrical stimulation therapy, balloon dilation, and other techniques are also

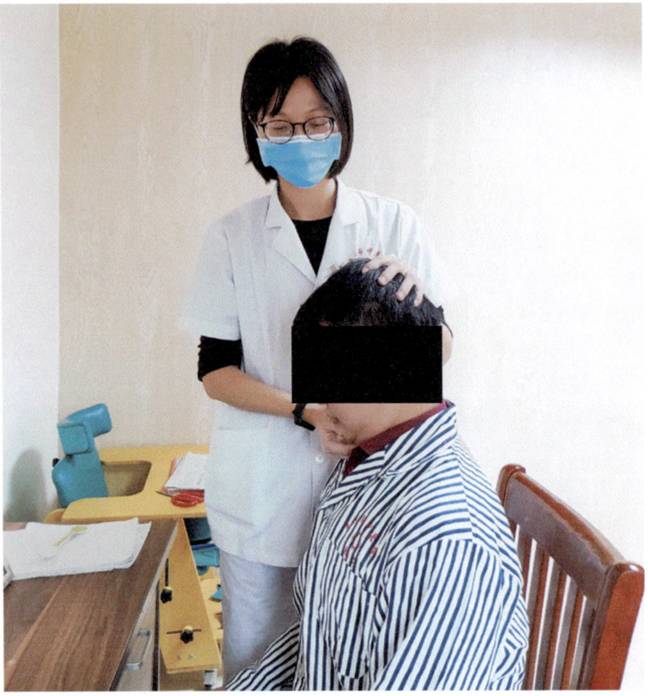

Fig. 23.15 Swallowing function training. Shaker training enhances strength of the submental muscles and increases pressure in the pharynx

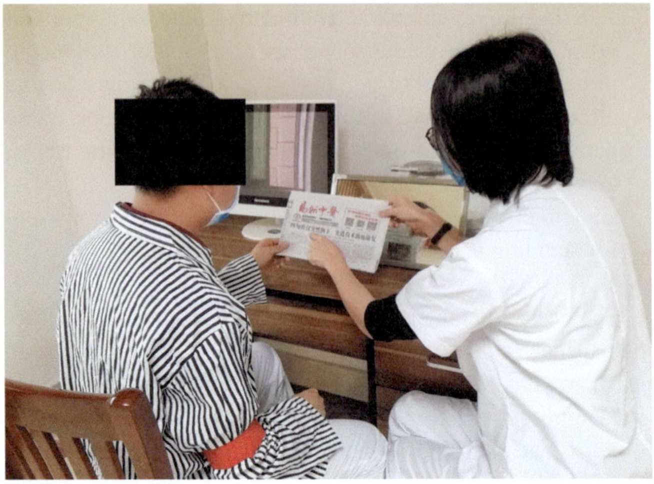

Fig. 23.16 Language training. Reading newspapers for fluent speech training

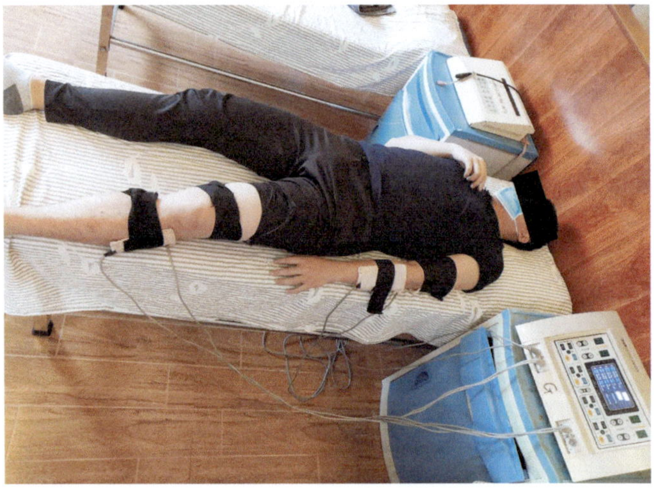

Fig. 23.17 Physical therapy. For patients in the recovery period, use low-frequency electrical stimulation to target extensor muscles of the affected upper limb and flexor muscles of the lower limb to improve their motor function

employed. Observing the presence of swallowing reflexes and minimal instances of aspiration, feeding training is conducted when the patient can voluntarily cough to expel.

Language and Speech Training: Aphasia and dysarthria are common in patients with brainstem hemorrhage. The rehabilitation goal is primarily to facilitate communication recovery, help patients develop compensatory strategies for communication barriers, and educate individuals around the patient to actively engage and reduce the patient's isolation, fulfilling their desires and needs. Early interventions may involve providing basic instruction training for auditory comprehension, speaking, reading, writing, and repeating. Training in imitation of facial muscles for speech production, as well as training in speech repetition, can be beneficial for patients with severe difficulties in oral comprehension. Patients with severe oral comprehension deficits may benefit from using written language, writing, or communication boards for interaction (Fig. 23.16). Necessary interventions aid in maximizing the restoration of communication abilities.

Physical Factor Therapy Physical factor therapy during the recovery period after brainstem hemorrhage primarily targets the extensor muscles of paralyzed upper limbs and flexor muscles of paralyzed lower limbs, aiming to improve functions such as elbow extension, wrist extension, finger extension, knee flexion, and ankle dorsiflexion. Additionally, appropriate physical factor therapies are utilized to treat various complications such as shoulder pain, shoulder-hand syndrome, and osteoporosis, improving patient symptoms and enhancing quality of life. Research has shown that low-frequency electrical therapy can stimulate neuromuscular activity and promote blood circulation. Devices such as low-frequency pulse therapy units and spasm treatment devices can be used to treat flaccid paralysis, muscle atrophy, spasms, etc. Care must be taken in electrode placement when using spasm treatment devices to select antagonistic muscles (Fig. 23.17). Compared to low-frequency therapy, medium-frequency therapy has a greater depth of action, better analgesic effects, and is more beneficial for skeletal muscle exercise. It can be used for symptoms such as flaccid paralysis, muscle atrophy, and shoulder pain after brainstem hemorrhage. Moderate warmth can alleviate muscle spasm.

Therapies such as infrared therapy, traditional Chinese medicine heat therapy, and paraffin therapy can be employed. Ultrasound therapy, extracorporeal shock wave therapy, etc., can improve circulation, release tissue adhesions, and effectively treat post-hemorrhage joint adhesions and restricted mobility during rehabilitation.

23.2.4 Rehabilitation Nursing

Rehabilitation nursing is an important part of post-brainstem hemorrhage recovery. Rehabilitation nurses are vital members of multidisciplinary treatment teams and need to undergo formal rehabilitation training. In addition to mastering basic nursing knowledge, rehabilitation nurses should also be proficient in basic rehabilitation nursing, including skin management for stroke patients, management and rehabilitation of bowel and bladder function, positioning and transferring of limbs into proper alignment, clinical assessment of swallowing disorders and swallowing rehabilitation guidance, nutrition management, training in feeding techniques, respiratory tract management, and basic respiratory function rehabilitation techniques. Effective rehabilitation nursing significantly improves functional recovery, reduces complications, and enhances activities of daily living for stroke patients.

23.3 Traditional Chinese Medicine Treatment for Postoperative Primary Brainstem Hemorrhage

In Traditional Chinese Medicine (TCM), brainstem hemorrhage is believed to be caused by imbalances in Yin and Yang, as well as the disorder of Qi and Xue, which results in the upward invasion of the brain. It is characterized by sudden onset and rapid progression and is a group of cerebrovascular diseases characterized by acute onset, focal or diffuse brain dysfunction. Brainstem hemorrhage corresponds to the category of hemorrhagic stroke, which can occur throughout the year, with a higher incidence in winter and spring, and a high mortality and disability rate. Once brainstem hemorrhage occurs, the condition is generally dangerous, and surgical treatment should be performed as early as possible for those who are eligible for surgery. TCM plays a significant role in the treatment of patients after brainstem hemorrhage surgery, functioning as either a supportive or leading therapy. After stabilizing the vital signs, patients should undergo TCM treatment to promote their recovery.

23.3.1 Etiology and Pathogenesis

Stroke occurs on the basis of Qi and Xue deficiency. It is caused by factors such as overexertion, emotional distress, and improper diet, which lead to imbalances in the Yin and Yang of the organs, disorder of Qi and Xue circulation, and direct invasion of the brain, resulting in cerebral artery obstruction or extravasation of blood outside the cerebral vessels. Clinically, the main symptoms include sudden collapse, hemiplegia, facial asymmetry, slurred speech or aphasia, and numbness on one side of the body. Other common manifestations include sudden dizziness, diplopia, unclear speech, inability to recognize objects or loved ones, unsteady gait, unilateral pain, or continuous tremors. The head is regarded as the residence of clear Yang and the convergence of all Yang energies, as well as the gathering place for the essence and blood of the five viscera and the clear Qi of the six fu-organs. If the body is weak due to old age, excessive fatigue, excessive emotional stress, improper diet, or excessive sexual activity, it can lead to imbalances in Yin and Yang, disorder of Qi and Xue circulation, stasis of cerebral vessels, and insufficient nourishment to the brain. Alternatively, deficiency of Yin in the lower body, excessive Yang in the liver, excessive transformation of Yang leading to wind movement, Xue counterflowing with Qi, accompanied by fire and phlegm, can obstruct the clear orifices, and in severe cases, result in extravasation of blood outside the vessels and the development of a stroke. The disease is closely related to the heart, liver, spleen, and kidneys.

1. Yin deficiency involves Yang, Yin and Yang weakness: The "Yellow Emperor's Inner Canon" states, "At the age of forty, Yin Qi is depleted, and one's daily activities decline." With old age and physical weakness, or long-term illness leads to Qi and Xue deficiency, while excessive fatigue further depletes Qi and Xue. The impaired Qi circulation hinders blood flow, causing stasis of cerebral vessels. Yin and Xue deficiency also results in the loss of Yin's control over Yang, leading to the excessive movement of wind and Yang, accompanied by turbid phlegm and stagnant blood obstructing the clear orifices, thus causing the disease.
2. Yin and Xue deficiency, internal liver wind: "Yang Qi is agitated by excessive fatigue." Excessive fatigue can cause the ascent and agitation of Yang Qi, which in turn induces internal wind. When Qi and fire are simultaneously elevated, Qi and blood, phlegm, and heat ascend to the brain, obstructing the clear orifices and leading to the onset of the disease.

3. Spleen dysfunction and production of phlegm: The "Yellow Emperor's Inner Canon" mentions "rich and noble individuals are prone to fatty and rich diseases." Overconsumption of fatty, sweet, and heavy foods impairs spleen function, leading to the accumulation of dampness and the production of phlegm. Phlegm and stasis can transform into heat, or excessive liver wood overacts on earth, resulting in spleen dysfunction and the generation of phlegm. Alternatively, liver fire can cause heat, refining fluids into phlegm. Phlegm and wind, carried by Yang, can spread through the meridians, resulting in the disease. This is what the "Danxi Heart Method" refers to as "dampness generating phlegm, phlegm generating heat, and heat generating wind."
4. Emotions causing harm: The "Suwen Xuanji Original Disease Patterns—Fire Category" states, "Many cases of sudden stroke are caused by excessive harm from the emotions of joy, anger, worry, sadness, and fear, which all result in excessive heat." Imbalances in the seven emotions, liver disharmony, stagnation of Qi circulation, and poor blood flow can occur. Alternatively, if the body is inherently deficient in Yin, water unable to contain Wood, and is further affected by emotional distress, liver Yang can suddenly become hyperactive. Excessive fire in the heart can lead to the exacerbation of wind and fire, counterflow of blood with Qi, and the invasion of the brain, ultimately resulting in a stroke.

23.3.2 Traditional Chinese Medicine Diagnosis and Differential Diagnosis

23.3.2.1 Key Points of Traditional Chinese Medicine Diagnosis

1. Sudden or rapid onset, progressive aggravation, or abrupt onset. The age of onset is often over 40 years, and there is often a history of smoking and alcohol consumption.
2. Often associated with factors such as overexertion and excessive alcohol intake. Prodromal symptoms may include dizziness, vertigo, headache, tinnitus, sudden transient speech impairment or limb numbness. Visual disturbances may occur, with multiple episodes within a day or recurring over several days.
3. Symptoms may include impaired consciousness, hemiplegia, facial and tongue deviation, incoherent or obstructed speech, or even aphasia. Additional manifestations can include limb numbness, choking or coughing while drinking water, and unsteady gait may also be present.
4. Typical global neurological symptoms or focal neurological signs.
5. Modern imaging examinations such as CT and MRI show corresponding abnormalities.

23.3.2.2 Key Points of Differential Diagnosis

1. Epilepsy: Presents with sudden loss of consciousness, but epilepsy is a paroxysmal disorder characterized by limb convulsions, foaming at the mouth, and peculiar sounds from the mouth. The patient regains normal consciousness afterward, without hemiplegia or aphasia. It is commonly seen in adolescents.
2. Syncope: Brief loss of consciousness, with no signs of hemiplegia, facial and tongue deviation, or aphasia upon awakening.
3. Tetanic spasm: Characterized by limb convulsions, stiffening of the neck and back, and opisthotonus. Although occasional loss of consciousness may occur, but there are no signs of hemiplegia.
4. Facial paralysis: Main symptoms include facial and eye deviation, drooling, and unclear speech. It is often caused by deficiency of vital Qi, invasion of wind pathogen, or stagnation of Qi and blood.

23.3.3 Traditional Chinese Medicine Syndrome Differentiation and Treatment

23.3.3.1 Key Points of Syndrome Differentiation

23.3.3.1.1 Differentiate Between the Involvement of Meridians and Collaterals and the Involvement of Zang-Fu Organs

Involvement of meridians and collaterals: Present in cases of stroke without impaired consciousness.

Involvement of zang-fu organs: Present in cases of stroke with impaired consciousness.

23.3.3.1.2 Differentiate Stages

Super-acute stage: Within 6 h of onset.

Acute stage: Within 2 weeks of onset. Impaired consciousness may persist for up to 4 weeks.

Recovery stage: From 2 weeks to 6 months after onset.

Sequelae stage: After 6 months of onset.

23.3.3.2 Principles of Treatment

Stroke is characterized by deficiency at the root and excess at the surface, with upper excess and lower deficiency. Although there is a deficiency at the root during the acute phase, the emphasis is on addressing the excess. Therefore, the principle is to treat the excess promptly, with expelling pathogenic factors as the main approach. Common treatment methods include soothing the liver and extinguishing wind, clearing and transforming phlegm-heat, promoting blood circulation and unblocking meridians, and awakening the mind and opening the orifices. For severe brainstem hemorrhage, treatment during the acute phase, especially after surgery, should primarily focus on addressing the acute phase management. During the recovery and sequelae stages, where deficiency and excess are often mixed and pathogenic factors remain partially unresolved while deficiency emerges, treatment should aim to nourish the body and expel pathogenic factors, supplemented by acupuncture, massage, and other rehabilitation therapies.

23.3.3.2.1 Traditional Chinese Medicine Syndrome Differentiation and Treatment for Severe Brainstem Hemorrhage

Acute Phase (Early Postoperative Period of Brainstem Hemorrhage).

Wind-phlegm-blood stasis obstructing meridians and collaterals.

Symptoms: Hemiplegia, deviation of the mouth and tongue, difficulty in speech or aphasia, limb numbness, dizziness, dark tongue with thin white or greasy coating, and wiry and slippery pulse.

Treatment principle: Extinguish wind and clear phlegm, promote blood circulation, and unblock meridians.

Prescription: The Decoction of Pinellia, White Atractylodes, and Gastrodia with modifications.

Composition: 12 g of Rhizoma Pinellinae Praeparata, 15 g of Poria cocos, 12 g of White Atractylodes, 9 g of Bile Arisaema, 12 g of Tabasheer, 12 g of Gastrodia elata, 12 g of Cyperus rotundus, 15 g of Salvia miltiorrhiza, 6 g of Rhubarb (to be decocted later). Take one dose daily, decocted in water.

Prescription explanation: The combination of Pinellia and White Atractylodes in this formula aims to dry dampness, transform phlegm, and alleviate nausea. Gastrodia, which enters the Liver meridian, excels at calming the Liver and extinguishing wind to alleviate dizziness. The synergy between these two ingredients achieves the effect of transforming phlegm and extinguishing wind. Poria and White Atractylodes strengthen the spleen and dry dampness, targeting the underlying cause of excessive phlegm production. When combined with Pinellia and Gastrodia, theses herbs enhance the formula's ability to transform phlegm and extinguish wind. Bile Arisaema and Tabasheer clear heat, resolve phlegm, and open the orifices. Cyperus and Salvia promote qi circulation, activate blood, and open the collaterals. Rhubarb stimulates bowel movements and revitalizes the spirit. The collective use of these herbs achieves the effects of extinguishing wind, purging phlegm, promoting blood circulation, and opening the collaterals.

Modifications: For cases with severe blood stasis and a tongue that appears dark purple or exhibits ecchymosis, add 10 g of Peach Kernel, 10 g of Safflower, and 15 g of Red Peony Root to promote blood circulation and dispel stasis. For individuals with a yellow and greasy tongue coating, restlessness, and signs of heat, add 15 g of *Scutellaria baicalensis* and 10 g of Gardenia Fruit to clear heat and drain fire. For those experiencing dizziness and headaches, add 15 g of Chrysanthemum Flower and 9 g of Prunella Spike to soothe the liver and calm wind. Due to the tendency for wind-phlegm intermingling and blood stasis obstruction, which can easily transform into heat over time, it is advisable to avoid excessive warm and drying herbs in the prescription to prevent exacerbating heat and fire.

Excessive liver yang and disturbance of wind and fire:

Symptoms: Hemiplegia, numbness on one side of the body, strong speech with obstruction or aphasia, dizziness, headache, red face, red eyes, bitter taste in the mouth, dry throat, irritability, easy anger, red urine, and dry stools. The tongue may appear red or crimson with a thin yellow coating, and the pulse is typically wiry and strong.

Treatment principle: Soothe the liver, clear heat, and open the collaterals.

Prescription: Gastrodia Rhizome, Uncaria Stem with Hooks with modifications.

Composition: 15 g of Gastrodia Rhizome, 15 g of Uncaria Stem with Hooks, 30 g of raw abalone shell (pre-decocted), 18 g of Achyranthes Root, 12 g of *Scutellaria baicalensis*, 12 g of Gardenia Fruit, 12 g of Prunella Spike, 15 g of Motherwort Herb, 15 g of Seaweed, 6 g of Scorpion (processed). Prepare one dose daily by decocting the herbs in water and consuming orally.

Prescription explanation: Gastrodia Rhizome and Uncaria Stem with Hooks soothe the liver and calm wind. Raw abalone shell suppresses liver yang. Achyranthes Root promotes blood circulation downward. *Scutellaria baicalensis*, Gardenia Fruit, and Prunella Spike clear liver fire. Motherwort Herb activates blood circulation and promotes diuresis. Seaweed resolves phlegm and promotes diuresis. Scorpion suppresses wind and stops spasms. The collective use of these herbs achieves the effects of soothing the liver, draining fire, and promoting meridian circulation.

Modification: For individuals experiencing dizziness and headaches, add 15 g of Chrysanthemum Flower and 15 g of Mulberry Leaf to clear and benefit the head region. For those with restlessness and irritability, add 15 g of Tree Peony Bark and 15 g of White Paeony Root to enhance the clearing and purging of liver fire. For dry stools and constipation, add 9 g of Raw Rhubarb (to be decocted later) to clear heat and promote bowel movement. Symptoms include confusion, mental haze, or clouded consciousness, indicating that the disturbance of wind and fire is affecting the clarity of the mind, with the transformation from the meridians to the organs. In such cases, pills like Niuhuang Qingxin Pill or Angong Niuhuang Pill can be administered to open the orifices and revive the spirit. If wind and fire pathogen obstruct the upward flow of blood, cooling and blood-descending herbs should be added to guide the blood downward.

Excessive phlegm heat, disturbance caused by wind-phlegm.

Symptoms: Hemiplegia, deviation of the mouth and tongue, slurred speech or aphasia, numbness on one side of the body, dry stools and constipation, dizziness, blurred vision, cough with phlegm or excessive phlegm. The tongue appears dark red, with a yellow or greasy coating, and the pulse feels wiry and slippery or the pulse on the affected side is wiry and slippery.

Treatment principle: Clear heat, resolve phlegm, and promote bowel movement to alleviate heat.

Prescription: Xing Wei Cheng Qi Decotion with modifications.

Composition: 10–15 g of Rhubarb (to be decocted later), 10 g of Natrii Sulfas (divided and added separately), 15–30 g of Trichosanthes Fruit, 6–10 g of Bile Arisaematis. Prepare one dose daily by decocting the herbs in water and consuming orally.

Prescription explanation: Trichosanthes Fruit and Rhizoma Arisaematis clear heat and transform phlegm. Rhubarb and Natrii Sulfas purge the bowel and stomach, promoting bowel movement and purging heat.

Modification: For individuals with prominent heat signs, add 10 g of Gardenia Fruit and 8 g of *Scutellaria baicalensis* to clear heat and purge fire. For elderly individuals with weak constitution and deficient body fluids, 15 g of Rehmannia Root, 10 g of Ophiopogon Tuber, and 10 g of Scrophularia Root should be added to nourish body fluids.

23.3.3.2.1.1 Phlegm-Fire Obstructing the Orifices

Symptoms: Sudden onset with profound confusion or unconsciousness, hemiplegia, snoring and phlegm rattling in the nose, strong spasms in the neck and back, limb rigidity, bodily heat, restlessness, and in severe cases, coldness in the extremities, frequent convulsions, and occasional hematemesis. The tongue appears red and crimson, the coating is yellow and greasy or dry and greasy, and the pulse is wiry, slippery, and rapid. This pattern belongs to the closure of Yang in the context of closure patterns.

Treatment principle: Clearing heat, transforming phlegm, awakening the mind, and opening the orifices.

Prescription: Modified Antelope Horn Decoction, combined with Angong Niuhuang Pills for treatment.

Composition: 30 g of Antelope Horn (pre-decocted), 30 g of Nacre (pre-decocted), 12 g of Bamboo Shavings, 15 g of Tabasheer, 9 g of Acorus Tatarinowii, 6 g of Polygala Root, 12 g of Prunella Spike, 15 g of Tree Peony Bark. Prepare one dose daily by decocting the herbs in water and consuming orally.

Explanation: Antelope Horn is the principal herb in the prescription, combined with Prunella Spike to clear the liver and calm wind. Nacre nourishes yin and suppresses yang. Bamboo Shavings, Tabasheer, Acorus Tatarinowii, and Polygala Root clear heat, resolve phlegm, and open the orifices. Tree Peony Bark clears heat and cools the blood. Angong Niuhuang Pill has the function of opening the orifices and awakening the brain. The combined use of these herbs achieves the effects of clearing heat, calming wind, nourishing yin, suppressing yang, and awakening the spirit.

Modification: For individuals with excessive phlegm, add 50 mL of Bamboo Juice and 15 g of Bile Arisaematis to clear heat and eliminate phlegm. For severe heat, add 10 g of *Scutellaria baicalensis* and 10 g of Gardenia Fruit to strengthen the heat-clearing effect. For heavy mental confusion, add 10 g of Radix Curcumaeto awaken the spirit and open the orifices.

23.3.3.2.1.2 Phlegm-Dampness Obstructing the Orifices

Symptoms: Underlying Yang deficiency, internal accumulation of phlegm-dampness, sudden onset of unconsciousness, hemiplegia, flaccidity of the limbs, limb paralysis with coldness, pale face and dark lips, and abundant phlegm and saliva. The tongue appears dull, the coating is white and greasy, and the pulse is deep, slippery, or slow. This pattern belongs to the closure of Yin in the context of closure patterns.

Treatment principle: Warming Yang, transforming phlegm, awakening the mind, and opening the orifices.

Prescription: Modified Ditan Decoction, combined with Suhe Xiang Pills for treatment.

Composition: 12 g of Rhizoma Pinellinae Praeparata, 9 g of tangerine peel, 15 g of Poria cocos, 12 g of rhizoma arisaematis, 12 g of bamboo shavings, 9 g of Acorus Tatarinowii. Prepare one dose per day, decocted in water and taken orally.

Explanation: In the prescription, pinellia, tangerine peel, poria, and bamboo shavings transform phlegm and dry dampness; bile arisaematis and acorus tatarinowii open the orifices and resolve phlegm; licorice strengthens the spleen, boosts Qi, and eliminates the source of phlegm production. Suhe Xiang Pills have the function of dispersing stagnation, opening the orifices, and relieving depression with their pungent and aromatic properties. The combination of these herbs serves to dry dampness, transform phlegm, awaken the mind, and open the orifices.

Modification: If there are prominent cold signs, add 9 g of cinnamon twig to warm Yang and transform fluids; if there are wind-related symptoms as well, add 10 g of gastrodia and 30 g of uncaria stem with hooks to soothe the liver and suppress wind.

23.3.3.2.1.3 Decline of the Ethereal Soul

Symptoms: Sudden collapse, loss of consciousness, profuse sweating, mouth agape, flaccidity of the limbs, hands dropping and limbs cold, excessive sweating, and involuntary urination and defecation. The tongue appears pale purple or withered, the coating is white and greasy, and the pulse is weak or barely perceptible.

Treatment principle: Supplement Qi, restore Yang, support the upright Qi, and stabilize leakage.

Prescription: Immediately use a large dose of Shenfu Decoction combined with Shengmai San.

Composition: 15 g of Ginseng (decoct separately and combine for consumption), 9 g of aconite (pre-decoct for half an hour), 15 g of schisandra.

Explanation: Ginseng greatly supplements the original Qi, aconite restores Yang and rescues collapse, and schisandra consolidates and stabilizes the leakage.

Modification: If there is excessive sweating, add astragalus, dragon bone, oyster shell, and dogwood fruit to stop sweating and stabilize leakage.

23.3.3.2.2 Traditional Chinese Medicine Injections

Qingkailing Injection: Add 40–60 mL to 500 mL of 5%–10% glucose for intravenous drip, administered 1–2 times daily. Indicated for hyperactivity of liver Yang and phlegm-heat obstructing the organs.

Xingnaojing Injection: Add 10–20 mL to 250–500 mL of 5% glucose for intravenous drip, administered 1–2 times daily. Indicated for hyperactivity of liver yang and phlegm-heat obstructing the organs, or zang-fu organs excessive pattern.

Xuesaitong Injection: Add 200–400 mg to 40–60 mL of 25%–50% glucose for intravenous injection, or add 250–500 mL of 5%–10% glucose for intravenous drip, administered once daily. Indicated for various patterns of disorders.

Salvia miltiorrhiza Injection or Compound Salvia miltiorrhiza Injection: Add 20–40 mL to 250 mL of 5%–10% glucose for intravenous drip, administered 1–2 times daily. Indicated for various patterns of disorders.

Xueshuan Tong Injection: Add 4–6 mL to 250–500 mL of 5%–10% glucose for intravenous drip, administered 1–2 times daily. Suitable for various patterns of disorders.

Shenmai Injection: Add 20–40 mL of 50% glucose for intravenous injection, or add 40–60 mL to 250 mL of 10% glucose for intravenous drip, administered 2 times daily. Indicated for stroke-induced collapse syndrome or critical conditions of sudden collapse and simultaneous injury to qi and yin.

Shenfu Injection: Add 5–20 mL to 40 mL of 50% glucose for intravenous injection, or add 20–100 mL to 500 mL of 5%–10% glucose for intravenous drip, administered 1–2 times daily. Indicated for collapse syndrome or critical conditions of sudden collapse and excessive yang escaping.

23.3.3.2.3 Acupuncture Therapy

23.3.3.2.3.1 Meridians and Collaterals

Treatment Method: Promote circulation and unblock the meridians.

Acupoints: Upper limbs: Jianyu, Quchi, Shousanli, Waiguan, Hegu.

Lower limbs: Huantiao, Yanglingquan, Zusanli, Xie Xi, Kunlun.

Additional Points according to the Syndrome: For tendon spasm, combine with Quze at the elbow, Daling at the wrist, Ququan at the knee, Taixi at the ankle. For difficulty swallowing, stimulate Jinjin and Yuye as well as both sides of the tongue. For speech impediment, use Yamen, Lianquan, and Tongli. For deviation of the mouth and tongue, use Dicang, Jiache, and Hegu. For numbness in the limbs, use superficial needling technique. For limb edema, perform bloodletting at the Shixuan points. Additionally, select acupoints based on the specific syndrome: for liver and kidney yin deficiency, use Taixi and Sanyinjiao; for excessive liver yang, use Taichong and Hangjian; for phlegm-heat, use Fenglong and Neiting.

23.3.3.2.3.2 Zang-Fu Organs

Treatment Method: Clear the mind and open the orifices.

Main Acupoints: Neiguan, Renzhong, Sanyinjiao.

Additional Acupoints: Jiquan, Weizhong, Chize.

Additional Points according to the Syndrome: For swallowing difficulties, add Fengchi, Yifeng, and Wangu; for clenched fingers, add Hegu; for speech impediment, add Shanglianquan and combine with bloodletting at Jinjin and Yuye; for strephenopodia, add Qiuxu and towards Zhaohai.

Technique: Bilateral Neiguan: first, insert the needle vertically 1.67–3.33 cm, using a combination of twisting, lifting, inserting, and purging techniques for 1 min; then, insert the needle obliquely 1–1.67 cm towards the nasal septum using a pecking technique until the eyes become moist or tears flow. Next, insert the needle at Sanyinjiao at a 45°along the inner edge of the tibia and the skin, penetrating 3.33–5 cm, using a combination of lifting and inserting techniques, with three contractions of the affected lower limb as the criterion. For Jiquan, move the original point 3.33 cm downward along the meridian, avoiding the axillary hair, and insert the needle vertically 3.33–5 cm, using a combination of lifting, inserting, and purging techniques, with three contractions of the affected upper limb as the criterion. For Chize, with the elbow flexed at 120°, insert the needle vertically 3.33 cm. Employ a combination of lifting, inserting, and purging techniques, using three contractions of the patient's forearm and fingers as the criterion. For Weizhong, position the patient supine with the legs raised. Insert the needle vertically at 1.67–3.33 cm, using a combination of lifting, inserting, and purging techniques, with three contractions of the affected lower limb as the criterion. For Fengchi, Wangu, and Yifeng, insert the needle towards the throat, penetrating 6.66–8.33 cm. Employ a small amplitude and high-frequency twisting technique for 1 min per acupoint. For Hegu, insert the needle towards the Sanjian points, penetrating 3.33–5 cm, using a combination of lifting, inserting, and purging techniques, with the second finger of the patient contracting or the fingers naturally extending as the criterion. For Shanglianquan, insert the needle towards the root of the tongue, 5–6.66 cm, using a combination of lifting, inserting, and purging techniques. For Jinjin and Yuye, use a three-edged needle to puncture and perform bloodletting, with a bleeding volume of 1–2 mL. For Qiuxu, penetrate towards the Zhaohai point, approximately 5–6.66 cm, until a local sensation of distension is achieved..

23.3.3.2.4 Tuina Massage

Based on the principles of warming the meridians, promoting qi circulation, and activating blood flow, acupoints are selected according to conventional acupuncture techniques. Common Tuina techniques include pushing, pressing, kneading, rubbing, stroking, tapping, and patting. Acupoints that can be targeted include Fengchi, Jianjing, Jianyu, Tianjing, Shousanli, Huantiao, Weizhong, and Chengshan. The areas of focus are the face, back, and limbs, with an emphasis on the affected side. It is advisable to avoid using stretching, twisting, and shaking techniques on joints, especially the shoulder and wrist joints, to prevent ligament and muscle injuries, and even joint dislocation.

Tuina treatment can be classified as follows:

23.3.3.2.4.1 Meridian Therapy

Basic techniques: Massage on Jianjing, acupressure on Fengchi, Fengfu, Jianzhen, and Tianzong, acupressure on Zusanli, Piguan, and Liangqiu.

Pattern identification and modification: For deficiency in the meridians and invasion of wind-cold, add kneading and lifting techniques on the three yang meridians of the hand, lifting and pressing techniques on the three yang meridians of the foot, and acupressure on Quchi, Hegu, Huantiao, Weizhong, and Chengshan. For liver and kidney yin deficiency with upward disturbance of wind and yang, add rubbing and pinching techniques on the spine, pushing and lifting techniques on Yintang, and acupressure on Ganshu, Shenshu, Yunmen, Chengfu, and Fenglong.

23.3.3.2.4.2 Zang-Fu Organs Therapy

Basic techniques: Acupressure on Renzhong and Shixuan, kneading on the three yin meridians of the hand.

Pattern identification and modification: For closure syndrome, add kneading on the three yang meridians of the hand, lifting and pressing techniques on the three yin meridians of the hand, and apply acupressure to Laogong, Taichong, Fenglong, and Yongquan points. For prolapse syndrome, add lifting and pressing techniques on the three yang meridians of the foot, tonify and purge Shenque, and apply acupressure to Neiguan and Zusanli points.

If the patient also presents with a sallow complexion, shortness of breath, a low voice, reduced appetite, a pale tongue, and a thin and rough pulse, it indicates qi deficiency and blood stasis. The treatment should focus on tonifying qi, nourishing blood, and promoting meridian circulation. Massage and acupressure should mainly target the Ren meridian and the points of the Spleen meridian of the foot Taiyin, supplemented by points on the affected limbs to promote the circulation of qi and blood in the affected limbs. If the patient also experiences stiffness and spasticity in the limbs, redness and heat in the face and ears, dryness and bitterness in the mouth, red tongue with yellow coating, and wiry and forceful pulse, it indicates liver yang hyperactivity. The treatment should focus on calming the liver, suppressing yang, relieving wind, and promoting meridian circulation. Massage and acupressure should mainly target the Liver meridian of the foot Jueyin, supplemented by points on the affected limbs, with emphasis on the wrist joints and fingers. Thumb manipulation can be used to improve flexion and extension functions. If the patient exhibits symptoms such as dullness and fullness in the epigastrium, phlegm rales in the throat, drooling at the corners of the mouth, purple and dusky tongue, white and greasy coating, and wiry and slippery pulse, it indicates phlegm obstruction and blood stasis in the meridians. The treatment should focus on eliminating dampness, transforming phlegm, promoting blood circulation, and unblocking the meridians. Massage and acupressure should mainly target the Stomach meridian of the foot Yangming and the Spleen meridian of the foot Taiyin.

23.3.3.3 Recovery and Sequelae Stage

23.3.3.3.1 Herbal Decoctions

23.3.3.3.1.1 Qi Deficiency and Blood Stasis

Symptoms: Hemiplegia, deviation of the mouth and tongue, slurred speech or aphasia, numbness on one side of the body, pale complexion, shortness of breath, fatigue, drooling, spontaneous sweating, palpitations, loose stools, and edema in the hands and feet. The tongue is pale and the coating is thin white or greasy, and the pulse is deep, thin and slow, or wiry and thin.

Treatment principle: Tonify qi, activate blood circulation, support the righteous qi, and dispel pathogenic factors.

Prescription: Buyang Huanwu Decotion with modifications.

Composition: 60 g of Astragalus, 12 g of Angelica tail, 12 g of Chuanqiong, 9 g of Peach kernel, 12 g of Earthworm, 12 g of Red peony, 9 g of Safflower, 9 g of Acorus tatarinowii. Prepare one dose per day, decocted in water and taken orally.

Explanation of the prescription: Astragalus in the prescription focuses on tonifying qi; Angelica, Chuanqiong, Peach kernel, Earthworm, Red peony, and Safflower nourish and activate blood circulation, and dispel stasis; Acorus tatarinowii transforms phlegm and opens the orifices.

Modifications: Astragalus can be used in large amounts, beginning with a small dosage and gradually increasing it to 120 g to avoid excessive warming. If required, add cooling and moistening herbs such as Anemarrhena asphodeloides and Trichosanthin. If phlegm symptoms are prominent, add 15 g of dried tangerine peel and 15 g of Rhizoma Pinellinae Praeparata to dry dampness and transform phlegm.

23.3.3.3.1.2 Yin Deficiency and Wind Stirring

Symptoms include hemiplegia, slurred speech and deviated mouth and tongue, strong tongue with difficulty speaking or silence, numbness on one side of the body, insomnia, and heat in the palms and soles. The tongue is red or dark red with little to no coating, and the pulse is thin and wiry or thin and rapid.

Treatment strategy: Nourish yin and subdue yang, activate blood circulation and unblock meridians.

Prescription: Hu Qian Pills.

Composition: 18 g of Rehmannia, 13 g of Tortoise Shell, 9 g of Phellodendron, 9 g of Anemarrhena, 12 g of White Peony Root, 12 g of Cynomorium, 12 g of Tangerine Peel, 9 g of Dendrobium, 12 g of Achyranthes Root, 12 g of Angelica, 12 g of Raw Dragon Bone and Oyster Shell, 9 g of Peach Kernel, 9 g of Safflower. Take one prescription daily, decocted in water.

Explanation: In the prescription, Rehmannia, Tortoise Shell, Phellodendron, Anemarrhena, and Dendrobium nourish the yin of the liver and kidneys and clear the deficient fire, achieving the effect of nourishing yin and subduing yang; White Peony Root, Cynomorium, Tangerine Peel, Raw Dragon Bone, and Oyster Shell nourish the blood and liver; Achyranthes Root guides the blood downward; Angelica nourishes the blood and promotes its circulation; Peach Kernel and Safflower activate blood circulation and remove blood stasis, unblocking the meridians. The whole prescription works together to nourish yin and subdue yang, activate blood circulation, and unblock meridians.

Modifications: For those with phlegm-heat, add 10 g of Tabasheer, Bamboo Juice 50 mL, and 6 g of Fritillaria to clear the phlegm-heat; for obvious deficiency heat, remove Angelica and add 30 g of Wolfberry Bark, 15 g of Sweet Wormwood, and 15 g of Bletilla to clear the deficiency heat.

23.3.3.3.1.3 Wind-Phlegm Obstructing the Orifices

Symptoms include a stiff tongue with difficulty speaking, numb limbs, or deviated mouth and tongue, a dark tongue with greasy coating, and a slippery and wiry pulse.

Treatment strategy: Calm the wind, dissolve phlegm, activate blood circulation, and unblock meridians.

Prescription: Jieyu Dan.

Composition: 9 g of Typhonium, 9 g of Acorus Tatarinowii, 6 g of Polygala Root, 12 g of Gastrodia, 6 g of Scorpion, 6 g of Auklandia, 6 g of Licorice, 15 g of Salvia miltiorrhiza, 12 g of Angelica, 9 g of Red Peony, 10 g of Earthworm. Take one prescription daily, decocted in water.

Explanation: In the prescription, Typhonium expels wind and dissolves phlegm to unblock the meridians; Acorus, Polygala, and Auklandia open the orifices, move qi, and unblock the meridians; Gastrodia, Scorpion, and Earthworm calm the liver and extinguish wind; Salvia, Angelica, and Red Peony activate blood circulation and remove stasis; Licorice harmonizes the other ingredients.

Modifications: For those with blood stasis, with purple or dark tongue and ecchymosis, add 10 g of Peach Kernel and 6 g of Safflower to activate blood circulation and remove blood stasis; for symptoms of yellow greasy tongue coating, restlessness, and heat signs, add 9 g of Scutellaria and 9 g of Gardenia to clear heat and purge fire; for dizziness and headache, add 9 g of Chrysanthemum and 15 g of Prunella to calm the liver and extinguish wind.

23.3.3.3.2 External Application of Traditional Chinese Medicine (TCM)

External application of traditional Chinese medicine (TCM) is commonly used in clinical practice, including methods such as herbal fumigation and washing, herbal steam therapy, herbal hot compress therapy, herbal acupoint plaster therapy, and ear acupressure with seeds. These methods promote blood and lymphatic circulation, improve local tissue nutrition, alleviate spasms, and aim to regulate organ functions, activate blood circulation, warm the body, promote smooth airflow, relieve pain, and reduce swelling. They also facilitate the recovery of limb functions. TCM external therapies offer several advantages including ease of operation, low cost, rapid efficacy, and safety without pain. The specific TCM external therapy is selected based on the patient's individual condition and functional impairments.

23.3.3.3.3 Acupuncture Therapy

Body Acupuncture: The conventional acupuncture method focuses on the main acupoints such as Neiguan, Jiquan, Chize, Weizhong, Sanyinjiao, and Zusanli. Depending on the syndrome differentiation, corresponding additional acupoints are used. For upper limb paralysis, additional acupoints may include Jianyu, Quchi, Shousanli, and Hegu. For lower limb paralysis, additional acupoints may include Huantiao, Yanglingquan, Yinlingquan, and Fengshi. For varus pedis, additional acupoints may include Juegu, Jiuneifan, and Qiuxu towards Zhaohai. For valgus pedis, additional acupoints may include Zhongfeng, Taixi, and Jiuwaifan. For foot drop, additional acupoints may include Jie Xi and Jingshang.

23.3.3.3.3.1 Staged Acupuncture

1. For flaccid paralysis, the treatment aims to quickly increase muscle tone and promote muscle strength recovery to help patients overcome the flaccid state. The main acupoints for upper limbs are selected from the Hand Yangming meridian, while the main acupoints for lower limbs are selected from the Foot Yangming meridian. For the lower leg, the main acupoints may include Foot Taiyang, Foot Shaoyang meridians. The main acupoints used are often Jianyu, Quchi, Shousanli, Waiguan, Hegu, Huan Tiao, Yanglingquan, Zusanli, Jie Xi, and Kunlun.
2. For spastic paralysis, the basic principle is to select acupoints that target the antagonistic muscles. For upper limbs, acupoints such as Jianyu, Jianzhong, Shousanli, Waiguan, and Hegu are selected. For lower limbs, acupoints such as Yinlingquan, Lougu, and Sanyinjiao are selected. The treatment can be adjusted based on the conventional acupuncture method by adding or reducing corresponding acupoints according to the specific symptoms.

23.3.3.3.3.2 Electroacupuncture

Acupoints selection: Jianyu, Quchi, Waiguan, Hegu, Huan Tiao, Fengshi, Yanglingquan, and Xuanzhong.

Procedure: Depending on the paralyzed area, 2–3 pairs of acupoints are selected each time. After needle insertion, the lifting and inserting technique is applied to spread the sensation to distant areas. Then, electrical stimulation is gradually introduced, with a duration of 30 s. After a short pause, the electrical stimulation is continued for another 30 s. This process can be repeated 3–4 times, inducing sensations such as soreness, numbness, or warmth in the relevant muscle groups with rhythmic contraction. It can effectively promote the recovery of limb function in post-stroke sequelae.

Head Acupuncture: For the treatment of stroke-induced hemiplegia, acupoints on the contralateral motor area, sensory area, and foot motor-sensory area are selected. After insertion, the needles are rotated for 3 min. For hemiplegia with motor impairment, the acupoints on the contralateral motor area are selected. For lower limb paralysis, the upper 1/5 of the contralateral motor area and the foot motor area on the contralateral side are selected. For lower limb paralysis, the middle 2/5 of the contralateral sensory area is selected. For facial paralysis, drooling, deviation of the mouth and tongue, and motor aphasia, the lower 2/5 of the contralateral motor area is selected. For sensory impairment on one side of the body, the contralateral sensory area is selected. For sensory impairment in the lower limbs, the upper 1/5 of the contralateral sensory area and the contralateral foot sensory area are selected. For sensory impairment in the upper limbs, the middle 2/5 of the contralateral sensory area is selected. For sensory impairment in the head and face, the lower 2/5 of the contralateral sensory area is selected. For aphasia, the lower 2/5 of the contralateral paralyzed side's motor area is chosen. For mental disorders, excessive crying or laughing, the needles are inserted along the midline above the chest cavity and horizontally. For limb edema, the acupoints on the contralateral vasodilation area are selected.

Eye Acupuncture: For the treatment of stroke-induced hemiplegia, acupoints in the upper and lower focal areas are selected to gradually restore autonomous movement in the affected limbs.

Moxibustion Therapy: Moxibustion has the effects of warming meridians, dispelling cold, resolving stasis, and strengthening yang. It is generally suitable for conditions with cold syndrome or yang deficiency syndrome.

For patients recovering after brainstem hemorrhage surgery, specific acupoints are selected according to the patient's condition, referencing the book "Acupuncture" edited by Academician Shi Xuemin. Techniques such as direct moxibustion, indirect moxibustion, moxibustion with a barrier, and heat-sensitive moxibustion methods are used to promote functional recovery or alleviate discomfort symptoms in patients after brainstem hemorrhage surgery.

Massage Therapy: Different techniques are used for different muscle groups to regulate the muscle and nerve functions of the affected limbs, induce the establishment of normal movement patterns, and facilitate voluntary and coordinated movements, thereby promoting overall functional recovery. The main massage techniques include kneading, grasping, pushing, and passive flexion and extension of various joints in the upper and lower limbs. Common massage techniques include kneading and rubbing, acupoint stimulation, One-Finger Zen Pushing Method, joint flexion and extension rocking technique, tapping, friction, and percussion.

24 Diagnosis and Treatment of Consciousness Impairment in Primary Brainstem Hemorrhage and Awakening Therapy

Shizhong Zhang, Hongbo Zhang, Mengqi Gao, and Baoyan Wang

24.1 Epidemiology

With advancements in clinical medicine, many patients with brainstem hemorrhage are now able to survive with effective treatment. However, a portion of these survivors develop chronic consciousness disorders. Statistics indicate that over 100,000 new cases of consciousness disorders are reported annually in China. The recovery process for these patients is typically lengthy and poses a heavy burden on both society and families. The transition from consciousness disorder to wakefulness occurs in several stages: coma, vegetative state, minimally conscious state, emergence from minimally conscious state, cognitive-motor dissociation, locked-in syndrome, severe disability, and in some cases, complete recovery. The prognosis for these patients varies, with some may eventually regain consciousness, while others may remain in a vegetative state. Since patients with consciousness disorders cannot communicate, healthcare professionals face difficulties in accurately assessing the degree of recovery. A retrospective analysis conducted by the "Vegetative State Treatment Center" in London found that at least 42% of patients diagnosed as being in vegetative state were misjudged by healthcare professionals and were able to regain consciousness independently. Among the 25% of patients truly in a vegetative state, one-third of them were able to regain consciousness with appropriate treatment. Recent advancements in understanding the brain's physiological mechanisms have led to the development of new methods for evaluating consciousness disorders caused by brainstem hemorrhage. Additionally, various techniques are now being explored and applied to promote patient awakening, offering hope for better recovery outcomes [1, 2].

Supplementary Information The online version contains supplementary material available at https://doi.org/10.1007/978-981-95-8942-5_24.

S. Zhang (✉) · B. Wang
Department of Neurosurgery, The Zhujiang Hospital of Southern Medical College, Guangzhou, China

H. Zhang
Department of Neurosurgery, The Second Affiliated Hospital of Nanchang University, Nanchang, China

M. Gao
Department of Neurosurgery, The Second Affiliated Hospital of Guangzhou University, Guangzhou, China

24.2 Assessment Methods

24.2.1 Scale Assessment

The most commonly used scales for assessing consciousness disorders include the Coma Recovery Scale-Revised (CRS-R), the Glasgow Coma Scale (GCS), and the Glasgow Outcome Scale (GOS). The CRS-R evaluates the level of consciousness in patients from six domains: auditory, visual, motor, verbal, communication, and arousal levels [3]. Based on the results of the scale assessment, it is possible to determine whether the patient is in a vegetative state, a minimally conscious state, or undergoing consciousness recovery (Table 24.1) [4].

24.2.2 Electroencephalogram (EEG)

EEG, as one of the earliest tools used for studying neuroscience, continues to hold a critical role in clinical practice, particularly in assessing patients with impaired consciousness [5]. By observing the patient's EEG waves, rhythms, and responses to external stimuli, clinicians can evaluate the electrophysiological activity of the brain and determine the degree of abnormal brain function. Literature suggests that the presence of sleep rhythms in the EEG, such as sleep spindles or changes in EEG rhythms, indicates a better prognosis for comatose patients. Conversely, patients who show sudden suppression of brain waves or continuous epileptic discharges

G. Chen, C. You (eds.), *Surgical Treatment of Primary Brainstem Hemorrhage*, https://doi.org/10.1007/978-981-95-8942-5_24

Table 24.1 CRS-R Scale

Score	Auditory	Visual	Motor	Verbal	Communication	Arousal Level
6	-	-	Use of objects	-	-	-
5	-	Object recognition	Purposeful reflexive movement	-	-	-
4	Following commands	Partial object recognition	Manipulation of objects	-	-	-
3	Following partial commands	Visual tracking	Localization to pain	Understandable language	-	Understandable language
2	Sound localization	Object localization	Withdrawal to pain	Vocalization	Functional (accurate)	Eye-opening
1	Startle response	Startle response	Abnormal posturing	Stereotypical vocalization	Non-functional (intentional)	Stimulus-induced eye-opening
0	None	None	None	None	None	None

Vegetative state Minimally conscious state Consciousness recovery

Table 24.2 Hockaday's prognostic grading for stroke patients

Evaluation	Grade	EEG presentation
Normal	I	Dominance of α activity with some θ activity
Mildly abnormal	II	Dominance of θ activity with some δ activity
Moderately abnormal	III	Dominance of δ activity
Severely abnormal	IV	δ activity with transient electrical silence
Extremely abnormal	V	Flat waveform

Table 24.3 Synek's prognostic grading for patients with impaired consciousness

Evaluation	Grade	EEG presentation
Favorable	I	Dominance of α activity with some θ activity
Good	II	Dominance of t θ activity with reactivity
	III	Sleep spindle pattern
	III	Frontal δ rhythm
Uncertain	II	Dominance of δ activity without reactivity
	III	Scattered δ activity (with or without reactivity)
	III	Scattered δ activity with epileptic discharges
	IV	α coma with reactivity
Malignant	III	Low-amplitude δ activity
	IV	Explosive inhibition
	IV	Explosive inhibition with epileptic discharges
	IV	α coma without reactivity
	IV	θ coma
Fatal	IV	Flat waveform ($<20\ \mu V$ δ activity)
	V	Electrical silence

often have a poor prognosis. Hockaday conducted studies on the EEGs of 39 patients with acute ischemic hypoxic brain disease. He tracked their prognosis and classified it into five levels based on background EEG frequencies (Table 24.2). Similarly, Synek, based on his clinical experience, provided a more detailed grading system to assess the prognosis for patients with impaired consciousness (Table 24.3).

In addition, the use of video EEG during EEG examinations provides valuable insights into the patient's responsiveness to external stimuli. This combined approach allows clinicians to observe changes in the EEG background that occur when the patient is exposed to specific stimuli, such as painful or auditory triggers (e.g., calling the patient's name). If the EEG background shows noticeable changes in response to such stimuli and can be repeatedly verified, it typically indicates a more favorable prognosis.

24.2.3 Evoked Potentials

Visual Evoked Potentials (VEP), Auditory Brainstem Responses (ABR), and Somatosensory Evoked Potentials (SEP) (Fig. 24.1) are electrophysiological tests that provide valuable information, although they have limited direct value in assessing consciousness levels [6]. These tests primarily help determine whether there is any impairment in peripheral neuronal function or disruptions in central conduction path-

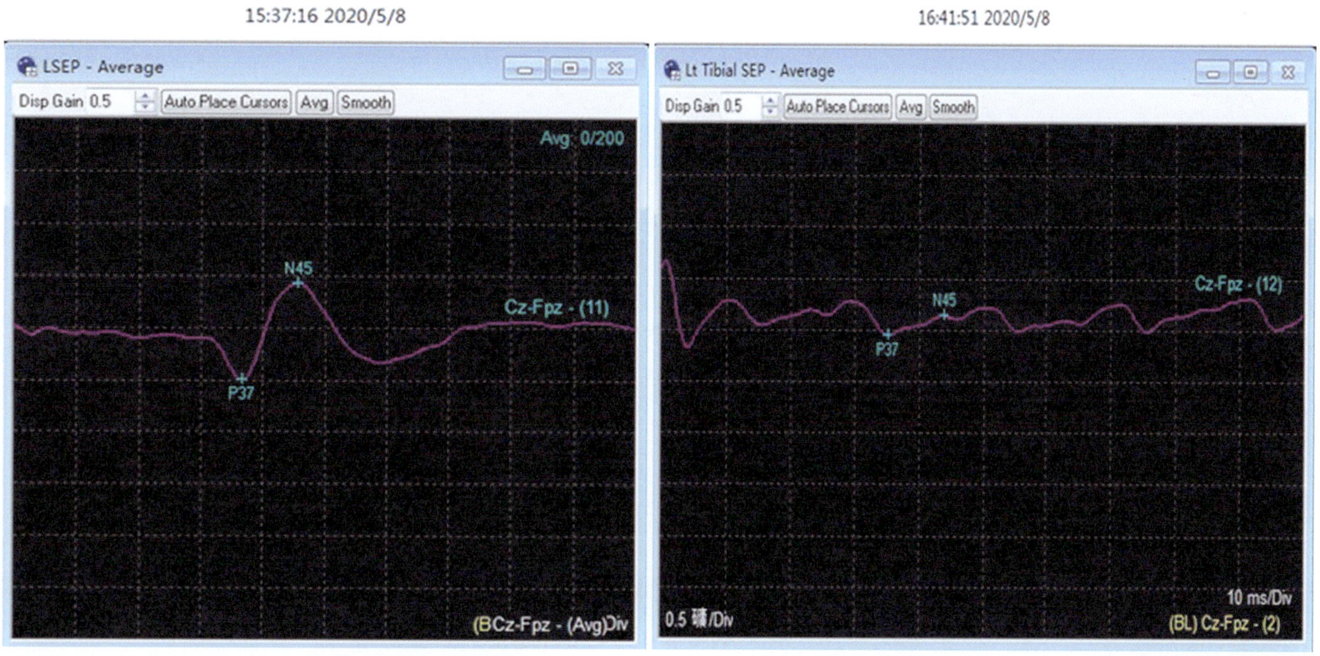

Fig. 24.1 Somatosensory evoked potentials in patients with brainstem hemorrhage

ways. For patients with brainstem injuries, these tests are especially useful as they offer a more sensitive evaluation of conduction bundle integrity compared to brainstem magnetic resonance diffusion tensor imaging (DTI).

24.2.4 Event-Related Potentials (ERPs)

The electrical signals captured by EEG arise from the synchronized postsynaptic potentials of numerous neurons within the cerebral cortex. However, EEG by itself can only detect the amplitude and rhythm of spontaneous cortical activities, which makes it challenging to pinpoint the exact onset, duration, and sequence of cognitive processes. Unlike EEG, which primarily captures the amplitude and rhythm of spontaneous cortical activity, ERPs capture the brain's electrical reactions at precise intervals following specific stimuli, with a resolution in the microseconds [4, 5]. By using computer algorithms to overlay and amplify these weak cortical signals (as illustrated in Fig. 24.2), ERPs provide a more sensitive tool to investigate whether coma patients retain the capacity to process stimuli and to gauge their responsiveness speed.

24.2.5 Magnetic Resonance Imaging (MRI)

Conventional magnetic resonance imaging (MRI) (T1/T2) is essential for identifying structural brain lesions, helping to locate and assess the severity of brain damage in patients. Functional magnetic resonance imaging (BOLD-fMRI) can help us understand the integrity of brain networks in patients with impaired consciousness [6]. Patients with brainstem hemorrhage often exhibit complete movement suppression due to damage to the pyramidal tracts, making it difficult to detect even after the patient regains consciousness. In Fig. 24.3, the clinical behavioral assessment of the patient indicates a vegetative state, but through functional MRI, we discover an effective connection between the ventral tegmental area (VTA) and cortical neurons. Consequently, the patient was diagnosed with locked-in syndrome.

24.2.6 Positron Emission Tomography-Magnetic Resonance Imaging (PET-MRI)

PET-MRI primarily measures the metabolic activity of the patient's brain to assess the degree of neuronal activity and determine the extent of neuronal damage in patients with impaired consciousness [7]. The closer the brain activity is to that of a normal individual, the better the prognosis (Fig. 24.4).

The above assessment methods each have their advantages and can mutually support and complement each other, forming a comprehensive evaluation approach that allows for a more accurate prediction of the prognosis of patients with chronic impaired consciousness. This is beneficial for clinical physicians in selecting further treatment strategies.

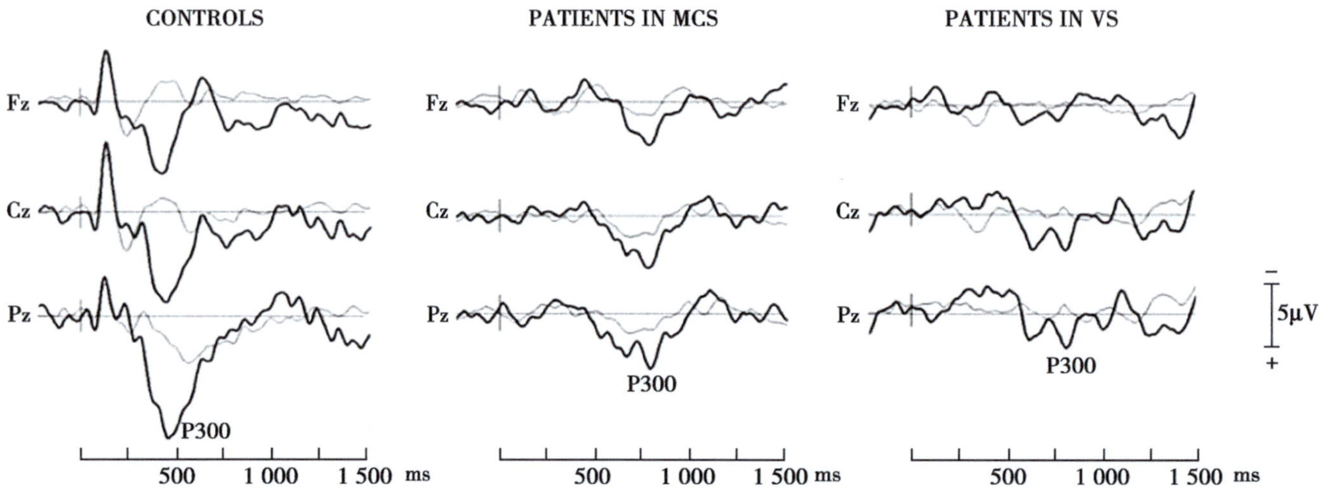

Fig. 24.2 Different detection results of event-related potential P300 in patients with different states of consciousness

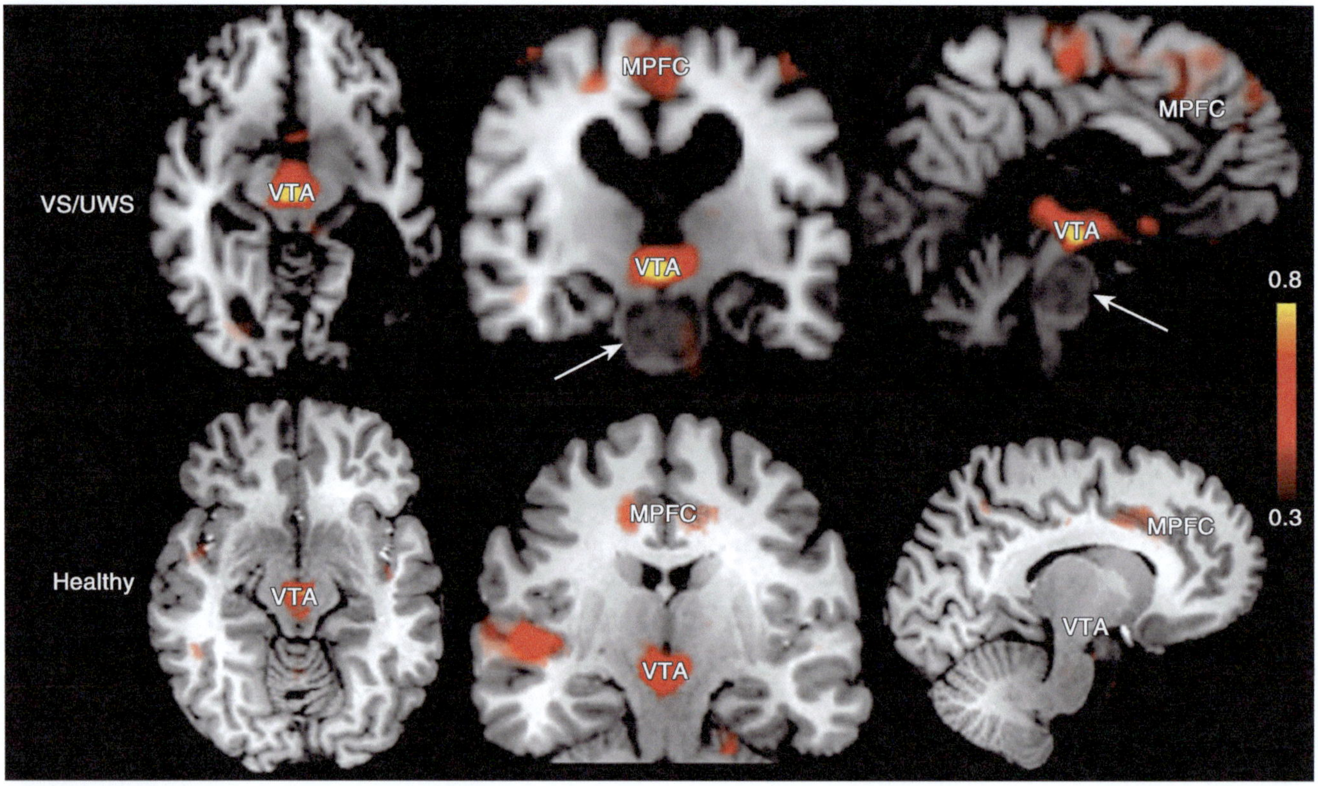

Fig. 24.3 Comparison of functional MRI between a patient with brainstem hemorrhage and a healthy individual

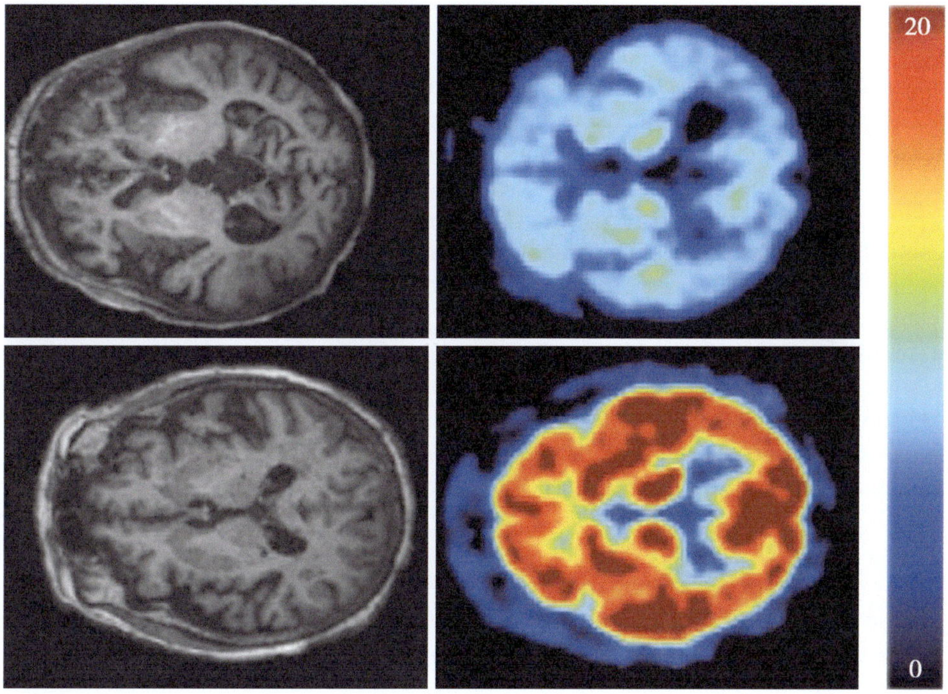

Fig. 24.4 Different brain metabolism patterns in patients with impaired consciousness as indicated by PET-MRI

24.3 Treatment of Consciousness and Cognitive Impairment After Brainstem Hemorrhage

24.3.1 Pharmacological Treatment

While the use of pharmacological agents to treat disorders of consciousness (DOC) is not backed by definitive clinical evidence, it remains a crucial aspect of clinical care. Currently, medications that stimulate arousal are primarily categorized into two types: those that target the dopamine system and those that affect the glutamate system. Commonly prescribed drugs include amantadine, bromocriptine, levodopa, naloxone hydrochloride, and zolpidem tartrate. In addition, traditional Chinese medicine also plays a role in the management of DOC. Clinical guidelines recommend amantadine as a standard arousal-provoking medication. In China, common treatments also include neurotrophic factors and vasodilators, such as nerve growth factor, naloxone/nalmefene, and extracts of Ginkgo biloba [3, 4].

24.3.1.1 Amantadine and Other Neurostimulants

To date, the most significant evidence supporting the use of amantadine in disorders of consciousness comes from a Class II randomized controlled trial. This trial involved 184 patients with prolonged disorders of consciousness resulting from traumatic brain injury. After 4 weeks of treatment with either amantadine or a placebo, followed by a 2-week follow-up, those in the amantadine group exhibited a quicker recovery as measured by the disability grading scale used throughout the treatment period [7].

In instances of non-traumatic brain injury, an uncontrolled case study suggested that amantadine had positive effects on the behavior of a patient who was in a deeply reduced state of consciousness, 16 months after sustaining a non-traumatic brain injury. Additionally, a controlled case study showed that amantadine treatment led to enhanced cortical metabolism in the frontal and parietal lobes of a hypoxic patient in a profoundly unconscious state. These case studies underscore the need for a randomized controlled trial to further investigate the effects of amantadine on patients with disorders of consciousness arising from non-traumatic brain injury.

In addition to amantadine, a retrospective study explored the use of various neurostimulants, including amantadine, bromocriptine, levodopa, methylphenidate, and modafinil), in 115 patients with consciousness disorders (within 180 days post-injury). This study showed no correlation between the frequency of neurostimulant use and meaningful behavioral improvement.

24.3.1.2 Zolpidem

Zolpidem is a hypnotic drug known to induce transient effects in rare cases of consciousness disorders. A double-blind crossover randomized controlled trial involving 84 patients with unresponsive wakefulness syndrome or in the lowest conscious state (more than 4 months post-injury) was conducted across 28 studies. The results showed that only 4 patients (5%) exhibited improvement after taking 10 mg of zolpidem.

24.3.2 Non-pharmacological Treatment

Non-pharmacological approaches also play an essential role in enhancing the recovery of patients with disorders of consciousness. These methods encompass a variety of interventions, including both invasive and non-invasive. Non-invasive brain stimulation techniques include transcranial direct current stimulation (tDCS), repetitive transcranial magnetic stimulation (rTMS), median nerve electrical stimulation, and percutaneous auricular vagus nerve stimulation. Invasive brain stimulation techniques are also employed, such as deep brain stimulation (DBS), vagus nerve stimulation (VNS), and spinal cord stimulation (SCS). Additionally, hyperbaric oxygen therapy, sensory stimulation therapy, and traditional rehabilitation therapies are utilized to aid in the recovery process.

24.3.2.1 Hyperbaric Oxygen Therapy

Hyperbaric oxygen therapy can increase cerebral tissue oxygen tension and improve blood oxygen diffusion radius. Early on, due to the vasoconstrictive effect of hyperbaric oxygen, it can reduce intracranial pressure, alleviate cerebral edema, and interrupt the vicious cycle of hypoxia-edema. At the same time, hyperbaric oxygen has a vasodilatory effect on ischemic and hypoxic brain tissue, improving local blood supply and oxygen supply. It can enhance vertebral-basilar artery blood flow, thereby promoting the excitability of the brainstem reticular activating system. It can also promote the opening of collateral circulation, conducive to nerve repair, and improve cognition. Given these effects, hyperbaric oxygen therapy is especially recommended early in the course of DOC, as it can be an effective intervention before patients enter the chronic state of VS or UWS.

24.3.2.2 Neurostimulation Therapy

24.3.2.2.1 Non-invasive Neurostimulation Therapy

Repetitive Transcranial Magnetic Stimulation (rTMS): rTMS is a non-invasive neurostimulation technique that generates electric fields in the brain through electromagnetic induction. This method can depolarize neurons and modulate cortical excitability, thereby indirectly influencing thalamic activity via the cortical-thalamic pathway [8]. rTMS is used for consciousness recovery therapy in patients with disorders of consciousness (DOC) following brain injury. It is recommended to initiate rTMS treatment early in stable patients without significant pulmonary infections, unstable lesions at the target site, a history of epilepsy, or metallic implants. MCS patients typically show greater overall benefits from TMS compared to those in a VS state. Parameters for rTMS therapy in DOC patients vary, but generally involve stimulation of the dorsolateral prefrontal cortex (DLPFC) or motor cortex (MI) at frequencies of 5–20 Hz, with a stimulation intensity of 90%–100% of the motor threshold, delivering a total of 300–1500 pulses over 1–20 days.

Transcranial Direct Current Stimulation (tDCS): tDCS modulates cortical excitability by applying weak direct currents, with anodal tDCS increasing cortical and subcortical excitability, and cathodal tDCS decreasing it. Research suggests that tDCS can enhance cortical excitability and connectivity in patients with MCS and induce consciousness-related clinical responses in VS patients, with MCS patients generally experiencing greater. tDCS is non-invasive, painless, and easy to administer, making it a viable option for consciousness recovery therapy in patients with disorders of consciousness (DOC). The treatment protocols are similar to those of rTMS. Both short-term and long-term stimulation methods are available, with long-term tDCS showing cumulative effects and the potential to reshape consciousness networks. However, there is currently no established consensus on the optimal stimulation sites, timing, parameters, or duration for tDCS therapy in DOC patients. Most studies have targeted the DLPFC or the posterior parietal cortex as the stimulation sites. Each session typically lasts 10–20 min with an intensity of 1–2 mA. The treatment course usually spans 10–20 days, with consistent stimulation parameters throughout.

Median Nerve Stimulation (MNS): MNS, a form of peripheral nerve stimulation, enhances the awakening effect on consciousness-impaired patients primarily by increasing bilateral cerebral blood flow, improving blood supply to the ischemic penumbra, boosting EEG activity, and stimulating neurophysiology processes. It directly stimulates the brainstem reticular formation and cortex, influencing neurotransmitter secretion, and thus improving clinical symptoms. Patients typically show improvements in arousal, awareness, and restoration of neural functions, such as consciousness, motor skills, speech, and other cognitive abilities. MNS is considered safe to use and is applicable to various causes of consciousness impairment, with earlier intervention often linked to a better prognosis. While there are no absolute contraindications, caution is recommended in patients with epilepsy, intracranial hypertension, or acute cerebral hemorrhage. The procedure involves placing one electrode above the median nerve point on the volar aspect of the forearm and another electrode at the thenar area. Typically, the right median nerve is stimulated with direct current at an intensity of 10–20 mA and a frequency of 40–70 Hz, once a day, for 30 min to 8 h, over treatment course of 7–30 days.

Transcutaneous Auricular Vagus Nerve Stimulation (taVNS): taVNS stimulates the auricular branch of the vagus nerve, modulating the central nervous system. Potential mechanisms include significant activation of areas such as the thalamus, posterior cingulate/precuneus, and default mode network, which may contribute to improved brain function [9]. While limited studies have been conducted on taVNS, one case report demonstrated a patient's improvement from VS to MCS following taVNS treatment. However, due to the lack of larger studies, caution is recommended regarding the specific treatment parameters.

24.3.2.2.2 Invasive Neurostimulation Therapy

Recent research has increasingly shown that neurostimulation can alter local cerebral blood flow and activate brain circuits involved in consciousness. Established neurostimulation methods, including deep brain stimulation (DBS), spinal cord stimulation (SCS), and vagus nerve stimulation (VNS), have been reported to have arousal effects on DOC. DBS, in particular, targets the activity level of consciousness-regulating neural circuits and is theoretically more effective due to its closer proximity to the core regions involved in central regulation [10, 11]. DBS is preferred when brain structural morphology allows. Patients with chronic cognitive impairments often experience malnutrition and thinning of the scalp tissues. To address this, a smaller intracranial electrode self-locking device (Scene Ray, Touch-loc, 0.43 ± 0.55 mm) can be utilized, reducing the risk of skin necrosis and other complications related to device exposure.

DBS is applicable for the rehabilitation of patients with chronic cognitive impairments when conventional treatment methods have proven to be ineffective. It is particularly beneficial for individuals who have been experiencing prolonged cognitive impairments. According to the "central loop hypothesis," the central thalamus-frontal-parietal loop is the core neural circuit for generating and maintaining consciousness. DBS can promote arousal by stimulating the central thalamus to excite the cerebral cortex. Several studies have confirmed the significant role of thalamic stimulation in consciousness recovery, with no unified standard stimulation nucleus currently available. The most commonly chosen targets are non-specific projection nuclei, which can induce widespread brain excitation. Commonly used nuclei in clinical practice include the bilateral central-medial/parafascicular complex (CM-pf) with specific parameters (Parameters: X: 7–9 mm, Y-axis: −8 mm, Z-axis: 0–3 mm). In China, leading experts in neurostimulation for chronic disorders of consciousness include Professor He Jianghong from the Department of Neurosurgery at the Seventh Medical Center of the Chinese People's Liberation Army General Hospital, Professor Zhang Jianguo's team from Beijing Tiantan Hospital, and Professor Zhang Shizhong's team from Zhujiang Hospital, Southern Medical University. In 2018, the Functional Neurosurgery Group of the Neurosurgery Branch of the Chinese Medical Association, the neurostimulation Professional Committee of the Chinese Medical Doctors Association, and the Consciousness and Disorders of Consciousness Branch of the Chinese Neuroscience Society jointly developed the first "Chinese Expert Consensus on neurostimulation Surgical Treatment for Chronic Disorders of Consciousness (2018 edition)" in China. This consensus provides important guidelines for neurostimulation treatment of chronic disorders of consciousness in China.

Patients meeting the following criteria are more suitable for DBS treatment of DOC:

- Moderate age, preferably between 10 and 65 years old.
- Duration of consciousness impairment exceeding 6 months with no expected short-term improvement.
- CRS-R score < 22 points.
- EEG recording for more than 1 h with <5% of desynchronized activity.
- Somatosensory evoked potentials induced on at least one side (N20 potential latency may be delayed up to 1 μs).
- Brainstem auditory evoked potentials induced on at least one side (V wave latency may be delayed by 1 μs).
- Cortical auditory evoked potentials induced on at least one side.
- Broca's area in the dominant hemisphere without injury, with at least one brain lobe injury degree <20%.
- The posterior two-thirds of the dominant hemisphere's temporal lobe without injury, with the remaining temporal lobe injury range <70% of the temporal lobe's total volume.
- Injury to one or both sides of the parietal lobe <30%.
- Injury to one or both sides of the occipital lobe <30%, with at least one visual cortex preserved.
- No injury to the thalamus.
- No injury to the bilateral central/parafascicular complex, with thalamic injury not exceeding 40% of bilateral thalamic volume.
- No injury to the area between the substantia nigra and subthalamic nucleus.
- No injury to the brainstem except for a single side and the ventral one-third of the brainstem.
- Cerebellar injury not exceeding 80%, with at least one side deep nuclear group intact.
- No injury to at least one side of the pyramidal tract.
- No injury to the cervical cord.

DBS treatment for consciousness disorders should be used with caution in patients with the following conditions:

- Secondary consciousness disorders due to neurological diseases.
- Concomitant diseases with a life expectancy of less than 1 year.
- Unresolved, persistent infections.
- Pregnancy.
- Untreated hydrocephalus.

Clinical studies have shown that DBS treatment of consciousness disorders can significantly improve outcomes in patients with consciousness disorders. Even when deep brain stimulation is turned off, patients' clinical status remains above the preoperative baseline. However, despite these promising results, there have been no sham-controlled trials on DBS for consciousness disorders. A standardized treatment protocol is still required to better define the parameters for treatment and to explore the generalizability of DBS effects. Additionally, there are several clinical and ethical challenges (such as infection risk and clinical deterioration) that need to be addressed.

SCS enhances arousal impulses at the brainstem's reticular activating system, promoting the regulation of cerebral blood flow and neurotransmitter release. However, its site of action is more indirect compared to DBS. SCS is considered an alternative option for patients who are not suitable for DBS surgery. In cases where there is severe damage to the thalamus or obvious brain atrophy leading to significant displacement of the third ventricle and thalamus, the accuracy of DBS implantation may be compromised. In such scenarios, DBS surgery should be cautiously selected.

The awakening effect of VNS has only been reported in individual cases and remains unclear, and its mechanisms remain unclear, warranting cautious use. While neurostimulation surgery is emerging as a significant research focus for treating DOC, several challenges remain, including limitations in understanding DOC diseases, practical regulation capabilities, and clinical experience. As a result, neurostimulation therapy must be approached with careful and scientific investigation. Detailed documentation of clinical efficacy, safety, and adverse events is essential before it can be considered a widely applicable clinical treatment method.

24.3.2.3 Sensory and Environmental Stimulus Therapy

Sensory and environmental stimuli help promote the connection between the cortex and subcortex, facilitating the restoration of cortical function in patients with consciousness disorders Various stimuli, including auditory, visual, tactile, olfactory, taste, and oral stimuli, as well as the use of neuro-facilitation techniques, and environmental stimuli, can be used to enhance this process. For example, by considering the patient's habits, preferences, and work situation, caregivers can design and provide tailored multisensory stimuli such as sounds, colors, smells, tactile sensations, and tastes that the patient likes or dislikes.

24.3.2.4 Traditional Chinese Rehabilitation Therapy

Common treatments for disorders of consciousness in traditional Chinese medicine include Chinese herbal medicine and acupuncture, such as Angong Niuhuang Pill, Zixue Dan, Zhibao Dan, Suhe Xiang Pill, and Annao Pill. Acupuncture has the effects of awakening the mind, improving cerebral blood circulation, promoting the recovery and regeneration of brain nerve cells, and stimulating dormant nerve cells to relieve the inhibitory effect of the cerebral cortex. By stimulating specific meridian acupoints, such as stimulating sensory areas, motor areas, Baihui, Sishencong, Shenting, Renzhong, Hegu, Neiguan, Sanyinjiao, Laogong, Yongquan, Shixuan, etc., acupuncture activate the brainstem reticular arousal system, promote the recovery of consciousness in patients with consciousness disorders.

24.4 Typical Cases

24.4.1 DBS Surgical Procedure

Preoperative installation of head frame; CT combined with MRI localization; target point and path design; patient enters the operating room, anesthesia, and connection of head frame fixation frame; sub-table simulation calibration of target point parameters; drill holes, opening of dura mater, electrocoagulation of cortical pathway; installation of head frame and simultaneous simulation of target point parameters twice on the simulator; installation of arc frame and microelectrode guide after stopping all anesthetics; dynamic positioning of nucleus with microelectrode from 10 mm above target to 5 mm below target; judgment of nucleus position based on microelectrode waveform, sound, and distance from target center; installation and fixation of microelectrode; intraoperative CT observation of microelectrode position; connection of microelectrode lead; resistance measurement; end of surgery (Fig. 24.5, Video 24.1).

24.4.2 Typical Case of DBS Treatment for Disorders of Consciousness

24.4.2.1 Summary of Medical History and Imaging Data

The patient is a 34-year-old male who lapsed into a coma for 5 months following a brainstem hemorrhage. He has a history of hypertension, managed with medication. Five months prior to admission, he experienced a sudden loss of consciousness, and a CT scan confirmed a diagnosis of brainstem hemorrhage (Fig. 24.6). He underwent tracheostomy for respiratory support and received medical treatment, after which his vital signs gradually stabilized. One month later, he began hyperbaric oxygen therapy and conventional rehabilitation at a local hospital; however, there was no improvement in his level of consciousness. Subsequently, he was transferred to our hospital for further assessment and treatment.

Upon admission, after correcting central fever, the patient spontaneously opened his eyes and demonstrated visual

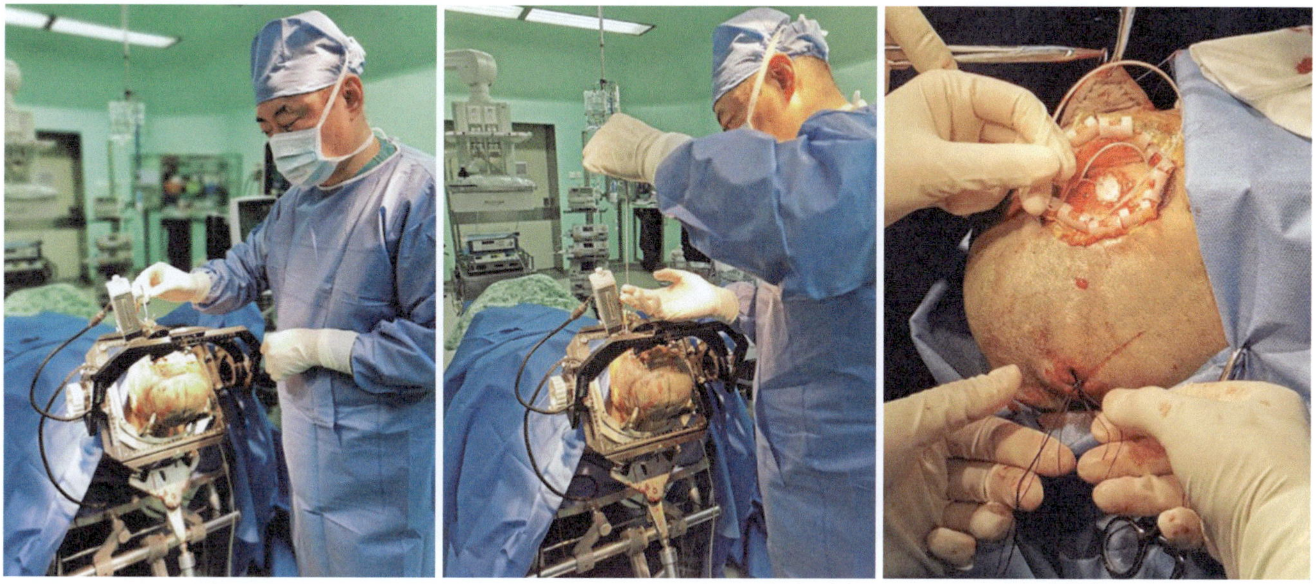

Fig. 24.5 Example of intraoperative rechargeable DBS. Provided by Professor Zhang Shizhong's team, Zhujiang Hospital, Southern Medical University

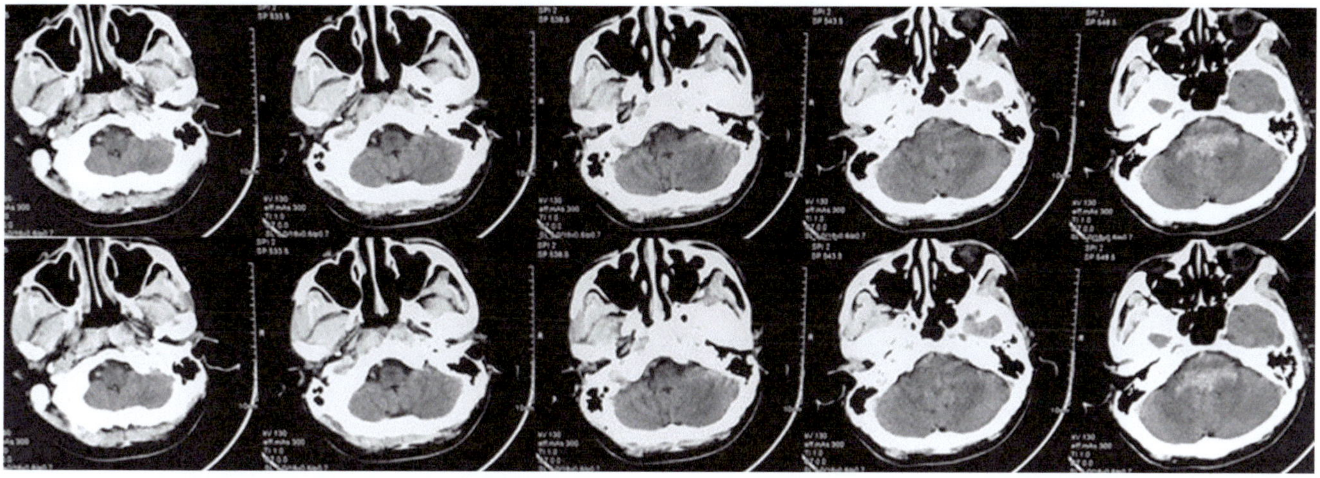

Fig. 24.6 CT of the patient on the day of disease onset

tracking in the vertical plane. His limbs exhibited slight flexion in response to painful stimuli, and he scored 8 points on CRS-R (1–1–3–1–0–2), leading to a diagnosis of MCS. A cranial MR examination performed at admission revealed residual changes in the brainstem, tegmentum of the midbrain, cerebellar peduncles, bilateral pontine arms, and bilateral cerebral peduncles resulting from the previous hemorrhage (Fig. 24.7).

Preoperative evaluations included electroencephalography, functional magnetic resonance imaging, transcranial magnetic stimulation electroencephalography (TMS-EEG), resting-state functional magnetic resonance imaging assessment, and prognosis prediction to determine the level of consciousness. Considering the patient's 5-month history, presentation of a minimally conscious state, comprehensive multimodal assessments, and the high likelihood of surgical benefit, DBS electrode implantation targeting the bilateral thalamic CM-pf nucleus was performed.

Postoperative re-examination of head MR, precise implantation of DBS, consistent with preoperative plan (Fig. 24.8).

One week after the operation, trial activation was conducted. Optimal stimulation parameters were determined based on clinical observations, EEG power spectrum topographic analysis, and near-infrared spectroscopy analysis, with a frequency of 100 Hz. Within 1 week after activation, the patient exhibited markedly increased responsiveness to external stimuli, followed by eye-tracking movements, voluntary mouth opening upon seeing food, and compliance with hand instructions, indicating significant improvement in

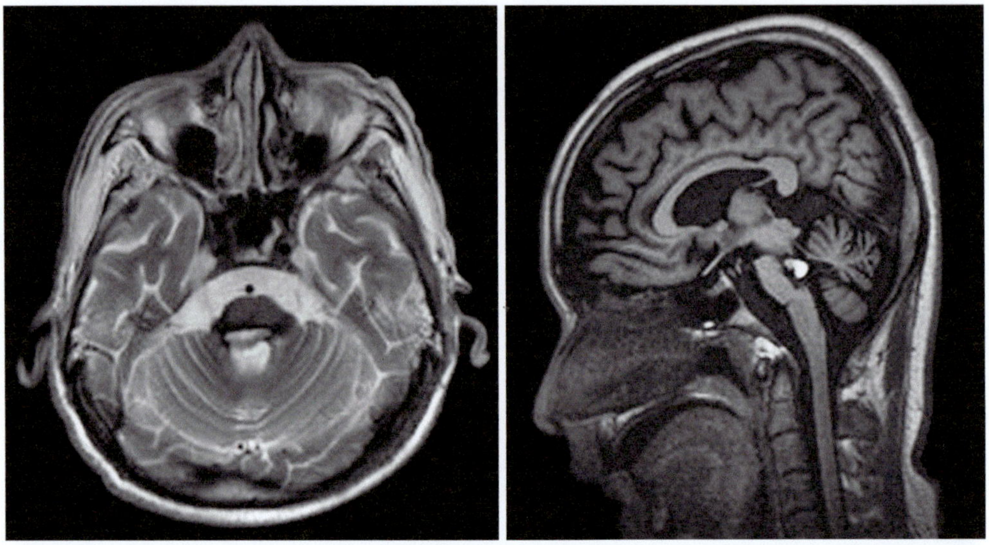

Fig. 24.7 MRI shows post-hemorrhagic changes in the brainstem, midbrain tegmentum, middle cerebellar peduncle, and bilateral cerebral peduncle

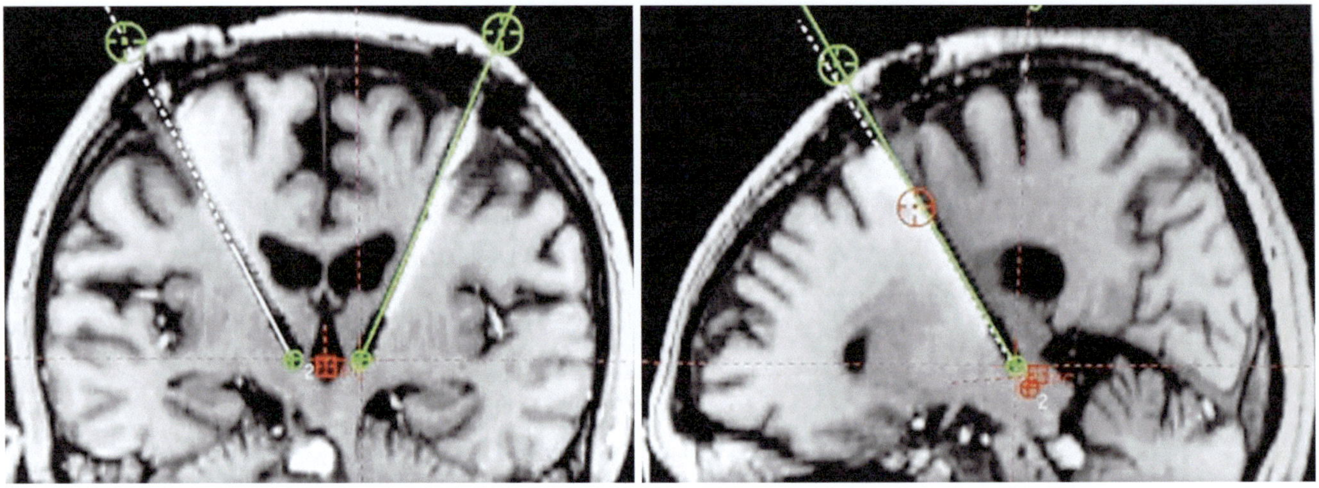

Fig. 24.8 Fusion image of postoperative MR and preoperative plan

consciousness level. TMS-EEG results demonstrated a notable improvement in consciousness level compared to assessments conducted before and 1 month after DBS treatment (Fig. 24.9). One month after discharge, the CRS-R score had increased to 15 points (auditory 0-visual 5-motor 5-oral motor 1-communication 1-arousal 3), and the patient was able to imitate gestures and engage in partial communication with family members (Fig. 24.10). The patient was discharged and continued rehabilitation treatment at a local hospital.

24.4.3 VNS Therapy for Consciousness Disorders

24.4.3.1 Brief Medical History and Imaging Data

The patient, a 41-year-old female, presented with "consciousness disorder for 4 months after cerebral hemorrhage." Clinical findings upon examination: deep coma, GCS 4, unresponsive to external stimuli, with limbs extended in response to stimulation, presence of tracheostomy.

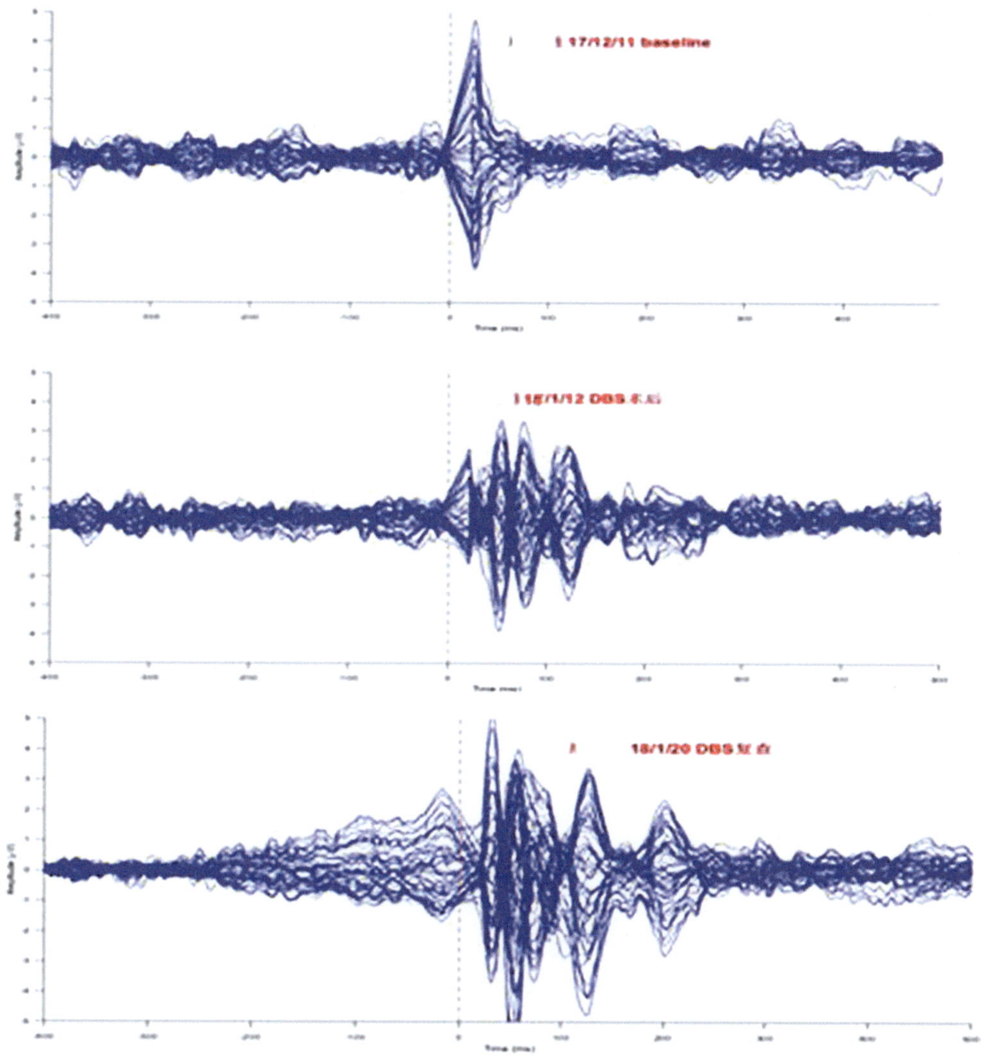

Fig. 24.9 TMS-EEG. The upper image is 4 days before DBS, and the middle and lower images are the results of 28 and 36 days after the operation, respectively

Preoperative CRS-R score was 6 (auditory 2, visual 1, motor 2, language 0, communication 0, arousal 1).

24.4.3.2 Surgical Procedure

Incisions were designed in the carotid artery area and chest. After routine disinfection and draping, a skin incision was made in the carotid artery area, and the left vagus nerve was exposed by opening the carotid sheath. Another incision was made in the chest, and the electrode wire was passed through a subcutaneous tunnel connecting the two incisions. The stimulating contact was wrapped around the vagus nerve and connected to the pulse generator, which was then inserted into the chest incision after verifying accurate data. The electrode wire's length and angle were adjusted, and the setup was secured with sutures. The incisions were closed layer by layer, completing the surgery (Fig. 24.11). One month postoperatively, the patient's CRS-R score improved to 10 (auditory 2, visual 2, motor 2, language 2, communication 0, arousal 2), with spontaneous eye opening observed, and a GCS score of 6.

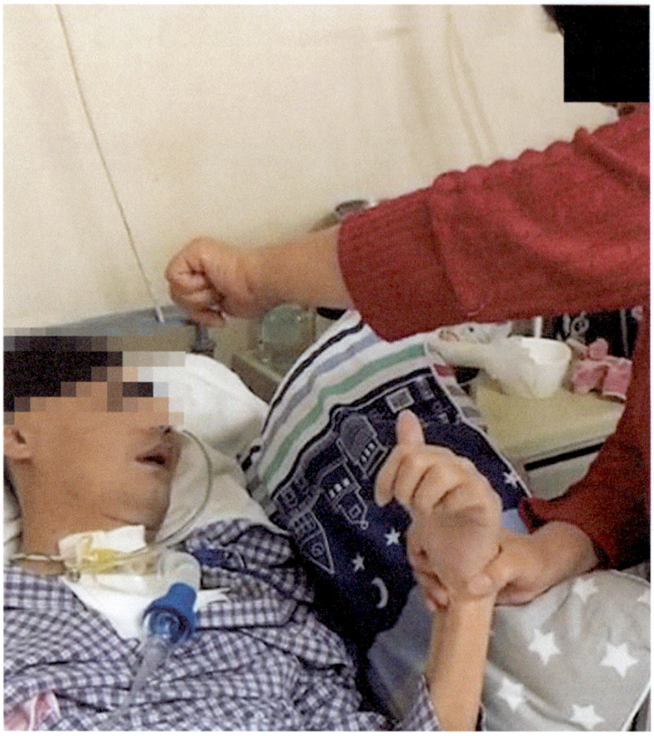

Fig. 24.10 The patient's improvement in consciousness at discharge

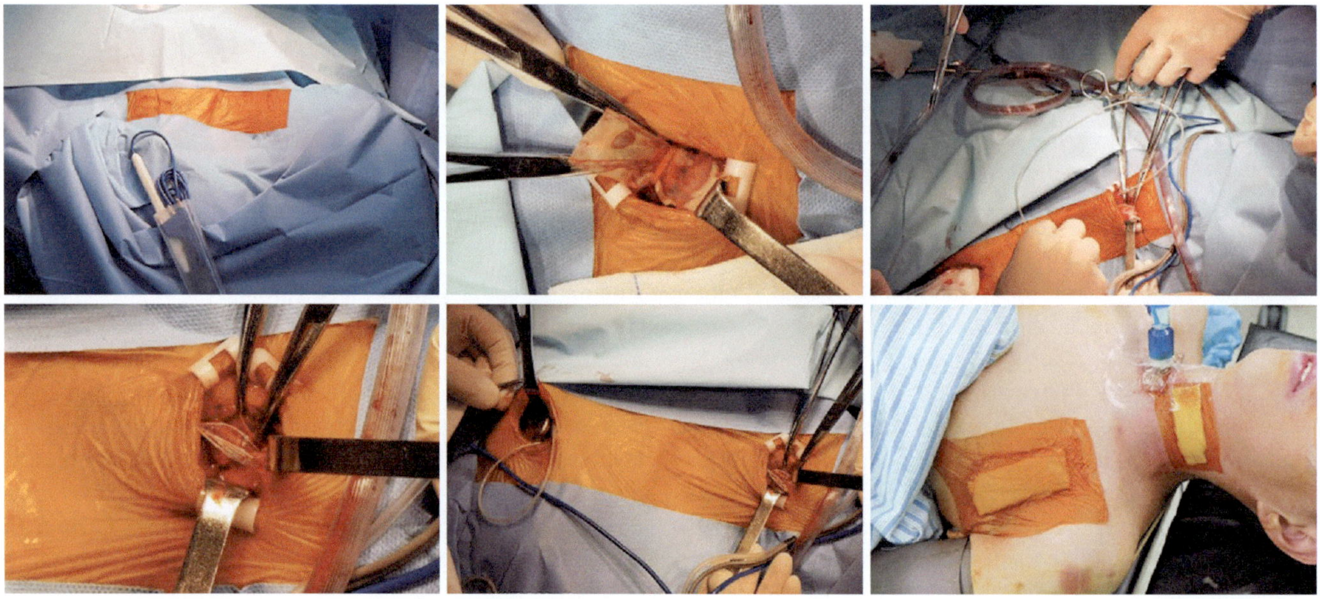

Fig. 24.11 Example of intraoperative VNS for disorders of consciousness

24.5 Conclusion

Proper preoperative assessment of consciousness levels, careful selection of surgical methods, and meticulous postoperative management are critical for the success of neuroregulatory surgeries. For patients with consciousness disorders resulting from brainstem hemorrhages, DBS can effectively improve consciousness levels when applied to appropriately selected candidates.

Acknowledgment Special thanks to the team led by Director He Jianghong, Department of Functional Neurosurgery, Bayi Brain Hospital, Seventh Medical Center, PLA General Hospital, for providing the above case data.

References

1. Lv W, He YB, Chen Y, et al. The relationship between thyroid hormone levels and prognosis in patients with chronic consciousness disorders after brain injury. Guangdong Med J. 2019.040 (022).
2. Thibaut A, Schiff N, Giacino J, et al. Therapeutic interventions in patients with prolonged disorders of consciousness. Lancet Neurol. 2019;18(6):600–14.
3. Giacino JT, Fins JJ, Laureys S, et al. Disorders of consciousness after acquired brain injury: the state of the science. Nat Rev Neurol. 2014;10(2):99–114.
4. Schnakers C, Vanhaudenhuyse A, Giacino J, et al. Diagnostic accuracy of the vegetative and minimally conscious state: clinical consensus versus standardized neurobehavioral assessment. BMC Neurol. 2009;9:35.
5. Lehembre R, Gosseries O, Lugo Z, et al. Electrophysiological investigations of brain function in coma, vegetative and minimally conscious patients. Arch Ital Biol. 2012;150(2–3):122–39.
6. Cologan V, Schabus M, Ledoux D, et al. Sleep in disorders of consciousness. Sleep Med Rev. 2010;14(2):97–105.
7. Sandroni C, Cavallaro F, Callaway CW, et al. Predictors of poor neurological outcome in adult comatose survivors of cardiac arrest: a systematic review and meta-analysis. Part 2: patients treated with therapeutic hypothermia. Resuscitation. 2013;84(10):1324–38.
8. Vanhaudenhuyse A, Laureys S, Perrin F. Cognitive event-related potentials in comatose and post-comatose states. Neurocrit Care. 2008;8(2):262–70.
9. Bodien YG, Chatelle C, Edlow BL. Functional networks in disorders of consciousness. Semin Neurol. 2017;37(5):485–502.
10. Golkowski D, Merz K, Mlynarcik C, et al. Simultaneous EEG-PET-fMRI measurements in disorders of consciousness: an exploratory study on diagnosis and prognosis. J Neurol. 2017;264(9):1986–95.
11. Magrassi L, Maggioni G, Pistarini C, et al. Results of a prospective study (CATS) on the effects of thalamic stimulation in minimally conscious and vegetative state patients. J Neurosurg. 2016;125(4):972–81.

Postscript

Gang Chen

In July 2015, by chance, I began to pay attention to the microsurgical treatment of brainstem cavernous malformations. Subsequently, I conducted an extensive review of both domestic and international literature, which deepened my understanding of therapeutic strategies for this condition. Through further study and clinical observation, I noted that the incidence of hypertensive brainstem hemorrhage substantially exceeds that of brainstem cavernous malformations. Hypertensive brainstem hemorrhage represents a critical neurological emergency, characterized by poor prognosis and high mortality. At present, conservative management remains the predominant treatment approach globally, while surgical intervention is often considered contraindicated. Consequently, standardized protocols for the surgical treatment of hypertensive brainstem hemorrhage are lacking, and no dedicated monographs on the subject have been published, leading to considerable uncertainty among clinicians devoted to its management. This clinical dilemma has stimulated my research interest, shifting my focus from brainstem cavernous malformations to exploring surgical interventions for hypertensive brainstem hemorrhage, with the aim of contributing preliminary investigative work in this area.

In March 2017, I established the first WeChat group for multidisciplinary collaboration in the diagnosis and treatment of brainstem hemorrhage in China. Through this platform, I became acquainted with several department directors who are primarily engaged in the surgical treatment of hypertensive brainstem hemorrhage, including Zhou Quan, Yang Jinhua, Mu Linsen, Sun Shujie, Zhang Hongtian, Liu Zhenchuan, Liu Fengqiang, and others, and gained insight into the current status of surgical treatment for hypertensive brainstem hemorrhage in China. With the joint efforts and assistance of these directors, three special forums on the surgical treatment and microsurgical anatomy of operative approaches for hypertensive brainstem hemorrhage were successively held in Suzhou, Yangjiang, and Shenzhen. All participants reached a consensus: Hypertensive brainstem hemorrhage carries the highest mortality and worst prognosis among all hemorrhagic strokes and has long been regarded as a contraindication for surgical intervention. Meanwhile, the management of hypertensive brainstem hemorrhage constitutes a systematic therapeutic program, encompassing surgery, intensive care, rehabilitation, and arousal therapy. Each component is critically important; in line with the "Barrel Theory," any weak link will compromise the final outcome. Patients with hypertensive brainstem hemorrhage often require a long treatment course with substantial medical costs, which are difficult for ordinary families to afford throughout the entire process of surgery, ICU care, rehabilitation, and arousal therapy. Abandoning treatment prematurely will also lead to unsatisfactory outcomes. Therefore, one of our key priorities is to carefully select suitable patients with a reasonable chance of favorable prognosis and to adopt optimal minimally invasive surgical approaches. The goal is to achieve maximal hematoma evacuation with minimal trauma, so as to accomplish both minimally invasive injury and sufficient brainstem decompression. When considering surgery for patients with hypertensive brainstem hemorrhage, surgeons must fully inform the family members of the possible prognosis, the prolonged recovery period, the high medical expenses, and the uncertainty of achieving a satisfactory outcome. Careful assessment of the patient's prognosis, the family's expectations, and financial status is essential. Accordingly, surgical treatment for hypertensive brainstem hemorrhage should not be performed blindly; it requires adequate theoretical, instrumental, and technical preparation. During the forums, the following consensus was reached: (1) Hypertensive brainstem hemorrhage is one of the most devastating forms of stroke. At present, there are no unified standards for its surgical treatment, which awaits rationalization and standardization. (2) It is planned to establish a Collaborative Research Group for minimally invasive surgical treatment of hypertensive brainstem hemorrhage. The group will hold 2–3 special forums annually to exchange views, revise and standardize diagnostic and therapeutic protocols, and gradually develop expert consensus. (3) A multi-

G. Chen
Neurosurgery Department, Zhuhai People's Hospital (The Affiliated Hospital of Beijing Institute of Technology, Zhuhai Clinical Medical College of Jinan University), Zhuhai, China

G. Chen, C. You (eds.), *Surgical Treatment of Primary Brainstem Hemorrhage*, https://doi.org/10.1007/978-981-95-8942-5

center study will be conducted to provide high-quality, evidence-based medical evidence for the surgical treatment of hypertensive brainstem hemorrhage.

In March 2019, during my communication with Director Yang Jinhua, we jointly recognized that, given the current domestic and international research status of hypertensive brainstem hemorrhage, compiling a monograph focusing on its surgical treatment would provide valuable reference for domestic clinicians engaged in this field. Following repeated recommendations from Director Yang Jinhua and in-depth discussions with several other directors who specialize in the surgical treatment of hypertensive brainstem hemorrhage in China, we formally decided to initiate the compilation of this book in April 2019.

The purpose of compiling this book is not to encourage colleagues to actively pursue surgical intervention for hypertensive brainstem hemorrhage, but rather to promote the advancement of diagnostic and therapeutic concepts and techniques for this disease—including enhancing collaboration among relevant departments, such as neurology and rehabilitation—thereby enabling all of us to learn from one another, exchange practical experiences, and make collective progress in this field.

I would like to extend my sincere gratitude to Director Yang Jinhua and all the contributors for their active support, invaluable assistance, and joint efforts in bringing this book to completion. During the entire writing process, I am deeply thankful to my wife, Ms. Hu Yanrong, for her tremendous dedication and countless efforts. I would like to present this book as the most precious gift to her, in heartfelt appreciation of her years of unwavering support, understanding, and care for both my work and life.

October 1, 2020